Health
Psychology

Health Psychology

Phillip L. Rice
Moorhead State University

Brooks/Cole Publishing Company

I(T)P® *An International Thomson Publishing Company*

Pacific Grove • Albany • Belmont • Bonn • Boston
Cincinnati • Detroit • Johannesburg • London • Madrid
Melbourne • Mexico City • New York • Paris • Singapore
Tokyo • Toronto • Washington

Sponsoring Editor: *Marianne Taflinger*
Marketing Team: *Lauren Harp/Alicia Barelli/Deborah Petit*
Editorial Assistant: *Scott Brearton*
Production Editor: *Tessa A. McGlasson*
Manuscript Editor: *Catherine Cambron*
Permissions Editor: *May Clark*
Interior Design: *John Edeen*
Cover Design: *Susan Horovitz*

Cover Photo: *Stephen Simpson-FPG International Corp.*
Art Editor: *Lisa Torri*
Interior Illustration: *John and Judy Waller*
Photo Editor: *Robert J. Western*
Typesetting: *Graphic World, Inc.*
Cover printing: *Phoenix Color Corp.*
Printing and Binding: *Maple-Vail Book Manufacturing Co.*

For more information, contact:

BROOKS/COLE PUBLISHING COMPANY
511 Forest Lodge Road
Pacific Grove, CA 93950
USA

International Thomson Publishing Europe
Berkshire House 168-173
High Holborn
London WC1V 7AA
England

Thomas Nelson Australia
102 Dodds Street
South Melbourne, 3205
Victoria, Australia

Nelson Canada
1120 Birchmount Road
Scarborough, Ontario
Canada M1K 5G4

International Thomson Editores
Seneca 53
Col. Polanco
11560 México, D. F., México

International Thomson Publishing GmbH
Königswinterer Strasse 418
53227 Bonn
Germany

International Thomson Publishing Asia
211 Henderson Road
#05-10 Henderson Building
Singapore 0315

International Thomson Publishing Japan
Hirakawacho Kyowa building, 3F
2-2-1 Hirakawacho
Chiyoda-ku, Tokyo 102
Japan

Printed in the United States of America

10   9   8   7   6   5   4   3   2   1

Library of Congress Cataloging-in-Publication Data
Rice, Phillip L., [date]-
    Health psychology / Phillip L. Rice.
        p.   cm.
    Includes bibliographical references and indexes.
    ISBN 0-534-33915-8
    1. Clinical health psychology.   I. Title.
R726.7.R5 1997
616'.001'9--dc21   97-11794
                                                                              CIP

To H. D. and Anna Weikal—
always, only, Grandma and Grandpa:

The years that separated us in life,
the time that now separates us
in death, cannot separate us from
your loving spirit.

About the Author

Phillip L. Rice is professor of psychology at Moorhead (MN) State University, a position he has held for more than 20 years. He has been recognized for excellence in teaching both early in his career as Outstanding Young Educator in 1972, and most recently as Moorhead State's nominee for CASE/Carnegie Professor of the year for 1996-1997. He also served as chair of the department for 9 years. For the past 15 years, his research and writing has focused on stress and its relationship to health and illness. He is the author of *Stress and Health* (2nd edition), also published by Brooks/Cole. The work stress scale published in *Stress and Health* has been used by many researchers in cross-cultural research including studies in England, India, and Africa. This work on *Health Psychology* is the culmination of nearly a decade of teaching and research on the topic, and the logical extension of his efforts to translate the many facets of theory, research, and application into exciting and accessible form.

Brief Contents

Contents

CHAPTER *3*

On Grief, Placebos, and Mind: Psychological Foundations of Health and Illness   56

CHAPTER 4

Social Networks: Social-Ecological Theories of Health and Illness 81

PART 3

Intervention and Research: Techniques in Health Psychology 109

CHAPTER 5

Four Therapies: Short-Term, Cognitive, Behavioral, and Pharmacotherapy 111

CHAPTER **6**

Biobehavioral Research: Experimental, Clinical, and Epidemiological Strategies   139

PART **4**

Stress, High-Risk Behaviors, and Health   167

CHAPTER **7**

Stress Models: Symptoms, Sources, and Coping   171

CHAPTER **9**

Substance Abuse II: Use and Misuse of Alcohol 237

CHAPTER **10**

Eating Behavior: Healthy and Unhealthy Habits 264

CHAPTER **11**

The AIDS Pandemic: A Behavioral Disease   293

PART **5**

Coping with Chronic or Catastrophic Illness   325

CHAPTER **12**

Heart Health: Silent Killers and the Hurry Sickness   327

CHAPTER **13**

The Problem of Pain: Headaches and Low Back Pain   355

CHAPTER **14**

Chronic Illness: Cancer and Arthritis   384

PART **6**

*Promoting Health in Children
and the Elderly*   411

CHAPTER **15**

*Pediatric Health Psychology:
Promoting Health and Coping
with Chronic Illness*   413

CHAPTER **16**

*Aging and Health: Myths,
Realities, and Actions*   445

Nothing sets the tone for life like health. Good health is the foundation of positive joy in living, while poor health is often regarded as the adversary of the soul. Contemporary society has expended tremendous effort to control illness and promote health, but only recently has society turned attention to the most important player: you. This book, then, reflects the growing recognition that promoting health transcends the boundaries of traditional medical science. An interdisciplinary effort is involved, which plays only a supporting role to the individual who is cast in the lead. In short, we each play a singularly powerful role in shaping our personal health through the attitudes and beliefs we hold and the health behaviors that become more or less habitual for good or ill. Health psychology tries to assemble a more clearly focused picture of how we can better shape our personal health to set the tone for a high quality life.

In the brief history of psychology, the rapid evolution and influence of health psychology is perhaps without precedent. Since its formal birth in 1978, it has flourished as a specialty within the discipline, attracted the attention of many people who were trained when health psychology did not even exist, and commanded the attention and respect of many people from other fields. The growth has been for the most part healthy, but not without certain tensions. In any case, it is one of the most vibrant fields of modern psychology. Also, its potential to help people change their lifestyles and achieve an overall higher quality of life seems nearly unlimited at this point. This book tells the story of how health psychology came about, critically recounts some of the tensions that have been part of its growth, and tries to present the

theories, principles, and applications that are part of this exciting new discipline.

Health psychology began with a threefold emphasis on research, teaching, and application. No one probably ever imagined at that time how important the latter emphasis would become to the current definition of the field. The development of the subspecialty—clinical health psychology—has occurred amazingly rapidly. It is tempting, as well as very easy, to allow that emphasis to dominate and say that the only really important issues are in the context of the practice of health psychology. I disagree with this notion and take the view that no matter how important the clinical emphasis may be, the other two faces of health psychology deserve even-handed treatment and are worthy of the reader's careful attention. I attempt, then, to present the practice of health psychology in the context of legitimate concerns over epistemology, methodology, and theory building.

The great aim of health psychology has been to bring humanity and science together in understanding the context of health and illness. In this book, I have attempted also to bring these two elements together in content and style. In regard to content, I tried to be true to the scientific traditions that underpin our discipline in general and current understanding of health in particular. This is reflected in the substantial body of empirical research and the theoretical intrigues summarized herein.

In regard to style, I have tried to convey something of real human dilemmas that present themselves when health seems to be slipping from one's grasp or fails completely. Toward this end, I have selected a different kind of biography than appears in many clinical texts. You will encounter many people—poets, writers, scientists, educators—whose lives exemplify something of the struggle we all go through to accomplish our life's goals as well as to keep a sometimes fragile hold on health. You will, I hope, learn something beyond the confines of health psychology about the rich web of literature, thought, and scientific discovery that has taken place in the cauldron of life's struggle to maintain health and cope with illness—such as that of Rosalind Franklin, whose battle with cancer took place during her important research that led to Watson and Crick's uncovering the mysteries of DNA.

Unique Features of the Book

This book has several features that set it apart from other health psychology texts:

- Treatment of women's issues is extensive across many chapters and includes information on biases in diagnosis, treatment, and medical research. Additional information is presented relevant to women's health concerns in chapters on addiction, coronary disease, and cancer, for example.
- Multicultural issues are addressed early in the chapter on social theory of health and illness. For example, the student will learn what happened to a group of Tarahumara Indians in Mexico when a high-cholesterol western diet was introduced. Later, substantial information is presented that is of concern to health status and health care among minority groups.
- Cross-cultural research is presented in many sections, showing how culture influences various lifestyle choices that subsequently influence health status. For example, comparisons across Finland, France, Great Britain, and Japan show how health status is influenced by customary eating patterns and food choices.
- Human interest stories are woven throughout the text, not just as chapter openers. These stories are based on the lives of real people, many well known, whose struggles with health have provided important object lessons for today's student.

- The new field of pediatric health psychology is introduced in a special chapter not found in other texts. Here, the student will learn about the special needs of children who struggle with various chronic ailments such as diabetes mellitus, asthma, and cystic fibrosis.
- Geriatric health psychology is the focus of another unique chapter, which discusses the special health problems confronted by the aging. Although a downside is shown in the decline in various physical and mental functions (such as Alzheimer's disease), the exciting upside is the great vitality displayed by many older people who make wise, healthy lifestyle choices.
- Critical analysis of the biopsychosocial model is presented, with its strengths and limitations highlighted. This model is reflected throughout the book by examining current thinking on the multiple pathways to illness and health. Each of the specific "disease" chapters (for example, cancer in Chapter 14) has space allocated for examination of what we know of the physical, psychological, and social influences in the onset, progression, and remission of the disorder.
- Physical systems (the biology of disease) are described in the context of a given disease with understandable language. Thus, cardiovascular pathology is presented in the chapter on heart health while the pathology underlying diabetes mellitus is presented when that disorder is discussed in Chapter 15.
- The book uses many visual aids to help tell the story of health psychology, including charts of notable research outcomes, photos of many researchers and clinicians who have contributed to our knowledge, and illustrations of concepts, physical conditions, and treatment interventions.

The Book's Plan and a Preview

Part 1

The first chapter introduces and defines the area of health psychology with a brief history of its origins. Then it describes what health psychologists typically do and where they work. Finally, to answer the questions many students have about the profession, the chapter ends with a discussion of how to become trained as a health psychologist.

Part 2

The second section presents information crucial to understanding the biopsychosocial model. This model is regarded by most as the central theoretical focus and rationale for health psychology's existence. Chapter 2 is unique among health psychology texts. It provides perspective on the sometimes tortuous progression of medical theory from the humoral notions of Hippocrates to the discovery of bacteria by Pasteur and others, to the quest for the magical bullet to treat syphilis, and on to the complex genetic theories entertained today. This study shows that the medical model is more than the unidimensional model its detractors often suggest it is. In my view, if we are to move to a truly integrative approach, the value of the medical model must be fully appreciated and nourished even as its limitations are recognized. Chapter 3 discusses the psychological foundations of health psychology. It examines the mind-body problem since current theory suggests that mental processes can alter body processes in profound ways. This chapter also uses data from stress and immune competence research to show how a psychological model can be built that integrates biomedical and psychosocial aspects. Chapter 4 presents the social side of the biopsychosocial equation, examining the social context of the practice of medicine. It shows how social networks (family, friends, and social agencies) are important to the maintenance of health and the prevention of illness. It is important to note that this part of the equation is not just social psychology, but the sociology *of* medicine and sociology *in* medicine. Social models of health and wellness are presented here as a background for understanding later research that focuses on large-scale systems variables.

Part 3

The third section presents information on two basic skills used by health psychologists, intervention (Chapter 5) and research (Chapter 6) strategies. Examples of both intervention and research are taken from current work in health psychology. Intervention strategies include various individual therapies, group interventions, and mass media educational programs. The goal is to change attitudes, control problematic emotional arousal (such as anticipatory anxiety for chemotherapy), and alter various health behaviors (compliance with a medical regimen or getting regular exercise, for example). We focus on four therapies widely used in practical settings: short-term therapy, cognitive therapy, behavior therapy, and pharmacotherapy. In Chapter 6, we consider the strengths and limitations of research designs in health psychology. This is intended to aid generalization from basic research classes, to provide a bridge for students who may not have a strong research background, and to illustrate some of the problems of doing research in such a complex area.

Part 4

Chapters 7 through 11 focus on lifestyle choices that affect health and illness. Chapter 7 begins with an overview of the stress model, one of the most powerful models suggesting how psychosocial processes may alter physical processes and affect health. Models of coping that may offset the effects of stress are also described. In Chapter 8, I introduce the topic of addictions in general and describe research on smoking addiction and smoking cessation programs in particular. Smoking is the most disastrous lifestyle choice that anyone can make, based on its ranking as the number one contributor to premature deaths—nearly 425,000 per year. Chapter 9 looks at alcoholism, the second most prevalent addiction in modern society. Important differences in women's metabolism of alcohol and consequent health risks are also described. Chapter 10 considers diet, obesity, and eating disorders. It reviews what is needed for a healthy diet, discusses the origins of eating disorders, and describes the interventions that may be useful to develop a healthy nutritional lifestyle. The closing chapter in this section deals with the AIDS epidemic, a disease that is largely spread through lifestyle choices involving high-risk sex and drugs. An important focus of this chapter is the attitudes that many people hold that lead to increased risk for exposure to HIV.

Part 5

Part 5 describes several chronic illnesses, the struggles of the patient to cope with disabling symptoms, and the impact of disease on caregivers, family, and friends. Chronic illnesses can go on over a lifetime in some cases, and typically exert a disturbing influence in family life and a debilitating effect on the person. The first chronic illness, discussed in Chapter 12, is coronary heart disease and other conditions related to heart health, such as hypertension. Recently developed models suggest how psychosocial events can hasten the onset of cardiovascular problems or contribute to better or worse prognosis following a coronary accident. Chapter 13 discusses the problem of pain. Pain is so common as to be a condition of existence, but its presence to the extreme in certain illnesses makes it the defining symptom. Here, I describe headache pain and low back pain, plus biomedical and psychosocial interventions to deal with pain. Finally, in Chapter 14, we take up the dread disease of cancer, and one crippling illness with a core of pain, arthritis.

Part 6

The last section of this book is something of a break from tradition as health psychology texts go. It presents information on two increasingly important areas, pediatric health psychology (Chapter 15) and geriatric health psychology (Chapter 16). As emphasis on preventive programs increases, more attention will be paid to educating children to make wise lifestyle choices. At the same time, children present special concerns in treatment for acute or chronic illnesses. On the other side of the age spectrum, as the life expectancy of the world increases, a much larger percentage of the population will be concentrated in the over-65 age range. This group also presents special concerns in maintaining a high quality of life. It perhaps goes without saying that the elderly also require special understanding as the spectre of personal mortality replaces the abstract notion of human mortality.

To the Instructor

A number of pedagogical devices have been included in this text to make the task of teaching and learning easier.

- End-of-chapter summaries highlight the important points, theories, and terms introduced in the chapter.
- Critical study questions help the student focus on core integrative concepts and become involved in a more active mastery of the material.
- A class projects section suggests ways in which students, with the assistance of the instructor, may introduce diversity into the classroom learning environment. My goal in these projects has been to provide various ways to encourage critical thinking about many of the pressing issues in health psychology.
- Suggested readings provide current research articles or integrative books that will help the motivated student move to more in-depth learning in each of the topic areas.
- A list of websites unique to the topic of the chapter provides the student with yet another way to access some of the best, most up-to-date information available on a variety of health issues. One word of warning that I encourage you to share with your students: In the midst of the great quantity and varied quality of information on the Web, many sites

are little more than forums for someone's pathology and rage (such as the prototypic "Barry's High-Anxiety Page"). Students increasingly want to use the web as a source for projects, but they may need help and sage advice in sorting the wheat from the chaff and avoiding reports turned in by suspect sources.

• Technical terms and concepts are boldfaced in the text and then compiled in an end-of-chapter "Key Words" list.

• A large number of visual aids (charts, graphs, tables, photos, illustrations, and artwork) is included to facilitate student engagement with the subject matter.

• A test bank of about 50 items per chapter is available in both paper and electronic form to assist in the evaluation component of the class.

Credits and Kudos

This work has benefited immensely from the guidance and patience of sponsoring editor Marianne Taflinger. There were times that I wondered whether this monumental undertaking would ever be finished, and I thought that perhaps the Biblical maxim was written as a sign to me: "And furthermore, my son, be admonished: of making many books there is no end; and much study is a weariness of the flesh" (Ecclesiastes 1:18).

A special thanks goes to the many reviewers who made extensive comments on strengths and weaknesses of the manuscript at various stages in its development: Andrew Baum, University of Pittsburgh; Joseph P. Bush, The Fielding Institute; Joan C. Chrisler, Connecticut College; Kathryn Graff Low, Bates College; Stephen H. Hobbs, Augusta College; Jeffrey Ratliff-Crain, University of Minnesota at Morris; and Theo B. Sonderegger, University of Nebraska, Lincoln.

In addition to the blind reviews, I have imposed on several colleagues and friends in the medical community to critically review several chapters. Dr. Anthony Bowman, former Director of Clinical Electrophysiology and Pacing at MeritCare Medical Center in Fargo and Clinical Assistant Professor of Medicine at the University of North Dakota School of Medicine, reviewed both Chapter 12 on the heart and Chapter 15 on diabetes. As a heart specialist, he made invaluable comments on Chapter 12. As a diabetic who has analyzed the strengths and weaknesses of current monitoring and lifestyle programs for diabetes management, he combined professional acumen with personal insights that I am sure made Chapter 15 much more focused. Dr. Carl Jensen, Medical Director of Radiation Oncology, Bay Area Hospital, Coos Bay, Oregon, reviewed Chapter 2 and Chapter 14. Dr. Jensen's professional expertise in treating cancer patients proved invaluable in regard to Chapter 14. Dr. Richard Kolotkin, professor of Clinical Psychology at Moorhead State University, made many helpful suggestions on the intervention chapter. Dr. Will Porter, in private practice in otolaryngology, reviewed Chapter 2 on the history of medicine.

I have also benefited from the work of several students who abstracted, collected articles and illustrations, rechecked resources, and managed permissions. In particular, I want to thank Nancy Waller who read Chapters 15 and 16 and commented on both clarity and style. Finally, thanks to Jeremy Holtgrewe, Andrea Beno, and Tammi Fortney for their work on this project and the many hours they spent obtaining resources and checking references.

Finally, if there were some way to fully recognize the contribution of public radio hosts Arthur Hoehn, Leigh Kamman, and Jim Wilkie, they would surely be entitled. I have written many, many pages accompanied by *Music Through the Night, The Jazz Image,* and *Jazz after Hours.* It seems in hindsight that the creative spirit of the composers and performers whose music lightened the long night hours lifted my own creative spirits and became an integral part of every page. Thank you all.

Phillip L. Rice

Note on Websites Feature

At the end of each chapter, a list of Internet sites is provided to help in furthering study, but also to guide individuals with health concerns (either personal or family) on where to find information and support sources. It is hoped that these Internet resources will prove valuable in many ways beyond the confines of the classroom.

A few words are in order regarding the selected sites. First, the amount of information on the Internet is now so voluminous that the issue is not whether you can find something, but how to narrow the choices. I tried to select websites that have been rated highly for quality and content. Second, I have opted for link sites in many cases rather than a long listing of individual sites. Link sites provide automated connections to many other sites with similar interests. Third, I tried to verify the operational integrity and currency of each site. At the same time, the Internet is a dynamic enterprise where some sites can disappear almost as fast as you find them, or they can be functional one day but not the next, or they are not maintained by their authors and thus become dated. There is no guarantee, then, that the sites will be functional or current by the time you read this. Still, if you learn some simple search strategies, you can generate your own list of important sites very quickly.

To this end, the list below shows some of the most powerful search engines available for searching the web, and also notes how individuals with disabilities can access the Internet. The Yahoo engine allows you to search by categories (such as health). Alta Vista tends to produce very broad searches. This is not very helpful when the topic is well represented on the Internet, but it can be helpful when you are having difficulty getting a lead. The Magellan site (Mckinley.com) is my favorite starting point because it allows a search on rated sites only if desired. This can produce a focused list of high-quality sites very quickly. In many cases, this is all that is needed to get started.

WEBSITES   *Internet Access*

ADDRESS	DESCRIPTION
http://www.yahoo.com	☆A general purpose, powerful search engine. Use the **Health** category to find virtually anything of interest.
http://www.altavista.digital.com	Powerful search engine
http://www.lycos.com/	Search engine with rated sites
http://searcher.mckinley.com	☆Powerful search with access to top-rated sites
http://www.c-cad.org/	Resource page for people with disabilities—links to disability websites and adaptive software

PART 1

Foundations and Definitions of Health Psychology

Psychology as a discipline has existed for little more than a century, yet events over the past quarter century testify to its surging vitality. In this short span of time, the timeworn black box models proposed by early behaviorists have been largely displaced by the emergence of cognitive psychology. Still, behaviorists left a rich legacy of techniques routinely used in various settings by different professional groups. Cognitive models provide new ways of viewing brain functions, abstract thinking processes, and possible links of psychopathology to disordered thinking. Physiological psychologists, functioning as the biologists of psychology, continue their quest to discover the relationships among body functions and behavior. Clinical psychology has an air of maturity, both in theory and technique, that is matched by practical gains. Clinical psychologists have gained recognition as licensed third-party pay providers. They are involved on more interdisciplinary treatment teams in various settings including hospitals. Medical specialists now are more likely to consult psychologists both to better understand and to treat their patients (Meyer, Fink, & Carey, 1988). Speciality fields continue to emerge as well, reflecting the diversity of interests and competence psychologists can bring to areas of practical and theoretical significance. Exemplary of this trend is psychoneuroimmunology, a field that overlaps neuroscience and biomedical research on the immune system.

As noteworthy as these events may be, this past quarter century may be most remembered for the birth of health psychology. Still in its infancy, this specialty field has established its own division and professional journal. It promises to make vital research contributions to complement our increasingly sophisticated database on health and illness. The focus of its theory building is the biopsychosocial model. This model suggests that although the onset of disease is typically triggered by physical insult to the body, the risk for illness, severity of symptoms, time course of the illness, and recovery from illness can be influenced by a complex matrix of psychosocial variables. Clinical interventions may be designed around this knowledge, and thus may help inform medical practice and reduce suffering. Educational interventions may also take advantage of knowledge that social attitudes and habitual patterns of acting can positively or negatively affect health. Then, education may become preventive medicine,

helping people avoid high-risk behaviors and thus reduce their vulnerability to illness.

The purpose of this book is to tell the story of health psychology—how it came to be and what it is about. Along the way, we will analyze the theoretical basis of this endeavor, in order to develop perspective on the interplay of forces that drew biomedical and psychosocial sciences together, and to clarify the strengths and limitations of current models. In time, we will discuss the background of research and clinical skills most often needed by health psychologists. Finally, we will look at health psychology applied to numerous problems such as heart health, pain, chronic illnesses, and in special populations such as children and the aging.

Here, we begin with defining issues. We consider how psychology came to have an interest in health issues, and how the field has been defined. Next, we discuss related fields that seem to share common themes and purposes. We will go inside common work sites and look at what health psychologists typically do, where they work, and what the future of health psychology might be. This is the story, then, of one of psychology's most dynamic new specialties.

CHAPTER 1

Health Psychology: A Growing Partnership in Health Care

Human Dilemmas: Questions for Biobehavioral Treatment

Consider for a moment this brief ledger of human ailments and physical miseries. The place is Hempstead, New York. It is a very warm day in the summer of 1987. An emergency rescue team is called to a small, nondescript apartment building, one of many like it in Main Street America's stereotypic row of tenements. Inside, a man, Walter Hudson, waist size *103 inches,* has become wedged in the doorway of his bedroom. Police, fire, and medical workers strain to rescue him. Workers estimate that Hudson must weigh at least 1000 pounds—this was *after* going on a diet to lose weight. By his own estimate, Hudson weighed around 1200 pounds at his peak. An exact weight was never established: no scale could be found to record a weight high enough. A follow-up investigation found that Hudson had not been out of his apartment since he moved to Hempstead 17 years earlier. At that time, he was a sleek 450 pounds. But after Hudson moved to Hempstead, he began consuming copious amounts of food. Breakfast and lunch, every day, he ate Thanksgiving-sized meals consisting of three or four ham steaks and six large bottles of soda. In the wake of intense publicity, the comedian Dick Gregory helped Hudson slim down to a svelte 520 pounds. Just three years later, during the holiday season of December 1991, Hudson died of a heart attack. Police had to cut a hole in the wall of his home. It took ten men and a forklift to remove his body. At the morgue, incredibly, he weighed 1120 pounds.

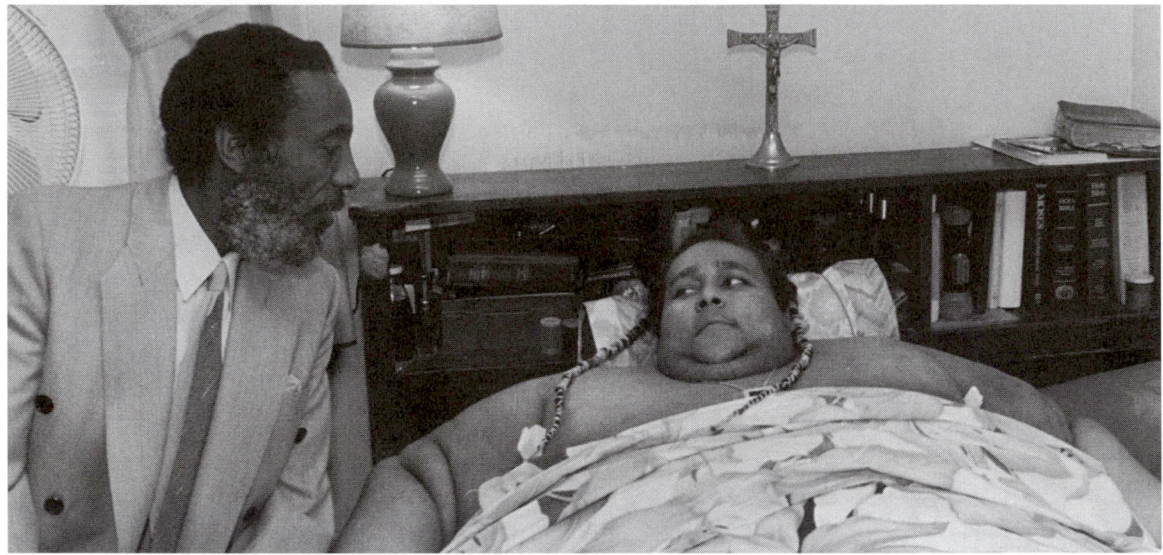

FIGURE 1.1   *Walter Hudson, whose 1200 pounds gained him national notoriety, visiting with Dick Gregory in New York (Associated Press photo).*

The place is rural Iowa. A 28-year-old man has been keeping doctors busy trying to find the cause of severe colitis, shortness of breath, and intense painful pressure in his chest. He has been to at least five of the best regional clinics including one of the world's best. He has had every relevant medical diagnostic test, plus some that were really placebos, given solely to convince the patient that the doctors were doing everything possible on his behalf. Still, medications provided no relief and surgery was not indicated. In spite of the fact that no medical explanation could be found for his symptoms, he remained convinced that there just had to be something physically wrong. That is, of course, the appealing answer. Not only does it fit our traditional belief system about causes of illness, but it also avoids the distastefulness we often associate with the notion that a physical disturbance might result from a psychological conflict.

Somewhere in Kansas, a bright, active young woman suffers from recurring painful and disabling migraine headaches. Her life has been turned into a shambles. Social activities are no longer open to her since she can never predict when another attack will occur. Family life has disintegrated. She feels cut off from her husband and children. They feel as if they are walking on eggs trying to hold on to a fragile peace that at any moment may be dispelled by another headache. All the sophisticated medical tests reveal no sign of an abnormal physical process. Pills provide only short-term relief. Her basic mood is one of despair because medical science seems to have offered no solution while the devastating headaches continue.

Picture a peaceful windswept bay near Boston. It was an early morning as a solitary figure walked the beach. These walks were not at all unusual, so there was little reason for concern when at first he did not return. But hours passed, and still there was no sign of him. Later, his body was found in the bay. This was no ordinary man, though. This was Lawrence Kohlberg, a man who devoted his life to the study of moral reasoning. Sadly, his health had changed dramatically after contracting a debilitating disease on a Central American trip (Rest, Power, & Brabeck, 1988). It may be that this solitary walk was a very private prelude to an existential suicide, but we will never know.

Medical science has taken gigantic strides to provide health preserving and health restoring services to humankind. But medicine is also coming to recognize that quality of life is as important as quantity of life. As good as his medical treatment was, Kohlberg was often disabled by nausea, pain, and depression. He tried to maintain his normal schedule of activities, but in the end found that he could not live as he once had. Perhaps he did not want to live his life so constrained. Perhaps he reached the moment when the solitude of death called more strongly than the echo of life.

Shared Themes: The Psychosocial Context of Health

On the surface, these cases do not seem to involve problems that are the primary concern of psychologists. The common link seems to be frailty of the body, pain, sickness, lab tests, medicine, surgery. In short, these problems seem to be the province of physicians and hospitals. Why should these dilemmas, then, be a topic for psychology? What place, if any, does psychology have in this arena?

The answer lies in society's incessant struggle to understand and control disease. Each case raises questions about **etiology,** the origin of disease and illness. The search for answers leads to one inescapable conclusion: We cannot conveniently divide disease into the physical and the psychological. Body and mind are not separate packages that can be bundled off to different healers. Disease has multiple causes, and illness results from many different forces acting in consort and collusion to alter body function and thus health status.

Think again of Walter Hudson. What could explain his extreme obesity? Surely, given the mass media blitz, people know that excessive weight poses serious health risks such as coronary disease. Was Hudson's problem, then, one of genes, or learning, or personality? Was he conditioned as a child to overreact to food cues, or was it a matter of willpower and self-

discipline? Did society shape attitudes toward slimness that made family and peers uncertain about how to respond to his largeness as a child? Each of these factors could reasonably be explored as contributing to Hudson's problem. As for treatment, was Hudson's condition to be remedied by drugs, by stomach surgery, by wiring his mouth shut? On the other hand, should it have been treated with behavioral therapy, cognitive therapy, or perhaps psychotherapy?

What forces conspired to produce the terrible colitis for the young man in Iowa or the dreadful headaches for the woman in Kansas? Did both occur because of problems in living, such as lack of coping skills to deal with life stressors? Even if stress played a role, might undiscovered physical factors still partly account for these disorders? Is it possible that some people are genetically less tolerant of stress than others? Where does one turn when the convenient and trusted medical explanations are no longer viable?

We are often reminded how brief the days of wine and roses are. Our social system values youth, health, and vitality above all else, and sometimes makes dying with dignity difficult. We may ask, then, about the physical, psychological, and social processes of aging—the erosion in quality of life—that often contribute to depressing, self-defeating views of retirement and old age. Matthew Arnold wrote of his despair to a friend:

The foot less prompt to meet the morning dew,
The heart less bounding at emotion new,
And hope, once crushed, less quick to spring
again.

As we shall see, the worldwide arena of health and wellness has been and is being redefined gradually but continuously to include issues, solutions, and providers that would not have been considered just a few years ago. In this arena, biomedical sleuths now wear a variety of disciplinary hats and probe many different dimensions of a person's environment to isolate factors believed to contribute to disease. As a result, traditional disease theories are being revised to include evidence of psychosocial influences in vulnerability to and risk for disease. There is evidence that the body's self-protective disease fighting tools may be impaired by chronic and intense stressors. Now, as a result, health care providers may be just as likely to provide treatments to influence the patient's mind and mood as to impact body structure and function. In this arena, illness behavior is just as important as a disease entity, and the positive quality of one's health is more important than the mere absence of disease.

Health Research and Treatment: Whose Business Is It?

Stop any person on the street and ask what psychology is and the answer might be something like "It's the study of the mind." If the person took a general psychology course recently, the response might be closer to "It's the science of behavior." For the most part, seasoned veterans in the discipline would recognize these informal ideas as close approximations to working definitions in vogue at one time or another in the history of psychology. Although there are important differences between informal and formal definitions, you would probably still feel you had a good idea of what psychology included and excluded. Indeed, psychology has built much of its reputation on practical successes with measures of intelligence, personality, and attitudes, and in treating the emotionally and behaviorally disturbed. These are all in some sense the province of mind and behavior.

Consider what your reaction might be, though, if that same person replied that "Psychology is a science of health and illness, how to keep healthy, how to prevent illness, and how to treat the ill." You would probably think the person had psychology confused with medicine. We go to medical doctors, not psychologists, when we are sick. When we are young, we get immunizations to prevent diphtheria, chicken

pox, and measles. The doctor gives us pills for high blood pressure. And when a heart goes bad, doctors may fix it surgically, or even replace it. Illness, in this conventional, socially approved way of thinking, is the province of medical science, not psychological science. Yet, the definition given at the beginning of this paragraph is very close to one adopted by the Division of Health Psychology (Division 38) of the American Psychological Association (APA).

How is it, then, that psychology has come to be concerned about questions of physical health and illness? The answer to this question lies partly within the history of psychology and partly within diverse social, political, and economic pressures that have emerged in the last quarter century. In the next few pages, we will retrace a few important steps leading to modern psychology's concern with health and illness. We will, of course, define the field and identify the boundaries that set health psychology apart from disciplines with similar missions.

Retracing Steps: What Do You Mean, You're Sick?

When the layperson says, "I'm sick," the phrase often means the same thing as "I'm ill." But in clinical circles, to be sick and to feel ill are not necessarily the same thing. I will discuss this issue more in Chapter 4, which considers social theories of disease and health. For now, we will focus on four basic questions and define terms. What does it mean to be sick or diseased? When one displays illness behavior, is that the same as sickness? Is health the opposite of being sick? How do health behaviors relate to being healthy?

Disease and Sickness: The System Malfunctions

Disease is a physical condition that results from a body malfunction. Disease may be due to a mechanical breakdown in a body organ (a defective heart valve, for example) or a malfunction in one of the body's systems (for example, the immune system). Disease may also occur because some toxin or microorganism invades the body, causing alterations in body tissue that lead to observable symptoms of distress. Sickness and illness, then, are technically equivalent terms that refer to a state of suffering from a disease. Note, however, that correct use of this terminology hinges on the presence of an identifiable pathological process.

Illness Behavior: Acting Sick or Being Sick

Symptoms are the first visible signs of disease. When they appear, you probably run through an internal check that evaluates and attaches meaning to the symptoms. In the process, you form a plan of action that may involve family members and a trip to the doctor's office. Upon reaching the clinic, you relate the details of your discomfort and describe your symptoms. You seek medical remedies and signs of support from medical staff, family, and friends. This process—evaluating symptoms, seeking medical help to bring relief, and seeking support from family—is the core of **illness behavior** (Mechanic, 1966). Foster and Anderson (1978) commented that "a medical doctor wishes to *cure disease* but he *treats illness,* for it is usually the impairment of function and not the presence of disease pathogens that causes us to seek aid" (p. 40).

Illness behavior can and does occur with or without physical indicators of disease. In fact, Barsky (1988) explained the rise in reports of illness between 1920 and 1980 as a result of our decreasing tolerance for even mild discomfort. Illness behavior is proper when a medical diagnosis or obvious symptoms (such as vomiting) occur. It is deviant, or at least frowned on, when it occurs in the absence of a diagnosed illness. Thus, disease refers to a physical condition of the body, while illness behavior defines a social role with expectations for both the sick person and the healer (Parsons, 1951).

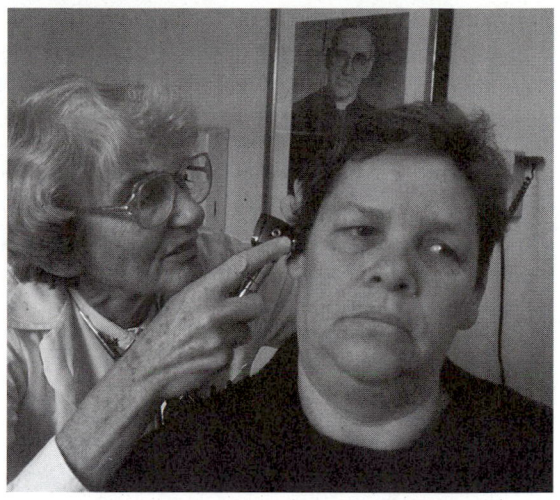

FIGURE 1.2   *Receiving care is often rewarding and may serve to maintain some illness behaviors.*

An important characteristic of illness behavior is that it often brings **secondary gains,** rewards or benefits obtained through the sick role. These gains include increased sympathy, attention, and special favors such as being waited on, and release from duty such as school or work. When health psychologists conduct research on psychosocial variables (such as stress) and health, the danger is that the social role of illness behavior (including unverified reports of sickness) may be confused with physical disease. This can lead to the erroneous conclusion that a psychosocial variable causes disease, when it may only increase the tendency to engage in illness behavior.

Health: The Opposite of Sickness?

We could define health as the absence of disease, but that defines health solely by reference to the negative. In other words, one could be free of disease but still not enjoy a full, wholesome, and satisfying life. Health entails quality valuations of physical soundness and mental vigor. The World Health Organization (WHO) defined health as "a state of complete physical, mental, and social well-being and not merely the absence of disease or infirmity" (cited in Seeman, 1989, p. 1100). On the physical side, it means the person enjoys a robust life with the energy needed to engage in satisfying pursuits and explorations of the environment. Simultaneously, the healthy person enjoys emotional fulfillment and self-esteem, both signs of positive mental health. Finally, social well-being is shown by the formation of close personal relationships.

Health Behavior: Positive Steps to Prevent Disease

Kasl and Cobb (1966) defined **health behavior** as activity undertaken by a person who believes himself or herself to be healthy for the purpose of preventing disease. It is estimated that 50% of premature deaths are a result of lifestyle risks and that lifestyle contributes 54% of the variability to cardiovascular disease (Institute of Medicine, 1979; Wilson, 1989). Health behavior may include reducing or eliminating high-risk behaviors such as smoking, poor diet, or unprotected sex. The person also may adopt positive behaviors such as regular exercise. Finally, health behavior may involve adhering to a distasteful though necessary medical regimen.

Marking Boundaries: Issues in Defining Health Psychology

Health psychology is still young—an infant as sciences go. Its birth as a discipline specific area within psychology is usually marked as 1978, when it was formally recognized as a division (Division 38) of the American Psychological Association with 1300 charter members. The first book to be named after the field was *Health Psychology,* a massive tome edited by George Stone and his colleagues (Stone, Cohen, & Adler, 1979), which notes in its introduction that "no book before this has borne that name" (p. 1). In 1982, the first official journal of the division was published, using the chosen name of the field as its title.

Health Psychology: A Working Definition

Division 38 still uses the definition first proposed by Joe Matarazzo (1982), a pioneer figure in health psychology: health psychology is

> the aggregate of the special educational, scientific, and professional contributions of the discipline of psychology to the promotion and maintenance of health, the prevention and treatment of illness, the identification of etiologic and diagnostic correlates of health, illness, and related dysfunction, and to the analysis and improvement of the health care system and health policy formation. (p. 4)

This definition contains several noteworthy features including recognition of three major pro-

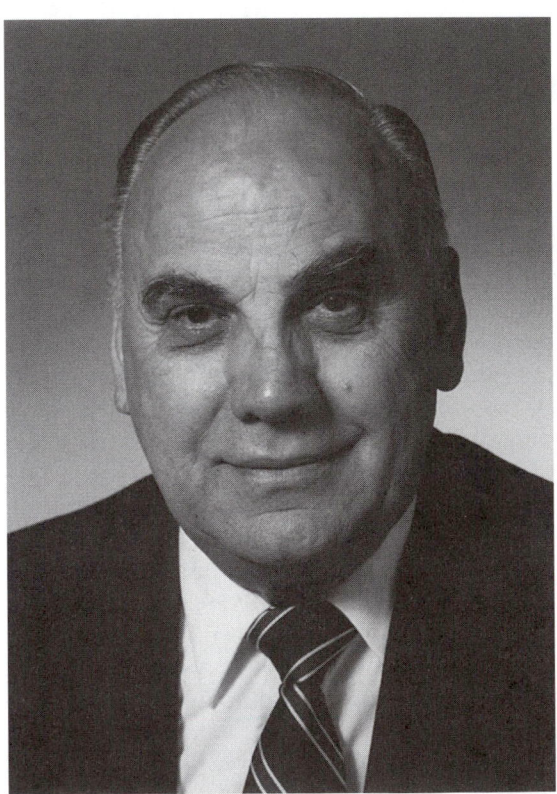

FIGURE 1.3   *Joe Matarazzo, past president of the American Psychological Association and one of the major figures in the development of health psychology.*

fessional activities: teaching, research, and intervention. These three roles will be discussed in more detail later.

First, although not explicitly stated, it is clear that the issue here is physical health and physical illness, not mental health and mental illness. Psychology clearly had no need to establish a new identity with a specialized division for issues of mental health and illness. That had been a central focus for nearly a century. Within this context, both health and illness are regarded as appropriate arenas for the work of psychologists.

Next, there is a strong emphasis on health promotion and maintenance, consistent with emerging societal concerns for the quality of life in general and the costs of health care in particular. Popular news sources are filled with reminders of astronomical increases in health care costs. Since 1980, when health care costs were $156 billion annually, costs skyrocketed to $989 billion in 1995 and may reach $1.5 trillion by the year 2000 (Health Care Finance Administration, 1997). The United States does not suffer alone; many industrialized nations have endured similar monumental cost increases.

In this context, one common theme of health promotion literature is changing lifestyles, based on numerous empirical demonstrations that behavioral and lifestyle risks are major contributing factors to illness and premature death (Institute of Medicine, 1979). About 50% of morbidity and premature mortality may be attributed directly to unhealthy lifestyles.[1] Since health behaviors arise from a multicausal matrix of emotions and motives, rewards and punishments, attitudes and beliefs, moods and traits, it seems natural that psychological research, theory, and intervention should make important contributions.

Further, the definition suggests that health psychology has a role to play in prevention and treatment of illness. In essence, the focus on promotion and maintenance of health is also a focus on preventing illness. Since the president's commission of 1962, mental health agencies have put increasing emphasis on preventive health care. The notion of preventive care has become even more important since it was noted that about 60% of patient visits to physicians are prompted by symptoms provoked by psychosocial stressors or by behavioral excesses such as smoking and overeating (Bohart & Todd, 1988).

Still, the treatment of disease was not traditionally recognized as appropriate territory for psychology. As subsequent chapters will demonstrate, though, many behavioral, cognitive, and attitudinal factors influence a patient's acceptance of medical interventions, recovery from illness, and compliance with vital medical and health maintenance regimens. **Compliance** is the patient's accepting the clinician's advice and, most important, actually engaging in the recommended behavior, whether that is taking pills, reducing weight, or increasing exercise. Compliance can be a significant problem, since 93% of patients fail to follow prescribed regimens properly (Taylor, 1990). In all these respects, health psychology has much to offer for treatment of the ill.

Fourth, the definition notes the concern for etiologic and diagnostic correlates of health, illness, and related dysfunction. **Etiology** is concerned with the origins or causes of disease, while **diagnosis** is concerned with accurately discerning the disease behind a cluster of symptoms. To the extent that psychosocial factors may contribute substantively to disease, health psychology has an interest in uncovering that etiology. Thus theories of disease may be refined to include not only the latest pathogens or toxins, but also malfunctions resulting from mood fluctuations or psychosocial stressors.

Psychosocial processes are also known to complicate diagnostic procedures. Shakespeare was aware of this as he wrote in *King Lear* (Act II, Scene 4):

We are not ourselves
When nature, being oppress'd, commands the
mind
To suffer with the body.

---

[1] Technically, morbidity is the presence of disabling symptoms, and mortality is death. Both are important measures in epidemiological research, which is described in more detail in Chapter 6.

Emotionality in the patient undergoing an invasive clinical test, or breakdowns in communication between doctor and client, can produce detrimental effects for diagnosis and treatment. The viewpoint of health psychology can add significantly, then, to uncovering variables that influence etiology or diagnosis.

Fifth, health psychology has a role to play in "the analysis and improvement of the health care system and health policy formation." Psychologists have, of course, had a long-standing interest in **program evaluation,** a branch of research that is primarily concerned with determining the value of service agency programs (Sechrest & Figueredo, 1993). In addition, psychologists now are actively involved in the arena of policy formulation at local, state, national, and international levels (Holtgrave, Doll, & Harrison, 1997). The effort has been to bring to policy formation the unique view of health as a multicausally determined process.

Health Psychology: What It Is Not

Finally, the definition leaves unstated what health psychology is not. Interest in health and illness does not mean that health psychology usurps medicine's prerogatives in diagnosis of physical disease, in prescribing medicines, or in medical practice. Those functions rightfully belong to medicine, although encroachments have already been made on this tradition. In addition, the development of health psychology does not deny the significant value of biomedical research and theory; but it does suggest that the time has come to add detail to disease theory by including the psychosocial context of disease.

As noted earlier, some of medicine's prerogatives are being challenged, and health psychologists may even lobby for autonomy in medical settings (Clayson & Mensh, 1987; Thompson, 1987). Within the domain of clinical psychology, for example, a concerted effort is under way to obtain prescription rights for psychologists working in medical settings. This effort assumes that psychologists will have both significant training in pharmacology and supervised experience before licensing. The debate on this issue is still going on in houses sharply divided both in the medical and psychological professions (Kingsbury, 1992; May & Belsky, 1992). At this time, it is not possible to say what the outcome will be, how it might impact clinical psychologists in general and clinical health psychologists in particular, or how it might affect the working relationship between medicine and psychology.

Marking Boundaries: The Difference in Health Psychology

In its brief life, health psychology has struggled for both identity and credibility. It has had to distinguish itself from several forerunners, such as psychosomatic medicine and medical psychology. These disciplines seemed concerned with similar issues, but initially they had different missions, and psychosomatic medicine has had a checkered history. At the same time, health psychology was, and often still is, confused with another specialty field, behavioral medicine.

On the theoretical front, health psychology comes down strongly on the side of the biopsychosocial model, a stance that requires some reconciliation with the biomedical view of disease. The biopsychosocial view holds that disease involves a physical cause, but psychosocial forces combine with physical forces to influence vulnerability to disease, success or failure in treating a disease, and success in maintaining health.

Further, even as health psychology has tried to carve out its unique domain as a discipline-specific enterprise, it has found itself involved with numerous collaborators and protagonists both within and outside the field of psychology. Within psychology itself, health psychology has provided many opportunities for new or renewed liaisons, such as the relationship between clinical and social psychology (Meyerowitz, Burish, & Wallston, 1986).

On the outside, health psychology collaborates with many health care specialties such as medicine, nursing, and neuroscience. Collaboration has led to true interdisciplinary efforts. While each specialty brings a slightly different viewpoint, the diverse theoretical notions increasingly are seen as supportive and integrative rather than divisive and competitive. And while our primary concern here is psychology's unique contributions to health care, it must be apparent that health care has been, is, and always will be an interdisciplinary effort.

I noted earlier that two forerunners were psychosomatic medicine and medical psychology. I will discuss contributions from these fields before considering related fields such as behavioral medicine, behavior therapy, and medical sociology. Even as we discuss these differences, I am reminded of George Stone's (1991) admonition that "any application of psychological theory or practice to problems and issues of the health system is health psychology" (p. xi).

Psychosomatic Medicine: The Psychogenic Theory of Disease

When people say an illness is all in the head, they are voicing the populist view of psychosomatic illness. But there is much more to it. The word *psychosomatic,* first coined by psychiatrist J. C. A. Heinroth (1773–1843), comes from two Greek words: *psyche,* which means mind or soul, and *soma,* which means body (Ackerknecht, 1982). **Psychosomatic illness** is physical disease caused by the mind; another term for this is *psychogenic illness.*

Psychosomatic medicine is the psychiatric treatment of the ill based on the theory of psychogenic origins of illness. Medical historians find evidence for the practice as early as the Golden Age of Greece (Lipowski, 1977; Schwab, 1985). In 1747, a medical professor by the name of Gaub said, "The reason why a sound body becomes ill, or an ailing body recovers, very often lies in the mind" (cited in Lipowski, 1977, p. 234). Helen Dunbar (1947), a noted psychosomatic theorist who was contemporary with renowned psychiatrist Franz Alexander, believed strongly that the time would come when medical teachers would find it necessary to come full circle to the wisdom of the ancients. She wrote: "They will explain that since the mind and body are one and indivisible, the same principle holds true in healing the breaks in human emotional fabric. They will teach that your mind is your body and vice versa" (p. 260).

Franz Alexander (1950) provided the most complete theory and developed many core assumptions of psychosomatic medicine. According to Alexander, psychosomatic medicine would allow physicians to integrate knowledge of psychosocial factors into treatment of patients. Above all, psychosomatic medicine was to be a bridge between the traditional practice of medicine and the then newly arrived Freudian view of psychic determinism. Alexander's theory stated explicitly that chronic emotional upheaval would lead sooner or later to changes in body functions and could lead to physical pathology. Even when organic changes did not immediately appear, insidious forces were still at work altering body process. Which organ or system would break down first depended on constitutional weaknesses that varied from person to person.

Alexander's theory suffered from two major flaws. First, it was heavily biased by Freudian psychoanalytic theory. Shepherd (1978) suggested that psychosomatic views were scientifically naive attempts to force physical illness into the mold of psychoanalytic theory in an attempt to demonstrate psychological causation. Second, Alexander's model was dualistic, defining some diseases as indisputably physical, requiring strictly medical treatment, and other disorders as mental and thus requiring psychotherapy. Health psychology does not accept Alexander's disease dualism. Ample evidence suggests that psychosocial factors influence most, if not all, disease processes in one way or another, and that treatment should also be multimodal.

In 1977, Lipowski tried to draw together what he called the general framework of psychosomatic theory. Two traits of this "new look" psychosomatic medicine are relevant here, but they stand in marked contrast to Alexander's views. First, in Lipowski's view, psychosomatic science studies the interactions among biological, psychological, and social causes of health and disease. These three factors "codetermine the timing of onset, course, and outcome of disease" (p. 235), and thus make up the multicausal matrix of disease. Second, psychosomatic science embraces a holistic approach to practice.

In Lipowski's framework, one core assumption is that symbolic activity alters body processes. All workings of the mind, including memories, thoughts, decisions, and imagery, can alter homeostasis (biological equilibrium), adaptation, and health. As an example, Lipowski used psychosocial stress to show that social, psychological, and biological forces interact to influence health. He concluded that "psychosocial stress may be . . . as injurious as extremes of temperature, pathogenic microorganisms, and physical trauma" (p. 237). It is interesting to note that this statement could just as easily have been made by a health psychologist. In the final analysis, there may be very few psychoanalytic ghosts to exorcise from Lipowski's new look psychosomatic medicine. However slow its transformation may be, it converges on the model adopted by health psychology. Defined in Lipowski's terms, psychosomatic medicine could be a sister discipline, sharing many of health psychology's interests and assumptions.

Medical Psychology: The Forerunner of Health Psychology?

We probably would not expect to walk into a hospital and bump into a psychologist. The stereotype is that psychologists work in mental health clinics, in counseling centers, or in private practice. Yet, between 1953 and 1976, the number of psychologists working in medical settings grew from 255 to 2336 (Gentry &

Matarazzo, 1981), and by 1986, there were about 3000 (Clayson & Mensh, 1987). There is even a name for this old and venerable group—medical psychologists. Still the impetus for medical psychology came, not from psychology, but mostly from medical schools. In the beginning of this century, medical schools sought to reintroduce the psychological component of clinical practice into medicine—in other words, to teach the *art* of medicine by having psychologists teach medical students something about the nature of being human.

People suffer from many fears and anxieties when they confront the unknown, when they face the first signs of trouble in a previously trustworthy body. They may not know how to express what they feel. They may not know how to ask the right questions of their doctors. Doctors may be so engrossed in their specialties they see only a weak heart, a diseased lung, or a malignant tumor. They might lose sight of the real person who suffers more than just physically when threats to health intrude. This understanding led to psychologists' first becoming involved in many issues of health care service and research.

In England, medical psychology is an old discipline more allied to psychiatry than to psychology. Even so, as Zilboorg (1941, p. 13) noted, medical psychology, or psychological medicine as it is sometimes called, is older and more comprehensive than psychiatry. As such, medical psychology is defined as the branch of medicine devoted to the "art" of handling patients as opposed to the "science" of diagnosis and treatment. The art of medicine involves tactfulness and intuition to fathom what might be behind patients' moodiness or reluctance to accept medical advice. Alexander (1950), seeking a more respectable vantage point, suggested that "modern scientific medical psychology is but an attempt to place medical art, the psychological affect of the physician upon the patient, on a scientific basis and to make it an integral part of therapy" (p. 18). Much later, Bohart and Todd (1988) defined medical psychology as a group of procedures concerned with the study and management of physical illness.

Unfortunately, these definitions do little to distinguish medical psychology from either health psychology or behavioral medicine. Prokop and Bradley (1981) edited an entire volume whose title, *Medical Psychology: Contributions to Behavioral Medicine,* implied that because it makes contributions to behavioral medicine, medical psychology is a subset of behavioral medicine. They also admitted that there is no consensus on what distinguishes medical psychology from behavioral medicine. To make matters worse, the terms *health psychology, medical psychology,* and *behavioral medicine* often have been used as though they are interchangeable. Gentry and Matarazzo (1981) even allude to the fact that pressure from a large group of medical psychologists played a role in formation of the APA's division of health psychology.

We will treat medical psychology as an early attempt to apply psychological concepts to the management of patients for the purpose of improving their health care while under medical supervision. In general, medical psychologists work in medical settings to provide diagnostic and counseling services (Gentry & Matarazzo, 1981). In addition, medical psychologists carry on research activities and teach classes on psychological components of illness and clinical services. From this vantage point, medical psychology is more an arena of activity than a formal discipline.

Behavior Therapy: Treatment That Made a Difference

Before describing the discipline of behavioral medicine, we must discuss one formative influence in the emergence of both behavioral medicine and health psychology—the development of behavior therapy. The history of behavior therapy may be as old as the history of

civilization itself (Franks, 1969), but here we are concerned only with its appearance in modern clinical practice. Adopting the definition from Masters, Burish, Hollon, and Rimm (1987), **behavior therapy** is a group of techniques that uses psychological principles, especially learning principles, to change behavior. The learning principles usually represent some combination of classical, operant, and modeling techniques. Wolpe (1958) is credited with bringing the classical conditioning approach to fear reduction with development of desensitization procedures.[2] Lindsley (1956), one of B. F. Skinner's students, was among the first to use operant techniques to treat mentally disturbed patients. Since then, a wide range of techniques has been developed with empirical data to support their efficacy and generality. Blanchard and colleagues (1982) and Agras (1984) made the case that the reliability of behavior therapy and the tradition of behavior research led to the acceptance of psychology as a legitimate partner with biomedical science in the treatment of medical patients.

Behavioral Medicine: Will the Real Health Psychology Please Stand Up?

Probably, more controversy has focused on the distinction between health psychology and behavioral medicine than any of the other related fields. The crux of the matter rests on one very simple point: Health psychology is discipline specific while behavior medicine cuts across several disciplines. For this reason, some still prefer the term *behavior medicine* to *health psychology,* feeling that it is more consistent with the emerging multicausal model of illness. At the core of behavior medicine practice is the group of techniques previously described as behavior therapy, consisting of the application of behavioral techniques to the treatment, management,

---

[2] A variety of behavior therapies will be discussed more fully in Chapter 5.

and rehabilitation of medical patients in various phases of their illness (Pinkerton, Hughes, & Wenrich, 1982). Some people believe there is more to behavior medicine than just management of illness. This can be seen by looking more closely at the concepts and people most involved in behavior medicine.

According to Doleys, Meredith, and Ciminero (1982, p. 83), the first use of the term *behavioral medicine* came when Birk (1973) discussed biofeedback in the treatment of medical disorders. As early as 1977, Yale University hosted a conference on behavioral medicine that set about developing a working definition of the field. Later, in 1978 (the same year that health psychology was formed as an APA division), two national societies were formed, the Society of Behavioral Medicine and the Academy of Behavioral Medicine Research, the latter with sponsorship from the National Academy of Sciences. The biobehavioral definition that follows was adopted at the Yale conference and was offered as an incentive to discussion, not an end in itself.

> Behavioral Medicine is the field concerned with the development of behavioral-science knowledge and techniques relevant to the understanding of physical health and illness and the application of this knowledge and these techniques to prevention, diagnosis, treatment and rehabilitation. Psychosis, neurosis and substance abuse are included only insofar as they contribute to physical disorders as an endpoint. (Schwartz & Weiss, 1978b, p. 249)

This definition makes several significant points. First is the explicit assumption that illness and health are states that cannot be understood solely by reference to medical theories of disease. This assumption was not intended in any sense to minimize the importance of medical theory, research, or techniques—just the opposite. The conference suggested instead that health and illness must be understood by reference to the integration of biomedical concepts with psychosocial constructs.

Almost before the dust had settled from the first conference, though, another conference was in progress at the National Academy of Sciences under the leadership of Neal Miller and David Hamburg. This group modified the first definition and in so doing showed more accurately the cooperative spirit of the endeavor. This spirit is also clearly revealed in the diverse fields represented. The amended definition reads as follows:

> Behavioral Medicine is the *interdisciplinary* field concerned with the development *and integration of* behavioral *and biomedical* science knowledge and techniques relevant to health and illness and the application of this knowledge and these techniques to prevention, diagnosis, treatment and rehabilitation. (Schwartz & Weiss, 1978b, p. 250; italics added)

The interdisciplinary emphasis shows that behavior medicine cuts across many boundaries and encourages collaborative efforts to help the patient. The Academy of Behavioral Medicine Research points out that anthropology, biostatistics, dentistry, epidemiology, health education, nursing, nutrition, pharmacology, physiology, and sociology are all likely collaborators in behavior medicine (Doleys et al., 1982, p. 5).

Now, the field is viewed as concerned with research on various factors contributing to the etiology and progress of illness. Much of what has been done is in keeping with Miller's challenge, delivered in the 1977 conference, to be "bold in what you try, but cautious in what you claim" (Schwartz & Weiss, 1978a, p. 6). Behavior medicine is concerned with substantive educational programs whose mission is the prevention or reduction of high-risk behaviors that contribute to illness. It seeks to develop and apply treatments that will serve clientele in various stages of coping with illness, including compliance with medical regimens. As Schwartz and Weiss (1978b) noted, the reference to physical disorders contained in the first definition was dropped from the amended definition because "mental vs. physical disorders are no longer described in purely behavioral vs. biological terms but rather are conceived and studied from a more integrated, *biobehavioral* perspective" (p. 250).

Numerous markers now reflect the rapid growth and widespread acceptance of behavior medicine. When it was founded in 1978, the Society of Behavioral Medicine was closely allied with the Association for Advancement of Behavior Therapy; by 1981, it was fully independent. Three journals have been founded to disseminate theory, method, and practice: the *Journal of Behavioral Medicine, Behavioral Medicine,* and *Behavioral Medicine Abstracts.* Further, more than 400 universities now offer courses in behavioral medicine, and specialized graduate programs are available leading to a doctorate and licensure.

This growth has led to a healthy debate on criteria for training in behavior medicine, a debate that has progressed to the discussion of essential components for a graduate curriculum (Dana & May, 1987). A set curriculum is not yet in place, but the components Dana and May suggested are consistent with the National Academy of Science's description of behavior medicine. The suggested curriculum includes (1) epidemiology; (2) anatomy, physiology, and psychophysiology; (3) pharmacology; (4) risk factors for coronary disease; (5) current treatments of choice for various illnesses; (6) skills in the use of various psychophysiological recording instruments and assessment procedures; (7) specialized clinical skills in biofeedback, autogenics, and imagery, among others, and (8) general clinical issues in treating medical patients (Dana & May, 1987, p. 263).

In retrospect, we can see that *health psychology* has on the one hand supplanted the older, vague term *medical psychology.* On the other hand, health psychology's primary mark of distinction from behavioral medicine is that it is more discipline specific. Though arguments are advanced that behavioral medicine focuses too narrowly on specific medical applications for behavioral techniques, these arguments do not appear to reflect either actual practice or the major developments in the field during the 1980s. Instead, behavior medicine can be regarded as a collaborator in current efforts to understand the interrelations between biomedical and psychosocial factors.

Rehabilitation Psychology: Prosthesis and Coping

As their title implies, rehabilitation psychologists work with patients to help them recover functional skills lost through accidents, strokes, or deteriorative disease processes. The goal is to help the patient retrieve or relearn as much as possible: to learn how to get the most out of available assistive technology and prosthetic devices that may restore only some functionality, or how to cope with the remnants of the affected skill (Millon, Green, & Meagher, 1982; Solarz, 1990). Rehabilitation psychologists often use psychodiagnostic skills, including psychophysiological assessment, to assess residual ability and suggest what reasonable expectations the patient can have for partial or full recovery. They are also likely to use a variety of behavioral interventions, including biofeedback strategies (Elliott & Gramling, 1990). Traditionally rehabilitation psychology has had a very narrow focus, covering only a small part of the total enterprise of health psychology.

Medical Sociology: Health and Illness in Social Perspective

The allied field that represents the sociological study of health and illness is medical sociology. In 1902 a medical doctor, Elizabeth Blackwell, was among the first to use the term in the title of a collection of essays on social work and public health. Just a few years later, James P. Warbasee foresaw the modern interest in health education with his book *Medical Sociology.* Later, in 1910, a few social workers and physicians organized a short-lived section on sociology within the

American Public Health Association. Suffering from a lack of active support among sociologists, the division was abandoned in 1921 (Mumford, 1983).

Later, medical sociology developed in two directions. First, the sociologists of medicine worked to clarify numerous questions about the social context of health care, medical settings, and medical professions. The second group of sociologists, in a tradition that most closely resembles that of medical psychologists, actually became faculty members in medical schools. They taught and researched issues such as the distribution and etiology of diseases, and attitudes and behavior that influence health and illness. One obvious variable of interest to medical sociologists was the relation between social class and illness, but they also developed influential theories of illness as deviance. Further, they considered the problem of labeling as a consequence of diagnostic procedures. Even today, there is a controversy about calling a person a patient, a label that may stigmatize, demean, and lower the person's sense of responsibility to assist in his or her own treatment. Some suggest that we should call the person a sufferer, not a patient. But as Atkinson (1993) argued, the term *sufferer* has its own negative connotations, including the notion of the person as a victim. Health education is still one of the major concerns of medical sociology. Unfortunately, the vested interests of the health care industry have erected many barriers, both political and economic, that discourage effective health education programs (Bartlett & Windsor, 1985).

Here and Now: Perspectives on the Profession

When anyone looks at a field for the first time, especially with an eye to a possible professional career, many questions require answers. Just what do health psychologists do and where do they work? What is the academic pathway to a

degree, and what type of training can the aspiring health psychologist expect to receive? It is also pertinent to ask what the future holds for a new discipline, especially one that is in such a state of rapid growth and change.

Typically, health psychologists engage in any of four activities: teaching, research, administration, and clinical services. In most cases, health psychologists wear more than one hat, though the proportion of time devoted to any area differs among settings.

The Health Psychologist as Educator-Teacher

At one time, teaching was largely done in medical, nursing, or public health schools. As traditional psychology programs continue to add health psychology courses, both undergraduate and graduate, health psychologists will find more opportunities for teaching combined with research or clinical activities in traditional academic departments. Teaching in medical and nursing schools has proved valuable because it offers these core health care providers valuable insights into many psychosocial factors that may affect the patient's interactions with the health care staff. Acceptance of painful diagnostic procedures, concern about risks in surgery, compliance with restrictive medical regimens—all may influence the success of treatment. Even bedside manner and office staff demeanor can affect the patient. Further, nurses have been trained in behavioral methods that help patients cope with illness, as well as research methods that help add knowledge about the relationship between behavior and risk for illness.

Educational efforts often take on an interdisciplinary flavor as the fruits of research and clinical developments are disseminated to different professional groups. Education also cannot be confined to the classroom, but reaches out to the community through efforts to educate people about the benefits of behavioral change. Finally, education may extend to government agencies as health psychologists provide information to influence health policy formulation and research funding (Carr, 1987).

Health psychologists have expended considerable effort to develop programs for preventing illness and maintaining health. These programs are very often of an educational nature, though the arena of delivery is not the conventional classroom. Health psychologists have worked in Employee Assistance Programs (EAPs) in business and industry, and in a variety of community health care agencies, to educate people about high-risk behaviors such as smoking, alcoholism, a sedentary lifestyle, and behaviors that may lead to exposure to AIDS. Health psychologists have helped develop programs to help people better cope with stress, develop more healthy lifestyles, reduce or prevent drug abuse, and reduce risks for coronary disease.

The Health Psychologist as Researcher

A second area of activity for the health psychologist is research. It sometimes puzzles undergraduate students that clinicians are required to master statistics and methodology. The educational philosophy for training clinicians comes from the Boulder Model, named after the conference held at Boulder, Colorado, in 1949 (Belar, Deardorff, & Kelly, 1987). This model suggested that psychologists should be trained as scientist-practitioners—that they should know both the basics of human behavior and how to think critically and evaluate hypotheses objectively. The model rejects the notion that clinicians (practitioners) can be competent while ignorant of the scientific basis for their profession. Although health psychology adopted this Boulder stance in principle, it did so only as the result of careful examinations of current needs, as exemplified in several recent health psychology conferences dealing with national training standards and licensure issues.

Health psychologists share with most psychologists a common core of methodological and statistical tools. Still, traditional psychological research and health psychology research differ in two major ways. First, the problems that interest health psychologists involve a complex matrix of biomedical and psychosocial variables. The problems also assume, at the outset, a multicausal answer. Second, because many problems concern the distribution and etiology of disease, some methodological tools are more important. For example, the health psychologist is more likely to use epidemiological methods than the traditional psychologist is. These research tools will be described in Chapter 6.

Altmaier and Meyer (1985) believe that health psychology focuses on three basic types of problems. The first problem is to identify psychological processes that may contribute to health maintenance or increased risk for illness. Current work on stress and the immune system exemplifies this approach (Kiecolt-Glaser et al., 1985). The second problem, related to health psychology's educational and intervention roles, is to develop and evaluate programs that persuade individuals to adopt a healthy lifestyle. For example, Richard Evans and his colleagues developed programs to educate juveniles about the dangers of smoking and hoped thus to deter them from smoking (Evans, Henderson, Hill, & Raines, 1979). Williams and Lund (1992) also noted that psychologists have an important role to play in injury control through both research efforts and educational strategies. The third type of research problem is direct evaluation of therapeutic interventions. Here, the intent is to improve overall quality of treatment programs. This emphasis is consistent with one trademark of behavior therapy: **outcome assessment,** or the objective assessment of treatment programs so that such things as success rate, permanence of change, and generalization of change are all known quantities instead of subjective estimates of success. We should add a fourth research problem to the three identified by Altmaier and Meyer—namely, program evaluation, when a complete institutional system, consisting of an entire group of health care providers and all the system's programs, is assessed for efficacy.

The Health Psychologist as Clinician

The newly defined field of clinical health psychology is the application of clinical skills to the problems of health and illness. For the interested reader, the work by Belar, Deardorff, and Kelly (1987) provides more detail on this field. As a clinician, the health psychologist may provide both indirect and direct services. A medical specialist might request a consultation to determine whether a patient has fears and anxieties, or even clinical pathologies (such as extreme depression), that bear on the medical treatment plan. Here, the psychologist provides indirect services to the medical team. Both assessment and diagnostic skills will be called into play in such situations.

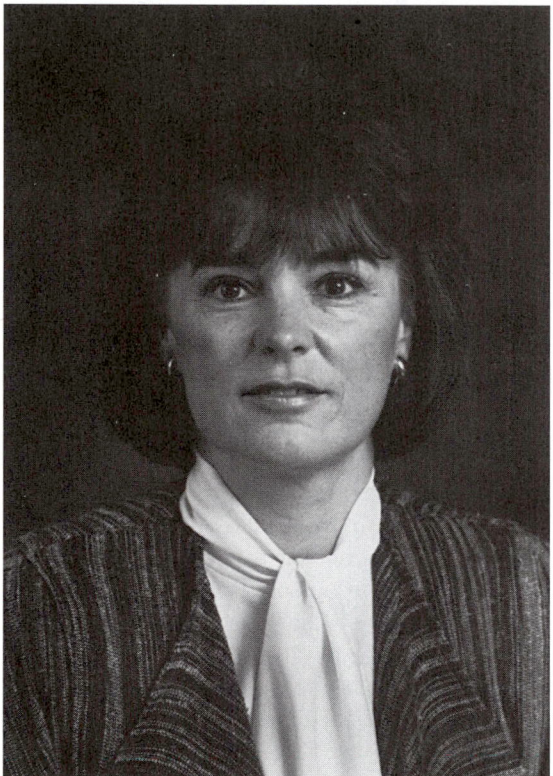

FIGURE 1.4 *Cynthia Belar, current president of Division 38, maintains that health psychology is not a practice division or a science division but both.*

At other times, direct interventions may be required. Clinical health psychologists might design a program to help a patient cope with chronic pain or adhere to a difficult medical regimen. They might provide biofeedback for migraine patients. They might counsel terminally ill patients and their families, or bereaved family members following the death of their loved one.

Thus, the clinical health psychologist requires the same broad base of training in assessment, diagnosis, and therapy that any clinician receives. In contrast to the traditional clinical psychologist, though, the health psychologist uses these clinical skills in a different setting and with different patients—people who have concerns with physical health. Further, the clinical health psychologist most often works in cooperation with a large group of health care professionals and can assume that primary responsibility for the patient's overall treatment program rests with one of the medical doctors.

Health Psychology's Work Settings: Where Is the Office?

Information about where health psychologists work changes as rapidly as the field itself. In an early study, Belar and her colleagues surveyed recent health psychology graduates and found that 41% were employed in university medical centers, 25% in universities, 17% in clinical treatment facilities, 7% in private practice, 4% in the federal government, and 2% in industrial settings (Belar, Wilson, & Hughes, 1982). An APA survey of 1993 doctoral recipients showed 47% of the health psychology graduates working in hospital settings, nearly 24% in a human service agency, 12% in an academic setting (including 6% in medical schools), and nearly 18% in business or government agency (Wicherski & Kohout, 1995). Among all graduates, more than 23% were employed in an academic setting, and another 5.5% were employed in medical schools. Nearly 18% were employed in hospitals, another 9% in managed care settings, and 12% in other human service settings.

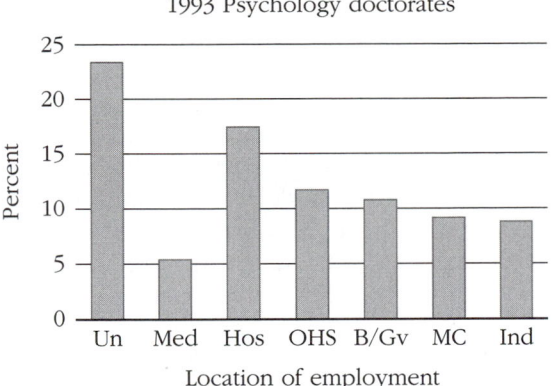

1993 Psychology doctorates

FIGURE 1.5 *Employment pattern of 1993 doctorate recipients across different settings (Data from Wicherski & Kohout, 1995). (Un = university; Med = medical school; Hos = hospital setting; OHS = other health service setting; B/Gv = business or government setting; MC = managed care setting; and Ind = independent practice.)*

Among the many possible work sites are hospitals, dental schools, nursing schools, neurosurgery and pediatric divisions of hospitals and medical schools, university undergraduate and graduate programs, medical schools (usually in a psychiatric division), health maintenance organizations (HMOs), and research agencies at various levels up to the national and even international level. HMOs generally emphasize preventive medicine. They recognize the importance of psychosocial factors in determining the rate and course of illness. It is, of course, in the HMO's best interest to promote wellness and thus reduce the use of medical services. To this end, HMOs may offer community education programs related to health and wellness.

Getting Ready: The Road to a Professional Career

From this brief description of the health psychologist's role, it may now be easier to understand the reasoning behind the specific require-

ments of graduate training programs. These standards are the result of several conferences that sought to define what health psychologists should know when they complete their formal education and what practical experiences they should have before beginning an independent practice. Although we refer to training standards, we should note that training for health psychologists is far from standardized. As will become obvious shortly, this lack of standardization reflects the newness and complexity of the field, not inattention to quality issues. Further, opinions justifiably differ when standards are devised for a clinical program as opposed to a teaching-research program. In either case, knowledge of graduate training guidelines may enable undergraduate students to select classes that will stand them in good stead for a graduate program in health psychology.

The first major conference to develop training standards for health psychologists was the Arden House conference, held at Harriman, New York, in May 1983. Officially, this was the National Working Conference on Education and Training in Health Psychology. The basic principles developed at this conference can be summarized briefly. First, the doctorate degree is the entry level degree for health psychology. Second, the goal of training is to develop scientist-practitioners. More explicitly, this means that the doctorate program must include both a scientifically based doctoral dissertation and a supervised internship before completing the degree.

The conference also identified the core components of an ideal graduate curriculum. Undergraduate training is generally not a concern where the entry degree is the doctorate. It is safe to assume that a broad liberal arts education, preferably including a psychology major, will suffice. Still, people may come into health psychology with training from other programs including biology, sociology, social work, education, or health education among others. Psychology's family tree is rich with influential people who have come to psychology with undergraduate degrees in other fields. The psychology major may be desirable, then, but it is not an absolute prerequisite for a psychology graduate program.

At the graduate level, the student can expect an analytic core of intensive training in general psychology, measurement, statistics, experimental design, and other methodological skills (for example, epidemiology and biostatistics) especially pertinent to research on health and illness. Although graduate programs continue to emphasize statistics and methodology, the breadth of coverage may not yet reflect the changes occurring in the last 20 years. One group concerned with the current quality of graduate teaching in statistics noted that many programs have not yet incorporated newer multivariate methods, causal modeling, multidimensional scaling, and meta-analytic techniques and that measurement and test theory have undergone some decline in emphasis (Aiken et al., 1990).

After this general background, the ideal program should contain a theoretical core pertinent to the three domains identified in health psychology's general approach, the biopsychosocial model. The first domain covers the bio-

logical bases of behavior and may entail work in physiology, anatomy, neuroanatomy, neuropsychology, and psychopharmacology. The second domain covers traditional elements of a psychology program, but the emphasis can vary depending on the type of program (clinical versus research) and the student's specialization. The courses usually cover content in affective, lifespan developmental, adaptive, and cognitive processes, plus theories of personality and psychopathology. The third domain includes the social bases of behavior, family theory, groups and ethnic systems, and social systems theory, but it also looks at all types of agencies involved in the distribution of health care services.

Beyond analytic and theoretical course content, the health psychologist receives instruction in a number of professional issues: for example, specialized courses in assessment, intervention strategies ranging from short-term individual therapy to family therapy to group interventions to systems interventions, consultation-liaison work, and interdisciplinary collaboration. Finally, many ethical, legal, and other professional issues will be discussed before the student is prepared. This training model is generally consistent with views on training clinical health psychologists (Belar, 1990).

Further, the conference discussed the need for postdoctoral training and provided recommendations for an adequate experience. Space does not permit full discussion here, but a thoughtful statement of the conference's rationale can be found in Sheridan et al. (1988). The conference recommended a two-year postdoctoral internship appropriate to either the research or the clinical-applied specialization of the student. Internships should, insofar as possible, provide experience with the type of problems, clientele, and setting most appropriate to the student's stated goals. This model adopts in principle the medical model for training including rotating internships and a supervised residency before being licensed to practice. APA's Division 38 now has available a listing of doctoral and postdoctoral training programs in health psychology.

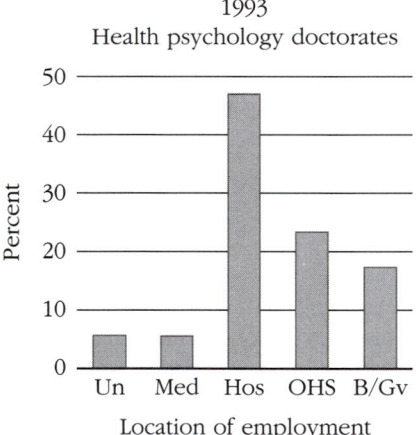

FIGURE 1.6   *Employment pattern of 1993 health psychology doctorate recipients across different settings (Data from Wicherski & Kohout, 1995). (Un = university; Med = medical school; Hos = hospital setting; OHS = other health service setting; B/Gv = business or government.)*

Further Down the Road: Health Psychology in the Future

Trying to predict the future is always a risky business. Any projections must be based largely on educated guesses and hunches based on trends that mix a wide range of professional, social, and economic factors. Still, the viability of health psychology must be a matter of concern to those who contemplate choosing it as a career.

First, it appears that some of the concern, even confusion, over name and identity is subsiding as *health psychology* has become the profession's chosen title. The development of training and licensure standards—though these standards have not by any means been uniformly adopted—goes a long way to establish health psychology as the umbrella organization under which psychology's concern with health and illness issues will be represented. The use of other terms, such as *medical psychology,* may gradually disappear, though the work of professionals already employed in those areas may change no more than would be expected by customary advances in theory and technology.

Second, it is likely that the newly recognized interdependence between medical and psychological personnel will continue to grow, including more complete integration into the national health network (Taylor, 1990). There will still be turf battles between medicine and psychology over such things as licensure and autonomy in medical facilities, third-party payments, primary responsibility for patient care, prescriptions, and so forth. But the progress made in the last 20 years gives every reason to expect continued growth in the two disciplines' mutual respect for the unique, valuable role each plays in the holistic treatment of patients. In addition, training in health psychology will probably increase its emphasis on medical and physiological background, which should enhance the health psychologist's acceptance in medical facilities. Medicine already faces a critical shortage of research

professionals to conduct basic research (Arias, 1989). The traditional employment of psychologists in medical settings to teach research design courses and participate in biomedical research could increase with these changes in graduate training for health psychologists.

Third, special populations will receive increasing attention as health psychology establishes a base of theory and research from which to work. There are already strong signs of this trend. The health problems unique to pediatric, geriatric, and minority groups and to women are the focus of many journal articles and specialized texts. Groups that share common health problems, such as coronary patients, anorexic and bulimic patients, AIDS patients, and cancer patients are also receiving more specialized attention. Research of this nature can be expected to produce more specialized assessment and intervention strategies as well.

Fourth, the profession will be forced to design new assessment methods appropriate for use with special populations in specific settings. These methods will likely go beyond paper and pencil tests to include a wide range of technologically sophisticated devices to measure physiological states either in clinical settings or in field settings with ambulatory patients. Some of these instruments will probably be better able to deal with the complex questions that must be asked in epidemiologic and etiologic research. Traditional psychometric measures will likely be discarded in favor of the new instruments, unless they can be validated and normed for use in these special applications (Bradley, Prokop, & Clayman, 1981). There is nothing to suggest, for example, that information about terminally ill patients can be compared to normative data from the general population. Diagnostic decisions will integrate biomedical and psychosocial data as research continues to add and refine knowledge. As medical technology continues to advance, psychologists may also play greater roles in helping patients understand and accept that technology. Descartes, writing centuries ago, said that science's bearing fruit in technology "is not merely to be desired with a view to

the invention of an infinity of arts and crafts-
. . . but principally because it brings about the
preservation of health, which is without doubt
the chief blessing and the foundation of all other
blessings in this life."

Finally, goals will be reevaluated to determine whether the outcomes normally deemed
appropriate for interventions are in fact the most
desirable outcomes. For example, in some substance abuse cases, temperance may be a
preferred goal, not total abstinence. A time will
come when we recognize that treating all
substance abusers as though they fit in the same
pigeonhole is inconsistent with the multicausal
model of health and illness. One goal that will
probably increase in importance is to influence
health and illness through primary prevention.
Pursuing this goal will involve increased research into risk assessment and screening,
evaluation of intervention programs whose sole
purpose is primary prevention, and implementation of more primary prevention programs in
field settings. Federal agencies will need to
reevaluate the premise of funding for health
research so that it is not dominated by problems
related to tertiary care on a long-term basis.

Summary

Customarily, psychology was defined as the
science of mind, behavior, or both. In the last
two decades, though, the field has been redefined to include issues of health and illness. This
redefinition, though departing from the conventional demarcation between the medical and
social sciences, nonetheless is true to psychology's historical roots in physiology, the starting
point to a science of human behavior. This
chapter has traced this history, defined the field,
compared it to several other fields that seem to
have similar names (perhaps even similar missions), and looked at several professional issues
in health psychology. The central points are
summarized here.

1. Crucial terms in health psychology include *disease, illness, illness behavior,* and
health behavior. Disease is a physical malfunction of the body. Illness is the resulting state of
suffering.

2. People may engage in illness behaviors
even when their bodies show no evidence of a
physical pathogen. Research that attempts to
establish a connection between an alleged cause
and a disease must be careful not to confuse
illness behavior with disease.

3. Health is a state of complete physical,
mental, and social well-being, while health
behavior includes positive steps taken to prevent illness and maintain health.

4. Health psychology formally came into
existence in 1978 when Division 38 of the
American Psychological Association was established.

5. Three major activities of health psychologists include teaching, research, and intervention. To a lesser extent, administration may also
be part of the health psychologist's role.

6. Psychosomatic medicine is a discipline
most often associated with psychiatry. Psychosomatic medicine used psychoanalytic notions
to try to explain disease; in other words, the
discipline gave psychogenic explanations for
disease. In its "new look," though, psychosomatic medicine has become markedly similar to
the biopsychosocial model used in health psychology.

7. Medical psychology was defined as an
attempt to apply psychological concepts to the
management of patients to improve their health
care while in medical settings.

8. Behavior medicine has similar goals but
is distinguished as an interdisciplinary field,
while health psychology is a discipline-specific
field.

9. The educational philosophy for health
psychology training is the Boulder Model, which
proposes that psychologists should be trained as
scientist-practitioners.

10. Training is becoming more standardized
but still varies in the emphasis placed on
research versus teaching versus clinical practice.

11. Most graduate health psychology programs emphasize courses that provide essential

background in the three components of the biopsychosocial model: the biomedical, psychological, and social bases of health and disease.

Key Words

behavior medicine	illness behavior
behavior therapy	outcome assessment
compliance	program evaluation
diagnosis	psychosomatic illness
disease	psychosomatic
etiology	medicine
health behavior	secondary gain

Study Questions

1. How is health psychology connected historically to such disciplines as physiology and neuroanatomy?

2. What are the defining characteristics of psychosomatic medicine, behavior medicine, and health psychology?

3. What are the three major activities that health psychologists carry out?

4. What are the core components of a graduate program in health psychology?

Class Projects

1. Discuss the strengths and weaknesses of the educational philosophy of health psychology based on the Boulder Model.

2. Consider inviting psychologists currently working in medical settings to describe and discuss their work.

3. Have a panel discussion on what professional psychologists typically do in different settings. Psychologists from the local department and community agencies may be willing to sit in to help the discussion.

Suggested Readings

Belar, C. D., Deardorff, W. W., & Kelly, K. E. (1987). *The practice of clinical health psychology.* New York: Pergamon.

Seeman, J. (1989). Toward a model of positive health. *American Psychologist, 44,* 1099–1109.

Taylor, S. E. (1990). Health psychology: The science and the field. *American Psychologist, 45,* 40–50.

WEBSITES   *APA, Health Psychology (Div. 38), and Related Sites*

ADDRESS	DESCRIPTION
http://www.apa.org	☆American Psychological Association. Check out the **PsychCrawler** search engine for information on many topics.
http://freud.apa.org/divisions/div38/	Health Psychology—Division 38.
http://socbehmed.org/sbm/sbm.htm	Society of Behavioral Medicine
http://is.dal.ca/~hlthpsyc/hlthhome.htm	Canadian Health Psychology Section
http://www.wp.com/accent/euro.htm	European Health Psychology Society

2

Theoretical Foundations of Health Psychology

In the next three chapters, we begin to build a theoretical foundation for understanding the etiology of health and illness. It will become clear very quickly that many diverse theories exist, each claiming that it can explain something about how health is maintained and illness occurs. Some models, such as the biomedical models of genetic and immune system influences, operate at the molecular level. Their scope may be limited but the particularity of detail also is very fine. Other models, such as social systems models, operate at or near the global level. Their scope may be very extensive—some may even attempt to be exhaustive—but the particularity of detail is crude. Although some people may see the different levels of analysis as competitive, each level has a role to play in science's quest to understand disease. The molecular level yields very important information without invalidating the global level.

Following the conceptual contributions of George Engel (1977) and Gary Schwartz (1982), health psychology adopted the biopsychosocial model of health and illness. This model suggests that health and illness are codetermined by the interaction of forces from the biological, psychological, and social spheres. Chapters 2 through 4 will treat theoretical models from these three perspectives each in its turn. Chapter 3 will examine the origins, elaborations, and criticisms of the biopsychosocial model: I suggest that the model serves useful integrative and guiding functions, but that it does not measure up to the criteria of a precise and directly testable theory. While the model should not therefore be abandoned, we are reminded that claims of integration must be supported with empirical tests. Testing integrative theory is not solely health psychology's responsibility. It is a task that requires continuing collaborative efforts from many disciplines.

At the biological level, a host of disciplines, often referred to as biomedical and life sciences, contribute relevant research and theory. Similarly, psychology has several branches, grouped under the generic title of biopsychology, that seek to understand the biological bases of brain-behavior connections (Davis, Rosenzweig, Becker, & Sather, 1988). A long-standing criticism of biomedical theory is that it has been dominated by single-cause models of disease, such as the germ theory, and the magic bullet notion of treatment. Indeed, this criticism is used as one justification, if not a rallying cry, to adopt the biopsychosocial model. As we will see later, far from being unidimensional and

simplistic, biomedical theory is both more complex and more multicausal than critics sometimes admit.

Chapter 3 will also trace the intellectual history of ideas that contributed to psychology's current interest and involvement in the health care enterprise. Folklore suggests that emotions can change body processes in positive or negative ways. Contemporary research provides evidence that some elements of folklore are accurate and suggests what systems may be involved. The issue of placebo healing also raises questions about the possible connections between mind (suggestions and beliefs) and body (altered physical functions). I will briefly retrace the mind-body debate and offer a solution that is consistent with views emerging from collaborative efforts of neuroscience and cognitive science. Finally, I will use the immunocompetence model as an exemplary research strategy. This model specifically tests the hypothesis that psychosocial stressors have the capacity to alter sensitivity in the immune system and thus either increase or reduce risk for illness.

Chapter 4 describes several sociological models of health and illness. The view of health and illness from a sociocultural perspective is often both exciting and illuminating. We are often reminded that all cultures, no matter how primitive or sophisticated they may seem, still have common needs to explain and control illness, to train and sanction legitimate medical expertise. In considering the sociocultural influences, we will look at epidemiological data describing the way in which health and illness are distributed differently based on such things as gender, race, and work. Then, we will discuss four theories that share a social perspective. In the end, the reader should have a broad perspective of the complex matrix of biomedical and psychosocial factors that influence health and illness.

CHAPTER 2

Of Germs and Magic Bullets: Biomedical Foundations of Health Psychology

Imagine what it would be like to live in the Middle Ages. Your house probably was heated with a single, central fireplace. The private nooks and crannies got precious little comforting heat. Most likely, the house had a thatched roof that leaked, grew molds, and harbored rats and bugs. There was no running water for cooking, toilets, and baths. Hot water did not come from gas or electric heaters but had to be boiled over an open fire. Bathing was more an aesthetic choice than a regular health habit. During cold and damp seasons, bathing could be difficult and uncomfortable if not death defying. You might wear the same clothes for months at a time, or even for years, until they simply wore out (Hudson, 1983). As a result, your body and clothes were breeding and feeding grounds for lice and bacteria.

People crowded together in conditions abominable by modern standards. As late as the early industrial age, dozens of people lived under the same roof, shared utensils, and slept side by side on the floor or in the same bed. Streets were littered with raw garbage and sewage (Ziegler, 1969). No water treatment plants removed bacteria and other pollutants from the water supply. No underground sewage system removed body wastes. You were fortunate indeed if your well was not polluted by your neighbors' wastes. Worse still, it was not uncommon to find the bodies of those who died during the night discarded on doorsteps or in a gutter. Hordes of rats infested with parasites and fleas roamed freely. The more people crowded into the cities, the faster the rats reproduced. As the rat population increased, so did the deadly

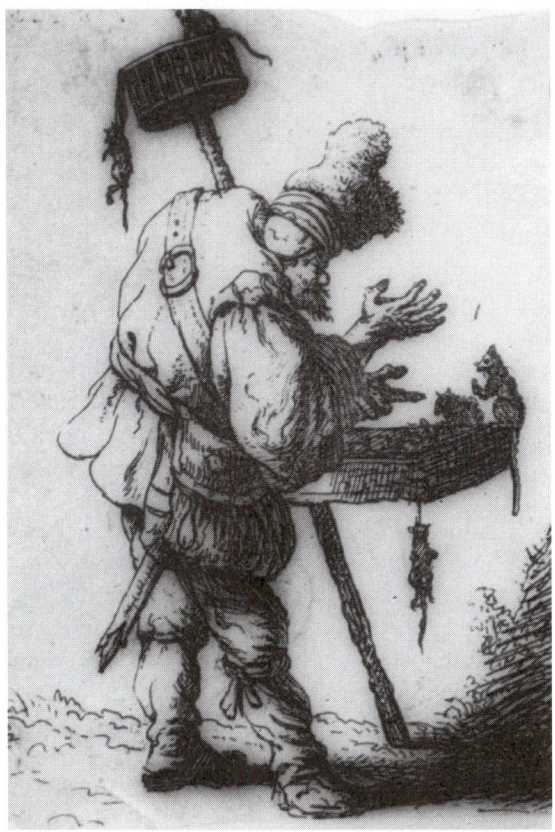

FIGURE 2.1   *The Rat Killer:* In this etching by Jan Georg van Vliet, a village resident works to control the messengers of bubonic plague, the flea-carrying rats (Associated American Artists, 1969, National Library of Medicine, Bethesda).

rat fleas, the harbingers of the ghastly black death, bubonic plague.

Bubonic plague was just one of three deadly recurrent diseases (including leprosy and syphilis) to ravage Europe during this time. How many people died is not precisely known. Cockerham (1982) reported that nearly 30,000 people died in London in just one month. 80,000 died in Milan (Lyons & Petrucelli, 1978), 55,000 in Florence, and perhaps 100,000 in Venice (Ziegler, 1969). Estimates suggest that if a town escaped with 10% of its populace dead, it was lucky. Some cities may have had death rates as

high as 60%. Overall, probably 25% of the populace of Europe died at the peak of the plague (Hudson, 1983).

We know now that the rat fleas were not the cause; they were just couriers for a bacterium first named *Pasteurella pestis* in honor of Louis Pasteur.[1] No one knew then about the existence of this microbe. Disease was still considered to result from moral sin, the fateful conjunction of the planets, or some particle (miasma) carried in the air (the closest ancient medical theory got to a physical explanation). Diagnosis was still an intuitive, artistic hodgepodge involving such methods as examining blood from bloodletting, urine examination (uroscopy), and taking the pulse (Taylor, 1981). General treatment consisted of herbal or chemical medicine, and bloodletting was used excessively. There were elemental notions of quarantine and some suggestions for environmental controls. Still, little in medical history suggests that those who guessed at the promise of quarantine understood the underlying mechanisms of disease transmission and cure.

Bubonic Plague: The Legacy of Gluttonous Fleas

Hudson (1983, pp. 31–32) provided a chilling description of how the bubonic germ moved from rats to humans. When a flea sucked blood from an infected rat, the germ began to multiply in the flea's stomach. After a short time, the flea's stomach became gorged and functionally blocked with bacteria. It was starving although full. The flea did what any hungry flea would do. It looked for another source of blood, the nearest rat or human. Finding a new meal, it would suck blood until it could hold no more. Then it would vomit the blood into the human

---

[1] The bacterium was later renamed *Yersinia pestis* after Pasteur's student Alexandre Yersin, the true discoverer.

host along with the bacteria growing in its stomach.

Further, the rat flea was very sensitive to the temperature of its host. When an infected rat or human began to die, its temperature dropped. Any respectable flea would immediately look for a new host with body heat. Whether the flea hightailed it to a rat or a human, the flea transported the deadly bacteria of bubonic plague from one victim to another.

Such assaults on human health and happiness did not go unchallenged by the medical community. Many attempts, however feeble, were made to understand and treat, if not control, disease. Most explanations of disease, though, were still variations on religious-supernatural or magical themes dating back to prehistorical eras. Hudson (1983) wrote that "supernatural belief provides the solace of explanation when the human mind cannot understand the nature of disease, or control its course" (p. 56). Some great minds of ancient medicine did try to give naturalistic explanations for certain disorders. Yet, most early theories were sullied by conventional thinking that integrated preternatural notions with the natural.

The history of these theories and treatments is much too involved to allow for any detailed account.[2] But the lessons for modern thinking about health in general and health psychology in particular merit some recounting. As we will see, these physical theories moved from the global humoral theory of Hippocrates to very molecular theories of today. Even the long-standing driving forces of medical theory and practice, the germ theory of disease and the magic bullet treatment are being elaborated if not replaced by multicausal theories. At the same time, the twin towers of medical practice, anatomy and physiology, have become increasingly refined and complex.

---

[2] Many marvelous accounts of medical history are available including the works of Ackerknecht (1982), Castiglioni (1947), Lyons and Petrucelli (1978), and Sigerist (1971).

Of Spirits, Stars, and Humors

It is often assumed that most, if not all, early medical theories were based on religious or magical notions, and that primitive thinking about the physical world had no empirical tendencies. The first part of this belief may be largely accurate, but the second part ignores various signs of empirical tendencies.

The Supernatural/Magical Approach to Disease

Supernatural explanation of disease had many variations but just a few central themes. Hudson (1983, pp. 59–60) identified five primitive disease notions:

1. *Disease results from sorcery.* It was widely believed that certain persons were skilled in so-called black magic that could be directed toward a human victim or could control supernatural events.

2. *Disease results from breach of social taboo.* This notion is exemplified by the psalmist (107:17) who wrote, "Fools, because of their transgression,/And because of their iniquities, were afflicted."

3. *Disease results from object intrusion.* Through magical means, objects such as bones, hair, splinters, or pebbles could invade a victim's body and cause disease.

4. *Disease results from supernatural possession.* Insanity might occur because a demon inhabited the person's body, epilepsy because a spirit had seized the person's soul. In the Vedas of ancient India, specific mental disorders were associated with specific demons. The Salem witch hunts of 17th century New England are an infamous example of demon possession used to explain behavior that actually might have resulted from rye grain poisoning (ergotism) (Caporael, 1976).

5. *Disease results from losing one's soul.* Losing one's soul could come about through magical potions or incantations or both.

Although the link between theory and treatment is seldom perfect, these religious/magical notions still prescribed treatments consistent with the alleged cause. Most often the goal of treatment was to restore peace among the offended gods. Breaching a taboo required confession or appeasing the gods. Object intrusion most often used magical sucking to remove the object. Demon possession required that the offending spirit be scared or driven off, perhaps with vile concoctions using animal excrement and body parts, incantations, or trepanning (see the following section). Loss of the soul could be countered by restoring the soul through a variety of magical rituals.

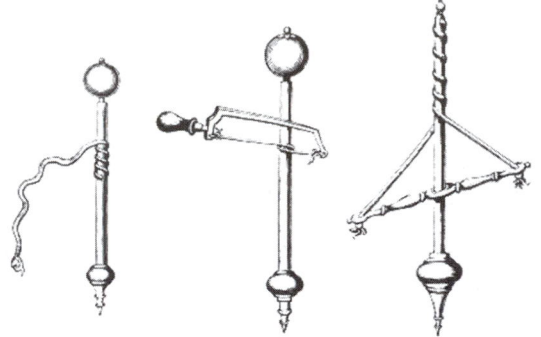

FIGURE 2.2   *Three augers or bone-drills (trypanon) of the type used by Greek physicians to trepan the skull.*

Trepanning: Magical or Natural Treatment?

Trepanning offers an interesting excursion into the mind and method of ancient medicine. **Trepanning**—a word derived from the carpenter's auger and the process of boring—is a technique for boring a hole through the skull. It was practiced on both the living and the dead, which suggests it may have been a religious practice as much as a medical procedure. Medical records from many cultures confirm its widespread use from India, to Egypt, Europe, and among the Aztecs and Incas of Central and South America. It was practiced as early as the neolithic period (late Stone Age); it was mentioned in the Talmud (Rosner, 1977); and it is still used by some South Pacific tribes (Hudson, 1983). That the practice reached a high level of precision and success is apparent. Recovered skulls show that many patients not only survived their operations but lived long enough for the hole to partly if not completely heal over.

What was the rationale of this operation? The prevailing supernatural/magical theory explained it simply: The patient was possessed by an evil spirit. Boring the hole allowed the spirit to escape. After the operation, the patient

behaved in a normal fashion. The theory must be correct since the treatment was a success.

Yet, there is evidence that ancient surgeons understood the link between injury, pain, and changed behavior. They could see the bone

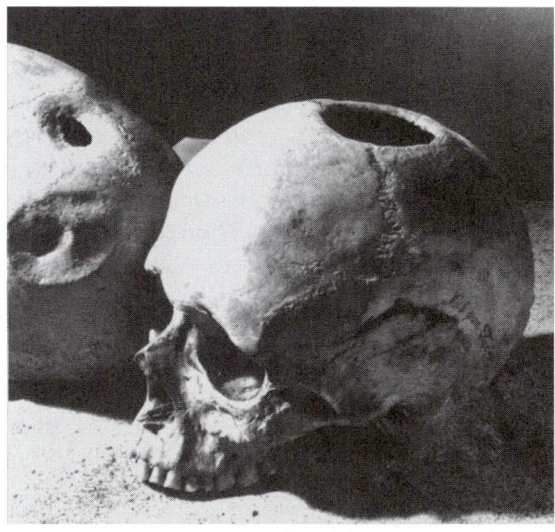

FIGURE 2.3   *This trephined skull from the Neolithic period shows the edges of the wound healed suggesting that the patient recovered from the operation (Nationalmuseet, Copenhagen).*

depression resulting from a head injury and they might have guessed that restoring the bones to correct position would solve the problem. Chipping and lifting the bones might allow blood (hematoma) at the injury site to gush out. This would relieve the pain and probably restore normal behavior. Success likely led surgeons to repeat the procedure (on completely empirical grounds) when another head injury patient came for help.

This scenario shows the extent to which medical theory and medical treatment can coexist comfortably while substantively disconnected. Even in modern medicine, treatments may be used with some success although the physician does not understand why. In practice, then, the connection between theory and treatment may be more a luxury than a necessity.

Hippocrates: Emergence of a Physical Theory of Disease

Even when a supernatural/magical tradition was present, several ancient societies exercised a type of crude **empiricism,** an approach to knowing that depends on experience and observation. Unlike the systematic empiricism of modern laboratories, where hypotheses are tested in controlled conditions, ancient empiricism was simple, pragmatic, and observational. If some herb or physical intervention had success, no matter how intuitively or serendipitously that success might have come about, the treatment was noted and used again. Then it found its way into the medical literature to be passed on to another generation. The emergence of acupuncture in China and the use of trepanning are examples of crude empiricism. The discovery in India of Ruwolfia serpentina (reserpine), the medicine of sad (depressed) men, and the use of rhinoplasty (plastic nose surgery after punitive removal for adultery) are also examples of empirical tendencies in ancient medicine (Majno, 1975).

Myths and Mysteries in the Life of Hippocrates

Nowhere was this naturalistic, empirical attitude more evident than in the work of Hippocrates (c. 460–377 B.C.E.), the venerable physician best known for the oath once taken by physicians before beginning to practice medicine (Sigerist, 1971). Very little is known about the life of Hippocrates. What we do know is that he made many notable contributions, including one of the first attempts to conduct a primitive epidemiological survey of gout (gouty arthritis) in the community (Brewerton, 1992).[3] In a sense, Hippocrates stood with one foot in the philosophical-religious quagmire of his day and his other foot on the brink of a natural science of medicine. Here, we will confine our attention to Hippocrates' theorizing about the natural cause of epilepsy and his theory of humors.

Epilepsy: The Sacred Disease

Epileptic seizures were as awesome and terrifying as they were mystifying. Imagine what it might be like to casually observe this sequence. A person, perhaps a friend, is in the marketplace engaged in a normal round of robust activities. Suddenly, he loses control. Convulsions take over, throwing him around as though a strange force grabbed and shook him. He falls to the ground moaning, perhaps drooling, and he loses bladder and bowel control. Just as suddenly as the seizure hit, it is gone. The person falls into a deep sleep. After awakening, he shows little or no memory for details of the event. Still, he seems confused, embarrassed, even distressed, as though there is a subconscious remnant of the experience. On the surface, he is physically none the worse for the experience. How could the ancient mind explain this strange event in rational terms?

---

[3] See Chapter 14 for more information on the nature and origins of arthritis.

Until the time of Hippocrates, the common explanation was that epilepsy, the "sacred disease," occurred because of supernatural intervention. Hippocrates (1952), however, took a very uncharitable view of those who advocated this view, calling them quacks and charlatans (p. 154). The ancient view of epilepsy did not consider host conditions such as damage to the brain, and it had little to offer as treatment.

Hippocrates changed all that. Boldly he declared: "It is thus with regard to the disease called Sacred: it appears to me to be no wise more divine nor more sacred than other diseases, but has a *natural cause* from which it originates like other affections" (p. 154; emphasis added). This statement is widely regarded as the origin of the view that disease is a natural phenomenon. When medicine was placed in the realm of the natural world, the door was opened to new ways of studying disease and to medical therapies that would not otherwise have been considered appropriate.

Humoral Theory: Of Essences, Airs, and Seasons

Hippocrates' second major contribution was a general theory of disease and treatment called **humoral theory.** Humors were body juices of varying colors and consistencies that flowed in different channels. Prior to the advent of meticulous dissections, microscopic examinations, and other high-tech probes into the structure and function of the body, these humors were the most visible elements of the body. They appeared to be directly related to disease. Blood flowed with injuries. Infected wounds gave off pus, and the nose dripped with fevers. Stools might be bloodied, loose, or both. Urine might be discolored or clouded with sediments, or it might change odor with disease. Stomach sickness usually produced vomit.

Hippocrates' unique contribution was to link symptoms to disorders. This may have been the true beginning of one mainstay of modern medicine: **symptom complexes,** or "images" of diseases as Sigerist (1971, p. 33) called them.

The most important feature in humoral theory was balance or equilibrium.[4] To Hippocrates, health existed when the body humors were properly balanced. A person could maintain balance by proper diet and lifestyle, including exercise, rest, and temperance. Disease existed when anything happened to disturb the natural balance—whether defects in physical, dietary, or medical regimens; particles in the air; or changes in the environment or the season.

According to Hippocrates, there were four humors: blood, phlegm, black bile, and yellow bile. (See Table 2.1.) Phlegm, like water, was wet and cold. Blood, like air, was wet and hot. Black bile, like earth, was dry and cold. Yellow bile, like fire, was dry and hot.

Each humor, when dominant over the other humors, had its specific effect on the person's mind and body. The **phlegmatic** person was impassive, sluggish, and dull. Colds, headaches, and strokes (apoplexy) resulted from an excess of phlegm (or mucus). The physician used allopathic (opposite) treatments such as hot baths and emetics. A person with an excess of blood was described as **sanguine,** or cheerful and optimistic. With an excess of blood, the person was more apt to suffer from angina, epilepsy, or leprosy. As one might expect, bloodletting was a common treatment for this excess, along with cooling agents or enemas. A **melancholic** person had too much black bile, and was supposedly sad, depressed, and brooding. An excess of black bile would most likely lead to ulcers, dropsy (edema), and fevers that may have been typhoid or malarial. They could be treated with cautery, emetics, and hot baths. Finally, the **choleric** person had an abundance of yellow bile and was described as fiery and excitable. The prominent diseases were cholera, jaundice, and stomach ailments. Treatment involved bloodletting, cooling agents, enemas, and pain medications.

---

[4] It is tempting to equate this balance with physiological homeostasis as represented in contemporary biomedical thinking. Still, the Hippocratic concept was very different from this modern notion.

TABLE 2.1   Parallels in the Hippocratic theory of the four humors.

HUMOR	ETYMOLOGY	SOURCE	TRAIT*	SEASON	DISEASE	TREATMENT	TEMPERAMENT
Phlegm	*pituita*	Brain	*Cold*	Winter	Colds/Pneu- monia Headaches Pleurisy Stroke Stranguary	Hot baths Warm gruels Diuretic medication Emetics	Phlegmatic
Blood	*sanguis*	Heart	*Hot*	Spring	Angina Arthritis Dysentery Epilepsy Leprosy	Blood letting Cooling agents Enemas	Sanguine
Black Bile	*melanchole*	Spleen and stomach	*Wet*	Autumn	Dropsy Hepatitis Sciatica Typhus/Malaria Ulcers	Ass's milk Cautery Emetics Hot baths	Melancholic
Yellow Bile	*chole*	Liver	*Dry*	Summer	Cholera Mouth ulcers Jaundice Stomach ailments	Blood letting Cooling agents Enemas Liquid diet Pain medication	Choleric

*Some writers suggest dual traits. Phlegm is cold and wet while blood is hot and wet. Castiglioni (1947) attributes this to the pneumatists and suggested that the true Hippocratic notion uses single trait descriptions.

Humoral theory survived for generations, largely through the efforts of such men as Galen, the Nestorians, and others (Majno, 1975). As late as the early 19th century, French medical scientists were humoral pathologists (Sigerist, 1971), and humoral theory continues in the folk medicine of many cultures (Cockerham, 1982). Personality correlates of humors continue to be discussed today (Merenda, 1987; Lester, 1990). Now, though, humoral theory is regarded as largely fanciful and speculative.

What Is Disease: Organ, Tissue, or Cellular Pathology?

According to religion and custom in ancient Greece, dissection of the human body was largely forbidden. As a result, physicians such as Hippocrates had little accurate knowledge of anatomy. What they could learn came largely from accident and tragedy: inner organs were exposed by the wounds of sport and war, or in domestic and market accidents. Even Galen carried out dissections only on animals. The taboo on human dissection served to consolidate errors in the medical literature, errors that were not recognized as such until the medical prodigy, Vesalius, corrected them nearly 1500 years later. By the 18th century, the taboo had been overturned to such an extent that people of all ranks and professions asked the great Morgagni to examine their bodies postmortem. To be dissected became both a badge of honor and a humane contribution to medical science.

As the human mind continued to grapple

with the mystery of disease causation, though, it naturally wanted—needed, in fact—to know more about **anatomy,** the systematic study of body structure and internal organs. Thus emerged the next step in conceptualizing disease: disease as organ pathology, also known as anatomical pathology.

Organ Pathology: Disease Attributed to Anatomy

Shortly after the time of Hippocrates, two well-known physicians established the first school of anatomy at the new Athens of learning, Alexandria, Egypt. The first, Herophilus (c. 300 B.C.E.) may have written his three anatomy volumes based in part on observing funeral embalmings (Sigerist, 1971), but he apparently openly dissected the human body as well (Singer, 1959). Herophilus identified the brain as the true nervous system center and the seat of intelligence. He noted that peripheral nerves were the sensory channels to the brain (Sigerist, 1971), and he gave an accurate description of the eye. Unfortunately, Herophilus proposed a preposterous theory of pulse based on musical rhythms. This led to numerous criticisms and may have slowed acceptance of anatomical observations.

Erasistratus and Plethora Theory

The second of these physicians was Erasistratus (c. 260 B.C.E.). He probably carried out dissections on animals and postmortem exams on human cadavers. He recognized that diseased organs appear markedly different from healthy organs. Erasistratus was first to recognize the distinction between sensory and motor nerves. He departed from tradition by stating that disease is no vague "corruption of the humors" (Sigerist, 1971, p. 48). As an alternative, he proposed **plethora theory,** the notion that disease results from blood and nutritive substances' stretching and tearing the vessels.

Anatomy in the Eyes of an Artist

From this legacy of great physicians, we must digress for a moment to the contributions of an artist, an engineer, a scientist, and a mathematician—not four separate people, but one great one, Leonardo da Vinci (1452–1519). Although he is best known for his mysterious, alluring *Mona Lisa,* da Vinci's interest in anatomy gave anatomical representation a great boost. He captured the natural endowments of the human body—its charm, grace, and beauty—while providing good detail. Still, his prints had little direct impact on mainstream medicine (Hudson, 1983).

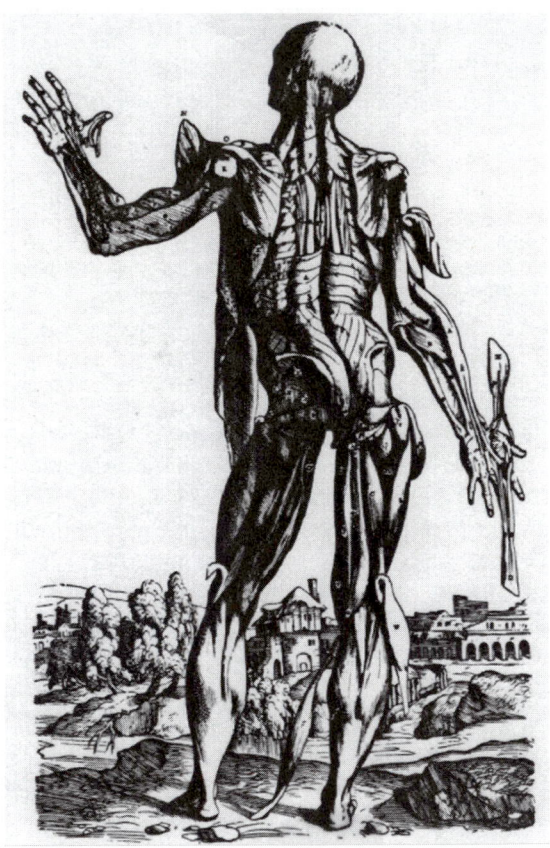

FIGURE 2.4   *An illustration from the work of Andreas Vesalius (from Saunders and O'Malley, plate 34).*

Vesalius: The Father of Modern Anatomy

Yet another artist, Vesalius (1515–1564), played a small role in bringing anatomy to its fullness. The career of Vesalius, like a meteor's, was exceptionally bright and equally brief. Vesalius began his ascent about the time Copernicus (1473–1543) published his heliocentric theory of the universe. Immediately after finishing his medical education in Padua, Vesalius was appointed professor, all before he was 23. In 1543, the same year that Copernicus published his monumental work, Vesalius published his *Fabrica,* otherwise known as *On the Fabric of the Human Body.* This seven-volume work became the foundation of modern biology and medicine (Sigerist, 1971). Human bones, joints, muscles, and internal organs, including the heart, were described with scientific clarity yet artistic sensitivity. In medical terms, Vesalius's work constituted the birth of **anatomical pathology,** the notion that disease might be localized in anatomy.

Morgagni: Anatomical Pathology

Later, Giovanni Morgagni (1682–1771) wrote the first textbook of pathological anatomy. His observations were the direct result of hundreds of autopsies done on the bodies of recently deceased people. He noted that the change in an organ was directly related to the appearance of symptoms of illness.

To summarize the small conceptual steps taken in this epoch, early medical theorists—knowing nothing of parasites, microbes, or teratogens—constructed theories that made sense to them and fit the available data. While basing much of their practice on crude empiricism, ancient medical theories nonetheless were largely absurd speculations. Yet continued study of the human body led to the emergence of the twin towers of medicine, anatomy and physiology. With this focus, medicine was ready to propose an alternative theory: disease as organ pathology.

TABLE 2.2   Time lines showing the emergence and duration of the major biomedical theories of disease below the time line and the theory's author-progenitor above.

400 B.C.E.	100 C.E. !!	1761 C.E.	1800 C.E.	1858 C.E.	1875–1885 C.E.
Hippocrates	Galen				
– – – – – – – – –	!!	– – – – – – –			
humoral pathology					
		Morgagni			
		– –			
		organ pathology			
			Bichat		
			– –		
			tissue pathology		
				Virchow	
				– – – – – – – – – – – – – – –	
				cellular pathology	
					Jenner Pasteur Lister
					– – – – – – – –
					germ theory

Tissue Pathology: Disease as Foul Tissue

The end of Morgagni's life coincided with the beginning of momentous events throughout the world. The American colonies had begun their war of independence, and France was being torn apart by its own revolution. Before it was over, France's internal bickering led directly to the deaths of 600 physicians and surgeons at the front lines. The beginning of the French Republic was a period of utter chaos for medical practice in France, with one consolation: The revolution also destroyed barriers in the medical establishment that had prevented it from becoming a modern enterprise. For the first time, medicine and surgery were united in a single curriculum, while new hospitals and research laboratories were provided for teaching (Sigerist, 1971).

Bichat: Tissue as the Fabric of Disease

In the midst of this political maelstrom, M. F. Xavier Bichat (1771–1802) began his medical career. As one of the lucky few to survive the wars, Bichat chose to work in anatomy, physiology, and pathology. Unfortunately, the wear and tear on his body, already weakened by poor health, proved too much, and he died in his 30th year.

Bichat's role in disease theory was to suggest yet a smaller body unit as the probable source of

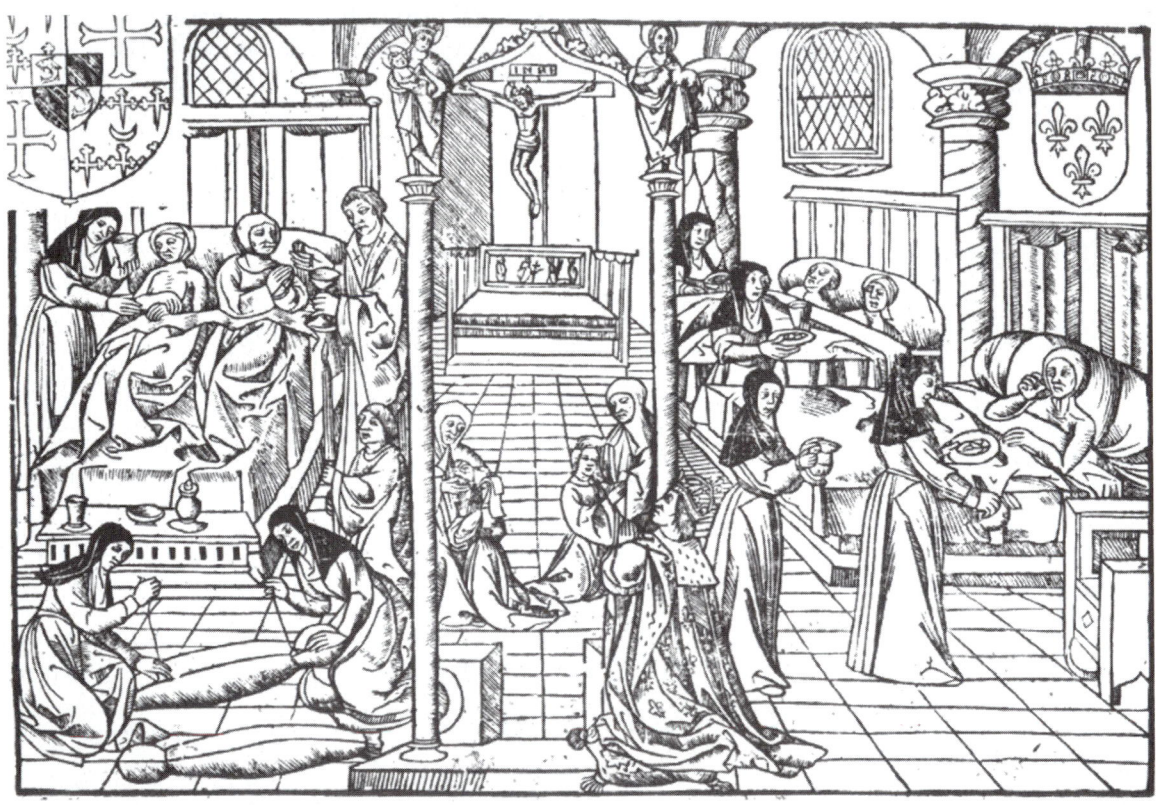

FIGURE 2.5   The Hôtel-Dieu, Paris, is shown in this engraving from about 1500. It depicts crowded conditions and familiarity with death, as corpses are routinely sewn into shrouds in full view of the patients (Ms. Ea 17 rés., Bibliothèque Nationale, Paris).

pathology. Following a suggestion from Philippe Pinel (the French reformer who released mental health patients from their chains) that organs were composed of several different tissues, Bichat proposed the idea of **tissue pathology.** Tissue of one kind could become diseased in an organ while nearby tissues could remain unaffected. Since the cell still was unknown, the idea that tissues might be made of yet smaller building blocks did not enter Bichat's mind.

Cellular Pathology: Disease Is in the Cell

In the years following Bichat's work, one of Johannes Müller's[5] pupils, Schwann, discovered that animal tissue consisted of nucleated cells. This discovery set the stage for the next development in disease theory—the notion that disease is **cellular pathology.**

With a 200-year legacy of cellular research, medical theory believed that all life resided in the cell. Therefore, the cell also must be the place to look for signs of disease. No one played a more prominent role in the development of the theory that disease is cellular pathology than Rudolf Virchow (1821–1902). Virchow, a savant with incredible knowledge of many subjects, was another student of Johannes Müller (De Kruif, 1926).

Among the most notable of Virchow's contributions to medicine was his study of phlebitis, or inflammation of the veins. Phlebitis gained attention when former president Richard Nixon suffered an acute and nearly fatal siege in the months following his resignation from the presidency (an episode that also reminds us of the role stressors may play in the appearance or the intensity of certain diseases). Virchow's work on phlebitis brought important insights into thrombosis and embolism, and introduced a new concept, leukemia, into morbid pathology.

In 1858, in his major work on cellular pathology, Virchow declared that the cell is the seat and sustainer of life and that illness is only life under modified conditions. The body is a "state in which each cell is a citizen," and disease is a civil war (cited in Singer, 1959, p. 344). Disease then is cellular pathology, the cell's response to abnormal stimuli. In response to these abnormal stimuli, the cell might malfunction, become malnourished, or be malformed. If the stimuli are strong enough, the cell could die.

Virchow's involvement in one social-political event is of interest. During the summer of 1847, famine fever—in modern terms relapsing fever—swept through Upper Silesia[6] in epidemic proportions (20 years later, Obermeyer

---

[6] Upper Silesia was a province in northeastern Germany on the border with Poland.

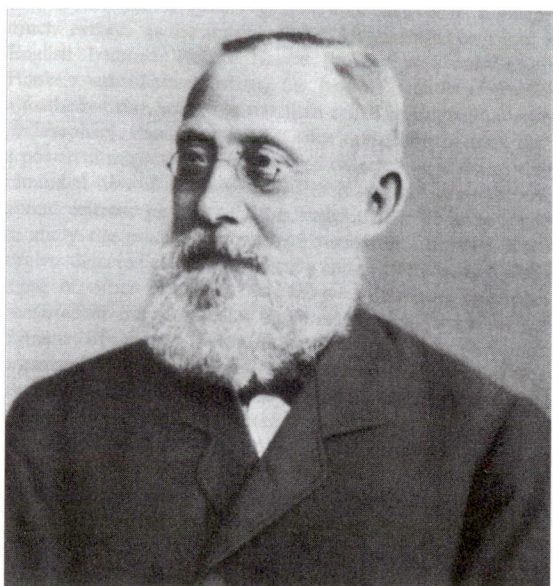

FIGURE 2.6   Rudolf Virchow, a primary contributor to the theory of disease as cell pathology.

---

[5] Johannes Müller is something of a legend in the history of psychology. He was a physiologist who promoted the doctrine of specific nerve energies, wrote influential works in physiology, and trained many important scientists for the 19th century.

located the cause of this disease, a spirochete [virus]). Virchow wrote an article about the fever that accused the state of using people as mere cogs on the wheels of an increasingly mechanized society. Life lost meaning as people lost jobs or saw their jobs changed beyond recognition and were deprived of cultural pursuits and free expression. According to Virchow, only prosperity, culture, and freedom could remove the source of the illness. Further, Virchow insisted that every worker, when disabled by illness, had the right to be cared for by the state. Even as his consuming passion was to find the cellular origins of disease, Virchow could still see disease as a social-psychological phenomenon. He also articulated, more than 100 years in advance, the modern platform that health care is the worker's right and the responsibility of business, industry, or government to provide.

The later discovery of bacteria significantly altered biomedical disease theory. But bacteriology superseded cellular pathology, complementing it without replacing it. Both hold prominent positions in contemporary disease theory.

The Semmelweis Tragedy: Iatrogenic Illness

There is little doubt that cellular and bacterial discoveries, tools that were decisive in the war against great epidemic diseases, dominated the medical news of the time. One important lesson of medical treatment, however—namely, that medical cures sometimes may be worse than the illness—was nearly ignored until its significance became inescapable. An **iatrogenic** treatment is any treatment that compounds a patient's medical problems. Molière provided perhaps the most pithy though caustic statement on this phenomenon when he wrote, "Nearly all men die of their remedies, and not of their illnesses." The lesson of iatrogenic illness is perhaps no more tragically detailed than in the life and work of Semmelweis, a man who wanted nothing more than to stop the terrible deaths of women after childbirth.

Ignaz Philipp Semmelweis (1818–1865) was a physician at a lying-in hospital in Vienna. This hospital engaged in training physicians who, as part of their training, had to conduct many postmortem examinations. The hospital also specialized in caring for women in childbirth. When Semmelweis took the position in 1846, the hospital was losing between 10% and 30% of its postpartum mothers to a terrible postpartum infection. Mothers coming to receive medical help from Vienna's best physicians instead departed the hospital in coffins, often just hours after delivering.

Meanwhile, across town at the second lying-in hospital, the death rate following childbirth was customarily low, at about 3% (Sigerist, 1971). There, midwives in training, not physicians, delivered the babies. This small, seemingly trivial bit of information contained the seeds of a solution that was tragically overlooked in favor of fatuous theories of atmospheric effects or overcrowding.

An unhappy accident led Semmelweis to recognize the still more unhappy truth—that the doctors were the couriers of death. A friend and colleague of Semmelweis, guiding a student in a postmortem exam, died suddenly after being cut by the knife used in the exam. Semmelweis noted the similarity of his colleague's dying symptoms to the women's symptoms. Immediately, he recognized that something in the dead tissue from cadavers caused the deaths of his friend and so many women. He guessed, correctly, that the postpartum uterus was like a great wound that became infected with rotten debris from the cadavers, debris transplanted by doctors. The end result was a lethal form of blood poisoning. The midwives across town, who did not frequent postmortems, were clean and safe.

Quickly, Semmelweis ordered the remedy: All personnel must disinfect their hands with chlorine water before they could examine women in labor. Just as quickly, deaths from puerperal fever plummeted to 1.2%, a rate below even the other hospital (Lyons & Petrucelli, 1978).

Instead of accepting the force of Semmel-weis's logic and data, the medical community generally ignored or categorically rejected his findings. Finding himself more or less ostracized from the company and respect of his medical peers, Semmelweis returned to his home city of Budapest. There, he practiced for a time under abominable conditions, but now with the added burden of bitterness and dejection. His mental condition deteriorated, at one time requiring restraint in a local asylum. In the end, at 47 years of age, like his friend before him, he pricked his finger accidently while performing an operation, and died of the same fever he had worked so hard to eradicate.

Of Wine, Silkworms, and Mad Dogs

While the great men of medicine struggled, diagnosed, and theorized, a chemist trying to save the wines of France began an improbable lifelong quest that ultimately led to a deeper understanding of disease. This quest, combined with parallel work of other bacteriologists, also established the **germ theory** of disease on a pedestal of medical honor.

Pasteur: The Industrial Chemist

The story is that of Louis Pasteur (1822–1895). After schooling in Paris and a brief teaching stint, Pasteur moved to Lille, a major alcohol produc-ing center. He became interested in fermenta-tion after a French physicist showed that alco-holic fermentation was caused by small living creatures called yeasts (Singer, 1959).

Pasteur surmised that yeasts added deliber-ately to produce alcoholic fermentation were the agents of change, not the result. Yet how could one explain the spoiling of wine or milk where yeasts were not deliberately added to the fluid? He had often heard wine makers talk about sick wine, wine that fermented in a way that made it bad. Aided by his observations of molds on the

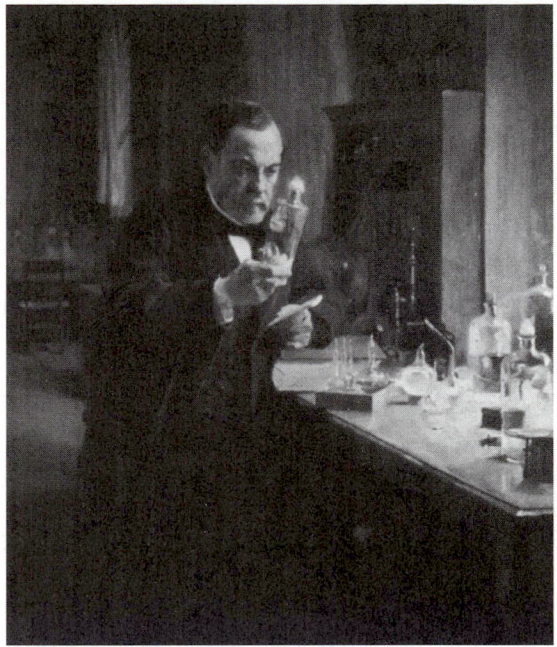

FIGURE 2.7   A portrait of Louis Pasteur in his laboratory, by Albert-Gustaf Edelfelt.

grape skins, Pasteur soon suggested a more concrete explanation.

In a series of well controlled experiments, Pasteur demonstrated that sterilized substances remained pure as long as they were protected, but became infected when exposed to air. He thus proved that bacteria were present in the air even though they could not be seen. Bad wine, then, came from bacteria causing decomposition and spoilage.

One other practical problem enabled Pasteur to take the next step from the origins of disease to treatment and prevention. The silk-producing worms in the south of France were dying from an epidemic of spotted disease. Bacteria be-lieved to be the infectious agents already had been identified and cultivated. Pasteur's next step was to introduce the bacteria in weakened form (technically, an inoculation) into the silk-worms. The response—in a culture, an animal, or a person—was immunity to that particular disease. In this case, the silkworms and the silk industry were saved, but the results were much more momentous than that.

Pasteur's work helped set in motion medical research that led to modern vaccination programs. Pasteur also discovered a vaccine—his name for the weakened viruses—for the fatal disease hydrophobia, or rabies. His work was just one part of a converging stream of data that gave rise to the germ theory of disease. Two of Pasteur's contemporaries, Jakob Henle and Robert Koch, also played a significant role in formulating the germ theory.

Koch-Henle Postulates: The Mentor's Logic, the Pupil's Method

During Pasteur's time, a teacher and his pupil laid the foundations for the logic of causal attributions in medical science. The teacher was Jakob Henle (1809–1885) and the pupil was Robert Koch (1843–1910).[7] At this time, disease theory still faced major confusion over the point that a given disease, the very same disease, could arise either from tiny unseen creatures in the environment (miasma theory) or from direct contact with small particles that existed on clothes or skin (contagium theory).

Jakob Henle recognized the solution to this conundrum: If an infectious disease can come about from either of these sources, then the agent of that disease must be one and the same, not separate entities. He concluded that the common denominator must be a living thing, a virus akin to yeasts or fungi. Henle's logic was superbly accurate, but he failed to support his arguments with concrete proof. His failure was due not to lack of effort as much as to the state of the art of laboratory instruments. Years later, Alfred Evans (1978) noted that "all of our concepts of causation are limited by the tech-

nology available to prove them and our understanding of the pathogenesis and epidemiology of the disease at the time of the investigation" (p. 250). Yeasts could be seen under the microscopes available to Henle, but the virus could not. As a result, he gained little recognition for his work on the cause of disease.

Henle's pupil Robert Koch provided the necessary and persuasive proof. Koch also was the first to formulate precisely the logic of disease causation, the Koch-Henle postulates. As a general practitioner in rural Germany, Koch observed many instances of splenic fever in livestock, a fever that also endangered human lives. A giant rod-like bacillus was discovered that upon inoculation transmitted the disease to uninfected animals. Still, a major medical riddle remained. The blood of infected animals injected into other animals could also produce the disease even when the blood was free of the bacillus. How could this bacillus, present sometimes but not always, be the actual cause of splenic fever?

Koch solved this riddle using mice infected with anthrax, in what may be one of the earliest instances of medical research using a substitute controlled subject population. Koch discovered that the bacillus, when exposed to air outside the body, grew into spores. Then the bacillus quickly died, but the spores retained their virulence for years. When the spores found a medium (such as food or air) for migration back into a host environment, the spores quickly grew again to bacteria, and the disease could be detected in the host. According to Sigerist (1971), this was the first time that the causal chain for infectious disease was conclusively demonstrated.

This decade, from about 1875 to 1885, proved to be a time of astounding discovery. During this time, microbes were identified for relapsing fever, gonorrhea, typhoid, leprosy, malaria, diphtheria, pneumonia, cerebrospinal meningitis, bubonic plague, and syphilis, diseases that had plagued the world for centuries. Traveling wherever diseases of unknown origin were most prevalent, Koch discovered the cholera vibrio

---

[7] We have met a number of Johannes Müller's students. Jakob Henle was among Johannes Müller's first pupils. Although not specifically involved in medical pursuits, then, Müller's teaching contributed greatly to the advance of medical physiology and knowledge of disease.

and the tubercle bacillus, the latter bringing him international acclaim and the prestigious Nobel Prize in 1905. In the same time frame, the German government adopted compulsory vaccination programs to prevent disease and maintain the health of its populace. Armed with this knowledge, a frontal assault began to bring under control the most terrifying diseases the world had known.

The Germ Model: Grand Unifying Theory or Myopic Simplicity?

Writing in a medical epidemiological context, Kleinbaum, Kupper, and Morgenstern (1982) summarized certain problems with the germ theory. First, because the theory established itself so quickly and with such convincing force, it led many researchers to assume that all one needed to know to explain the etiology of a disease was the identity of the offending microorganism. Second, in spite of the phenomenal growth and sophistication of modern medical theory and treatment, there is still evidence that the germ theory adversely affects both theories of what should be studied and strategies for carrying out the study. Finally, germ theory was largely a single-cause, single-effect model of disease etiology. Still, such oversimplification is not an inherent limitation of the theory itself, only an unfortunate side effect of its application in research and treatment.

As Mumford (1983) noted, even as the germ theory evolved, medicine was moving toward a multicausal model of health and illness. Medicine began long ago to consider how environmental change and social stress might impact mental and physical health. Additionally, medical research showed that germ theory can be successfully elaborated and integrated with multicausal models of disease. However criticized, then, germ theory, has more than justified its existence in millions of lives saved and in suffering relieved. No one, not even the most ardent critics, would now suggest that we banish germ theory entirely. Instead, the criticisms

sound a warning: We should not be limited by the notion that we have explained everything about a disease when we have identified the pathogen.

Paul Ehrlich: The Magic Bullet Is Cast

The first pedestal—the germ theory of disease—had been erected. The second pedestal—the magic bullet for the treatment of disease—was still more than a decade away. The term **magic bullet,** attributed to Rene DuBos (cited in Cockerham, 1982), referred to the notion that medical research is prone to look for the cure, the specific medicine that, in a figurative sense, would restore a sick person to health with one shot. One foundation for this hope and practice was the work of Paul Ehrlich. Ehrlich's toil is an epic tale of dogged tenacity against many odds,

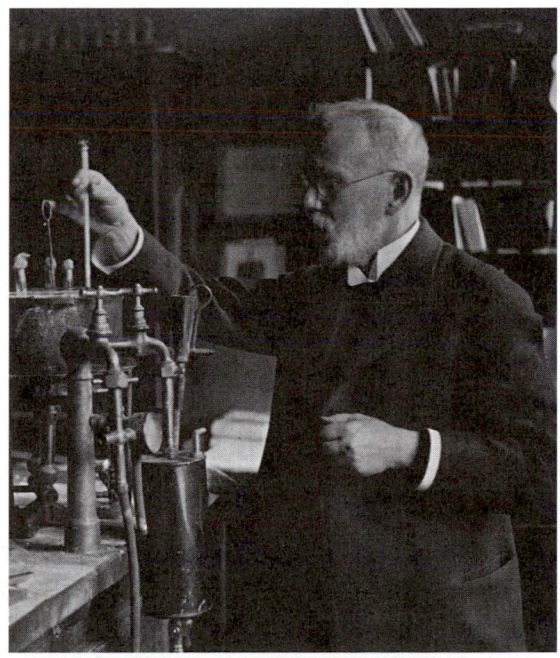

FIGURE 2.8   Paul Ehrlich, the histologist who discovered a "charmed bullet" to cure syphilis.

a tale that began about 1880 and only reached first fulfillment in 1909 when he found his "charmed bullet," as he preferred to call it.

Although Ehrlich is symbolically enshrined in medicine's hall of fame, he was not a physician, but a histologist and chemist by training. His contribution came about, not through the altruistic pursuit of clinical treatment, but through more mundane efforts to advance laboratory cell stain techniques (Sigerist, 1971). He reasoned that since different cells stain differently, there might also be some way to inject a substance into the cell that would attack the bacteria leaving the cell not only unharmed but protected against the bacteria. Ehrlich began his tedious work using syphilis as the model disease and an arsenic compound as the medicine of promise. Systematically he changed the molecular structure of the arsenic compounds, following each molecular change with careful testing on animals. This work took nearly 20 years, but Ehrlich finally obtained a compound effective against syphilis, although it had toxic side effects.

The medicinal concoction, cryptically labelled compound 606, was so designated because it came after 605 failures. The medicine was first called arsphenamine, otherwise known as salvarsan (Hudson, 1983). It was used to treat many people over the next few years, including the noted author of *Out of Africa,* Isak Dinesen (Thurman, 1982).[8]

Ehrlich had established an exceptionally effective way to treat diseases that corrupted body processes at the cell level without the treatment's doing harm to the cell itself. Given the social context of his discovery, the decades during which millions of people had died from epidemic diseases, and the epidemic of syphilis then sweeping the world, it is no wonder the notion of magic bullets should be so forceful and captivating for both the medical profession that dispenses them and the eager populace that demands them.

---

[8] More will be said in Chapter 13 about Isak Dinesen's struggle with the pain of syphilis.

Modern Biomedical Theory and Pathology

Over the past quarter century, many critics of medicine have suggested, either implicitly or explicitly, that medical theory is unidimensional, dominated by a germ theory of disease and a magic bullet notion of treatment while singularly ignorant of psychosocial influences in the etiology and course of disease (for example, Ullman & Krasner, 1965; Engel, 1977). Additional criticisms of the medical model suggested that it had little concern for positive health values, that it defined health simply as the absence of illness and the physician as the healer. Finally, medical practice has been criticized for being less concerned with prevention than with **tertiary care,** treatment of the sick after the illness has already progressed significantly.

Although these statements may contain kernels of truth, the more extreme assertions are largely self-serving, if not factually wrong. To say that biomedical theory is represented by a single germ model is somewhat like saying that psychology is represented by a single stimulus-response model (London, 1972). To say that medicine is typified by a magic bullet notion of treatment is like saying that psychological treatment is only psychotherapy. These statements do not accurately represent theory or therapy in either profession.

Medical theorists and medical epidemiologists have long recognized that numerous factors interact to predict disease. Among the contributing factors to the etiology of a disease are host factors of the organism, including genetic-constitutional characteristics and some mood-dispositional traits. In addition, environmental factors could influence the onset, course, duration, or severity of disease (Evans, 1978). This triad—an agent interacting with a host organism in a unique environmental context—became the more accepted model of disease. In this model, germs are just one component in the class of agents that could lead to disease.

As for prevention, medicine has increased its attention to early screening and diagnostic procedures. Finally, worldwide vaccination programs that have controlled or eradicated many diseases attest to the impressive role of prevention in modern medicine.

Modern medical theory, then, is more accurately viewed as concerned with a wide variety of biological factors that contribute to illness. In addition to the cellular and germ models previously described, biomedical theory considers genetic, biochemical, musculoskeletal, hormonal, and immune system pathologies. Later chapters will give more details of the biological etiology of certain disorders as needed. Here, I will describe the genetic model of disease to illustrate the complex nature of modern biomedical theory.

Genetic Contributions to Health and Illness

The contribution of genetic endowment to disease continued to be a beguiling though impenetrable mystery until recently. Admittedly, some genetic influences were guessed at in ancient civilization. The Talmud, for example, shows some understanding of the genetic origins of hemophilia (Rosner, 1977). Development of the genetic model, however, was delayed in part due to limitations of technology. Causal models could not be developed until adequate instrumentation was created, and enough information accumulated to allow researchers to probe the inner recesses, even the nucleus, of the cell. Only in the last 100 years has real progress been made in identifying diseases with genetic etiologies and in understanding the mechanisms whereby the **genotype,** the genetic code, is translated into the **phenotype,** the physical or behavioral expression of the code. Now possibly as many as 3000 diseases have been traced to genetic sources.

The Genetic Code

Buried within the each person's genes is the genetic code, the blueprint that regulates how each body is built, how it physically matures, and how it operates. This code controls external appearance, making some tall and some short, some fat and some thin, some beautiful and some plain. The genetic code contributes to temperament, personality, and intelligence. It contributes to disease directly through organ disorders or biochemical imbalances, and indirectly by increasing vulnerability to disease. It is believed that mapping of the human genome may be complete in the next 10 to 15 years (D'Alton & DeCherney, 1993). Briefly told, the story of this genetic central command begins with the chromosomes.

Humans have a total of 46 chromosomes arranged in 23 pairs, a fact that was not established until 1956 (Tjio & Levan, 1956). The first 22 pairs are called autosomes, while the 23rd pair determines the sex of the new child. Sex cells from both parents go through reduction division, a process called **meiosis,** when the number of chromosomes in each cell is reduced to just half the usual number (Plomin, DeFries, & McClearn, 1980). After a sperm penetrates (fertilizes) an ovum, the new cell, now called a **zygote,** again has the customary 46 chromosomes. When all goes normally, a natural symmetry exists in that exactly half the chromosomes come from the mother and half from the father. The new cell then begins the normal growth process of somatic division, called **mitosis,** when the cell divides first into two "daughter" cells, then into four, and so on.

Chromosome Abnormalities: Supermen and Superwomen?

Unfortunately, things do not always go normally in this genetic lottery. Irregularities can occur at different stages, leading to **chromosomal anomalies**—in other words, abnormal chromosomes or pairings of chromosomes. About half of the chromosomal anomalies are related to the sex (23) chromosome, and about half occur in the autosomes (Plomin, DeFries, & McClearn, 1980). The most common sex chromosome anomalies are Turner's, Triple-X female, Kleinfelter's, and XYY-male syndromes. The most common autosomal anomaly is Down's syndrome, a trisomy of the 21st chromosome (Groër & Shekleton, 1983).

In **Turner's syndrome** (written as 45,X), a female lacks the second X chromosome. She appears to be female, of normal intelligence, short in stature, but with immature genitalia and no ovaries. The **Triple-X female** (47,XXX) appears to be like any other woman outwardly and follows a normal course of sexual maturation with fertility. But she is more likely to have lower intelligence than average, and she may have an increased tendency to psychotic and antisocial behavior.

In **Kleinfelter's syndrome** (47,XXY), a male child receives an extra female sex chromosome. He is outwardly male, but his genitals are usually smaller and he is infertile. There is an increased prevalence of lower intelligence with IQs in the 60 to 80 range, but most will function in the normal range. The **XYY male** (47,XYY) occurs when a male receives an extra Y male chromosome. XYY males are typically tall with no physical abnormalities; they may in fact be physically handsome, though they are generally infertile (Roberts & Pembrey, 1985).

The XYY syndrome achieved notoriety in 1968 due to speculation about associated violence after Richard Speck, an XYY male, killed eight nurses in Chicago. A survey suggesting that a disproportionate number of prison inmates had the syndrome added more fuel to this fire. This misconception was subsequently dispelled through a project that used data on 31,436 males from the Danish Population Register (Witkin et al., 1976). As it turned out, only 5 of the 12 XYY males identified had been imprisoned; 4 had been convicted of property crimes, but only 1 had a record of violent crime. Further, XYY males may have been detected and caught more easily than criminals with other genetic profiles, not because there were more of these males to catch among the criminal populace, but because of their markedly lower intelligence.

The Problem of Causal Attribution in Chromosomal Abnormalities

I noted earlier that one common autosomal abnormality is Down's syndrome, named after Langdon Down, who first described the symptom complex. Down's syndrome expresses itself in both mental and physical traits. The condition is characterized by a mild to moderate level of retardation and an unusually sunny, happy disposition. Down's children are typically short and stocky, and they walk with a shuffling gait. Their skulls are often small, faces round, and their eyes almond shaped and slanted.

These features are obvious, but another facet of the phenotype is more problematic, even life threatening. Down's children experience heart problems, are at increased risk for respiratory infections, and are more than 15 times likely to have leukemia compared to normal children (Groër & Shekleton, 1983). These risks translate to a much shorter average life span for Down's children, often no more than 20 years. Modern medicine now makes it possible to control some of the infections that earlier would have taken the child's life probably before late adolescence. If they are fortunate enough to survive, the genetic load still may rear its ugly head, because any Down's person who lives past 45 will develop Alzheimer's disease (Rosenhan & Seligman, 1989). This is especially noteworthy since recent research has implicated the 21st chromosome pair in Alzheimer's disease.

Although Langdon Down described the mental and physical symptoms of this syndrome quite accurately in 1886, it was not until 1959 that the genotype was identified. Then, Lejeune, Gautier, and Turpin (1959) showed that Down's syndrome results when three chromosomes exist, in what is called a **trisomy,** at the 21st chromosome location. 95% of the time, the trisomy occurs during meiosis because the cell fails to divide correctly, a defect called **nondisjunction** (Plomin, DeFries, & McClearn, 1980). In fact, all the chromosomal anomalies that have been described here are believed to be errors in disjunction. Normally, each parent contributes

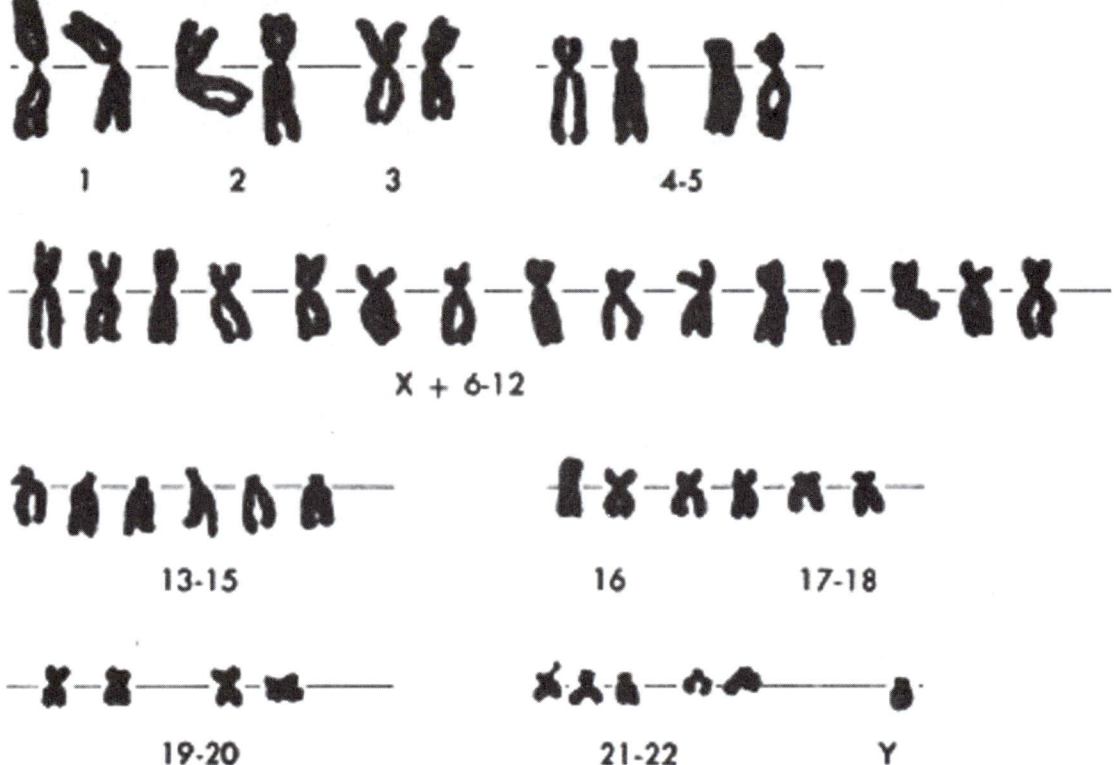

1   2   3   4-5

X + 6-12

13-15   16   17-18

19-20   21-22   Y

FIGURE 2.9   *An abnormal arrangement with 47 chromosomes showing the trisomy at location 21, the karyotype of Down's syndrome (from Reisman & Motheny, p. 69).*

one chromosome, but in Down's, one parent contributes two chromosomes because of a failure of the two cells to divide. These two cells then combine with one chromosome from the other parent. Taylor (1981) pointed out that it grossly misstates the complexity of Down's to say that it is merely a trisomy of the 21st chromosome, since nondisjunction may occur in at least three or four ways. In addition, Down's may occur from **translocation,** when the extra chromosome occurs at location 14 or 15.

At one time, it was thought that nondisjunction must be a flaw on the mother's side because the prevalence of Down's children increases dramatically when the mother's birth age is 35 or older. For mothers over 35, the rate is three times that in mothers under 35; for mothers over 40, it is nine times the rate; and for mothers over

45, it is more than 19 times the rate of mothers under 35 (Plomin, DeFries, & McClearn, 1980). This belief turned out to be an example of the logical fallacy of reasoning from mere correlation. For some inexplicable reason, people seemed to forget that women over 35 are also frequently married to men over 35. It is now known that the syndrome may occur due to nondisjunction on either the mother's or the father's side (Roberts & Pembrey, 1985) and that nondisjunction may stem from subtle age-linked biochemical changes.

This notion of disease as faulty genetics is quite different from models that assumed that a diseased organism had been invaded by an external pathogen, a germ. In the genetic model, the process is one that appears entirely due to subtle, infinitely complex biochemical processes that influence the reproductive sequence.

At the Heart of the Chromosome: Dissecting the Gene

Each chromosome contains many **genes,** which are coded sequences of the double helix, DNA or deoxyribonucleic acid. How many genes the chromosomes contain is somewhat conjectural. The estimated range is from 10,000 to 100,000 per full (diploid) set (Plomin, DeFries, & McClearn, 1980), but Roberts and Pembrey (1985) stated that each half (haploid) set of chromosomes contains around 50,000 expressed genes.

Some traits are controlled by single genes with a major effect such as sickle cell anemia. Other traits may be determined by polymorphic variations. Still other traits may be **polygenic**— that is, determined by two or more genes (Plomin, 1990). This variation makes it all the more difficult to identify the relationship between the marker genes (genotype) and the physical expression (phenotype). Among the more common disorders linked to genetic defects are diabetes milletus, galactosemia, Tay-Sachs disease, phenylketonuria (PKU), and cystic fibrosis. It is also thought that hypercholesterolemia and body weight may be genetically determined. Other genetic diseases are shown in Table 2.3.

The condition in which a gene occurs at the same location in two or more forms is called **polymorphism** (Roberts & Pembrey, 1985). Certain blood disorders, such as abnormal hemoglobin disorders, are examples of clinical disorders that appear to have polymorphic gene determinants. One polymorphic disorder in-

TABLE 2.3   *A list of genetic diseases grouped according to the primary body system that malfunctions and is responsible for the appearance of symptoms (adapted from Groër & Shekleton, 1989).*

Disorders of carbohydrate metabolism	**Disorders of metal metabolism**
Diabetes mellitus	Wilson's disease
Pentosuria	Hemochromatosis
Glycogen storage diseases (types II, III, and IV)	
Galactosemia	
Disorders of lipid metabolism	**Disorders of connective tissue, bone, and muscle**
Familial lipoprotein deficiency	Familial periodic paralysis
Familial lecithin-cholesterol acyl-transferase (L-CAT) deficiency	Muscular dystrophies
	Mucopolysaccharidoses
Tay-Sachs disease	Hunter's syndrome
Gaucher's disease	Hurler's syndrome
Sandhoff's disease	**Disorders of the hematopoietic system and blood**
Disorders of protein metabolism	Sickle cell anemia
Familial goiter	Glucose 6-PD deficiency
Phenylketonuria	Thalassemias
Albinism	Hereditary spherocytosis
Alkaptonuria	
Tyrosinosis	**Disorders of exocrine glands**
Disorders of purine and pyrimidine metabolism	Cystic fibrosis
Gout	
Lesch-Nyhan syndrome	
Disorder of kidney?	
Huntington's disease	

volves the inherited deficiency of a serum protein called −1-antitrypsin. Absence of this protein was first detected in Scandinavian workers with pulmonary emphysema. In **homozygotes,** those who received the same gene from both parents, carbohydrate side-chains of the protein are abnormal, leading to faulty processing in the liver and inhibited passage into the serum. The protein then accumulates in the liver, leading to cirrhosis of the liver and possible death. Those who do survive are at greatly increased risk for pulmonary emphysema, especially if they smoke (Roberts & Pembrey, 1985).

Sickle Cell Anemia: Silent Savior or Insidious Killer?

Sickle cell anemia is a genetically inherited disease that appears in about one of every 400 African American newborns in the United States (Consensus Conference, 1987). It is thought to be caused by a single mutated gene that controls the coding of amino acids in the blood cell (Groër & Shekleton, 1983).

The disease is one of nature's Jekyll and Hyde paradoxes. In the heterozygous state, some patients may experience mild anemia but most are asymptomatic: They show none of the usual symptoms associated with sickle cell anemia, although there are still concerns for both diagnosis and treatment (Witkowska et al., 1991). The heterozygous state may even have been of great benefit in tropical climates because those who carry it have increased resistance to malarial fever. In the homozygous state, though, the disease is symptomatic and potentially lethal.

The symptoms of sickle cell anemia include chronic anemia and acute pain (Platt et al., 1991). The pain is usually a result of the blood's failing to pass through the capillaries for return to the heart. Surrounding tissue then lacks necessary oxygen and nutrition for normal maintenance. If blood volume is sufficiently reduced, shock may occur, followed by death. Multidisciplinary treatment may include both medical intervention and intensive counseling

for the debilitating effects of chronic pain (Vichinsky, Johnson, & Lubin, 1982).

The disease is classified as a blood pathology, specifically a hemoglobinopathy, because it alters one of the amino acids in the hemoglobin molecule. This change is illustrated in Figure 2.10, which shows that one amino acid, valine, displaces glutamine at position 6 in the hemoglobin molecule. This slight change greatly alters the ability of hemoglobin to carry and transport oxygen (Groër & Shekleton, 1983).

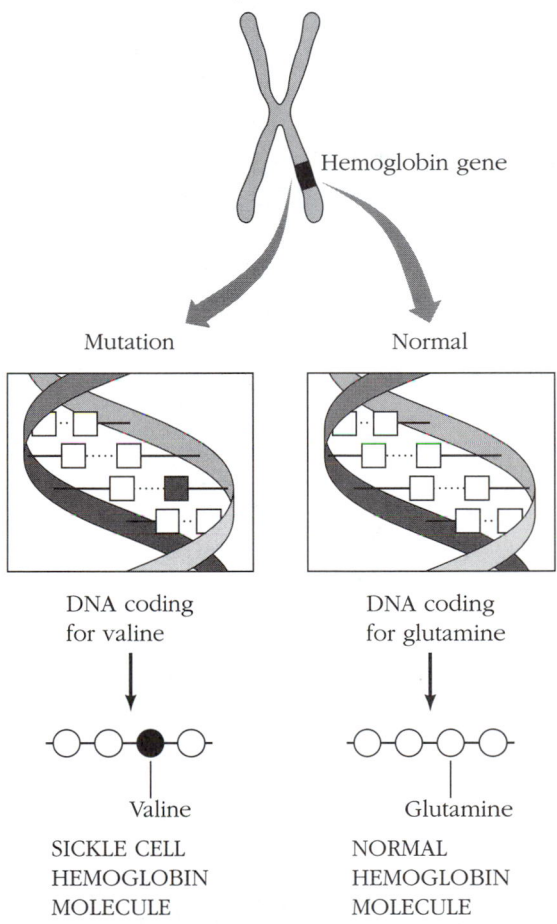

FIGURE 2.10   A substitution of valine for glutamine at position 6 leads to abnormal hemoglobin and the appearance of sickle cell anemia (from Groër & Shekleton, 1983).

Genetic Screening and Genetic Counseling

Newly developed prenatal genetic screening techniques, including amniocentesis and a blood test, now make it possible to determine the likelihood of giving birth to a Down's syndrome child or one with any number of other genetically determined conditions (American Academy of Pediatrics, 1989). Genetic diagnostic procedures may determine the probable existence of a genetic defect either before conception or *in utero* (McCormack, 1981; D'Alton & DeCherney, 1993). Further, some suggest that genetic screening should be extended to the workplace to monitor the possible mutagenic effects of numerous agents used in a work environment (Khoury, Newill, & Chase, 1985; Office of Technology Assessment, 1990).

Perhaps the best known method of genetic screening for defects is the test procedure called **amniocentesis.** Amniocentesis is considered a low-risk procedure when carried out at 16 to 17 weeks. One time in 150, a miscarriage may occur that otherwise would not have occurred, and in rare instances structural damage to the fetus may occur (Roberts & Pembrey, 1985). Such risks increase when the test must be repeated. This procedure removes amniotic fluid from the womb, fluid that contains cells from the fetus and thus provides a genetic map of the fetus. The procedure is shown in Figure 2.11.

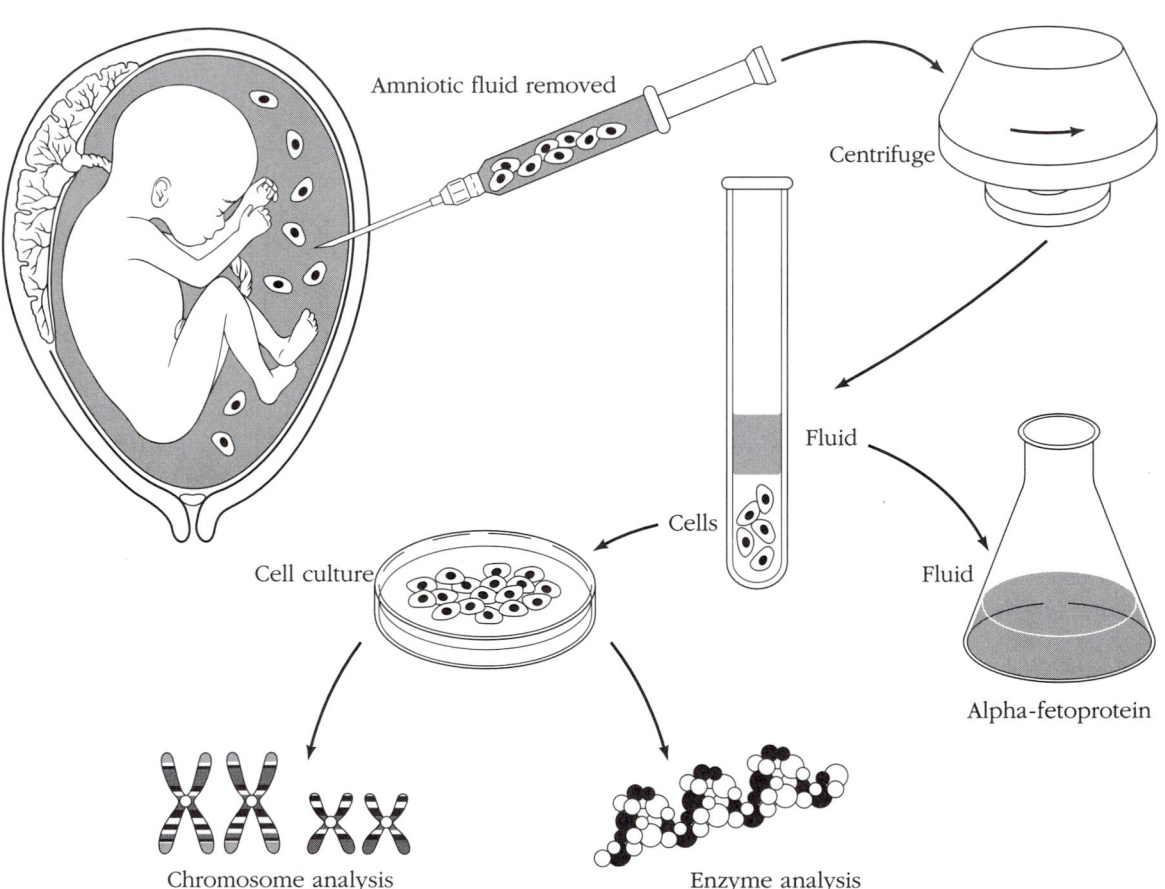

Amniotic fluid removed

Centrifuge

Fluid

Cells

Cell culture

Fluid

Alpha-fetoprotein

Chromosome analysis

Enzyme analysis

FIGURE 2.11   A description of amniocentesis (from Heller et al., 1996).

Through cytology, cell culture techniques, and biochemical analysis, clinical geneticists can determine such things as chromosomal abnormalities (for example, Down's syndrome), fetal sex (which may be linked to important recessive traits), neural tube defects (for example, anencephaly), and biochemical disorders or imbalances (for example, Tay-Sachs disease). An important adjunct to detect larger structural defects is ultrasound. Some conditions, such as anencephaly and hydrocephaly, may be detected through ultrasound without exposing the woman to the risks entailed in amniocentesis, however slight those risks may be.

The effect on parents of giving birth to a child with a genetic defect can be devastating, psychologically and socially (in terms of family structure and function). Consider the emotional reactions that might occur when parents receive the shattering news that their long-awaited child may be one of the 3% of babies to be born with a genetic defect. Add to this the fact that about 20% of infant deaths occur because of genetic defects (Plomin, DeFries, & McClearn, 1980).

Genetic counseling attempts to help people deal with emotional reactions to the prospect of the birth of a child with a genetic defect. Further, it plays an important role in providing information and advice to parents, both after the unexpected happens and in planning for the future with knowledge of the chances of conceiving another child with a similar defect. Conveying medical information about the risks involved is usually the province of a clinical geneticist. The medical counselor may dispel mistaken notions about risks by giving accurate probabilities. Further, some disorders, such as phenylketonuria (PKU), may be readily managed through other means. PKU, for example, can be managed effectively through a diet that is low in phenylalanine.

Still, counseling may include other members of an interdisciplinary team, such as a health psychologist, especially when the parents begin to openly express questions loaded with the potential for psychological damage. For example, biological parents quite often begin to

ask questions that imply fault: Which partner was the guilty party? One partner may assume undue responsibility, adding a great weight of guilt to what may already be an overwhelming load of grief. Finally, if the child is likely to survive but with greatly diminished capacity, there may be endless questions about whether the parents have the emotional, physical, cognitive, and financial resources to meet the child's needs without diminishing their capacity to provide for other family members. In all of these areas, families may benefit from a patient, sympathetic counselor.

Teratogens and Mutagens: Uncontrolled Genetic Engineering

The first trimester is regarded as a critical period in the development of the embryo. Very early in the somatic division process, three layers of cells are formed that presage major body structures. One layer, the ectoderm, differentiates into skin and nervous system. Another layer, the mesoderm, differentiates into muscles and skeletal structure. The third layer, the endoderm, differentiates into the gastrointestinal tract and internal organs. During the division process, the embryo is vulnerable to numerous **teratogens,** agents that cause damage to developing tissues. Either structure or function may be changed in a harmful way as a result of these teratogens, a condition called a **congenital anomaly.** Later in the gestation period, the fetus can also be negatively affected by teratogens.

Approximately 1% of all infants are born with a congenital heart defect (Horovitz, 1988), but more females are thus affected than males. These defects range from minor to potentially lethal. They may affect resistance, oxygenation, or other processes that are important to blood circulation. Examples of teratogens that have damaging effects on the embryo include rubella during the first trimester (central nervous system damage and congenital heart defects), tranquilizers such as thalidomide (limb and organ defects), alcohol (fetal alcohol syndrome), chemotherapy (central nervous system defects), or diagnostic radiation (central nervous system and skeletal abnormalities) (Groër & Shekleton, 1983). Changes may also occur across generations because of spontaneous mutation or because of **mutagens,** agents that physically alter the structure of the gene that is then passed on to offspring.

The Sweet Smell of Success: The Critics Unconvinced

As models of disease, these genetic disorders (sickle cell anemia in particular) are instructive in a variety of ways. First, it is clear that no external entity, no germ, invades the body to produce sickle cell anemia; the disease instead results from an endogenous malfunction at the molecular level. Second, it is apparent that the search for the origins of disease progresses to infinitely smaller units, much smaller than was imagined even when cells and bacteria were discovered. Third, the issue of cause is still obscured. The description of the general process is certainly sophisticated; it sounds very precise. We are, sadly, lured by the sophistication into a false complacency. We tend to believe too readily that we have provided a causal explanation of the disease when all we have done is described another malfunction. What leads valine to displace glutamine, for example, is not known. In this sense, searching for an ultimate cause is like walking a path of infinite regress, always pushing back further and further to find a cause. Still, each step along that path reveals clues to how the deviant process and its disease consequences may be corrected.

In the end, even this great promise of medical research is used by its critics to confirm what they had suspected, that medicine continues its headlong slide to reductionistic models, models that become ever more fine grained as issues of psychosocial context are ignored. Biomedical research somatizes disease, looking for the cause of disease in an abnormal physical process, a deviant cell structure, or biochemical imbalances. And in spite of this increasing complexity, the medical model is still viewed as a single-cause model (S. E. Taylor, 1986), although it should be clear by now that this criticism lacks significant sting when considered in the context of the disease triad of an agent interacting with a host organism in a unique environmental context.

Finally, the critics charge that this reductionism perpetuates an unhealthy mind-body dualism, in which disease is viewed as something confined to details of anatomy and physiology, having nothing to do with the mind. In the next chapter, though, as we revisit these criticisms and begin to consider psychological theories of health and illness, we will see that the attempt to construct an integrative model is fraught with many unresolved problems. But the pursuit of plausible answers is also beguiling and promising. As our efforts continue, we would do well to recall Engel's (1977) admonition that the challenge for today is "to include the psychosocial without sacrificing the enormous advantages of the biomedical approach" (p. 131).

Summary

This chapter approached the biological nature of health and illness first by exploring the historical development of disease theory. Biomedicine usually does not have the luxury of developing in isolation from necessity, in the detached halls of ivy, as a few other sciences do. Biomedical progress has, more often than not, had to respond to social necessity, even extreme urgency, to thwart some natural holocaust. In so doing, it has provided an enormous amount of theory and technique, most of which must be recognized as having had the most salutary effect on health and the quality of life.

The chapter's second approach to this topic involves understanding the logic required to establish causal explanations for disease—a sometimes difficult, though I hope not odious, task for the student. The intent has been to show the complexity of the biological part of the biopsychosocial equation, which, however much it may be superseded by the discoveries of tomorrow, must nonetheless be appreciated and accommodated in proposed integrative alternatives. The following items, then, highlight crucial points made during this lengthy construction project.

1. Although early medical thinking was often limited by notions of supernatural causation, simple empiricism was already at work building a practical base for understanding relations between disease symptom complexes and modes of treatment.

2. Theory and treatment seldom, if ever, perfectly correspond, but even primitive theories of disease prescribed treatments consistent with their view of the disease; trepanning is one example.

3. The earliest systematic theory of disease, the four humors theory proposed by Hippocrates, is often viewed as a holistic theory of health and illness. It incorporated both mental and physical aspects of health and illness and proposed natural lifestyle treatments such as diet and exercise.

4. Hippocrates' declaration that epilepsy is no more sacred than any other disease is usually taken as the beginning of a natural approach to medicine.

5. Important departures from speculative theories, such as humoral theory, occurred when medical researchers began a more systematic study of anatomy and physiology.

6. As a model of disease, anatomical (organ) pathology assumed that disease resulted from damage to a body organ, or malfunctioning of a set of interconnected organs. It failed as a sufficient theory of disease when it was noted that disease in widely separated organs could still present similar symptoms. Even so, anatomy and physiology became the cornerstones of informed medical science.

7. Tissue pathology emerged as the successor theory to correct the flaws in organ pathology theory. This theory stated that different diseases occur because of selective damage to different types of tissues. This theory was also

short-lived, since medical science already had a smaller unit to propose for causal analysis.

8. Cell pathology theory suggests that disease occurs when the cell responds to abnormal stimuli in such a way that the cell malfunctions, is malformed, or becomes malnourished. Cell theory continues to be an important part of contemporary notions of disease.

9. Even as physical-somatic theories of disease continued to be developed and refined, there was growing recognition that psychosocial factors could, in some unknown fashion, influence disease—as illustrated in the life and work of Virchow.

10. The Semmelweis tragedy exemplifies iatrogenic disease, caused when a cure produces a fate that is worse than the illness.

11. During the time that the theory of cell pathology was being developed, the elusive pathogen that could cause cells to respond abnormally continued to escape detection. Louis Pasteur played a significant role in finding that germs—bacteria, or microbes as they are sometimes called—are the culprits that may cause the cell to malfunction. Pasteur's work contributed to the process of vaccination that ultimately led to the control or eradication of the worst epidemic diseases.

12. The notion that a disease can be treated with a magic bullet—a pill or a shot—is usually traced to the work of Paul Ehrlich, who developed the first successful treatment for syphilis.

13. Modern medical theories of disease are criticized for focusing primarily on somatic malfunction, ignoring psychosocial influences; for being largely concerned about sickness and not about positive health; and for emphasizing tertiary care instead of preventive care. These criticisms are used to argue in favor of a biopsychosocial model.

14. Theoretical models of disease today cannot be regarded as limited solely to a germ model. There are many disease theories, just as there are many learning theories or personality theories.

15. The genetic model of disease shows that medical theory has become increasingly sophisticated and molecular, producing increasingly

sophisticated diagnostic techniques and treatments. Amniocentesis is an example of a genetic
screening method that may help couples make
informed decisions about the risks of having a
child with a genetic defect.

16. Even when description of a disease
occurs at the level of the chromosome, the
chromosome abnormality may have multiple
causes. Down's syndrome is an example; the
disjunction that causes the syndrome can occur
in a number of different ways.

17. The biopsychosocial model may be considered as an alternative to biomedical theory,
but the enormous benefits of the biomedical
model should not be discarded.

Study Questions

1. Critique the notion that medical theory
and treatment are of necessity always linked.
(Hint: To what extent is it necessary that a
successful treatment should have an accurate
theory behind it?)

2. Critics of contemporary medical practice
and theory base their criticisms largely on the
notion that germ theory and magic bullets are
dominant approaches in biomedicine. To what
extent is this criticism justified or not justified?
Can germ theory be eliminated from biomedical
theory? If so, what would take its place? If not,
why not?

3. The genetic model was presented as a
view of pathology. Is this model compatible
with a germ theory of disease? If not, how is it
incompatible? What logical adjustments should
be made in biomedical theory if it is incompatible? If it is compatible, in what way is this so?

4. Biomedical theory recognizes that an
agent interacts with a host organism in a given
setting. How is this the same as an integrative
approach? How does it differ? Is this a true
multicausal model of health and illness?

5. To what extent, if any, is there room in
the agent-host-environment biomedical model
for psychosocial influences in health and
illness?

Key Words

amniocentesis	mutagens
anatomical pathology	non-disjunction
anatomy	phenotype
cellular pathology	phlegmatic
chromosomal anomalies	plethora theory
choleric	polygenic
congenital anomaly	polymorphism
empiricism	sanguine
gene	symptom com-
genotype	plexes
germ theory	teratogens
humoral theory	tertiary care
homozygotes	tissue pathology
iatrogenic illness	translocation
Kleinfelter's syndrome	trepanning
magic bullet	Triple-X female
medical model	trisomy
meiosis	Turner's syndrome
melancholic	XYY male
mitosis	zygote

Class Projects

1. Consider conducting an informal survey,
or a formal field study if class objectives and time
permit, of both general health screening and
genetic screening techniques used by local
medical facilities and physicians. At the informal
level, you might contact your personal physician
for a short interview. Ask few but clear questions
about when counseling patients includes information on lifestyle, nutrition, and exercise. Ask
how much time is customarily available to
pursue this type of discussion with patients. Ask
how medical training and practice is changing, if
any, to incorporate these skills in the physician's
area of competency.

2. Look for current news items that show any
breakthroughs in medical science research. Both
disease theory and specific clinical interventions
may be of interest.

3. Look for journal articles or news items that
bear on the issue of whether medical practice is

becoming more concerned about primary prevention as opposed to tertiary care.

Suggested Readings

Evans, A. S. (1978). Causation and disease: A chronological journey. *American Journal of Epidemiology, 108,* 249–258.

Herman, C. E. (Ed.). (1997). Special issue: Psychological aspects of genetic testing. *Health Psychology, 16.*

Hudson, R. P. (1983). *Disease and its control: The shaping of modern thought.* Westport, CT: Greenwood Press.

Sigerist, H. E. (1971). *The great doctors: A biographical history of medicine.* Freeport, NY: Books for Libraries Press.

WEBSITES   Medicine, Genetics, and Genetic Counseling

ADDRESS	DESCRIPTION
http://www.arcade.uiowa/hardin-www/md.thml	☆ Hardin's Meta-Directory of Internet Health Sources
http://www.gen.emory.edu/MEDWEB/	☆ Medical Index Website—excellent and extensive index for health/disorder topics
http://www.ama-assn.org/	American Medical Association with news, information, advocacy, and links to other sites
http://www.nlm.nih.gov	U. S. National Library of Medicine
http://www.nhgri.nih.gov/	National Human Genome Research Institute at NIH—technical information, public policy, and news related to human genetics

On Grief, Placebos, and Mind: Psychological Foundations of Health and Illness

Physicians hold a place of honor, even reverence, in most societies. The best of the best may become part of that great tradition of worried care bestowed on presidents and prime ministers. In ancient China, for example, it was the custom for each king to have a personal court physician. Unfortunately, a court physician in ancient China might live a precarious existence compared to modern doctors, as the following—possibly apocryphal—story shows.

A certain king was very sick and confined to bed for many days. He would not eat, and his sleep was terribly restless. The king's court watched and became ever more anxious as his health declined. His physician had been regular in attending to the king, giving the best medical treatment possible. But nothing seemed to work.

One day when the king was desperately ill, the staff again summoned the king's physician. Although palace police carried out an intensive search, he was nowhere to be found. Three days later, unannounced, the doctor barged into the king's quarters and hurled a string of crude and ugly insults at the king. The king was so outraged at the doctor's uncouth behavior that he leaped from his bed and ordered his palace guard to boil the doctor in a vat of oil. From that day, the king quickly regained his health and good spirits. He resumed his kingly duties with vigor, showing few if any of his previous symptoms. Sadly, he also showed no remorse for executing the doctor in such a summary fashion.

Love's Sorrow: The Illness of a Yearning Heart

Centuries after this story took place, medical literature in the Mediterranean world contained teaching stories, informal case studies for practicing physicians. These stories were about doctors who recognized their patients' maladies as **psychogenic**—in other words, caused by psychological processes. Early writers did not use that term, but their thinking was nonetheless explicit. One writer put it this way: "It is impossible for the mind to suffer without the body becoming sick also or the body to be ill without the mind being associated with it in the distemper" (George Baker, 1755).

Perhaps the most celebrated such story appeared in the work of Galen (Jackson, 1969). Galen reported that he went to see a woman suffering from insomnia, but he could find no evidence of fever, no physical symptoms with which to confirm a physical basis for her distress. He postponed his diagnosis to the next day, determined to explore whether a disturbance in black bile caused her melancholy or some trouble that she would not admit was behind her malaise. The next day, accident came to Galen's rescue.

As Galen examined his patient, a family member returning from the theater announced that he had just seen Pylades dancing. Galen noted that the woman's expression and color changed dramatically. Quickly taking her pulse, he found her heart rate much accelerated. He inferred that the woman's illness had no physical cause but came from unrequited love.

Galen kept his suspicion to himself in order to conduct an informal experiment. The following day, by design, one of Galen's friends came by and announced that he had just seen Morphus dancing. Galen saw that the woman did not change expression, color, or heart rate. The next day, he had another announcement made about the third member of the troupe, again with no effect. But the next day, when Galen's friend reported that he had seen Pylades dancing, the woman's expression, color, and pulse suddenly changed, confirming Galen's theory.

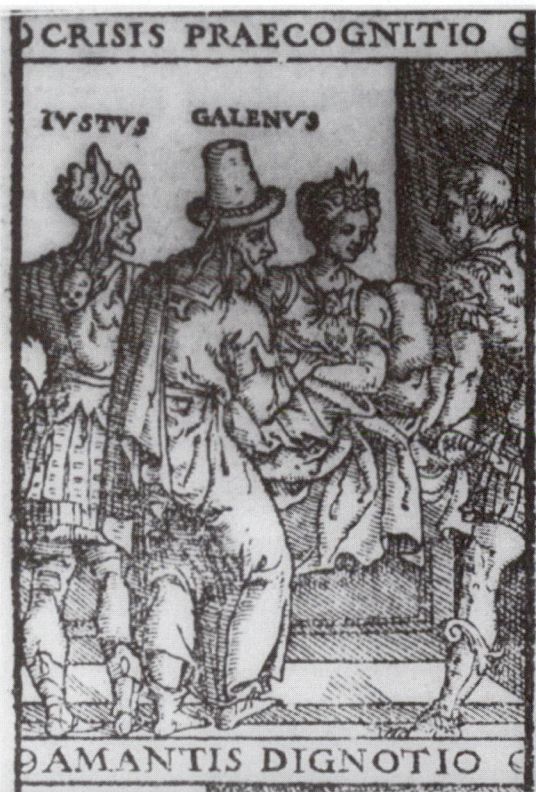

FIGURE 3.1 From a 1586 edition of works by Galen, depicting the tale of the doctor's correct diagnosis of the woman's illness as due to unrequited love (National Library of Medicine, Bethesda, MD; Frame 16387, side A).

Taboos and Black Magic: The Issue in Death Delayed

Magic is an ancient art, the name itself coming from occult practices of the Persian Magi. It may (forgive the pun) conjure up images of exciting, wonderful, even fantastical powers. But when it becomes black magic, it summons up very different, sinister connotations, as in so-called voodoo death.

The Harvard physiologist Walter Cannon (1942) collected stories of voodoo death from Brazil, Africa, Australia, and Haiti, among other countries. In one such story,[1] a young man from Jamaica attended a small high school graduation dinner given by a dear family friend. During the sumptuous dinner, several guests asked about a meat dish, one that was very delicate in texture and subtle in flavor. The host steadfastly resisted telling them: It was a very secret family recipe.

Later that year, the young man left the island to attend college. On a visit to his home two or three years later, he decided to call on his old friend, the dinner host. Prompted by the young man's wistful remembrance and thankfulness, their chat turned to the dinner—and again, the question about the meat. At this time, for whatever reason, the host decided to confide in his young friend the true nature of the dish: It was a taboo meat, even as some of the original guests had feared but dared not believe. But the host observed the young man had survived unharmed these years. Surely, then, the host surmised, all these notions of taboo must be just so much nonsense. Unconvinced, certainly feeling betrayed, the young man left his host's presence, still pondering the question of the meat. Within 24 hours he was dead, presumably the victim of his innocent violation of a taboo three years earlier.

Super Pills: The Healing Power of Suggestion

Each of us probably has some story, perhaps part of our family oral history, that tells of a friend (or a friend of a friend) who repeatedly went to the clinic. Almost always, they described the same symptoms, always asked for medications but almost always never got better—until some doctor gave them a wonder drug. Usually, the drug was nothing more than a **placebo,** a pill with no active medical ingredient.[2] Whenever a patient's physical status improves because of a placebo, questions arise about purely physical theories of disease and treatment. Placebos raise fundamental questions about the relation between mental processes and body function. Adolf Grünbaum (1985) told a story relayed to him personally by an English physician, Jennifer Worrall, that captures the essence of this tradition.

In the course of her practice, Dr. Worrall treated a middle-aged woman who suffered from a superficial leg ulcer. The woman was known as an extremely difficult patient. Her pain was always the worst possible pain, even though the trained medical eye could find little if any physical evidence of pain. Dr. Worrall prescribed a variety of mild to moderate pain-relieving medicines. Still, the patient belittled the medicines as useless and ineffective.

At this point, Dr. Worrall turned to her superior for advice. He agreed to see the patient, and after discussing her pain said that he wanted to try a "completely different sort of treatment" (p. 31). Disappearing into his office for a few minutes, the supervisor then reappeared, walking slowly and solemnly down the corridor. He carried in his outstretched arm a huge white pill clamped in equally large tweezers as though to keep the pill as far from his body as possible. He deposited this pill in water, and admonished the patient that she should sip the potion slowly but only after the fizzing stopped. This completely different sort of treatment immediately and effectively removed the pain. Unknown to the patient, the pill was nothing more than a large vitamin C capsule. The power of the placebo has been attributed to the human capacity for self-deception. Guy Saperstein, a placebo researcher, said "how people think about [medication] may influence improvement

---

[1] I have taken some license with this story, but the themes and essential factors are accurate.

[2] The word *placebo* comes from a 12th century Latin word that means "I shall please."

more powerfully than the chemical substance itself" (Bower, 1996, p. 123).

Common Threads: The Role of Mind and Emotions in Illness

These short stories illustrate how mind and body are connected in illness as in health. The story of the Chinese doctor suggests a view of health and illness very different from the biomedical germ notion. Presumably, the doctor guessed that the king's condition was beyond physical medicine, which is not to suggest that the physical symptoms were unreal or meaningless. Recognizing that the problem, physical symptoms included, was in the king's mind, the doctor sought a means to reverse the king's negative thought process. The cure was simple: Anger the king, give him a cause to live for and action to take for the cause. The physician was absolutely correct, though he paid the dearest price for the remedy. Thomas Ots (1990) noted that the Chinese people still have great appreciation for the power of emotions to influence physical disorder.

The story of the young woman craving love beyond reach implies that thoughts can alter physical function quickly and dramatically. An extreme case of this effect is voodoo death. Cannon argued that extreme grief caused voodoo death, not some supernatural effect nor mere somatic disorder. Cannon also argued that voodoo phenomena were largely restricted to primitive societies, a notion that is disputed by evidence of sudden inexplicable deaths in modern societies (Kamarck & Jennings, 1991; Natelson, 1983).

The Problem with Placebos: Suggestion or Natural Healing?

The story of the pill so powerful it could not be touched except by tweezers contains much material for thought. The most positive interpretation is also an uplifting view: Healing power lies within oneself. Some have suggested this healing from within is simply a matter of belief: If the patient believes in the cure, healing will take place. Research continues to accumulate, however, showing that placebos are not so simple as believing, that placebos activate the body's resources for healing. Further, a person with strong belief may also show increased **compliance,** or willingness to follow the doctor's prescription. Epstein (1984) concluded that greater compliance led to better treatment outcomes, whether the medication was active or a placebo.

There is another related interpretation: If the doctor gives medicine with great conviction for its efficacy, the healing effect in the patient will be greatly enhanced whether the medicine was intended for the disorder or not. Writing at the turn of the century, the physician William Osler (1901) noted, "We [physicians] should use new remedies quickly, while they are still efficacious" (p. 189). By implication, new remedies were more potent because they were more believable. Thus both the patient's positive belief and the physician's strong conviction may combine to produce healing.

On the negative side, cure by placebo is taken by some to mean that the sickness was only in the patient's head. If the cure was not real, then the sickness must not have been real either. Unfortunately, this view is confused both about the link between mental processes and physical symptoms and about the complex nature of the healing process. Physical symptoms, including organic insult, are just as real when they result from emotional distress as when they result from physical distress.

The basic issue raised by these stories is the connection between mind and body. Is the mind distinct from body? Is the mind a mere physical entity, nothing more than the brain at work? This problem has plagued thinkers for thousands of years, and it persists today in a lively debate among philosophers, cognitive psychologists, and neuroscientists.

Some health psychologists suggest that the issue is irrelevant to health psychology. This may be true, but only if one believes that health psychology is defined solely by clinical practice and pragmatic issues. It is my bias that health psychology should be as much concerned about theory and research as practice.

The following discussion suggests how cognitive science is grappling with the mind-body problem. It is impossible in so short a time and space to resolve this dilemma; still, highlighting certain issues might serve to inform the enterprise of health psychology.

The Mind-Body Problem Revisited: A Pointless Journey to the Absurd?

Much has been written about the mind problem: the issue of how the mind, a seemingly nonmaterial entity, can cause a physical event (the act of sitting down), or change a physical process (the alteration of heart rate). Indeed, the rationale for health psychology is that mental events can and do modify physical health. It is important, then, that we understand the prevailing arguments about the mind-body problem.

In one sense, much of what has been said about the mind-body problem is pointless if not absurd. We may not even have adequate tools to resolve the dispute, at least as yet. Wiliam Uttal (1978) implied that empirical data may actually be irrelevant to the debate, which quite often has depended on softer criteria, including emotion and values, combined with judgments of consistency and completeness.

The issue may be more a pseudo-problem (Churchland, 1986), reflecting the anemic quality (or the historically loaded, if not muddled, connotations) of the concepts and language we have to describe an extremely complex process. Yet the issue will not be discharged so easily for several reasons. The mind-body problem suffers first from an egocentric, and perhaps self-serving, myopia; we are too close to—we are part and parcel of—the phenomenon we seek to understand. We also have an inescapable subjective sense that we possess our bodies and that

we are masters of our fate. The self, the mind, myself as subject, *I,* must be the possessor. The body, this physical fabric I wear, must be some object *I* possess; the body must be merely the tool of my intentions. We believe firmly that we could lose a leg or an arm and still be ourselves. But we could not lose our minds and save our selves. From this perspective, mind is superordinate and body subordinate.

To come to grips with this issue, I will briefly retrace its origins. We will consider a select few typical solutions that lie on a dimension from dualism to interactionism to monism (Rakover, 1989). **Dualism** argues that mind and body are separate entities but still might influence each other in numerous ways. **Interactionism** believes that mind and body exist independently but interact somehow. **Monism** argues that mind and body belong to the same realm, but again there are numerous monistic proposals. Several solutions are presented in Figure 3.2.

Descartes the Dualist— Or Is That Interactionist?

It is widely believed and often pronounced that the villain behind our contemporary dilemma, the progenitor of dualism, was the French mathematician-philosopher René Descartes (1596–1650). The fact that Descartes's views were the product of his intellectual and cultural history is often conveniently overlooked. Compounding Descartes's dilemma, knowledge about the human body was still scarce. Descartes attempted to deal with intense conflicts between science and religion—between the reality of material existence and mortality on one hand, and belief in spiritual existence and immortality on the other. Descartes's solution provided a way, however dubious, for science to advance at that time with minimal threat from religion (Schwab, 1985). Even so, many of his peers regarded Descartes as a dangerous and heretical thinker (Hergenhahn, 1986).

Descartes divided human nature into two very different types of existence (Kenny, 1989). To appease the clerics, he posited that the rational soul—*mind*—was immaterial and could

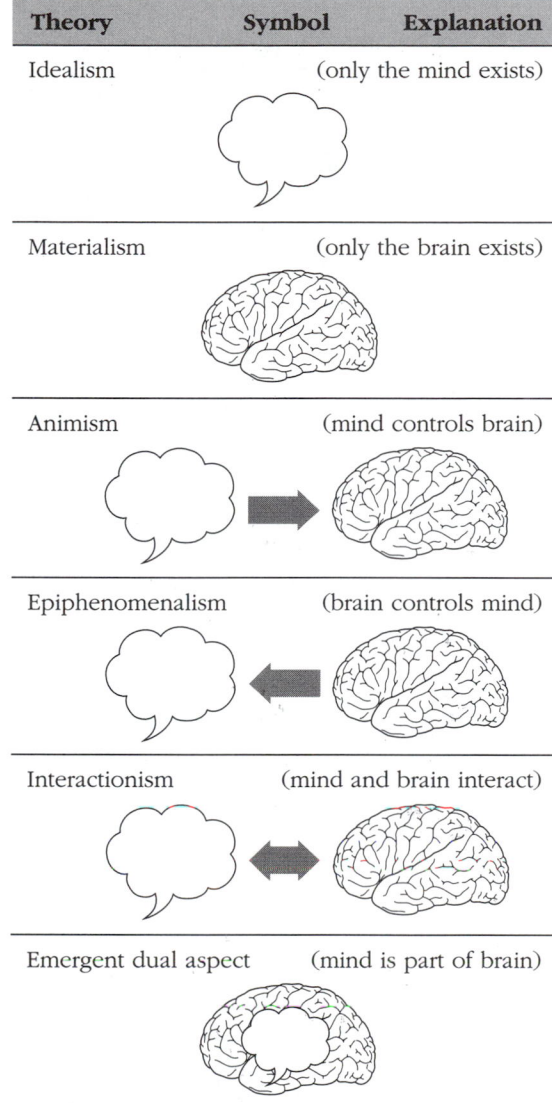

Theory	Symbol	Explanation
Idealism		(only the mind exists)
Materialism		(only the brain exists)
Animism		(mind controls brain)
Epiphenomenalism		(brain controls mind)
Interactionism		(mind and brain interact)
Emergent dual aspect		(mind is part of brain)

FIGURE 3.2 *A comparison of several mind-body solutions proposed over the centuries (adapted from Bunge, 1980).*

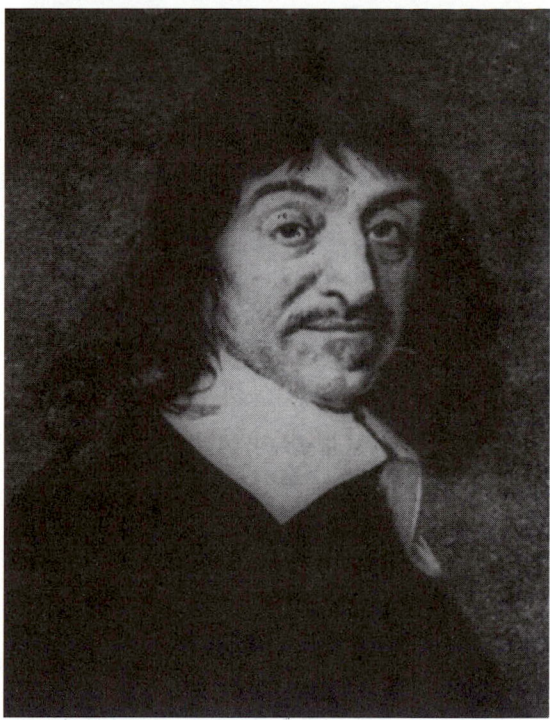

FIGURE 3.3 *Descartes's mind-body solution has often been regarded as a barrier to correct thinking about mind-brain unity. (National Library of Medicine, Bethesda, MD.)*

exist independently of the body, even separately from the brain. To comport with the growing scientific climate, he proposed that *body* was part of and subject to all the laws of the physical world, including the same mechanisms that governed animals' reflexes. Mind and brain interacted in a little known and misunderstood part of the brain, the **pineal gland.**[3] These ideas are the core of dualistic interactionism as proposed by Descartes.[4]

Successive generations continued to be unkind as many joined the parade of those damning Descartes's dualism. Gilbert Ryle

---

[3] Until just recently, it was assumed that the pineal body was vestigial—that it served no useful purpose. It is now known that this body synthesizes melatonin from the neurotransmitter serotonin and, further, that melatonin mediates the body's response to light-dark cycles. Melatonin is now the hot new natural sedative, marketed in capsule form to help with sleep disturbances. The pineal body, then, may be an important natural clock that helps regulate circadian rhythms (Binkley, 1979).

[4] Other terms for Descartes's theory include *psychophysical interactionism* and *substance dualism* (Churchland, 1986).

(1949) put it bluntly when he wrote, "I shall often speak of it [mind], with deliberate abusiveness, as 'the dogma of the Ghost in the Machine'" (pp. 15–16). According to Brown (1989), criticisms of Cartesian dualistic interactionism are based on only the most casual reading and shallow understanding of Descartes. Such criticisms overlook the basic role assigned in his theory to passions and their action on the body. These criticisms also minimize the basic interdependency Descartes assigned to mind-body interactions. No matter how much the language conveyed an impression of different entities, the mind and body were not literally two distinct entities, but parts of an integrated system in which the force of passions could effect dramatic body changes.

Neither was fate kind to Descartes in death. Summoned to Sweden to tutor the queen, Descartes suffered from the harsh winter conditions and died barely four months later. Buried in Sweden only temporarily, his body was later exhumed for return to his homeland. Unfortunately, the casket brought for the purpose would not accommodate his lengthy body. And so, in a most macabre twist of fate, his head was cut off and his body returned alone for burial. Then, as the ultimate insult, his head was stolen and passed as a curiosity among collectors for nearly 150 years until it was placed in a museum (Boakes, 1984).

The Philosopher: A Commonsense View of the Mind-Body Problem

John Searle (1984) felt the mind-body problem could be solved using simple notions from everyday language. He even defined mind in conventional fashion as "the sequences of thoughts, feelings and experiences, whether conscious or unconscious, that go to make up our mental life" (pp. 10–11). In support of his commonsense approach, Searle raised the rhetorical question: Why do we even have a mind-body problem and not a digestion-stomach problem? To Searle, the digestion-stomach relation, like the mind-body relation, is a relationship between a function and a structure.

To answer his own question, though, Searle pointed to four core features that make mind events seem so very different from physical events: consciousness, intentionality, subjectivity, and causality. **Consciousness** is more than just primitive awareness of stimuli; it extends to the notion of self-awareness and the capacity to reflect on our internal states. **Intentionality** describes the way we direct cognitive processes to some end: We intend to be better persons; we know we can change our spouses; we plan and effect changes in our world. **Subjectivity** describes the very private and deeply personal nature of our mental states, which cannot be directly observed or meaningfully shared with others in any but the most superficial way. Finally, **causality** refers to the notion that we believe our thoughts have a real causal influence, first in direct observable effects in the external world and second in the less observable, but no less real, inner world.

In the final analysis, Searle believed there is no mind-body problem. Mental events are only features of neurons firing, just as wetness is a feature of hydrogen and oxygen molecules' combining in a certain way. No one asks about an implicit dualism in this arrangement, and no one accuses the physicist of reductionism.[5] Why should we be so concerned, then, that neural firing gives rise to thoughts that we can detect? Why should we believe that the monist statement "mind is the brain at work" reduces mind to the activity of a single neuron? Why should we accuse monists of reductionism when they say that mind is a feature of the way neural activity sums? According to Searle, then, it is only a matter of time until everyday language integrates the mind-body relationship as naturally as it now accommodates the relationship between digestion and the stomach.

---

[5] Searle did not raise the issue of reductionism, but this is a logical extension of his point.

The Functionalist View: Riddles for the Mind-Body Problem?

Searle introduced the notion that mind may be viewed as function. On the philosophical side, functionalist theory is frequently supported with riddles, or "thought problems," such as the Turing (1950) imitation game or the brain in the vat problem (Dennett, 1991). Some riddles try to guess how a mind event, some thought, could enter into brain and cause physical change. The riddle usually begins with an unstated assumption: The thought is—in other words, the thought exists in and of itself. Then, the solution, constructed as a coup against an alleged reductionist program, shows that there is some problem in getting from the mind event to the body event, or that mind is unmistakably different from body because it deals with meaning, intentions, values, or beliefs.

Unfortunately, these thought problems are treated as though they provide some definitive test of what the mind is or how mind-body relationships can or cannot be conceived. Speculative mind theorists seem convinced that they can build a model of mind based largely on rational armchair analysis of an arbitrarily constructed thought segment, which itself is isolated from the continuous dynamic and endless stream of brain-mind events. Such methods are not usually regarded as creditable to verify or refute theory, yet they are almost pandemic among this group. In a comment that touched on both functionalist psychology and philosophy, Patricia Churchland (1986) wrote, "My guess is that it [functionalist psychology devoid of neuroscience] shares a flaw with many other philosophical thought-experiments: too much thought and not enough experiment" (p. 363).

The Cognitive Psychologist: Mind as a Semantic Engine

On the scientific side, cognitive scientists in the functionalist camp accept the idea that mind must arise from brain as opposed to being a spiritual entity. They view mind as a language engine that runs on semantics or meaning. Mind works through logical manipulations of symbols, and it is rule-based. In other words, it does not depend on absolute mechanical connections between stimuli and responses (Churchland, 1986). Mind is able to use abstract symbols, including words, to represent a vast array of objects and events. Symbols function as images of knowledge and experience. They are the seeds of values, attitudes, and beliefs; the fuel of expectations and hopes; the ground of intentions and plans; the fountain of hypotheses and theories. Incredibly, the mind can even represent, think about, events that have never been directly observed and probably never will be directly observed, only inferred. This brings into focus that mind, according to the functionalist, consists of contents, not merely of mechanics.

In this view, neurobiological theories that relate mind to the firing of neurons will never provide an adequate explanation for how we manipulate abstract symbols in reasoning (Eimas & Galaburda, 1989). Such theories will never be able to come to grips with issues of meaning, how we come to hold precious beliefs, how we rule-govern human behavior over an incredibly diverse set of environmental and social conditions, how we are inventive and creative, and how moods or beliefs influence health. In the final analysis, though, functionalists offer little or no insight into the means whereby thought can influence the body for better or worse.

The Neuroscientist: Mind as a State of Brain

Identity theory, also called brain state theory or eliminative materialism (Eimas & Galaburda, 1989), suggests that mental events do not possess brain states—they *are* brain states. In a most thoughtful analysis of the mind-body problem, Patricia Churchland (1986) attacked the notion that neuroscience cannot deal with logical relations, the functionalist's semantic engine, in terms of causal connections between neural elements. She stated that various disciplines—neuroscience, cognitive science, and psychology—need to work as collaborators, not competitors, to uncover the mystery of how mind-brain events occur.

Churchland also believes that structure-function distinctions are relative not absolute. For example, we may talk about the structure of the brain as a whole, or the structure of a neuron as an individual unit, or the structure of a molecule involved in synaptic transmission. We may talk about the function of the cerebral cortex, the function of a neuron, or the function of a neurotransmitter. Most important, if current research in neural networks is correct, clusters of neurons, or neural modules, may be defined by involvement in a computing function, not by some morphological similarity or proximity—so that distinctions between structure and function become essentially meaningless.

Finally, Churchland suggested that models already under development in the neurosciences show promise of resolving mind-body dilemmas. She gave no credence to the idea of "grandmother" cells, cells that house a memory for a single person or event. She noted, however, that the brain, through the joint activity of its billions of connections, has the capacity to construct complex representations, to manipulate symbols, and to generate and elaborate abstract concepts.

In Pursuit of Closure: The Mind-Body Problem Revisited

Given the history of the mind-body debate, there is little reason to believe that everyone will be satisfied with the solution offered here, which is neither wholly unique nor, in any sense, the final word. Still, I conclude, as others have, that *mind is what brain does*. All operations of the mind—including thinking, remembering, planning, intending, feeling pain, being angry—are operations of the brain in all its extraordinary diversity and complexity. Further,

consciousness is no mysterious or quasi-spiritual mode of existence. It is the operation of self-sensors: the brain's monitoring and thus being aware of its internal functions. This latter notion is admittedly speculative and may be proved wrong, but it is consistent with research showing the brain has a variety of specialized sensor cells. Dennett (1991) came to much the same conclusion, though he couched it in different language. Further, it appears that the brain contains such complex computational networks that self-awareness is not only possible, but a highly likely function.

In support of the first proposition, evidence shows that mind functions deteriorate progressively with progressive damage to brain. Korsakoff's psychosis and Alzheimer's disease are two examples, although many more could be cited. With severe brain damage, mind appears to cease altogether. Without brain, mind ultimately ceases to exist.

Against the charge of reductionism, consider the following. Technology made it possible to measure brain activity at the cellular level. This measurement provided information about how neurons function in changing states and transmitting knowledge of that change[6] to another neuron. This information, however, was and still is mostly useless when it comes to understanding the summative processes of perhaps hundreds of thousands of neurons involved in a single, simple thought. To say, then, that mind is what brain does does not reduce mind to a neuron's firing. The software of the brain is exceedingly complex and permits, indeed probably demands, a variety of higher-order explanatory constructs to represent what occurs when the brain is thinking, planning, or reflecting.

---

[6] We are inclined to say transmitting information, but use of the term *information* often connotes much more complexity than is necessary. The information transmitted is not in the form, or even the sense, of (for example) "John's phone number is 587-9683." It is information only in the sense of "I am active." Propagating that information to another neuron provides the basis only for an adjacent neuron to become "active" or "inactive."

Given that mind is what brain does, the fact that thoughts and feelings can and do alter body states, a fact that has been repeatedly demonstrated empirically (John, 1967; Kiecolt-Glaser et al., 1985), should not be so mystifying. The mind so conceived has many pathways for operating in (not on) the body. The greater mystery is that we are conscious of ourselves, conscious of aches and pains, of tiredness and sickness, of joys and sorrows, of thoughts and intentions. And yet even that mystery may not really be so mysterious.

As evidence for the second proposition, then—that consciousness is the operation of self-sensors—we turn to two pieces of relevant data. First, evidence exists that elements of self-awareness are split off when brain damage occurs. Most to the point is Milner's (1966; Milner, Corkin, & Teuber, 1968) classic case study of H. M., a patient who underwent surgery for intractable seizures and subsequently suffered severe amnesia. H. M. could then solve very complex puzzles while completely unaware of what he was doing or why. This case suggests that consciousness is a function of an intact healthy brain and that it becomes disturbed or fractured, or may disappear entirely, with damage to the brain. The second fact supporting this proposition is that many neurons (or neuron modules or neuron networks) function as sensors for one type of process or another, such as touch, pressure, and pain.

Why should we readily accept the notion of pain sensors and visual edge sensors and then, knowing what we know about the marvelous capacity of the human brain, seldom consider that the brain can sense what it is now thinking? It certainly has enough built in power to do exactly that. Current neurobiology research suggests that the brain may comprise 10^{11} neurons and 10^{15} connections (Eimas & Galaburda, 1989). Self-monitoring would be just what we would expect of an intelligent system. Yet most arguments that treat mind and consciousness as exceptionally mysterious seem to adopt the implicit notion that, where thought is concerned, the brain cannot sense itself at work.

To construct, as an alternative, a model of brain devoid of self-sensors would require a model of human behavior that is essentially machine-like and unconscious to the ultimate degree. Further, such a model would be built on a premise of paradoxical stupidity in so magnificent and accomplished an organ as the brain.

In this view, then, we need not relegate consciousness to the mysterious-spiritual realm, as did one writer who stated that "consciousness will always be one degree above comprehensibility" (Ehrensvard, 1965). Just as mind is what brain does, consciousness is what brain does in monitoring its own activity. Mind acts in body as a consequence of brain activity, activity that does not end with the thought but is part of a dynamic continuous stream. Mind has full rights of passage; it is part and parcel of the same system. That it should have the capacity to alter physical states should seem not the least bit surprising, but wholly and perfectly natural.

On Facts, Theories, Models, and Integrations

Whatever mind-body position it adopted, psychology entered the health arena with vested interest in an explanation that grants an important role to mind. Psychology seized on the critical stance toward medicine taken by psychiatrist Georg Engel (1977). It too condemned medicine's myopic view of disease as nothing more than somatic malfunction and chided medicine's failure to consider the psychosocial context of disease and to promote positive health (Schwartz, 1982; S.E. Taylor, 1986).

In place of biomedical theory, Engel informally proposed the biopsychosocial model (BPS model). According to the BPS model, understanding health and disease must include more than physical (biomedical) explanations for disease. It must also include understanding the patient (psychological factors), the patient's context (social factors), and the health care systems erected to help deal with the disease (social systems). This view had already been endorsed at the 27th World Health Assembly in May 1974 (Lipowski, 1977). Still, the model was little more than a catchword (Kimball, 1986), a slogan that encompassed three major forces operating in a complex systemic health network. Engel (1977) also admitted, "Not all models are scientific" (p. 130). Then, ten years later, Engel (1987) abandoned his own notion and suggested that what was needed was simply better communication between patient and therapist. Still, what he set in motion could not be stopped, and the BPS model continues to provide an integrative view for health psychology.

What does it mean to say that psychology is using the BPS model? What are the requirements, from a scientific stance, of good theory? When proponents say that their model provides a framework to explain complex interactions, what constitutes proper tests of those interactions? These questions—along with refinements, however superficial or incomplete, of the BPS model—will be the focus of the discussion that follows. In the end, we must agree with Churchland (1986) who noted that "it is of course no defense of the truth of a theory that it's the only theory we've got" (p. 386).

The Nature of Theories: Bank Vaults or Road Maps?

Although development in any science requires some period when we make deposits in the information bank (Thomas, 1980), it has seldom suited psychology to just fill intellectual vaults with bare facts. Raw data must also be summarized and integrated, which is one vital function of good theory. Psychology's enterprise, its stated mission, is much like drafting a blueprint to explain connections between the numerous factors that influence human behavior. This map should then enable us to make useful and accurate predictions. If constructed carefully, the map should serve to guide others into unexplored areas. Thus, the map, theory, may serve a **heuristic** purpose—in other words, it may generate activity that fills in missing detail.

Theories are maps of knowledge domains. In the classical sense, a **theory** is an integrated statement, only partly confirmed, that serves to explain a set of events. In spite of the fact that a theory is only partly confirmed, we require a good fit between the data and the propositions that make up the theory. After we test a theory extensively and prove that it is largely without error, the theory may gain most favored status as a law of science. First, however, good theory must meet four essential criteria.

First, *a theory must be testable;* that is, it must be subject to empirical rebuttal or confirmation. If no test of the theory is possible, it is essentially useless.

Second, *theories must adequately account for most relevant data.* A theory of cognitive appraisal, such as Lazarus and Folkman (1984) proposed, should be able to explain how personal evaluations lead to stress, challenge, passivity, or other outcomes. This same theory, however, would have to explain how the immune system responds to prolonged stress. That would be a task for some other theory.

Third, scientists accept the principle of **parsimony.** This principle states that, all other things being equal, *a simple theory is preferable to a complex theory,* although as Einstein said, "I like to keep things as simple as possible, but not simpler" (cited in Ader, Cohen, & Felten, 1987, p. 1). Note the qualifier: "all other things being equal." An example will illustrate. Theorists once accepted a simple mechanistic model of classical conditioning, explaining conditioning largely by frequency of association and contiguity between the unconditional stimulus (UCS) and the conditional stimulus (CS). A number of observations, however, did not fit this notion. As a result, Rescorla and Wagner (1972) developed a cognitive model of conditioning that incorporated expectancies and the probability that the CS predicts the UCS. This model is, without doubt, more complex than the earlier frequency-contiguity theories, but it is also better able to handle more data.

Finally, *a theory should have heuristic value:* that is, it should generate interesting and useful hypotheses about events not previously considered. It should fill in gaps or enlarge the window of our view.

We also talk about theories as educated guesses or intuitive hunches—for example when we say we have a theory about why the car stalled, why a friend betrayed us, or why the stock market crashed. In the technical language of science, though, an educated guess is a **hypothesis,** a tentative answer to the researcher's question. Rosenthal and Rosnow (1991) suggested that theories are large-scale maps, whereas hypotheses are small-scale maps, focusing only on a very small area of detail that the larger map may have omitted.

Theories and Models Compared: Models as Belief Systems

The term *model* has been used in three distinct ways. In one view, modeling is an attempt to build an exact replica of something (Chaplin & Krawiec, 1979). If, in order to better understand the eye, we built a sensory device that worked exactly like the eye, that would be a model.

In the second view, a model is an "as if" statement. It does not concern itself with whether the two things being compared work exactly the same way as long as the copy produces the same result as the original. One model of the brain, for example, suggests that the brain works *as if* it were a computer. Artificial intelligence, exemplified by computers that play chess, has made extensive use of this approach (Chase & Simon, 1973). Yet no one seriously suggests that the computer's solution is exactly the same as the human's.

Third, a model may be viewed as a belief system used to explain puzzling or disturbing natural phenomena. When we refer to Engel's BPS model, it is primarily as a belief system: We have reason to believe that biological, psychological, and social forces interact to influence health. But the propositions that make up the model are only loosely connected. With few exceptions, they are not formally developed or expressed with the precision expected of good theory, which presents a danger. As one writer put it, "A theory has only the alternative of being right or wrong. A model has a third possibility: it may be right, but irrelevant" (Eigen, cited in Mehra, 1973).

Finally, to this point the BPS model has seldom been tested systematically, with the full complement of the three factors that we believe interact (although we will examine one research program that exemplifies how such testing may be done). Sullivan (1990) stated that the model "offers us no common conceptual ground on which these very different types of causes can interact." Further, "its unity exists only at the most superficial level" (p. 272). We cannot say, then, that the BPS approach is rigorous theory or as yet a truly scientific model. We have even less justification for saying that we are going through a paradigm shift (Sheridan & Radmacher, 1992), an unfortunate misuse of Kuhn's (1972) idea.

Testing the model is most often done indirectly: Researchers test narrowly focused hypotheses that fill in pieces of the puzzle. They begin to build small-scale theories to integrate the three domains. Gradually, through a wide range of research tactics, we may gain evidence of the model's usefulness. With this caveat in mind, then, we will consider the BPS model in more detail.

The Need for a New Biomedical Theory

Without a model such as the BPS model, psychology would have little justification for involving itself in the health arena. The model grew out of Engel's (1977) concern for a crisis he perceived in psychiatry and medicine. On the medical side, the crisis involved adherence to a model of disease no longer adequate for either the science or practice of medicine. Medicine gave precious little time, at best only begrudging recognition, to the role of psychosocial influences in disease. Physicians could readily admit that someone survived a life-threatening illness through the force of their indomitable spirit or, conversely, that a patient died from grief. They might reluctantly concede that the patient's belief, not medicine, cured. Confronted with an inexplicable healing that transcended even the most artful surgeon's skills, for example return to life after clinical death, they might even propose that a higher power was behind the patient's recovery. Still, when Engel published his paper, physicians faced considerable pressures to quit the battlefield of theologists and philosophers, to leave the psychosocial morass to others and attend to their true calling—healing the sick by correcting body malfunction.

On the psychiatric side, the crisis had to do with whether emotional disturbance could be conceptualized as disease in the medical sense. The dilemma for psychiatrists was considerable. Either they could treat only emotional disturbances with a known physical etiology (for example, emotional disturbance following brain damage), or they could treat any and all emotional disturbances as long as they admitted that psychiatry was not consistent with and not part of medical theory and practice.

To escape this impasse, Engel argued that every age and every culture has used a wide range of behavioral, psychological, and social criteria to diagnose disease. Western medicine's obsession with somatic deviation as the primary, if not sole, criterion of disease has certainly been practical and beneficial. It has led to enormous gains in medical technology, which in turn has reduced suffering, improved quality of life, and increased longevity. Further, Engel diplomatically argued, every science at one time or another has had to arbitrarily exclude certain variables that time, knowledge, or technology prevented incorporating in efforts to build theories. It should come as no surprise to anyone, then, that medicine excluded psychosocial variables in favor of physical-somatic variables.

To further support his contentions, Engel noted that most health phenomena are inexplicable in the absence of psychosocial constructs. He identified several medical problems that tacitly admit the importance of psychosocial variables, only four of which will be mentioned. First, many medical tests indicate only a *potential* for disease, not the *presence* of disease. Patients often provide test samples with pathogens present, yet they are free of symptoms. Individual differences, including constitutional integrity, psychological moods, and social learning of illness behavior, may codetermine one person's becoming sick while another person stays healthy despite testing positive for pathogens. Second, numerous diseases (colds, for example) respond to life-stressors in terms of onset, severity, duration, and remission. Third, treating somatic symptoms alone does not necessarily restore a person to health. Medical treatments may, in other words, require support from psychosocial therapies. Finally, the psychosocial context of treatment, including the relationship between doctor and patient, can powerfully influence the success of medical treatment. Unfortunately, aside from common sense bolstered by anecdotal evidence, Engel provided no support for his view.

Engel concluded with a note that general systems theory has had great utility in biology, as well as other disciplines. In an almost offhand way, then, he admitted that his model is more commonly known as systems theory. Engel's service was to narrow the focus from all possible systems to the three hierarchically related systems of the BPS model. Unfortunately, systems models are difficult to test because of their enormous complexity and global scale. It may be a matter of evolutionary necessity, then, that several disciplines have spent great time and effort developing independent knowledge foundations in their respective domains. It may be evolutionary coalescence that now, and only now, allows integrative work to begin in earnest. Other systems may yet be added to the equation, but this is an issue for time to judge.

A Systems Trio: Biology, Psychology, and Sociology

Despite Engel's brevity, we can logically amplify the three areas of the BPS model. The *biological* component requires detailed study of no less than three subsystems. First, we must have detailed knowledge of the physical system, which includes predisposing factors, such as genetic and constitutional variability, combined with anatomy and physiology. Second, we must know what precipitates illness; that is, we must understand germs, teratogens, mutagens, and toxins. Finally, we must understand behavioral risk factors that influence health (exercise and nutrition); that increase vulnerability to illness (smoking and drug abuse); or that increase compliance with medical regimens (taking medications for hypertension).

The *psychological* component is also very complex. The person, the psychological system, is the crossroads of biological and social influences. We need to understand how the person, through various behavioral, emotive, and cognitive systems, combines these forces in unique ways. Behavioral processes include all the ways in which the person learns to adapt to changing demands. Emotions are the subjective feelings aroused by environmental transactions. Lazarus (1991b) stated that the study of emotions also requires a systems analysis that reconciles biological universals and sociocultural variations. Cognitive components include, among other things, beliefs about health and illness vulnerability (Janz & Becker, 1984); attributions of causation (Peterson & Seligman, 1987); perceptions of personal efficacy (Bandura, 1989); and perceptions of control (Rotter, 1990; Strickland, 1989).

Further, complex decision processes are involved when people calculate the risk of contracting a disease (such as AIDS) or accept medical advice. The same is true when they decide to accept or reject risky medical treatments with some known chance for success but also some risk of death (Gigerenzer, Hoffrage, & Kleinbölting, 1991). One example is the dilemma faced by parents who must decide whether or not to have a bone marrow transplant for their child with sickle cell disease. The success rate can be as high as 90%, but the death rate can also be as high as 50% (Kodish et al., 1991). How does the parent decide what to do?

Finally, another integrative construct of great interest is **personality:** "the dynamic organization within the individual of those psychophysical systems that determine his characteristic behavior and thought" (Allport, 1961, p. 28). While modest support exists for the notion that personality variables may be related to illness, we still know little about whether and how personality variables can cause body malfunctions. It is more likely that affective tones, such as depression (Friedman & Booth-Kewley, 1987) or anger (Wright, 1988), are related to increased health risks than are specific personality profiles.

The *sociological* component requires study of support networks, including family, schools, church, and other support systems that buffer against stressors. Further, the distribution and delivery of health care services and the relationship between health care personnel and the patient are very important. At a broader level, social policy, tacit or otherwise, that supports or reduces high-risk behavior (for example, cigarette ad campaigns on the one hand, and mandatory seat belt or helmet laws on the other) can have significant health consequences. Finally, social policy can influence national health care goals and priorities.

The Biopsychosocial Model in Psychology: Making Predictions

Probably no one has done more to gain acceptance for the BPS model than Gary Schwartz (1982). He provided a thoughtful extension from systems theory and suggested, as one prediction from the model, that medical diagnosis should *always* consider the interaction of the three

TABLE 3.1   The Patient Evaluation Grid suggests that the three factors contained in the BPS model interact to influence illness (from Leigh & Reiser, 1980).

| | CONTEXTS | | |
DIMENSIONS	CURRENT (CURRENT STATES)	RECENT (RECENT EVENTS AND CHANGES)	BACKGROUND (CULTURE, TRAITS, CONSTITUTION)
Biological	Symptoms	Age	Heredity
	Physical examination	Recent bodily changes	Early nutrition
	Vital signs	Injuries, operations	Constitution
	Status of related organs	Disease	Predisposition
	Medications	Drugs	Early disease
	Disease		
Personal	Chief complaint	Recent illness, occurrence of	Developmental factors
	Mental status	symptoms	Early experience
	Expectations about illness	Personality change	Personality type
	and treatment	Mood, thinking, behavior	Attitude to illness
		Adaptation, defense	
Environmental	Immediate physical and	Recent physical and	Early physical environment
	interpersonal	interpersonal	Cultural and family
	environment	environment	environment
	Supportive figure, next	Life changes	Early relations
	of kin	Family, work, others	Cultural sick role expectation
	Effect of help-seeking	Contact with ill persons	
		Contact with doctor or	
		hospital	

forces both in making the diagnosis and in recommending treatment. This is really more a prescription than a prediction, but Leigh and Reiser (1980) took a step in this direction with their Patient Evaluation Grid (PEG), shown in Table 3.1. Unfortunately, little medical or psychological research has made use of this model in the decade since Schwartz published his article. In fact, Antonovsky (1989) observed that no substantive changes have occurred in medical practice because of the BPS model.

Second, the BPS model predicts that treatments will interact with patients, with other treatments, and with the social context of treatment to produce different outcomes. In other words, a single treatment cannot be expected to produce the same outcome in each and every patient in each and every situation. Research should be able to assess the success of treatments interacting with other treatments and with

different types of patients in terms of morbidity, mortality, and cost-effectiveness, among other things. Psychology in general, and health psychology in particular, should be active in testing hypotheses of this nature. Once again, however, testing has been more indirect than direct.

Testing Interactions: Brain, Behavior, and Immunity

As noted earlier, the customary approach is to test narrow hypotheses or small-scale theories to build support for the model. For our purposes, then, we can look at research that combines the three variables in appropriate fashion, and then judge whether the outcomes confirm or do not confirm the model's belief system. One of the most exemplary current integrative programs is based on the immunocompetence model. This work is carried on by scientists in a new field called psychoneuroimmunology, a discipline dedicated to research on the intricate relations between psychosocial stressors and neural-immunologic systems that govern adaptive biologic response to stress (Jemmott, 1985). We will only sketch the outline of the model here and leave more detail to Chapter 7, which provides a more in-depth view of stress and health.

The immunocompetence model is concerned with causal connections between psychosocial variables such as grief following loss of a loved one and biological variables such as immune efficiency (Jemmott & Locke, 1984). One explicit hypothesis is that psychosocial stressors lower immune system efficiency, which leads to an increase in medical symptoms (either morbidity or mortality). The model suggests that risk for disease, the course of illness, and remission of symptoms may all be related to the interaction of psychosocial factors with the potency of biological threat.

Before we can detail the logic and method of this model, though, we need some elementary knowledge of the immune system itself. The information provided is highly selective and cursory; it is in no sense intended as an extended analysis of this very complex system. Later, I will review early research that provided the first

supporting evidence, and finally, we will preview how stress may alter the immune system itself.

Searching for the Mechanisms of Action: The Immune System

The immune system has one primary function: to help the body resist disease. **Immunity** is the organism's ability to resist or overcome the effects of disease or harmful foreign agents (Memmler & Wood, 1977). We will focus on two forms, humoral immunity and cellular immunity. **Immunocompetence** is the ability of the immune system to protect the body at any given time. The immune system may be highly active and effective or suppressed and less effective. The immune system's effectiveness depends on various factors, including the person's current health status and the potency and duration of an infectious agent. One possible psychosocial source of lower immunocompetence is the presence of severe chronic stress.

The body is vulnerable to a wide range of potentially harmful microorganisms, such as viruses, bacteria, and toxic substances. The surface of invading microorganisms carry proteins that are different from the body's proteins.

PEANUTS reprinted by permission of United Features Syndicate, Inc.

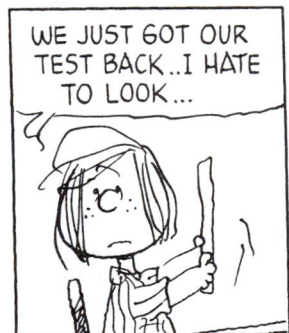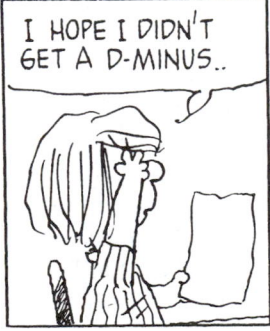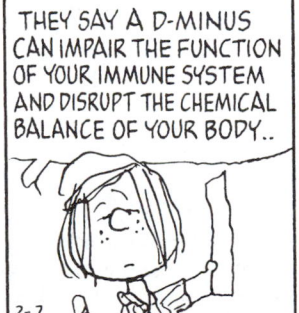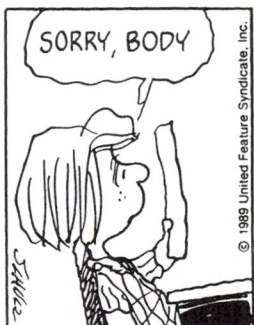

FIGURE 3.4 *Peanuts and psychoneuroimmunology: Even the cartoons are aware of stress and immunocompetence.*

The body recognizes that these proteins, called **antigens,** are foreign. The immune system, then, begins a defense through humoral immunity, a process that involves producing **antibodies** or **immunoglobulins** (Ig) to attack and destroy the antigens it has recognized as "notself" (Jemmott, 1985; Nossal, 1987).[7] The factory for antibodies is in the bone marrow, and the assembly line is in the B-lymphocyte cells (Nossal, 1987), most commonly known simply as **B cells.** The antibodies bind to the antigens, in so doing both neutralizing the antigens and tagging them for destruction. The destruction process is carried out by phagocytes (Johnston, 1988). **Phagocytes**—aptly named from the Greek words *phagein,* to eat, and *kytos,* cells—have one function, to eat the deactivated tagged microorganisms. Another type of cell, called the natural killer cell, is a specialized lymphocyte that recognizes and kills tumor cells and virus-infected cells (Shavit, Lewis, Terman, Gale, & Liebeskind, 1984). Figure 3.5 shows one simple view of interactions within this system.

The thymus gland, the "master organ" of the immune system, produces **T cells,** also called helper cells because of the way they work with B cells. They provide cellular immunity, fight bacterial infections (such as tuberculosis), and combat some viral infections. They also attack cancer cells, fungi, and cells from transplanted organs (Royer & Reinherz, 1987). Both T cells and B cells multiply and undergo structural changes when stimulated by antigens (also called mitogens). Under certain conditions, however, the body may not be able to produce enough B cells or T cells to protect itself. In this event, the body is more vulnerable to disease if exposed to it.

Until recently, scientists regarded the immune system as an autonomous system, operating only to recognize what is self and what is not-self. The immune system's sole purpose was to attack and kill what is not-self. In his review of scientific literature, though, Robert Ader (1983) argued that "the immune system is integrated with other physiological systems and, like all such systems operating in the interests of homeostasis [in other words, biological equilibrium], is sensitive to regulation or modulation by the brain" (p. 251). Ader also provided evidence that conditioning influences immune function and that factors such as life-stress may alter the body's immunocompetence. Rabin and his colleagues summarized a large body of data on bidirectional interactions between the central nervous system and the immune system (Rabin, Cohen, Ganguli, Lysle, & Cunnick, 1989). They concluded that it is no longer in question that the central nervous system can alter immune function; remaining questions are largely technical, addressing the range of influence. This context frames the work on stress, immune competence, and illness.

The Stress-Illness Connection: First Steps to a BPS Model

Beginning with the work of Hans Selye (1956), a vast body of stress research accumulated supporting the notion that stress and disease are connected. Selye suggested that chronic unremitting stressors lead to exhaustion of the organism's adaptive reserve. The term *adaptive reserve* glossed over the remarkably subtle and complex body mechanisms involved in resisting stress, mechanisms that involve interconnections between brain, hormones, and immune system response. Selye argued that given sufficient time, the body wears down and becomes vulnerable to physical insult such as ulcers and even death. These extreme insults would not occur, though, if stressors naturally ceased or the organism used adequate adaptive coping behavior.

---

[7] The body has many immunoglobulins; the most commonly identified are IgA, IgE, IgG, IgM, and IgD (Groër & Shekleton, 1983). IgE is involved in allergic responses (Bochner & Lichtenstein, 1991). IgG is the major blood antibody, and since it can cross the placenta, it provides an infant with any maternally acquired immunity. IgM appears to be the major immunoglobulin produced during infancy, protecting the child until acquired immunities develop.

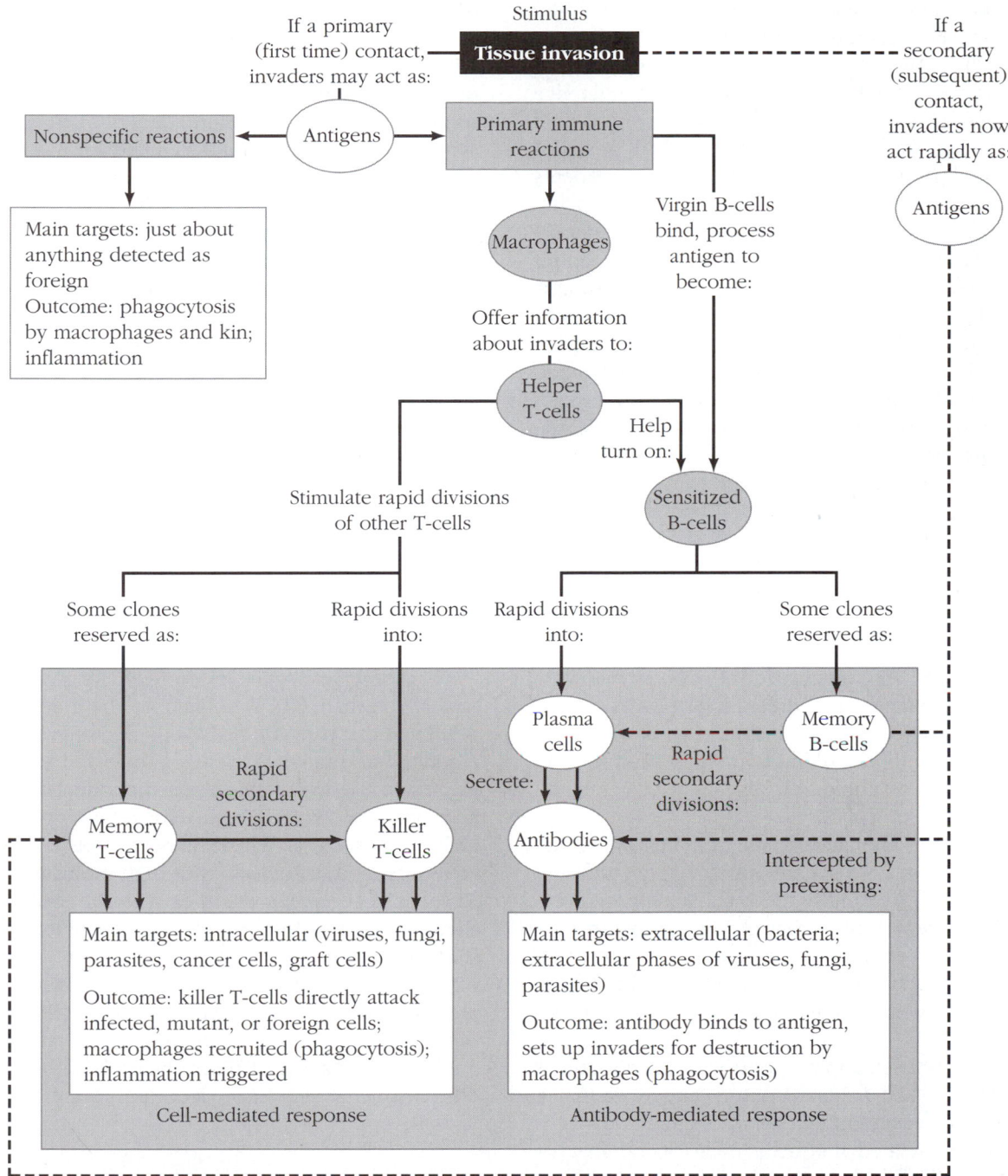

FIGURE 3.5 *Primary and secondary immune pathways involved in the body's defense and immunocompetence (from Starr & Taggart, 1987).*

The threads that connect stress and the immune system were provided at first only by indirect evidence. As one example, Langer and Rodin (1976) wondered whether psychosocial factors in retirement homes might influence health. They noticed that many residents lacked involvement in meaningful activities. Accordingly, Langer and Rodin asked some residents to carry out a chore: simply care for a plant. Months later, gardener residents were generally healthier and had fewer deaths than a control group with no such responsibility. Responsibility is probably a complex variable with both psychological (motivational-emotional-attitudinal) and social (commitment to values beyond the self) components. Still, the simple task of caring for the plant seemed to provide the gardeners with life-sustaining meaning, whereas the absence of meaningful involvement for others may have induced subtle changes detrimental to health.

A classic line of research on life-stress adjustment (Holmes & Rahe, 1967; Dohrenwend & Dohrenwend, 1982) and daily hassles (Kanner, Coyne, Schaefer, & Lazarus, 1981) showed that increased frequency of illness often follows a prolonged period of stress. The stressors encompass numerous social changes (marriage, divorce, and job promotion, for example) and resulting psychological states (such as grief and frustration).

Due to the state of the research art at that time, most of the early work lacked sufficient precision to identify the mechanisms involved. Yet it repeatedly pointed to a probable connection between higher stress and increased morbidity, if not mortality. More refined techniques were needed to continue this line of inquiry.

As one example, Stone and his colleagues (Stone, Cox, Valdimarsdottir, Jandorf, & Neale, 1987) measured the level of one antibody (IgA) and correlated this measure to mood fluctuations. The antibody response was lower (there was less immune resistance) on days when the subject had a strong negative mood. Conversely, on days when the subject had a highly positive mood, the antibody response was stronger (there was more resistance).

Totman and Kiff (1979) inoculated adults with two rhinoviruses, just two culprits among the many that cause the common cold.[8] Then, using a prospective design, they looked for symptoms of upper respiratory infection over a six-month period. A **prospective design** conducts tests or introduces a variable at one time, and then waits until specified later dates to repeat the tests or determine whether the previously introduced variable has caused any change.[9] Totman and Kiff tested their subjects with five life-change scales (including Totman's Loss Index, a measure of gain or loss in social activity, and Totman's Change Index, a measure of absolute change in social activity) plus neuroticism and introversion-extraversion scales. Loss of social activity during the prior three months was the only measure able to predict upper respiratory infection. Absolute activity change during the previous three months, though, was able to predict virus shedding, a measure of the extent of infection as the body gets rid of the rhinovirus.

In another prospective study, Kasl, Evans, and Niederman (1979) looked at the role of academic pressure and achievement motivation among 1400 military cadets. They found a greater incidence of infectious mononucleosis and longer hospitalization in subjects with poor grades, in subjects whose fathers were overachievers, and in subjects with high motivation for a military career. Another research group (Jemmott et al., 1983) studied first-year dental students, also using a prospective design. The psychosocial variables of interest were academic pressure and inhibited power motivation (IPM). They found greater rates of upper respiratory infection after stress in IPM subjects but not in other subjects. Further, Plaut and Friedman

---

[8] About 120 viruses are known to produce colds, so it is clearly impossible to speak of *the* cold virus.

[9] We will examine research designs in more detail in Chapter 6.

(1981) showed that stress increased risk for contracting infectious diseases, allergic reactions, and autoimmune disease in humans.

Animal models of psychosocial factors in disease also proved useful in this quest. Robert Ader (1983) summarized a large amount of relevant data showing that avoidance conditioning, restraint, and manipulation of social interactions could all modify response to or risk for infectious disease. Sklar and Anisman (1980) showed that abrupt changes in social contact increased tumor growth in laboratory mice. This finding is important since it confirms observations of human reactions to stress (Locke, Hurst, Heisel, et al., 1978). Also, Bovbjerg, Cohen, and Ader (1987) found that immune system response to antigens could be altered by Pavlovian conditioning to either enhance or suppress activity. Shavit's research group (Shavit, Lewis, Terman, Gale, & Liebeskind, 1984) found that a stressor such as inescapable shock can suppress natural killer cell activity in rats.

To summarize this section, these studies generally provided support for the notion that psychosocial processes are related to increased risk for illness. Social factors (such as social activity) and psychological factors (such as classical conditioning, mood, or stressors) were all found to be related to increased risk. Most of the diseases under investigation were immune system diseases—in other words, related directly to the operation of the immune system. As much evidence as these studies seemed to provide, they still did not reveal how the psychosocial processes change immune system response. To establish this causal link, more controlled studies were needed.

Stress, Bereavement, and Immunocompetence

One of the most widely talked about issues in immunocompetence is the alleged link between bereavement and immunosuppression. Early work suggested that bereavement was often followed by increased incidence of deaths among the bereaved. According to the immunosuppression hypothesis, though, grief might lead to a change in morbidity but probably not in mortality.

A classic early study was done by Bartrop, Lazarus, Luckhurst, Kiloh, and Penny (1977) on depressed lymphocyte function and bereavement. Bartrop's group studied 26 people ranging in age from 20 to 65 years. Each person had lost his or her spouse to illness or fatal accident in the weeks prior to the study. The control group included 26 hospital staff members who were matched to bereaved subjects on age, sex, and race. Subjects were screened for health history to eliminate those who had recent infections, allergic reactions, or blood disorders. Control subjects were also screened to ensure that no control member had lost a spouse in the prior 24 months.

About two weeks and six weeks after the spouse's death, blood samples were taken to provide evidence on endocrinological and immunological change. As an added level of experimental control, immune response was challenged with varied dosages of both Concanavalin A and P.H.A.[10] Bartrop's team found T cell function, but not B cell function, significantly depressed relative to the control group after challenge by P.H.A. both at two weeks and six weeks. T cell function was significantly depressed only at six weeks in response to Con A. This effect was most pronounced at low doses, suggesting a type of immune system insensitivity that could be reversed only with major antigen assault.

Additional studies provided evidence that psychosocial factors can influence immune system function in a positive fashion. Janice Kiecolt-Glaser's group (Kiecolt-Glaser et al.,

---

[10] Researchers often use mitogens such as Concanavalin A (Con A) and phytohemagglutinin (P.H.A.) experimentally to stimulate T and B cells. Use of such substances gives researchers much better control over exposure (Stein & Miller, 1993).

1985) used social contact and relaxation to intervene with geriatric residents in an independent living center. They found a significant increase in natural killer cells and decrease in antibodies in the relaxation group, but not in the social contact or control groups. They also found enhanced T cell response to P.H.A., with the greatest enhancement occurring at lower doses. These results suggest increased immune system sensitivity in response to types of social intervention, an outcome that contrasts markedly with Bartrop's bereavement results.

In spite of these promising beginnings, research on grief and immune suppression must be viewed with caution. First, many of the studies lacked adequate controls to eliminate alternative hypotheses. For example, few studies controlled for changes in lifestyle that often follow bereavement. Diet, exercise, sleep, and social activities may change drastically for good or ill. Without careful control of these variables, it is difficult to attribute the outcome to grief alone. Second, most grief studies take grief at face value, with no apparent attempt to opera-

tionalize or scale severity. Third, most deaths after bereavement are related to cardiovascular failure, not to immune diseases (Stein & Miller, 1993).

A large scale epidemiologic study questioned the notion that bereavement is linked to higher death rates and provided insights into the complexity of this issue. In this study, Levav, Friedlander, Kark, and Peritz (1988) compared mortality in a group of parents whose sons died in war or in auto accidents. Death rates among the bereaved parents were different from the general population, but in an unexpected direction. Fathers who lost sons in war had *lower mortality rates* than those who lost sons in accidents.

The outcome of this study supports the idea that a psychosocial variable such as grief may influence mortality. Yet, it also sounds a warning about simplistic interpretations of complex processes. Grief does not invariably produce the same result, because it is embedded in a rich web of contextual factors involving the personality of the griever (psychological process) and the social context of the grief. Also note that most of the studies on grief did not answer the important question of the pathway of operation.

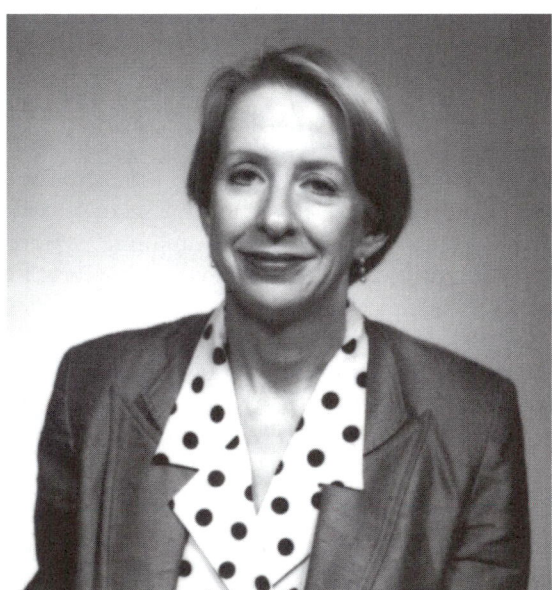

FIGURE 3.6   *Janice Kiecolt-Glaser has conducted extensive research on psychosocial influences on the immune system.*

Stress and the Immune System

Recent research has begun to build a more complete picture of how stress alters immune system efficiency (Baker, 1987; Jemmott & Locke, 1984; Locke, 1982). The brain, hormone, and immune systems are connected in ways far more complex than we can detail here. Some appreciation of this complexity may be gained by considering these few links: Damage to the hypothalamus, the brain's motivation control center, influences the immune response;[11] lymphocytes have surface receptors for hormones and neurotransmitters;[12] and hormones and

---

[11] See Chapter 7 for more detail concerning the hypothalamus.

[12] Neurotransmitters are chemicals that mediate communication among neurons.

neurotransmitters influence the immune system (Stein & Miller, 1993). When the organism encounters a stressor, the brain initiates an arousal response through the hypothalamus-pituitary-adrenal (HPA) complex. This includes the release of adrenocorticotropic hormone (ACTH), which prods the adrenal cortex to action. Shortly after ACTH release, the adrenal cortex secretes several hormones called glucocorticoids. One glucocorticoid, cortisol, works primarily to provide more energy to the body through conversion of body stores into glucose.

There is now evidence that glucocorticoids can suppress mitogen-induced lymphocyte stimulation and also lead to a redistribution of T cells and helper T cells from blood to bone marrow (Stein & Miller, 1993). The net effect is to reduce the number and potency of lymphocytes, at least in response to acute stressors (Dantzer & Kelley, 1989). As a result, the body is less able to resist infections and disease. At one time, immune suppression was the primary, if not sole, model of immune immunocompetence, and the regulatory influence of the glucocorticoids was believed to be the primary pathway. Now it is clear that this view was far too simplistic.

Robert Dantzer and Keith Kelley (1989) believe the immune system's interactions with stressors is just one part of an extensive regulatory system that includes information feedback among the components as well as reciprocal influences. This complex communication network includes brain neurotransmitters, endogenous (naturally occurring) opioids, and hormones (Taylor & Fishman, 1988). Further, since stress can either suppress or enhance immune function, it is important to understand the conditions under which either suppression or facilitation may occur. One organismic trait under study is genetic. Irwin and Livnat (1987) showed that genetic factors influence immune response to stress, making some organisms more vulnerable and others more resilient.

Finally, stressors interact with a dynamic immune system; that is, the immune system's status changes over time, so that the timing of stressors is important (Dantzer & Kelley, 1989). In sum, the results present a major argument for a stress-immune response interaction, and the research suggests that immune function is influenced by an interacting set of biopsychosocial variables.

The Biopsychosocial Model: A Retrospective

We have seen through this intellectual history that the BPS model is not a rigorous theory, but primarily a statement of beliefs about the factors that influence health. The model does not have the precision expected of theory and has not yet generated the type of direct confirming tests that would also be expected of theory. Current research in health psychology may be characterized first as making many deposits to the storehouse of information. Second, numerous small-scale maps—in some cases even larger-scale theories—are emerging to provide evidence in support of the BPS model, particularly in immunocompetence research.

Perhaps the most positive sign is that growing interdisciplinary efforts, in one fashion or another, give tacit support to the model. While tensions over power and authority related to the social conventions of medical practice remain, the evidence of converging efforts is encouraging. There is more collaboration than antagonism, and more interdisciplinary exchange than disciplinary isolation. In the final analysis, we do well to recall Engel's plea that we find a way to integrate the psychosocial context of health without minimizing or discarding the enormous benefits of the biomedical model.

Summary

While biomedical research focused primarily on somatic and environmental (physical) sources of illness, health psychology has begun to examine psychosocial influences on health. There is increasing awareness that several disciplines have important things to say about health, and thus there is growing acceptance that the enterprise is truly interdisciplinary. Use of the biopsychosocial model, then, does not deny the important contributions that biomedical research has made and continues to make. Use of the BPS model also does not usurp causal prerogatives: In other words, it does not assume that psychosocial forces are necessary or sufficient in and of themselves to cause disease. The BPS model suggests only that such things as illness behaviors, risk of disease, severity, duration, and recovery are influenced through an interconnected matrix of forces, an extended system that includes the biological, psychological, and sociological.

In this chapter, we have reviewed the intellectual history of ideas leading up to psychology's current approach to health and illness.

1. The histories of civilization in general and medicine in particular are filled with stories showing a long-standing awareness that mental-emotional processes exert a powerful, even sometimes physically debilitating, influence on the body. This influence is sometimes minimized or discarded on the grounds that the stories are mere folklore, but contemporary research suggests otherwise.

2. Placebos provide some proof that psychosocial influences play an important role in health processes. Even though a growing body of research suggests the final mechanism may be alteration in body process, the fact that it is stimulated by a psychosocial process cannot be ignored.

3. Both the influence of emotions and placebos raise important questions about the mind and its connection with the body. Indeed, the practice of health psychology to some extent depends on the notion that mental processes have a real and substantial influence on body process.

4. The issue of mind-body relations historically is as old as thinking itself. Numerous theories have been proposed that try to explain how mind and body cooperate.

5. Dualistic theories suggest that mind and body exist as separate entities, but the solutions vary concerning how they influence each other. Some dualistic theories even suggest that there is

no causal interaction between the two, which distinguishes these dualist theories from all interactionist theories.

6. Interactionist theories are also dualist theories, but they hold that mind and body interact in some causal fashion. The interaction, though, may or may not be two-way.

7. Descartes is often accused of responsibility for mind-body dualism. Descartes's solution to the issue of mind-body relations was a dualistic interactionism in which the mind and body interact through the pineal gland.

8. John Searle used a commonsense approach to state that mind is the action of the brain. He suggested that the digestion-stomach relationship is similar to the mind-body relationship and that everyday language will one day be as comfortable with the notion of mind as a function of brain as it is with the idea of digestion as a function of stomach.

9. Functionalists in the cognitive sciences usually view the brain as the physical base of mind, but they believe that mind transcends brain. In their view, mind is a semantic engine that works with abstract symbols, attaches meaning, and considers values—activities that cannot be explained by the mere firing of neurons.

10. Neuroscientists such as Patricia Churchland believe the inherent complexity of the brain makes it fully possible for the brain to operate with symbols and values. They believe that mind is what brain does.

11. The biopsychosocial model grew out of concern in psychiatry and medicine for a missing human element in the practice of medicine.

12. A theory is a map of a knowledge domain. It summarizes and integrates information in that domain.

13. A hypothesis is a small-scale map. It is a tentative answer to a research question, or an educated guess about what the correct answer may be.

14. A model is more an "as if" statement, but it may also be simply a set of beliefs. The biopsychosocial model is more like a set of beliefs. It does not have the rigor and formal properties of a theory, and it has not been directly tested.

15. The biopsychosocial model is being evaluated mostly through indirect research tactics. Narrow hypotheses, small-scale theories, or some large-scale theories are providing confirming evidence for the essential correctness of the model.

16. One exemplary approach to testing the model has emerged in immunocompetence research. Immunocompetence research assesses the relationship between psychosocial stressors, alterations in immune system efficiency, and the appearance of symptoms.

Key Words

antibodies	intentionality
antigens	interactionism
B cells	law
biopsychosocial model	model
	monism
causality (mental)	parsimony
compliance	personality
consciousness	pineal gland
cortisol	placebo
dualism	prospective design
heuristic	psychogenic
hypothesis	psychoneuroimmu-
identity theory	nology
immunity	subjectivity
immunocompetence	T cells
immunoglobulin	theory

Study Questions

1. Discuss the significance of the placebo to the notion of illness as a biogenic versus a psychogenic outcome.

2. Compare and contrast the different theories of mind-body interaction.

3. What point of view is taken by the neuroscience group, especially as represented in the work of Patricia Churchland?

4. Define the term *theory,* and discuss what special features distinguish a theory from a model.

5. This chapter suggested that the biopsychosocial model can be tested only indirectly. What does this statement mean? How can the model gain strength if this statement is true?

6. Describe the rationale and procedure of immunocompetence research as a test of the biopsychosocial model.

Class Projects

1. Find current information on placebos and what body processes may be stimulated by placebos. Then discuss the implications of this evidence in terms of competing assertions that (1) healing is a matter of belief; and (2) the role of the body in placebo healing adds strength to the biomedical theory of disease as somatic process.

2. Have a formal debate, with one group taking the cognitive functionalists' position that mind is a semantic engine and one group taking the neuroscientists' position that mind is what the brain does.

3. Discuss the implications of the biopsychosocial model for a multicausal approach to health and illness. Does this approach suggest that people can get sick without the presence of some physical pathogen?

Suggested Reading

Churchland, P. S. (1986). *Neurophilosophy: Toward a unified science of the mind-brain.* Cambridge, MA: MIT Press.

Engel, G. L. (1977). The need for a new medical model: A challenge for biomedicine. *Science, 196,* 129–136.

Jemmott, J. B., III, & Locke, S. E. (1984). Psychosocial factors, immunologic mediation, and human susceptibility to infectious diseases: How much do we know? *Psychological Bulletin, 95,* 78–108.

Nossal, G. J. V. (1987). Immunology: The basic components of the immune system. *The New England Journal of Medicine, 316,* 1320–1325.

White, L., Tursky, B., & Schwartz, G. E. (Eds.). (1985). *Placebo: Theory, research, and mechanisms.* New York: Guilford Press.

WEBSITES   Psychological Theory

ADDRESS	DESCRIPTION
http://www.coil.com/≈grohol/web.htm	Psychology Web Pointer—goldmine starting point for general support and psychology resources
http://cctr.umkc.edu/user/dmartin/psych2.html	CyberPsychLink—very useful for information in psychology and behavioral medicine
http://www.lycaeum.org/drugs/other/brain/	Devoted to epistemology, consciousness, and the mind—links to institutes, newsgroups, journals, and the Neuroscience-Net
http://www.psy.aau.dk/bobby/pni.htm	Resource page for bibliographies, articles, and books on psychoneuroimmunology
http://www.yorku.ca/dept/psych/orgs/apa24/apa24.htm	Division 24 of the APA—Theoretical and Philosophical Psychology

CHAPTER 4

Social Networks: Social-Ecological Theories of Health and Illness

Picture a jungle setting in the highlands of New Guinea. Women and children are sitting around a fire eating meat that looks a lot like brains. This is no ordinary meal. It is a funeral wake after the death of a kinswoman—and the beginning of a grim story of how social custom and illness intertwine. In this chapter, we turn our attention to social forces and illness, the last part of the biopsychosocial equation.

Of Kuru, Keepers of the Priestcraft, and Curanderas

The connection between culture and disease is illustrated by a mysterious disease unknown to modern medicine until the mid-1950s. The disease, *kuru,* was discovered in a single linguistic group, the South Fore in New Guinea (Foster & Anderson, 1978). The name comes from the typical staggering gait and shivering tremor the disease causes (Hudson, 1983). Kuru attacks the nervous system, leading to motor paralysis and death within three months to one year. At first, there were few leads to guide medical investigators, few clues to explain what caused kuru. But there were many theories. Kuru was thought to be genetic, or infectious, possibly immunologic, or nutritional if not behavioral, or perhaps social.

Gradually, pieces of the puzzle fell into place. First, the disease, while almost epidemic among women and children, rarely affected adult males, who lived in marked separation from the women and children. Second, women practiced ritual cannibalism following the death of a kinswoman. They ate the deceased's half-cooked body, notably the brain tissue. The men did not share in this practice.

In 1959, an epidemiologist noted that kuru showed striking similarity to a sheep disease called scrapie. This disease, caused by a virus infection, requires a very long incubation period, possibly as long as a year. In laboratory studies, chimpanzees were inoculated with brain tissue taken from South Fore kuru victims. The chimpanzees also died of the disease after a long incubation period.

Another research team learned that kuru had first appeared about 1910, nearly the same time the cannibalistic practice was adopted by the South Fore. The explanation then was clear. When the women ate the half-cooked brain tissue of a kuru victim, they unwittingly acquired the kuru virus. The men, who did not practice ritual cannibalism and who lived apart from the women and children, were protected from the disease—an example of social custom's having a reverse quarantine effect that protected the healthy.

Under government pressure, the South Fore abandoned this ritual in the 1960s. Kuru went into a dramatic decline, even though its origin had never been fully explained. Kuru provides an example of how social factors interact with physical agents to influence the emergence of disease. The history of the disease also shows how social policy (government pacification and intervention) may control a disease even when its cause is imperfectly known.

The Way of Curanderas: Of Green Medicine and Vision Quests

Long before contemporary society began training and licensing doctors, long before hospitals and laser surgery, people had their own commonsense theories of illness. They also had very special folk healers. These healers, sometimes called medicine men and women,[1] are marked by special traits that may be evident at birth or seen in an elder's dreams.

In Hispanic communities, a special group of women healers, *las curanderas,* minister to the needs of the sick. In one Native American group, the healers are called the keepers of the priestcraft (Perrone, Stockel, & Krueger, 1989). They are trained by the older healers and in due course become the repository of the culture's medical wisdom and skill. In the end, though, no medical association says they can be doctors; societal custom provides the sole recognition needed for their practice.

Their tools include **green medicine,** pharmaceuticals not obtained from Upjohn, but from roots and herbs native to their region. They know their drugs have curative power from having seen them work over many years. Now, nearly 200 indigenous drugs attributed to Native Americans are part of the U.S. pharmacopoeia. Their procedures bear little resemblance to the sanitized practices carried out in modern hospitals. Healing is more often part of a ceremony carried out in the patient's home.

The ritual might include family and friends in communal prayer, invoke friendly spirits to assist the ill, or try to drive off unfriendly spirits. The ceremony might involve a touch that transmits healing energy, massage (acupressure) to correct bone alignment, or pricking with bone needles (acupuncture) to restore tonal balance. The noted anthropologist Margaret Mead used a Chilean *curandera* to recite prayers and massage her diseased body during the last four years of her struggle with cancer. This fact was not widely known, apparently because the family tried to suppress public knowledge of it (Scheper-Hughes, 1990). That they should have

---

[1] Dhyani Ywahoo (in Perrone et al., 1989) observed that the terms *medicine men* and *medicine women* are anthropologists' terms to try to make the Native American tradition somehow more compatible with Euro-American medical tradition.

TABLE 4.1   *Use of unconventional therapy for the ten most frequently reported principal medical conditions (from Eisenberg et al., 1993).*

CONDITION	PERCENT	USED UNCONVENTIONAL THERAPY	SAW PROVIDERS OF UNCONVENTIONAL THERAPY	THERAPIES MOST COMMONLY USED
Back problems	20	36	19	Chiropractic, massage
Allergies	16	9	3	Spiritual healing, lifestyle diet
Arthritis	16	18	7	Chiropractic, relaxation techniques
Insomnia	14	20	4	Relaxation techniques, imagery
Sprains or strains	13	22	10	Massage, relaxation techniques
Headache	13	27	6	Relaxation techniques, chiropractic
High blood pressure	11	11	3	Relaxation techniques, homeopathy
Digestive problems	10	13	4	Relaxation techniques, megavitamins
Anxiety	10	28	6	Relaxation techniques, imagery
Depression	8	20	7	Relaxation techniques, self-help groups
10 most common conditions	73	25	10	Relaxation techniques, chiropractic, massage

done so may be both a product of the time and the person that Margaret Mead was.

Now, public use of unconventional medicine occurs at a much higher rate than previously believed, as Table 4.1 shows. In one study, 34% of the sample used unconventional therapies for such disorders as cancer, arthritis, chronic back pain, and AIDS, among others (Eisenberg et al., 1993). Just as it did years ago, the accuracy of these healers' diagnoses and cures often amazes the most cynical medical practitioners.[2]

These healers' practice is always consistent with their beliefs about health and sickness.

Their views are holistic: Spirit, mind, and body are one; humans, animals, and nature must live in harmony; healing is equally religious, psychological, and physical. Healers must believe as strongly in God and their ability to heal as they do in the medicine itself. The sufferer must believe just as strongly.

On Common Themes: Causes, Theories, and Agencies

These brief excursions into culturally different medical systems highlight three points about the sociocultural context of health and illness. First, society's values and behavior patterns may influence the appearance and distribution of disease. In the case of kuru, the value attached

---

[2] Of course, contemporary medical practitioners are also often quick to point out that some folk healers bypass proven methods and produce disastrous results for their clients.

to the cannibalistic grieving ritual cost many lives. Local groups that did not follow this custom were untouched by kuru. The presence of a germ may be necessary but not sufficient for the appearance of an illness.

In addition to differences between cultures, differences within cultures may influence the distribution of illness. These include ethnic group differences, socioeconomic status (SES), occupational risks, and traits such as age, sex, and gender. Social roles (gender) assigned to South Fore men, for example, isolated them from exposure to the virus that killed so many of the women and children.

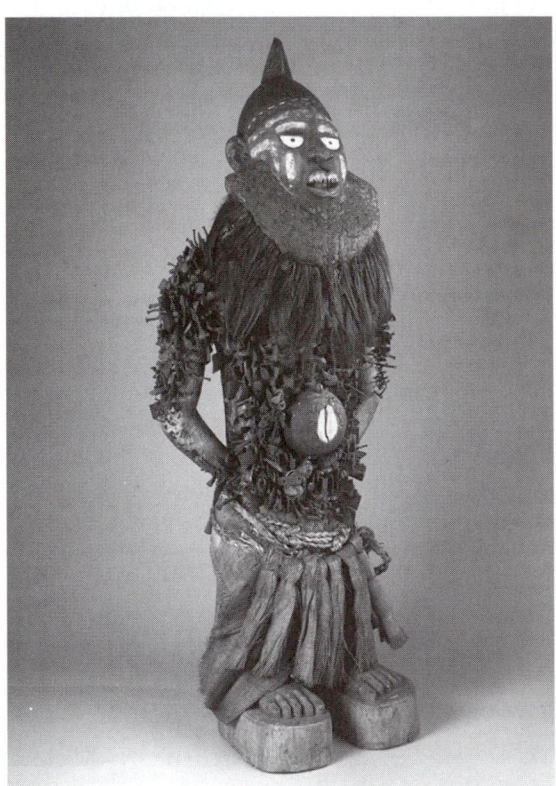

FIGURE 4.1   *Bakongo nail fetish used in the Congo for either aggressive or protective magic, as directed by a witch doctor; a nail is driven into the figure each time its powers are called on (Field Museum of Natural History, Chicago).*

Second, in every age society has sought a way to come to grips with illness through explanatory systems. Society attaches meaning by trying to explain the origins of illness. The corollary hope is that understanding the disease may enable society to control disease's harmful effects. Whether we dub these explanatory systems theories, beliefs, or myths—whether they evolve through deliberate science or informal pragmatic empiricism—they are a vital part of the sociocultural context of healing. Pelligrino (1963) noted: "Medicine is an exquisitely sensitive indicator of the dominant cultural characteristics of any era, for man's [sic] behavior before the threats and realities of illness is necessarily rooted in the conception he has constructed of himself and his universe" (cited in Foster & Anderson, 1978).

Finally, society formalizes treatment rituals in one way or another by according privileges to health-care providers who meet established criteria, sanctioning illicit attempts to cure, and establishing the means to transmit its medical wisdom and lore to the next generation of healers. In a broad sense, society also carries out educational activities to convince group members that the assumptions of its medical system are accurate. These formalized rules, then, exert a type of quality control over the practice of medicine. They also establish, implicitly or explicitly, social policy and goals for the group.

Cross-Cultural Sleuths: From Anthropology to Sociology

Over the past century, three groups have emerged that share an active interest in sociocultural variables affecting health and illness: medical sociologists, medical anthropologists, and medical epidemiologists. Medical sociologists are interested in how people define themselves as sick and the behaviors and emotions they display when sick. Medical sociologists study social customs that define people's responses to illness and sick people's access to medical services, as well as how social structure in medical settings affects the quality of health care. Medical sociologists also are concerned with issues of health education, especially how a large group may be persuaded to adopt new positive health habits or health services. When the primary focus is research and theory development, the custom is to use the term **sociology of medicine.** When the focus is on how sociological knowledge may be used to improve health and manage disease, the custom is to use the term **sociology in medicine.**

Medical anthropologists study such things as human evolution, anatomical variations and change, and what I choose to call **cultural pediatrics**—cross-cultural variations in treatment of children and their diseases. Medical anthropologists study cultural variations in the formation of medical policy, the evolution of medical bureaucracies, and differences in medical training. In each instance, anthropologists seek clues to the appearance of disease, the severity or duration of disease, the use of medical services and technology, or variations in doctor-patient relations that impact treatment and recovery (Foster & Anderson, 1978). Anthropologists also divide their attention between research—called anthropology of medicine, and application—called anthropology in medicine (Scheper-Hughes, 1990). Earlier when I spoke of the keepers of the priestcraft and the *curanderas,* we were technically in the arena of **ethnomedicine,** a branch of anthropology concerned with indigenous health beliefs and practices.

Medical epidemiologists are interested in the occurrence of disease by time, place, and person (Lilienfeld & Lilienfeld, 1980). They look for patterns in the distribution of disease that may offer clues to **etiology,** the origins or causes of a disease. Medical sociologists and anthropologists may define their research in such a way that it is the same as medical epidemiology. This research method will be described in more detail in Chapter 6.

Here, we are concerned with three major issues. First, epidemiology: How are sociocultural factors related to the appearance and distribution of disease? Second, social explanatory systems: What theoretical models explain health and illness from a social perspective? Third, health care systems: How does society govern its medical services and health care providers, and how does it formulate goals for its members?

Medical Epidemiology: Of Gender, Race, and Work

At a much too tender age, Karen Carpenter died suddenly from a heart attack. Later, her family revealed that she had been a victim of a condition called anorexia nervosa. Nearly 90% of anorexia nervosa cases are women (American Psychiatric Association, 1994). Is this difference due to biology, or is it fallout from the way we socialize women into a particular role? Why do women live on average seven years longer than men (Kaplan, Anderson, & Wingard, 1991)? Several cultural groups, both primitive and industrialized, have healthier diets than residents of Great Britain and the United States. What special benefits or risks do different eating habits confer? What happens to people who change their diets to the rich foods of affluent societies? What occupational health risks do workers face? These are some of the questions that connect sociocultural variables to possible health outcomes. Here we will review a select few findings that bear on these concerns.

Sex and Gender: On Morbidity and Mortality

Men should marry women who are on average four to seven years older. Women pay lower auto insurance premiums. Implicit in these and other facts and pieces of folk wisdom is the assumption that men and women differ in health, longevity, and risk-taking. Now researchers have taken up these issues, comparing differences in both mortality and morbidity. The

TABLE 4.2   Death rates by age, sex, and race: 1988 preliminary census data (number of deaths per 100,000 population; data from U.S. Bureau of the Census, Statistical Abstract of the Unites States: 1990).

AGE	WHITE MALES	WHITE FEMALES	BLACK MALES	BLACK FEMALES	COMBINED M/F RATIO
–1	938	693	2197	1860	1.22
1–4	52	43	83	49	1.46
5–14	29	19	39	38	1.19
15–24	144	52	214	74	2.84
25–34	170	61	405	143	2.81
35–44	255	123	704	287	2.33
45–54	573	314	1294	596	2.05
55–64	1557	866	2416	1399	1.75
65–74	3534	1993	4527	2887	1.65
75–84	8235	5145	9360	5998	1.57
85–	18934	14728	15343	12260	1.27

amount of research on this topic alone justified several recent reviews, notably those by Lois Verbrugge (1986) and Judith Rodin and Jeannette Ickovics (1990). The journal *Health Psychology* (1991) devoted an entire issue to the topic of gender and health.

This work confirms that girls and women have fewer deaths and longer life expectancy at every age across the life span compared to boys and men (Strickland, 1988). The estimated life expectancy in 1990 was 72.1 for males and 79.0 for females (U.S. Bureau of the Census, 1991). Recent statistics from the U.S. National Center for Health Statistics, summarized in Table 4.2, show this effect is most pronounced between the ages of 15 and 34, when nearly 300 males die for every 100 females. These differences come largely through deaths due to accidents, homicide, suicide, and chronic obstructive pulmonary disease (Wingard & Cohn, 1990).

When we consider morbidity data, however, a different picture emerges. Women suffer a higher rate of morbidity although their symptoms are typically less serious than men's. In practice, this means women have more acute disabling symptoms that disrupt their comfort, life style, and work. Each year women restrict their activities for health reasons about 25% more than men, and they spend about 40% more

days in bed than men (Verbrugge, 1985). Several morbidity measures are shown in Table 4.3. Women also obtain and use a larger percentage of prescriptions than men.

Although morbidity differences are largest during childbearing years, a significant difference in morbidity still remains when maternity symptoms are removed. A new quality of life model estimates an index called **well-life expectancy,** a measure that combines mortality and morbidity statistics. Even with the combined statistic, women show an advantage of nearly three well-life years compared to men (Kaplan et al., 1991).

To understand differences in morbidity and mortality between males and females, we must separate health problems that are sex-linked from those that are gender-linked. **Sex-linked disorders** result from the specific biological variations between men and women. Certain health problems are unique to women, such as dysmenorrhea and breast cancer, and thus may be viewed primarily as biological variations in illness.

Gender-linked disorders are ailments caused by socialization processes that put men and women in different roles with different expectations. Verbrugge (1985) argued that differences in mortality and morbidity are "the

TABLE 4.3   *Morbidity indicators by sex and sex ratios in the United States in 1987 (from Rodin & Ickovics, 1990).*

INDICATOR	FEMALES	MALES	SEX RATIO
Restricted activity day			
Total days of disability (millions)	1984	1464	1.35
Days/person	16.1	12.7	1.28
Bed disability days			
Total days of disability (millions)	879	595	1.48
Days/person	7.1	5.2	1.36
Work loss days			
Total (millions)	304	299	1.02
Days/person	6.1	4.8	1.27
Hospital utilization rates			
Patients discharged per 1,000 persons	159	116	1.37
Days of care per 1,000 persons	968	860	1.20
Average stay (days)	6.1	6.9	0.88
Physician visits			
Total (millions)	765	523	1.46
Visits/person	6.2	4.5	1.38

outcome of differential risks acquired from roles, stress, life styles, and preventive health practices" (p. 156). Gender-linked disorders may affect both sexes but tend to affect one group more than the other (Rodin & Ickovics, 1990). Ailments in this category include eating disorders, rheumatoid arthritis, osteoporosis, and lupus.

Several theoretical models emphasize biological variations, as occur in sex-linked disorders. In this view, differences in morbidity and mortality result from a selective advantage that women have because of genetic codes, structural differences, biochemical differences, or some combination of these factors. In regard to genetic differences, women may have an advantage because of their double X chromosome. Men have the XY code which contains little

additional information beyond that needed for the male reproductive system (Travis, 1988). Biochemical theories focus on several body processes, for example differences in estrogen and testosterone. Estrogen appears to provide women some advantage in cardiovascular processes by keeping HDLs (the good lipoproteins) high relative to LDLs (the bad lipoproteins). Even here, more than biology may be at work, since women who smoke and take oral contraceptives do not seem to share the estrogen advantage. These women are at increased risk of coronary heart disease, peripheral vascular disease, and stroke (Matthews, 1989).

Other theoretical models emphasize the psychosocial factors that influence gender-linked morbidity and mortality. These theories usually focus on such variables as behavioral risk-taking, environmental hazards, work environments, job stressors, and role strains, among other things. Examples that support this argument are readily available, including the cultural obsession with slimness and multiple roles at home and work.

First, undue pressure on women to be slim puts them at increased risk for nutritional and dietary disorders (Rolls, Fedoroff, & Guthrie, 1991). Women use more than 90% of weight-loss pills, increasing women's risks for negative side effects up to and including death (Rodin & Ickovics, 1990). This differential use, perhaps even abuse, of diet pills is already evident among high school females (Gritz & Crane, 1991). Conversely, men tend to be less concerned about nutritional standards and diet risks. Yet men tend to engage more frequently in dangerous behaviors, especially high-risk sporting activities, and drinking and driving (Verbrugge, 1985; Lex, 1991).

The second example concerns multiple roles. People with multiple roles, regardless of sex, tend to have better overall health (Verbrugge, 1986). Specifically, employed, married parents tend to enjoy the best health while unmarried and unemployed people tend to have more health problems (Umberson, 1987). Marital status as a predictor of health, though, is strongest for men and weak or nonexistent for women, a fact that may be related to social support networks. Irregular hours, heavy time constraints, high family dependency (preschool children, chronic illness in a family member, or elderly dependents) contribute to poorer health. In dual-career homes, women may suffer more only when traditional values lead to a disproportionate load on the woman. In egalitarian dual-career homes—that is when the household chores are more evenly divided and support exists for the woman's career—there is little objective difference in health between women who work outside and those who work in the home (Barnett, Davidson, & Marshall, 1991). Verbrugge (1986) concluded that when roles are similar, health is similar.

Rodin and Ickovics (1990) noted recent epidemiological trends supporting the notion that lifestyle may be behind some advantages women enjoy. Women made a significant move into the work force after World War II. Now, close to 40% of married women work outside the home, and no more than 11% of families are composed of the traditional working father and mother at home with children (Zedeck & Mosier, 1990). If multiple roles and life satisfaction are important to good health as some suggest, then women who work outside the home should have better health than those who do not; and as noted earlier, they do. Further, women locked into powerless, mundane, and dead-end jobs suffer poorer health compared to women who are in positions of higher status and power.

Evidence suggests that health differences between men and women may be related to social support (Cohen, 1988; Cohen & Syme, 1985; Cohen & Wills, 1985). Men tend to have more extended social support networks than women, but women have more intimate and intensive supports than men (Shumaker & Hill, 1991). The man's intimate and intensive support system is most frequently his spouse, which may explain why unmarried men fare much worse than unmarried women. Further, during crises, women are more likely and men are less likely to use their support systems.

Women in the Health Care System: Labeling and Treatment

Another level of social analyses focuses on sex differences in labeling of symptoms and differences in health care. Women tend to respond more actively to symptoms and seek care early. Men tend to ignore symptoms longer and are more reluctant to seek care. This difference may be related again to differences in socialization: It is acceptable for women to report discomfort, but men are supposed to endure suffering in silence. Still, the fact that women customarily obtain earlier care for health problems undoubtedly has a positive effect in reducing the risk of serious illness in the future.

In spite of the ease of reporting and early treatment, women may receive lower quality treatment in the health care system. It appears that women tend to receive more psychologically loaded diagnoses, perhaps an unfortunate carryover of the sex bias found in psychoanalytic theory (Hare-Mustin, 1983). Women are given more prescriptions and, up to a point, are put through more unnecessary diagnostic services compared to men (Verbrugge, 1985), in what is called physician sex bias. A recent study also showed that women are not as likely to receive the same quality of medical service for coronary accidents as men (Ayanian & Epstein, 1991; Steingart et al., 1991). Problems in this area, and the underrepresentation of women in clinical trials in general, led the Board on Health Sciences Policy (Institute of Medicine) to begin formulating a policy that may guide researchers on the inclusion of population subgroups in research (Bennett, 1993). In 1994, the National Institutes of Health (NIH) issued rules on inclusion of women and minority groups in clinical trials (Burd, 1994).

As one example of this bias, consider the sex differences in treatment for coronary artery disease (CAD).[3] CAD is the leading cause of death among women as well as among men,

---

[3] See Chapter 12 for an extended discussion of heart health.

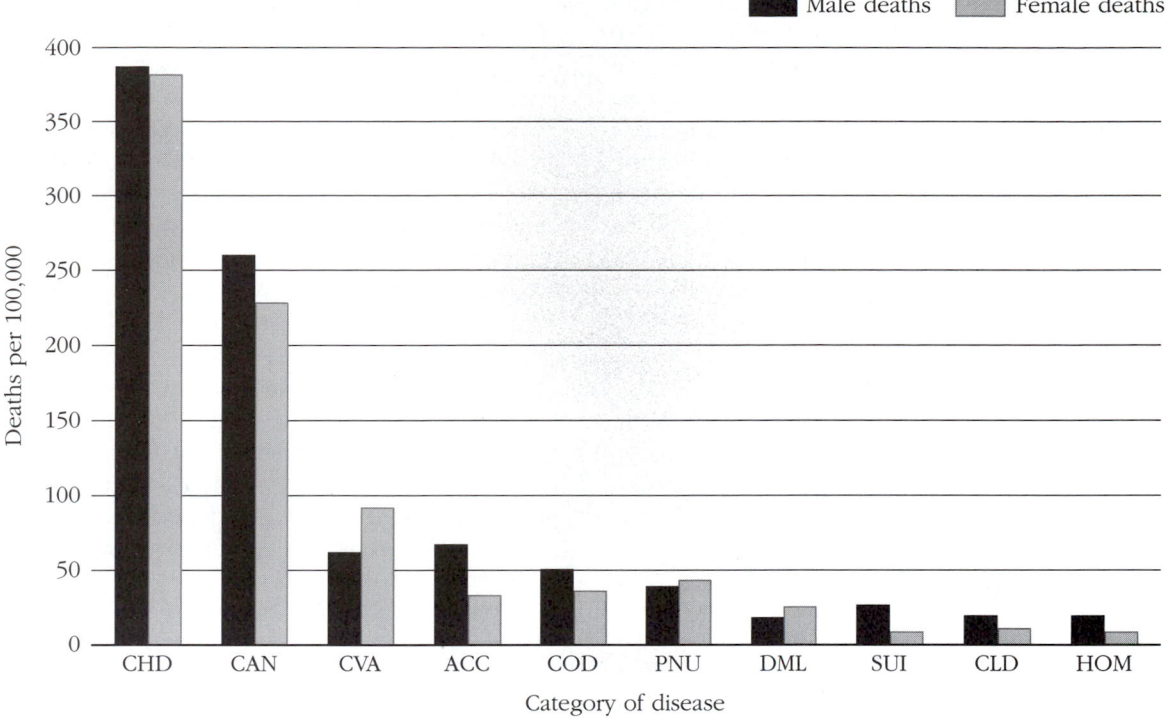

FIGURE 4.2   *The ten leading causes of death listed by sex (data from 1991 U.S. Bureau of Census Statistics).*

killing nearly 500,000 women each year. Yet physicians pursue a less aggressive approach to managing the disease in women. Following reported chest pains, fewer women are referred for more sophisticated diagnostic and surgical procedures, such as catheterization and coronary bypass surgery. This occurs in spite of the fact that, in Steingart's sample, the angina symptoms reported by women were more severe and disabling than the men's symptoms. Another disturbing piece of information came from this study: the efficacy of many diagnostic and surgical procedures is tested most extensively in and for men. Thus the efficacy for women is not well-known.

One healthy sign of change in this area is the recently launched Women's Health Initiative, under the auspices of the NIH (Kirschstein, 1993; Matthews et al., 1997). The largest clinical trial ever attempted in the United States, it will involve 45 clinical centers across the country, enrolling more than 160,000 postmenopausal women in a study that will take nearly 15 years to complete. The focus of the study will be on the determinants, and ultimately the prevention, of disability and death in older women. Specifically, the WHI will look at both breast and colorectal cancer, osteoporosis, and coronary heart disease. Additional issues addressed will be the value of hormone replacement therapy, dietary habits, and the value of vitamin supplements in preventing health problems in women.[4]

Epidemiological and biomedical research must break the bounds of convenience, perhaps

---

[4] Note, though, that criticisms emerged almost immediately, contending that the study's purpose was being subverted by too narrow a focus on the issue of cancer at the expense of other issues, especially coronary heart disease (Shaffer, 1993).

even funding politics, to ensure that women and minorities are represented. Biases such as those reflected in research (disproportionate use of male subjects), diagnoses (more psychological diagnoses for women), and patient management (less aggressive treatment of women's coronary disease) have actual and potential negative outcomes that reflect poorly on the medical establishment and social policy.

Race and Disease: On Coronary, Tay-Sachs, and Hypertension

On the high plateaus of the Sierra Madre Mountains, in a small region of northwestern Mexico, live a group of Indians called the

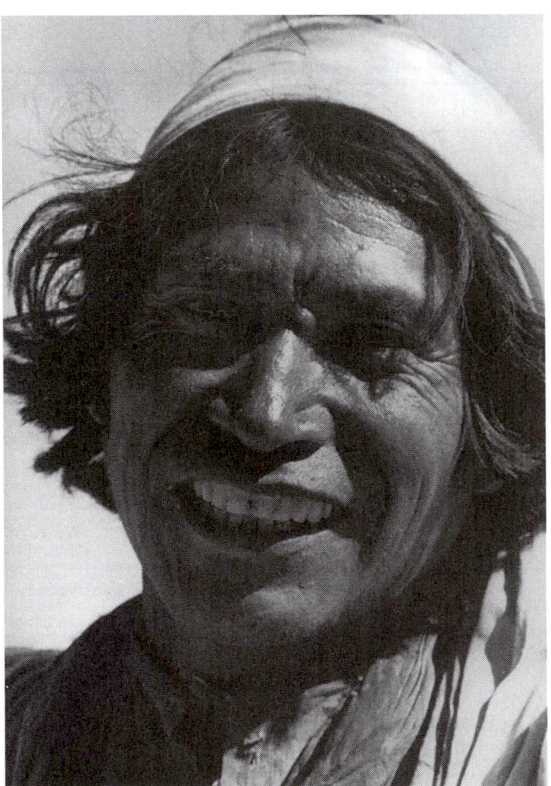

FIGURE 4.3   *The Tarahumara, from Mexico, are known for their running and low incidence of coronary disease.*

Tarahumara ("foot runners"), whose prowess in running is legendary (Fontana & Schaefer, 1979). The Tarahumara are best known in medical circles because of their very low risk for coronary heart disease. Their diet, typically composed of low-fat and high-fiber foods, has long included corn and beans, fruits and vegetables, and small amounts of game, fish, and eggs.

Now, however, industrialization and globalization of the economy may have brought hidden, potentially disastrous results to the Tarahumara as well as other groups. The unhealthy nutritional habits of affluent societies—with rich, tasty foods in liberal quantities—can be overwhelming in their allure. The facts are alarming: Switching the Tarahumara from a bland and limited diet to a rich and plentiful diet can quickly produce major changes in medical indices of coronary risk.

This conclusion comes from study of a small group of Tarahumara volunteers (McMurry, Cerqueira, Connor, & Connor, 1991). McMurry's team observed 13 women and men for a period of one week while on their traditional diet. This allowed the study team to establish baselines of cholesterol concentration. Then they asked the group to eat an "affluent" diet. For the next five weeks, the Tarahumara group ate meals comparable to those consumed by people in societies with abundant rich foods. Comparisons between the Tarahumara and the affluent diets are shown in Table 4.4. During both the baseline diet and the affluent diet, volunteers provided two blood samples each week. The research team also monitored activity levels and noted that the subjects did not alter their running activity during the study period.

The results were clear: Cholesterol levels increased from 121 mg to 159 mg during the study period. Almost 75% of that increase came after only four days on the affluent diet, and the balance came in the next three days. Triglycerides increased significantly, as did both LDLs (39%) and HDLs (31%). Even though LDLs and HDLs went up, they both went up about the same amount so the ratio did not change

TABLE 4.4   *Composition of diets during each study period among 13 Tarahumara Indians (from McMurry et al., 1991).*

	TARAHUMARA DIET		AFFLUENT DIET	
	CALORIES	% TOTAL	CALORIES	% TOTAL
Energy (kcal)	2700		4100	
Protein (g)	101	15	101	10
Total fat (g)	61	20	198.2	43
Monounsaturated	28.6	10	84.7	19
Polyunsaturated	12.8	4	16.5	4
Saturated	19.5	7	97.0	21
Carbohydrates (g)	438	65	479	47
Complex	419	62	314	31
Simple	19	3	165	16
Dietary fiber	102		33	
Soluble fiber	49		13	
Cholesterol (mg)	Trace		1020	
Cholesterol-saturated fat index	20		149	

significantly. The Tarahumara continued their physical (running) activity even as they indulged in the affluent diet. That the ratio of LDLs to HDLs did not change, then, may be due in part to this important aspect of lifestyle. Finally, as one might expect from the nature of the diet, all subjects gained weight, approximately two pounds each week. While this study has much to teach us, we must be cautious about generalizing from a six-week diet to diets that may last for years.

Ethnic groups may also have genetic differences that place one ethnic group at increased risk compared to others. We noted in Chapter 2 one such illness, sickle-cell anemia, a blood pathology that afflicts blacks in greater proportion than other ethnic groups. **Tay-Sachs disease,** or infantile amaurotic idiocy, is an error in lipid metabolism caused by an autosomal recessive gene. This disease afflicts Ashkenazi Jews more often than other groups: About 1 in 3,600 of these children will be affected compared to 1 in 360,000 in the general population (Gelehrter & Collins, 1990).

An infant with Tay-Sachs appears perfectly normal at first. But then vision deteriorates

(nystagmus), normal mental functions fail to develop (retardation), and the body deteriorates as well. There is no known treatment, and death usually occurs between two to four years of age. Although prevalence among the Ashkenazi Jews is not great, that the disease occurs as often as it does suggests the importance of premarital counseling and genetic screening, and led Congress in 1976 to enact a law (PL94-278) to control genetic diseases including sickle cell anemia and Tay-Sachs (Office of Technology Assessment, 1990). Tay-Sachs carriers can be identified by an inexpensive blood test. In the fetus, Tay-Sachs can be detected using amniocentesis at about the fourth month of gestation. Tay-Sachs thus presents a situation in which public information and use of services can influence the actual appearance of the disorder. Because of such screening, the disease has been virtually eliminated in this high-risk group during the last 20 years (Gelehrter & Collins, 1990).

Biomedical research has invested enormous effort and money to understand and treat cardiovascular disease. As sophisticated as much of the research is, much has been left unexplained (Saad et al., 1991). For example, many questions remain unanswered about the greater prevalence of hypertension among blacks. Some believe that we must look to social structure and cultural customs for additional pieces of the puzzle (Rostand, 1989). Hypertension among blacks is related to a variety of social ills, including income, work, and access to health care, combined with nutrition standards and cooking customs. Among rural blacks, there is a tendency to cook food for long periods of time (Heyden, 1981). The effect is that potassium salts are pulled from the food cells into the water, which is subsequently thrown out. As a result, blacks in three states (Georgia, Louisiana, and Mississippi) and Washington, D.C., may consume 50% less potassium than whites in the same areas. Low potassium intake is a risk factor for hypertension, and if combined with high sodium intake, can increase risk for hypertension dramatically.

Work and Disease: Of Toxins, Stress, and Sick Buildings

Unless we specifically work in a job known for high risks, such as handling radioactive materials, we probably do not think much about connections between work and illness. But an emerging medical field called occupational medicine devotes substantial time to the issue (Frank, 1990). One case study illustrates the insidious forces that may operate in certain jobs.

A 50-year-old mortician had suffered loss of sexual drive, reduced testicular size, and marked breast growth (Finkelstein, McCully, MacLaughlin, Godine, & Crowley, 1988). He had seven children by his first wife but he had divorced and was now remarried. In the process of embalming, he applied base creams and pigments to corpses, their last makeup in this world. Although the supplier suggested that gloves should be worn while handling the cream, he had never done so. Still, nothing in the ingredients caused any suspicion. The medical group in charge of his treatment conducted a number of

tests and found that an organic compound from the cream acted as an estrogen. The compound caused an excess estrogen reaction in his system. Estrogen, a female hormone, had the expected biologic effects—effects opposite to those of the male hormone testosterone.

In contrast to this unusual case, we are probably more familiar with highly publicized dangers in the work place. A variety of manufacturing methods create unsafe work environments as well as spillover that endangers health and habitat. The National Institute for Occupational Safety and Health (NIOSH) lists the ten leading work-related diseases or injuries as follows (Levi, 1990):

1. occupational lung diseases
2. musculoskeletal injuries
3. occupational cancers
4. severe occupational traumatic injuries
5. cardiovascular disease
6. disorders of reproduction
7. neurotoxic disorders
8. noise-induced loss of hearing
9. dermatologic conditions
10. psychological disorders

About 270,000 workers in the U.S. are exposed to a gas, ethylene oxide, commonly used to sterilize medical supplies. Although these workers do not show greater mortality rates overall compared to the general population, men have a slightly increased risk for cancer and death after exposure, a risk that increases as exposure time and latency increase (Steenland et al., 1991). Low sperm counts occur in men working with pesticides. Women in certain jobs become infertile and suffer spontaneous miscarriages, and their infants more often have birth defects. The jobs likely to produce reproductive problems typically involve exposure to anesthetic gases, lead, mercury, irradiation, and solvents. NIOSH estimated that 1 million women from the work force of 16 million women in their childbearing years work in jobs with the potential for exposure that could produce birth defects or miscarriages (Institute of Medicine, 1979).

Management and social policy affects the appearance of these disorders. Safety standards that are too lax or not enforced could be changed and more strictly enforced. Ergonomic design of workstations could reduce physical strain and alleviate many disorders related to work on computer terminals. Better education of workers with incentives to adhere to safety standards might reduce unnecessary exposure and lower accidental exposure. Behavioral methods are at least partly beneficial in reducing exposure (Hopkins et al., 1986), but the need to alter unsafe production environments is still apparent. Management might reassign workers to other jobs based on specific screening standards. Pregnant women could be relocated from areas where known risks for birth defects exist to areas that are safer. Decision latitude, work rewards including salary, and work concerns including hazards also are related in a predictable fashion; that is, when the job allows some degree of decision latitude, when rewards are adequate and salary satisfactory, and when work hazards and hassles are low, people report the fewest symptoms of illness (Barnett et al., 1991).

Unfortunately, many factors work against the ideal. Management often is not willing to incur the costs for a redesigned work environment, for increased in-service training, or for job relocation. Workers may be bored, careless, or ill-informed. They may refuse reassignment because of perceived loss of status, lower pay, or disruption in friendships.

Then, there are cases when the best intentions produce an unforeseen health hazard. An interesting example of iatrogenic policy came when business instituted well-intentioned conservation measures following the 1970s energy crunch. At that time, many new buildings were built to extremely high energy standards. The buildings were made so tight they sealed in many byproducts of human and electromechanical activity. Cullen, Cherniack, and Rosenstock (1990a, 1990b) called these "sick buildings" because of the marked rise in upper respiratory infections, central nervous system dysfunction, and low morale associated with living or working in them.

Sociological Theory: Of Deviance, Beliefs, and Altruism

One does not have to look far to find social theories of health and illness. They are all around in folk wisdom and popular sayings. Even in Garrison Keillor's (1985) fictional Lake Wobegon, illness could still have as much to do with laziness, sin, and guilt as with any physical germ. Centuries after Martin Luther, one of Keillor's whimsical characters wrote his own *95 Theses 95*, in which he seemed to lament the injustice of his parents' theory of disease: "Your illnesses were the result of exhaustion by good works, mine the result of having disobeyed you and not worn a scarf, not taking vitamins" (p. 264). Social scientists built their theoretical models on a number of sociological constructs. These include sick-role theory, the health belief model (HBM), social integration theory, and sociobiology.

Sick-Role Theory: Of Deviance, Doctors, and Patients

Few people have influenced sociological theory as long and as extensively as Talcott Parsons. Nowhere has his influence been more evident than in the view that social norms place constraints on both the sick and their healers.

Role theory suggests that society develops norms to specify the expected and accepted behaviors for people who occupy a certain position at a certain time and in a certain place. For Parsons (1951), the same notion could be applied to the sick. Parsons' sick-role theory holds that sick people adopt typical, normative behaviors. These behaviors are normative because society regards them as customary and accepted for a sick person. They are, in essence,

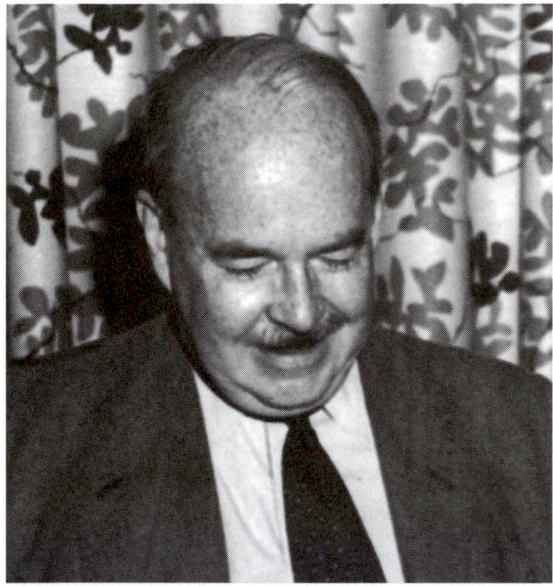

FIGURE 4.4   *Talcott Parsons, sociologist, originated the theory of sick-role behavior.*

the person's badge of legitimacy in an otherwise wholly distasteful situation. People probably come to adopt these behaviors through a social learning process that begins in the family and leads to internalization of a cognitive script or set of rules that tells the person what behavior is expected in what situation.

In sick-role theory, being sick is undesirable for both the person and society. It is, in a word, deviant. It departs from an ideal that can still be measured in tangible coin. The person has to endure at least discomfort with mild illnesses, perhaps unbearable pain with severe illnesses. While illness prevails, work, social and leisure activity, family companionship, and conjugal bliss may all suffer. Being sick may threaten family solidarity, income, and job security and plunge the family deep in debt.

These adverse effects seem all too obvious. But how is a person's illness undesirable for society? The rationale parallels biology's notion of homeostasis. Just as all living organisms work to maintain a state of internal balance, social organisms—families, cities, and nations—must preserve order and stability. A sick person destabilizes social units in various ways.

A sick person loses personal wages from work, but also costs the employer productivity. Extended illnesses entail huge costs for private or federal insurance agencies. Family members, especially those caring for the sick, undergo excessive strain, both physical and emotional. To preserve order, to discourage rampant deviancy, society sets standards, providing rewards for those who adhere to them and imposing sanctions on those who violate the social trust. One can be ill and escape these sanctions only if one meets society's criteria for appropriate sick-role behavior.

Parsons built his sick-role theory on four core assumptions. First, sick people are exempt from normal social roles. Legitimate illness is grounds to relieve a person from work, social, and family responsibilities. Second, society does not hold people responsible for being sick. We customarily give people the benefit of the doubt, assuming they have not knowingly or deliberately contrived an illness. Third, sick people should try to get well. This depends on the sick person's accepting the social norm that being sick is undesirable. If the person displays behavior that violates this norm—in other words, does not seem anxious to get well—then support for exemption from social responsibility may be withdrawn and sanctions applied. Assuming the person accepts the notion that getting well is desirable, the fourth assumption of Parson's sick-role theory is that sick people should seek technically competent help and cooperate with the physicians. Medical authority also has its constraints and normative behaviors; society is obligated to provide care through legitimate medical agencies. Doctors, as agents of society, seek to return the sick to a healthy and productive life as quickly as possible.

Although Parson's theory has intuitive appeal, it has also received much criticism. One such criticism is based on the view that medicine has unlimited authority to define illness and to control the distribution of (thus the access to) medical treatment. After reviewing more than

500 articles on sick-role theory, Gold (1977) suggested that Parson's theory perpetuates this dangerous notion.

The Health Belief Model: On Barriers and Vulnerability

Many families have their rock of Gibraltar: a member who is a pillar of stone against the onslaughts of sickness and disease. They defy the odds by running around on cold damp days with inadequate clothing. They chain-smoke, believing that cancer only happens to other people. They ride motorcycles barefoot and without a helmet, believing that helmet laws are just another example of government's trying to

take away fundamental rights. When flu hits, digestion nags, or chest pains develop, they are the last to think that going to the doctor might be a wise thing to do. If you are familiar with any of these scenarios, you already have some sense of what is at issue in the Health Belief Model (HBM).

This model, shown in Figure 4.5, is the offspring of field theory and value expectancy theory (Rosenstock, 1966). It proposes that health behavior results from the joint influence of psychosocial factors, including demographic traits and social cues aimed at changing risk behaviors. At the core of the cognitive system is a set of personal beliefs about illness. These beliefs mediate the perception of threat and thus affect the likelihood of taking action against

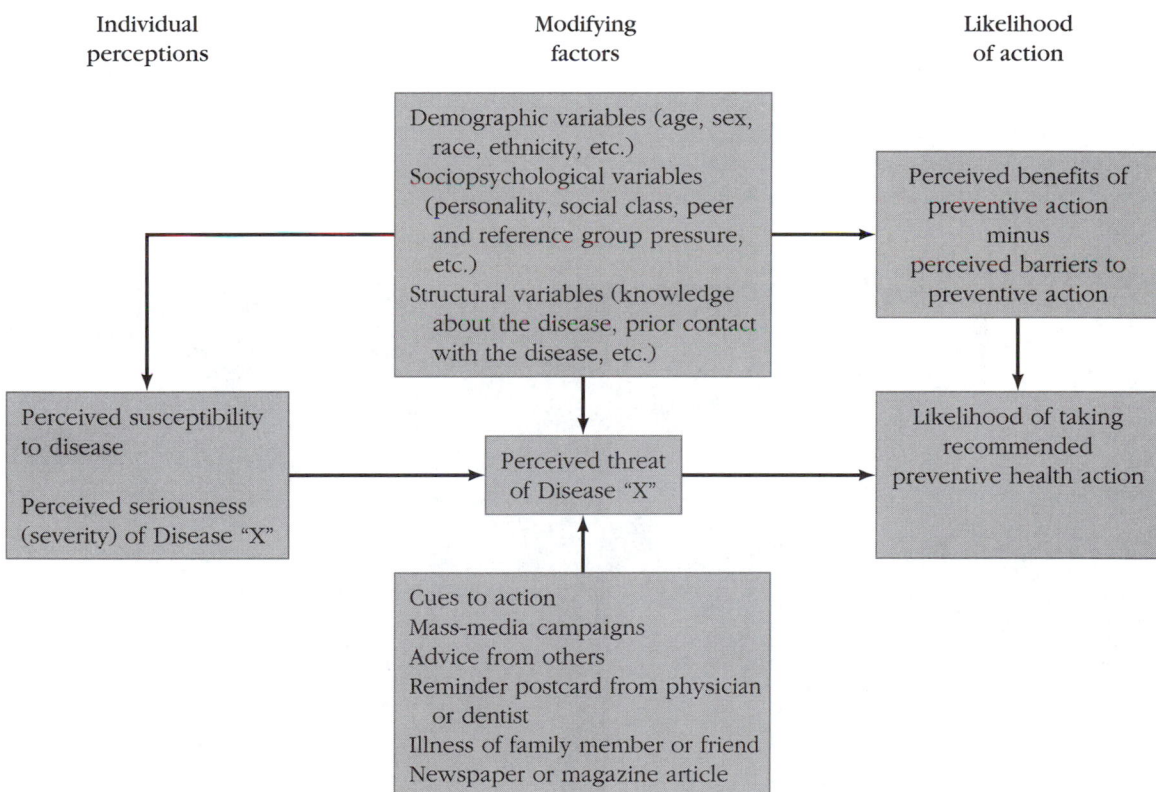

FIGURE 4.5   *The Health Belief Model suggests that perceptions of vulnerability and severity are linked to actions that may prevent illness (from Becker & Maiman, 1975).*

illness. At the core of the social system are various forms of policy formation and mass media campaigns designed to convince the public that the risks are real but that preventive behaviors—changes in lifestyle—can have beneficial effects.

To elaborate, the model assumes that people hold beliefs about the perceived severity of disease. **Perceived severity** is a very private, subjective evaluation of the consequences of sickness (Janz & Becker, 1984). This evaluation cuts across two dimensions. First, we evaluate personal consequences, including severity of pain, likelihood of disability, and chances of death. Second, we judge social outcomes, including impact on immediate family, loss of work, and emotional suffering in the extended family and network of friends. This belief system is presumably the motivating factor that makes health issues important. Someone who believes that death from lung cancer is a likely outcome of smoking should be motivated to quit, though this belief alone does not appear to be enough to guarantee quitting.

Support for this component is not strong when it comes to changing high-risk behaviors; that is, people do not seem to engage in a higher rate of preventive health behaviors based on their perceptions of the seriousness of a disease. Yet this belief is strongly related to sick-role behaviors. The more serious the illness, the more legitimate is the person's release from social responsibility and winning care and attention (Janz & Becker, 1984).

Next, each person has some belief about risks, their perceived susceptibility for disease. **Perceived susceptibility** is our personal estimate of the chances that we will contract a disease. Perceived susceptibility includes our degree of belief in the doctor's diagnosis, and the chances, after having had a disease and recovered, that we will get a disease again. Some people worry constantly about getting sick. Others think of themselves as invulnerable, immune to illness. The AIDS epidemic is a case in point. Many people, including prominent figures such as Magic Johnson, believed HIV could never happen to them. This kind of belief usually leads to reduced efforts to avoid risks.

In the general population, perceived susceptibility is strongly related to personal health behaviors (Janz & Becker, 1984). One study

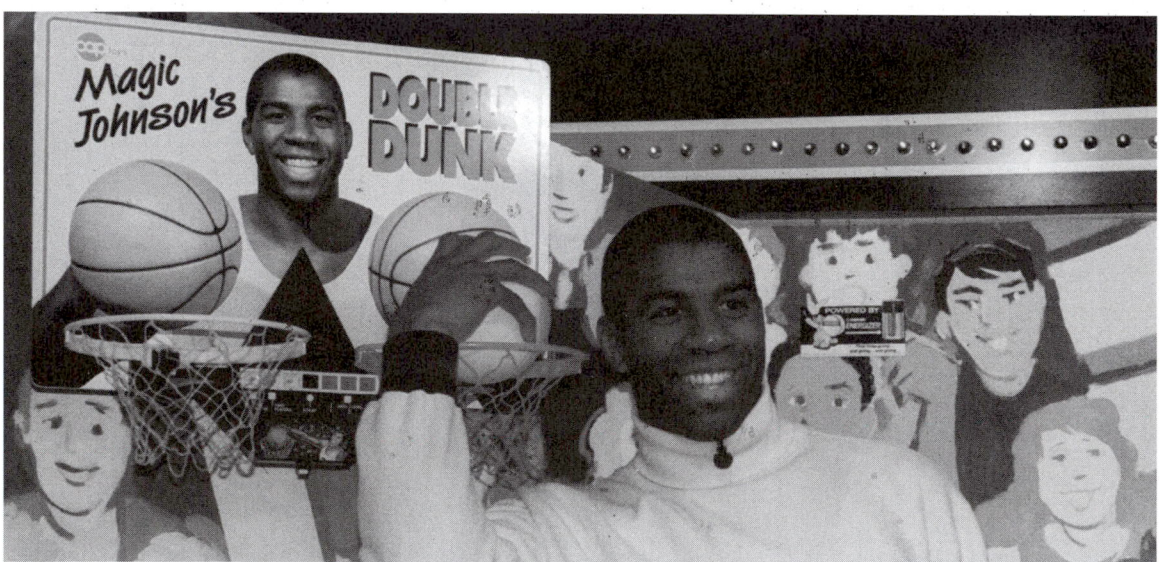

FIGURE 4.6   *Magic Johnson, all-star guard of the Los Angeles Lakers, announced that he had contracted the AIDS virus.*

by Becker's research team aimed at distinguishing participants in a screening program for Tay-Sachs disease. A group of at-risk Jewish residents from the Washington-Baltimore region received educational information on risk, screening methods, and availability of testing. The study revealed that the people who participated later had a higher level of perceived susceptibility than those who did not.

In addition to these subjective estimates of severity and susceptibility, we also have beliefs about the perceived benefits of health actions. **Perceived benefits** include personal estimates of the costs of some action plus estimates of the likely success of the action. A friend of mine had high familial risk for coronary disease, but he continued to drink and smoke excessively even after a major heart attack. For him, the costs of giving up his lifestyle were greater than the risk of death. He stated in a matter-of-fact way that he would rather die than change.

Finally, people have beliefs about the perceived barriers to health behaviors. **Perceived barriers** involves a type of cost-benefit analysis that weighs the costs of an action against the likely return. Smokers might feel that the risk of lung cancer warrants quitting and that they are personally at risk. Still, they might not be willing to endure the effects of smoking withdrawal. They might calculate that quitting would lead to undesirable weight gain. They might fear loss of companionship with friends who smoke. These would be barriers to quitting. Barriers to other health action might be the time involved, the monitoring required, or the actual risks entailed by surgery or treatment. People suffering from cancer may benefit greatly from radiation treatment, but costs may include severe nausea, hair loss, and constraints on social life. Victims of coronary artery disease may benefit from bypass surgery, but the surgery also creates a small risk of death. Recent evidence suggests that information emphasizing costs is most likely to motivate illness-detection behaviors while information emphasizing gain is most likely to motivate health-affirming behaviors (Rothman & Salovey, 1997).

Early surveys of health beliefs provided descriptive support without testing the model's predictive power (Kirscht, Haefner, Kegeles, & Rosenstock, 1966). Since then, many investigators have elaborated and tested the model with different populations (Calnan & Moss, 1984), in varied settings, and with various health-illness behaviors (Cockerham, 1982). Later research, including prospective research, continued to show the strength of the approach (Janz & Becker, 1984). The model probably is most applicable to upper socioeconomic groups with above average education. Research on children's beliefs about health is notably absent, although this absence may be short-lived (Peterson & Harbeck, 1988). The model still enjoys popularity, as we shall see in several later chapters.

Social Integration Theory: On Control and Compliance

Debra Umberson's (1987) work fits in the framework of Durkheim's social integration theory. Social integration theory suggests that marriage and parenting are social relationships intended to integrate the individual into society and provide a sense of meaning and purpose as well as social obligation. For Umberson, though, the issue is whether marriage and parenting confer any beneficial effects in encouraging positive health behaviors and reducing morbidity and mortality. Umberson suggested that health behaviors are positively influenced by marriage and parenting through the mechanism of social control. The notion of social control is that social systems provide ways of influencing people to engage in socially desirable behavior and to avoid unconventional and deviant behavior. Social control may become internal if and when the person assimilates society's norms. On the other hand, social control may be largely external, exercised through incentives and sanctions.

In principle, the complete process should work as follows. High-risk behaviors increase morbidity and mortality. Any illness or death resulting from high-risk behaviors, then, may be viewed as deviant and socially detrimental (à la

Talcott Parsons) since it deprives society of that person's creativity and productivity. As primary agents of society, families work to encourage healthy behaviors and discourage high-risk behaviors. Families remind their members to watch their diets and get exercise or stimulate exercise through play activities. Families devise orderly meal and bedtime routines for young children. Families usually impose penalties for improper activities such as substance abuse. By implication, lack of a family network should increase the likelihood of engaging in health-compromising behaviors.

Umberson found general support for the model by comparing three family configurations: families with children at home, families with children who lived separately, and families who were childless. The strongest effects were observed in the area of substance abuse and drinking and driving. Apparently, having children in the home serves as a major deterrent to substance abuse. In addition, marital status appears to be significantly related to positive health behaviors. Widowed and divorced subjects engaged in negative or self-defeating health behaviors more often then their married counterparts. Once again, men seem to benefit more from marriage than women, although women do benefit somewhat. Women are more likely to maintain a similar lifestyle regardless of marital status, whereas single men do not maintain as orderly a lifestyle as married men. Divorce in particular appears to contribute to much higher likelihood of drinking behavior in men than in women.

Although Umberson's analysis makes intuitive and logical sense, there are certain problems with the study. For example, no baseline measures of prior alcohol use were taken in any of the families. In part, this problem results from the study's being archival and static, not prospective and dynamic. A longitudinal approach that assesses changes in health behaviors as families change, with births, deaths, divorces, and empty nests, would be more convincing. Finally, many of the coefficients (from a standard regression analysis) were significant but

very small, suggesting that the model may have little explanatory power (explained variance).

Sociobiology: On Genetics, Investments, and Social Behavior

Darwin's theory of evolution suggested that physical traits were genetically selected and transmitted through the survival of the fittest. E.O. Wilson (1975) tried to add social traits to the equation. Wilson's approach is called **sociobiology,** which he defined as the study of the biological bases of social behavior.

Many authors have applied sociobiology theory to issues of health and illness. For example, Rushton (1987) argued that health and longevity are part of a reproductive strategy that includes intense nurturing of few offspring. Another example of social behaviors with relevance to health and illness is food cultivation and diet. Lumsden and Wilson (1981) argued that the connection between cuisine and genetic fitness is already extensively detailed. In support, they cited research on cultivation of maize among North, Central, and South American indigenous groups. The importance of maize to the diet depends on a chemical, lysine, and an alkali cooking method that releases it. The amino acid lysine is a chemical the body cannot produce; it must be obtained from food sources. Maize is a cereal that contains large amounts of lysine but in a locked-up form. One simple way to unlock the lysine in maize is through alkali cooking.

Among 51 societies of the Americas, there was a strong association between maize cultivation, use of alkali cooking, and population density. Yet these ancient societies did not have agricultural research stations. The connection between lysine, alkali cooking, and physical health could not have been observed directly by these groups. Sociobiologists assume, then, that it was a social trait that was genetically selected, propagated, and culturally diffused.

Other examples are used to support the sociobiologists' position, including a preference for sugar consumption to obtain high calorie intake taste preferences for foods that combat different types of illness, and genetic traits such as sickle-cell anemia that are protective in some environments (Freedman, 1979). As many critics continue to point out, however, alternative explanations exist for many of these examples, and so the position of sociobiology can only be described as tenuous at best.

Health Care Systems: Providers, Trainers, and Policies

When most people think of health care, they tend to think of their doctor's office, a community clinic, or the hospital. But medical systems are complex extended networks with health agents, health organizations and regulations, and still more people to interpret or misinterpret the rules. Foster and Anderson (1978, p. 36) wrote that a medical system embraces all the health-promoting beliefs, actions, scientific knowledge, and skills of the people who subscribe to the system. These medical systems also include policies formulated by government on behalf of its citizens. The German writer-philosopher Goethe worried that the modern world might turn into one giant medical institution. In a more contemporary analysis, Arnold Relman (1991) expressed concern for the commercialism in the new medical-industrial complex. He said that "we are witnessing a pervasive change in the ethos of the voluntary hospital system in America from that of a social service to that of a business" (p. 856).

The moral dilemma quietly concealed in these statements is deepened with a modern medical practice called joint-ownership, in which doctors own special service facilities to which they refer patients. As one study showed, such practices increase costs for patients and have adverse effects on access (Mitchell & Sunshine, 1992). Robert Kaplan (1992) echoed this theme when he pointed to three major problems: lack of affordable health care, lack of access to health care, and poor accountability in the health industry.

No Room at the Inn: Rejection, Selection, and Negligence

Although we continue to believe that modern medical systems work with a high degree of efficiency, it is apparent that systems also can fail. A young woman, Andrea, was near the end of her term, eagerly looking forward to the birth of her second child.[5] She had good prenatal care, and there was no need for concern. But, since babies do not make appointments, one early fall day when Andrea's baby decided its time had come, Andrea's husband was gone and Andrea had no one else to turn to for help. Her contractions were so close, she believed the baby could come at any moment. She quickly dialed 911 and got a swift response. The paramedics felt they could get her to the local hospital in time, and they did. Then, the system reared its head. There was no room in the obstetrics ward, so the doctor refused admission. There in full view of the public, watched

---

[5] This anecdote is based on an AP news wire report from New York on September 27, 1991.

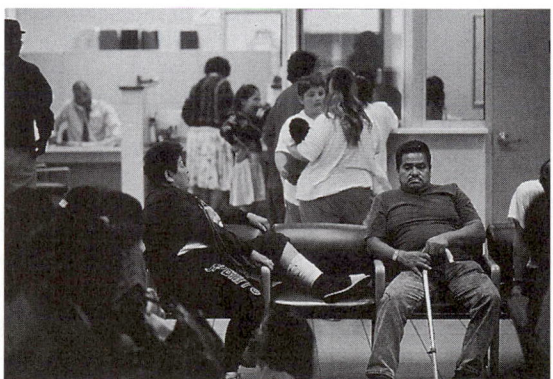

FIGURE 4.7   *A crowded inner-city hospital admissions area such as Andrea might have encountered.*

but never assisted by doctors or hospital staff, the two paramedics delivered Andrea's baby.

Is this merely an isolated instance or a symptom of a more pervasive problem in the health care industry? From a mere statistical point of view, such extreme cases as Andrea's are rare. But they highlight the way a system, or staff interpretation of system regulations, can become impersonal and detached from the immediate concern of giving care to a person in need. Among the many problems that must be confronted in the complex network of our health care system, three stand out: rapid change, differential access, and patient management in the health setting.

First, both medical technology and system regulations may change so rapidly that systems, providers, and consumers may be hard pressed to keep up. Belar, Deardorff, and Kelly (1987) noted that health care policy is changing so quickly that any reference more than five years old should be regarded as obsolete.[6]

Second, there is a problem in differential access to health care. Even after considering all sources of health benefits, more than 36 million nonelderly people (including 10 million children) do not have health coverage (Frank, 1993). Cockerham (1982) spoke of the de facto dual health care system that exists in America, one a type of private health care system that is utilized by the middle- and upper-income groups, the second a public care system that is used largely by lower-income groups. As one might expect, members of ethnic groups that are disproportionately represented in the lower-income groups depend much more on public health care. Patients who depend on the public sector generally wait longer to see a doctor and probably never will have a personal physician. In turn, the patient is less likely to be counseled about preventive health behaviors that could reduce future health problems. Finally, more than likely these patients will return to living conditions that do not promote good health. In

turn, the patient is less likely to be counseled about preventive health behaviors that could reduce future health problems. More than likely these patients will return to living conditions that do not promote good health. Even in government financed programs, race and income appear to influence treatment. Black and low-income medicare beneficiaries have fewer visits to physicians yet are hospitalized more often and have higher mortality rates compared to whites and middle- and high-income groups (Gornick et al., 1996).

More evidence to support this argument comes from studies of hospitals like the one Andrea went to, a public hospital in Harlem, New York City. In spite of the fact that overall mortality rates have fallen in the United States, mortality rates are still extremely high in inner-city communities such as Detroit, Los Angeles, and Harlem (Geronimus, Bound, Waidmann, Hillemeier, & Burns, 1996). Based on a survival analysis, McCord and Freeman (1990) concluded that black men in Harlem were even less likely to reach the age of 65 than men in Bangladesh (see Figure 4.8). Statistics for similar inner-city areas in Boston tell much the same story. Most revealing is the fact that current death rates in Harlem are equivalent to the death rates among whites in 1930. Hospitals cannot be blamed for all these mortality and morbidity differences. Instead, these differences reflect the combined effect of many variables that lower quality of life and restrict access to treatment over a person's life span.

Third, health care professionals confront many problems that are directly related to patient management—decisions to admit to the hospital or treat on an outpatient basis, decisions to use tiered diagnostics or to carry out shotgun diagnostics right away, decisions about surgery, and decisions about early or delayed release from the hospital. Each of these decisions has economic effects for both the system and the patient and creates risks for both as well. Medical systems typically benefit by increased payments from third-party payers when more admissions, more diagnostic procedures, and more surgeries are done, and when patients stay

---

[6] Apparently, then, even Belar, Deardorff, and Kelly's advice is obsolete—a point that is not completely facetious since the rate of change tends to escalate as well.

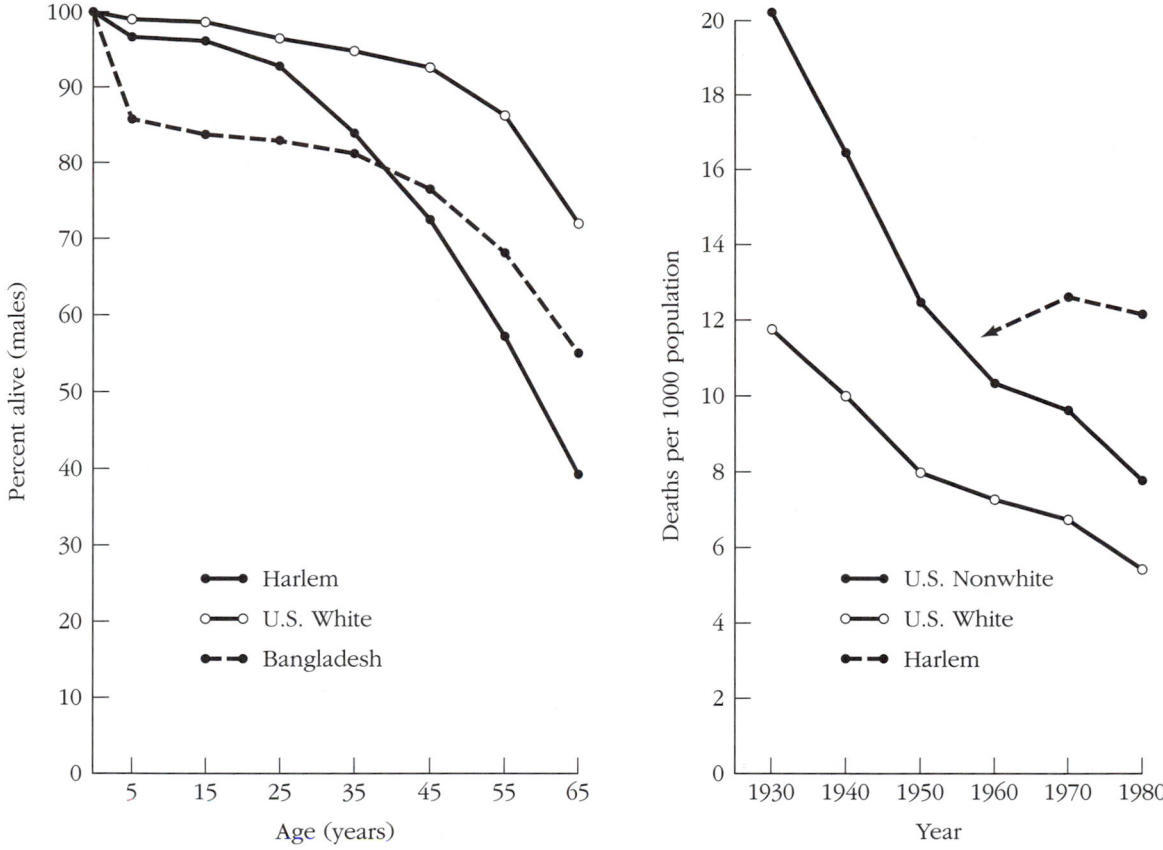

FIGURE 4.8   *Death rates in some inner-city areas are not much better than in some less developed countries (from McCord & Freeman, 1990).*

longer. Arnold Relman (1991) commented: "The medical-industrial complex had developed mainly as a response to the entrepreneurial opportunities afforded by the expansion of health insurance coverage. . . . " (p. 854). This entrepreneurial abuse may have been behind criticisms that doctors were overusing the cesarean section for delivering babies, a practice that pays doctors and hospitals handsomely but may not be necessary for many births. This type of situation builds in inflationary factors for the health care industry that feed back negatively to the entire social system (Kiesler & Morton, 1988).

Patients are caught in a system that is complex, forbidding, sometimes unfriendly, even ominous. They must balance costs against risks in a situation where they are highly dependent on medical authority. Yet some patients may not even ask for a second opinion, feeling that it would simply add to the costs, that it would produce the same outcome, or that it would be impolite.

Finally, there are issues of negligence or substandard care in a variety of health care facilities. In an extensive study called the Harvard Medical Practice Study, the data showed that adverse outcomes—in other words iatrogenic treatments—were associated with hospitalization in 1278 of the 30,121 cases reviewed (Brennan et al., 1991). Negligence was involved in 306 cases, and substandard care in the remaining 972 cases. Technical errors in performance (35.2%) or prevention (21.9%) were the most common, but diagnostic errors (13.8%) and drug reactions (8.9%) also contributed (Leape et al., 1991). Although 70.5% of the cases involved less than six months of disability, 33 (2.6%) resulted in permanent disability, and 174 (13.6%) led to death.

Health Service Training: Teach the Science, Preach the Art

Hall and Beresford (1983) related the case of a 60-year-old diabetic woman whose leg was amputated because of gangrene. The woman was most upset about the fact that she would no longer be able to care for herself, go out shopping, and get around town. The medical student, after reviewing results from medical tests, concluded that she was in excellent metabolic balance and allowed her to go home. The student thus fulfilled his responsibility to the patient and to his sophisticated medical science training. For all the judicious use of medical knowledge, though, no one thought to follow up to see whether the woman could manage the complex diet that had been prescribed. Several days later, the woman returned in a deep diabetic coma.

Medical students must absorb tremendous amounts of technical information to ply their trade. Apparently this load takes its toll; one study showed that 1 in 8 medical students suffers major depressive symptoms. In this four-year study of medical students at Rush Medical College in Chicago, David Clark and Peter Zeldow (1988) reported that 12% could be diagnosed as clinically depressed at any time during their progress through the program, partly because medical education offers little support for students' emotional needs.

Many years ago, Flanders Dunbar wrote that the doctor's bedside manner is a vital element in the treatment of the sick. Hall and Beresford (1983) cautioned: "The danger medicine faces today is that we will be seduced by our science and forget our art" (p. 112). An effort is under way in modern medical schools to retrieve the art, an area where health psychologists have been increasingly utilized in medical education.

Public Health Education: Of Tractors, Cars, and Motorcycles

January 11, 1992: National headlines report a shocking story. A young man, John Thompson, alone on the family's North Dakota farm, becomes caught in the tractor's power take-off. Caught by the legs first and whipped around twice like a rag doll, he still manages to get loose, only to be caught again, this time by the arms. Both his arms are ripped off, right arm at the shoulder, left arm at the elbow. No one is there to help. His father and mother, in nearby Bismarck visiting a hospitalized friend, hear of the accident only later by phone.

Somehow, John has the strength and the presence of mind to get to the house, only to encounter the first new obstacle: He cannot open the house door with the remaining stump. Mustering what reserves he has left, he manages to turn the door knob with his mouth and get to a phone. There, with a pencil in his mouth, he dials a nearby cousin to call for help and to come and stay with him. While waiting for the ambulance, he sits in the bath tub to keep blood from

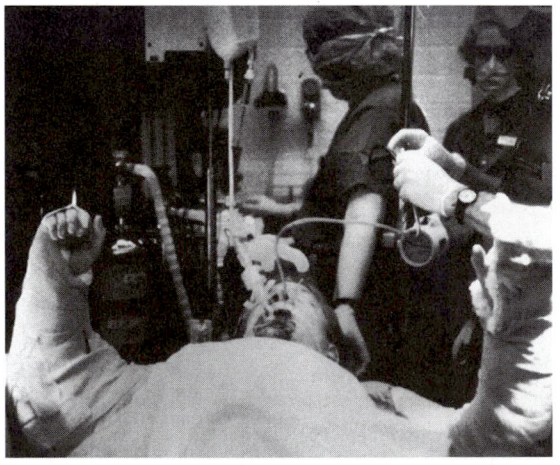

FIGURE 4.9   *The courageous teenager John Thompson lost both his arms in a farm accident.*

running on the carpet. Even after the emergency team arrives, he is still thinking: Get my arms, pack them in ice, bring them along. After six hours of surgery, his arms are reattached, and the long road to recovery begins.

In the aftermath of this story of personal courage, there were pleas for improved educational programs about the precautions needed when working around dangerous equipment. This danger is not unique to large farm machinery, but can be a life and death issue every day for many people, in many walks of life, in virtually every corner of the globe. The house is still a major site for serious injuries, and most auto accidents occur within a short distance of home. Many deaths occur on the road because people bypass safety measures, disconnect warning signals for car seat belt use, equip their cars with radar units to defeat speed control measures, or refuse to wear helmets. These actions may be done in the name of self-determination and personal freedom (Lorion, 1991), but it is small consolation to the families who are left to grieve the premature, unnecessary deaths of family members. As science has provided more convincing evidence that health and behavior are connected, more energy has been expended to increase public awareness of the benefits of lifestyle change.

Florida, for example, developed a simple program to promote seat belt and helmet use among state employees (Rogers, Rogers, Bailey, Runkle, & Moore, 1988). Although there are many approaches to increase use, such as engineering methods, legal sanctions, and media persuasion, Florida elected to use a behavioral approach. The state contracted with its employees to read a sheet with the state regulation on it. After reading the sheet, employees signed a statement that they understood the consequences for noncompliance. Employees' cars were also equipped with dashboard stickers reminding them to use seat belts. Baseline data showed that only about 10% of the employees used their seat belts before the program. In the group exposed to both the sticker and the signature sheet, compliance went up to about 52%. In another group, exposed only to the dashboard stickers, compliance still went up to 38%. The program also had another very beneficial effect: It reduced the costs for accident claims from a little over $2000 to just under $1000. In another study, investigators used a buckle-up sign at the exit of a parking lot plus a human prompter. They obtained increases from a baseline of about 43% to about 71% (Williams, Thyer, Bailey, & Harrison, 1989). Mandatory seat belt laws in Australia, Belgium, and Canada increased use from 20 to 90% and resulted in as much as a 54% reduction in deaths and injuries (Rogers et al., 1988).

Still, there are numerous impediments to mass health education. Socioeconomic forces at work within the medical establishment are not completely supportive of a broad-based health education program. Bartlett and Windsor (1985), writing from a medical sociology perspective, pointed to five problem areas that often work against cooperation between medicine and allied health service disciplines. These are the distribution of medical power; accountability to patients; fear of potential reduction in use of medical services; tension over professional autonomy and dependence; and substantive changes in the cultural authority of medicine to control the health industry. I will briefly explain the significance of these barriers to health education.

First, doctors have the power to control much of their work conditions, the flow of knowledge, and the regulation of their incomes. They are not likely to give up powers that may be perceived as weakening their position or hurting their incomes. Second, an informed citizenry can place doctors in the uneasy position of being second-guessed and second-opinioned. Further, education might lead more patients to self-controlled practices, even self-medications. To the extent that these practices, correctly applied, reduced patients' use of medical services, it could have disastrous economic consequences for many medical facilities. Fourth, doctors enjoy a great deal of autonomy with power that includes the dependence of many medical service personnel on direct orders from the doctor. Establishing a number of health service professionals as fully autonomous and independent providers, including those in the health education arena, would erode the physicians' customary autonomy and control. Fifth, the educational approach assumes that health and illness are influenced by multiple factors. This decentralizes medicine's role in the prevention of illness. It also means that numerous forces affecting the course of an illness may be under the control of people other than medical professionals. Thus, according to Bartlett and Windsor, a broad health education program is an assault on the power and economics of the medical industry.

Health Care Policy: The Failure of Our Success

Critics of the medical establishment and national health policy point to reasons our nation needs to rethink health goals. Since the turn of the century, the pattern of deaths has gradually changed from epidemic diseases to diseases with substantial behavioral components. The "failure of our success" is that we have increased longevity at the cost of increased exposure to chronic, disabling illnesses (Barsky, 1988). The cost of health care has skyrocketed and soon could make reasonable care inaccessible for many families, if it has not done so already. Expenditures for all medical costs in 1991 were over 13% of the GNP, or $752 billion per year, more than a 200% increase from $359 billion in 1983 (U.S. Bureau of the Census, 1993).[7] Health care costs could reach $1.5 trillion by the year 2000. Finally, the misplaced emphasis on high-tech medicine for tertiary treatment ignores the positive benefits of preventive medicine and, at the same time, misdirects vast financial resources that could be used to develop preventive programs.

Faced with similar stinging indictments, many countries set to work formulating national health policy. In the United States, the most recent effort directed by the surgeon general's office has been to formulate goals for the year 2000. Three major goals are to increase the average healthy life span, to reduce disparities between different groups within society, and to provide equal access to health maintenance services for all Americans (Sullivan, 1990). About 80% of the states already have implemented actions to further these goals (McGinnis, 1991).

These goals have some interesting lessons to teach us. First, the goals show that disease is now being considered in a biopsychosocial context. This suggests that contemporary policy and to some extent medical practice have already assimilated the basic tenets of the BPS

TABLE 4.5   *National health goals for 2000 (from McGinnis, 1991).*

Health promotion
   Physical activity and fitness
   Nutrition
   Tobacco
   Alcohol and other drugs
   Family planning
   Mental health and mental disorders
   Violent and abusive behavior
   Educational and community-based programs
Health protection
   Unintentional injuries
   Occupational safety and health
   Environmental health
   Food and drug safety
   Oral health
Preventive services
   Maternal and infant health
   Heart disease and stroke
   Cancer
   Diabetes and chronic disabling conditions
   Human immunodeficiency virus infection
   Sexually transmitted diseases
   Immunization and infectious diseases
   Clinical preventive services
Surveillance and data systems

---

[7] Compare these figures to the paltry $75 billion spent for health care in 1970—7.4% of the GNP.

model. Second, the goals show that we have taken major steps toward rewriting folk theories of disease. The translation of the BPS model from a laboratory icon to a national policy that has captured the imagination of many segments of the population says much about how far we have come.

Society generally values discovery. It assumes that new investigative techniques will be developed to probe deeper and deeper into the mysteries of illness. We must understand, though, that even as we gain increased confidence in the model currently being tested, new discoveries will challenge, perhaps even displace it. In reality, science's love affairs with theory are often one-night stands, not permanent relationships. The process of refining is never done; the theory is never finished. It is only revealed at a given moment in one of its stages of evolution.

Summary

The biopsychosocial model currently being tested suggests that health and illness must be explained in the matrix of biomedical science, psychological science, and sociocultural science. We constructed the rationale and theoretical issues for the biomedical sciences in Chapter 2, and the same for psychological science in Chapter 3. Here, we have concentrated on several important contributions of social science, including the work of medical sociologists, anthropologists, and epidemiologists. In sum, these disciplines have provided a richly textured quilt of information showing a variety of ways in which social customs and traditions, beliefs and values, and policy and systems contribute to health and illness.

1. The disease kuru shows that the presence of a physical germ is not always sufficient to produce illness. Social custom in this case provided a context in which the germ could be contacted and transmitted.

2. The existence of special healers within many cultures points to the fact that virtually every society has attempted to explain and control illness through a systematic view of disease and training of specialized healers.

3. Green medicines used by many cultures across the centuries suggest that a healthy, pragmatic, informal empiricism has been used to develop ways to relieve symptoms and cure illnesses.

4. The great thrust of cross-cultural research in health and disease has been supported by the emergence of new research specialties such as medical sociology, medical anthropology, and medical epidemiology.

5. Ethnomedicine is a branch of anthropology that studies the health beliefs and health practices of indigenous groups.

6. Women have lower mortality and longer life expectancy than men, but they have higher rates of morbidity. Still, women enjoy three well-years more than men when mortality and morbidity are combined.

7. Differences between men's and women's health problems are explained both in terms of biology, as in sex-linked disorders, and in terms of psychosocial processes, as in gender-linked disorders.

8. Sex-linked disorders are illnesses specific to one sex, such as breast cancer in women.

9. Gender-linked disorders result from socialization processes that put different role expectations and pressures on women than on men.

10. Multiple roles, instead of adding stress and reducing health, appear to benefit people as measured by lower rates of morbidity.

11. A physician sex bias exists in that women are likely to receive more psychologically loaded diagnoses and less aggressive diagnostic strategies and treatment than men.

12. Culture may instill good health habits, in terms of both nutrition and physical activity. The study of the Tarahumara shows conversely that when pressure is put on a group of people, such as immigrants, to adopt a new lifestyle, there may be negative effects, such as the increased risk for coronary associated with affluent diets.

13. Some diseases also occur at a higher rate among certain ethnic groups. The example of Tay-Sachs disease shows how such information can be used to provide screening and counseling to control the disorder.

14. Although biomedical science continues to probe the genetic and biochemical environment of the host organism for clues to hypertension, among other disorders, it is likely that sociocultural factors also explain many such disorders.

15. Work sites expose many workers to toxins with potentially negative effects. A variety of environmental design strategies and behavioral strategies can be used to reduce risk.

16. Sick-role theory suggests that society develops norms for behaviors that sick people are expected to follow. They are expected to desire to get well and to seek legitimate medical help to get well.

17. The Health Belief Model assumes that people hold certain beliefs about personal vulnerability, the severity of disease, and the costs and benefits of taking action. These beliefs presumably motivate the person to a greater or lesser degree to seek help or to modify high-risk behaviors.

18. Umberson's social integration theory suggests that the family operates as a type of social control agency to provide support for health behaviors and sanctions for inappropriate high-risk behaviors.

19. In the context of Wilson's sociobiology theory, health-related behaviors such as cooking methods and dietary choices may have social components that are genetically selected. Still, the evidence is weak, and alternative explanations exist for the same phenomena.

20. Health systems are extended networks of agencies, agents, and clients, who have some beliefs about the way the system should work and vested interests in the system's efficient operation.

21. Health systems confront numerous problems because of the rapid pace of change in both technology and policy. They are not equally accessible to all segments of the population because of costs, and they sometimes lead to adverse outcomes.

22. Medical training may be too narrowly focused on technical competence at the expense of interpersonal skills. Still, there are numerous signs that medical education is coming to grips with the issue by reintroducing more of the art of medical practice into the modern medical curriculum.

23. Health education focuses on the use of current knowledge to achieve changes in high-risk behaviors. Increasing the use of seat belts could reduce deaths by as much as 50%. Still, there are barriers to implementing mass education programs, some of which come from vested interest groups that could suffer economic and power losses from widespread educational activities.

24. National health policy is now focused on three objectives: to increase the average healthy life span, to reduce disparities between different groups within society, and to provide equal access to health maintenance services for all Americans.

Key Words

cultural pediatrics	perceived barriers
culture	perceived benefits
curanderas	perceived severity
ethnomedicine	perceived susceptibility
etiology	physician sex bias
gender-linked disorder	role theory
green medicine	sex-linked disorders
medical anthro-pologist	sick-role
medical epidemi-ologist	sociobiology
medical sociologist	sociology in medicine
	sociology of medicine
	Tay-Sachs disease
	well-life expectancy

Study Questions

1. What lessons can we learn from the story of kuru?

2. Compare and contrast biological views of sex

differences in health and disease with psychosocial views of gender differences.

3. What social factors may be involved in such diseases as hypertension and Tay-Sachs? How may behavioral or lifestyle factors influence such diseases?

4. Outline the core features of the Health Belief Model. What psychological processes are believed to be related to preventive health behaviors?

5. Health systems are important because they regulate the distribution of health care, train doctors and nurses, educate the public, and help formulate policy. Discuss possible positive and negative outcomes in each of these four areas.

Class Projects

1. Find current articles on ethnomedicine and compare the medical systems, theories, and beliefs of several cultures.

2. Delve deeper into aspects of sex and gender.

Consider in more depth the issue of physician bias in medicine. Find more current information, and consider the extent to which physician bias is a serious problem in medical practice and distribution of health services.

3. Prepare classroom reports on educational programs designed to impact health behaviors. Consider both the cost and the efficacy of such programs.

Suggested Readings

Baer, H. A (Ed.). (1987). *Encounters with biomedicine: Case studies in medical anthropology.* New York: Gordon and Breach.

Dutton, D. B (1988). *Worse than the disease: Pitfalls of medical progress.* Cambridge: Cambridge University Press.

Rodin, J., & Ickovics, J. R (1990). Women's health: Review and research agenda as we approach the 21st century. *American Psychologist, 45,* 1018–1034.

WEBSITES Social, Women's Health, and Minority Health Issues

ADDRESS	DESCRIPTION
http://asa.ugl.lib.umich.edu/chdocs/womenhealth/womens health.html	☆ Women's Health Resources on the Internet—with index to many topics
http://www.pitt.edu/~ejb4/min/	☆ Minority Health Network—grouped by minority group and by specific diseases
http://www.gen.emory.edu/MEDWEB/alphakey/Alternative medicine.html	☆ Emory University's MedWeb Page with huge index to alternative medicines
http://www.healthwire.com/women	Forum, news, and browser for women's health issues
http://www.omhrc.gov/welcome.htm	Office of Minority Health Resource Center
http://www.exit109.com/~zaweb/pjp/	☆ Guide to Internet resources for health economics

Intervention and Research: Techniques in Health Psychology

This part of the text lays the foundation for two crucial skills in health psychology: intervention and research. Health psychologists often are called on to design and implement clinical interventions for mental and physical health problems. The range of interventions developed over the past 50 years is extensive, including many different forms of psychotherapy, behavioral and cognitive-behavioral techniques, and pharmacotherapy. These interventions may help people cope with stress, alter high-risk behaviors, accept invasive medical tests and surgeries, cope with news of terminal illness in a family member, or comply with a medical routine that involves a substantial adjustment in lifestyle.

While some interventions may be viewed as theoretically biased—that is, originating in and committed to a theoretical model—it is probably more useful to take an eclectic view toward interventions (Lambert, Shapiro, & Bergin, 1988). In fact, the percentage of therapists espousing an eclectic point of view has increased to around 50% (Garfield, 1989). In simple terms, eclecticism means using the best interventions regardless of theoretical origins. That one is eclectic, however, does not mean that one is also uncritical. It has now become standard practice to test the outcomes of therapies carefully and thus establish their effectiveness before they are put into widespread use (Garfield & Bergin, 1986). Further, interventions are more often being carefully linked to models of mental and physical illness that detail the origins of the illness. There is little room any longer for therapies whose sole justification is logical consistency, and even less room for therapies that reflect little more than the forceful personality of the originator. Several intervention methods will be described in Chapter 5.

Health psychologists also need to know how to design research that will provide unambiguous answers to important questions. Quite often, research design requires that investigators combine assessment and intervention skills in the project. Research methods include the traditional case study, experimental designs that manipulate causal variables in well-controlled settings, quasi-experimental designs using existing groups in field settings, and highly sophisticated epidemiological studies that may use thousands of subjects. The methods most commonly used in health psychology will be reviewed in Chapter 6 with the assumption that most readers have already had an introductory research course.

CHAPTER 5

Four Therapies: Short-Term, Cognitive, Behavioral, and Pharmacotherapy

The years from 1980 to 1985 saw the beginning of America's black plague, the epidemic of AIDS—a disease that did not itself kill but was almost certainly fatal (Batchelor, 1984). Even as the epidemic grew, many agencies—both public and private—were seeking ways to provide therapeutic support to the victims. They sought ways to minimize damage to families and friends, and to help caregivers better understand how to help manage the course of the disease. Last but not least, these agencies worked, sometimes at a frenetic pace, to develop methods to intervene in the community to stop the spread of AIDS.

The prevailing notion, supported by much scientific data, had it that AIDS was the disease of down-and-out drug derelicts sharing needles in seedy crack houses and ghetto alleys. If it wasn't that, it was the disease of gay males, especially minority males, engaging in unprotected sex. Data collected even after the middle 1980s continued to show 90% of the victims were gay males, intravenous drug abusers, and African American and Hispanic men (Batchelor, 1988; Peterson & Marín, 1988). Often, a combination of unprotected sex and high-risk drug use compounded individuals' risks.

But this common knowledge proved to be only a temporary protective facade for a populace unwilling to believe that it too might be vulnerable. This facade, now described as an epidemic of denial, prevented people from transforming abstract risk statistics into an awareness of personal vulnerability. These facts were not wrong; but they were incomplete. Since then, little by little, the facade has been destroyed.

Heterosexual activity was supposed to be safe. But startling new facts first revealed after the mid-1980s began to destroy this myth. Studies of prostitutes in several countries (Calabrese & Gopalakrishna, 1986) showed that AIDS could be transmitted by heterosexual contact. Now, evidence presented in a WHO report at the 1992 European AIDS conference suggests that women may be the high-risk group of the 1990s (Chase, 1992). They are the single fastest growing patient group, and worldwide, 70% of new AIDS infections occur through heterosexual contact. One piece of the protective facade is gone.

Next came headlines that read like a roll call of Hollywood's notables: first Rock Hudson, then Liberace, Magic Johnson, Arthur Ashe, Anthony Perkins. Each in turn became identified with the AIDS virus. The message was clear: If the heroes of society, role models for youth, the wealthy elite who could afford the best in

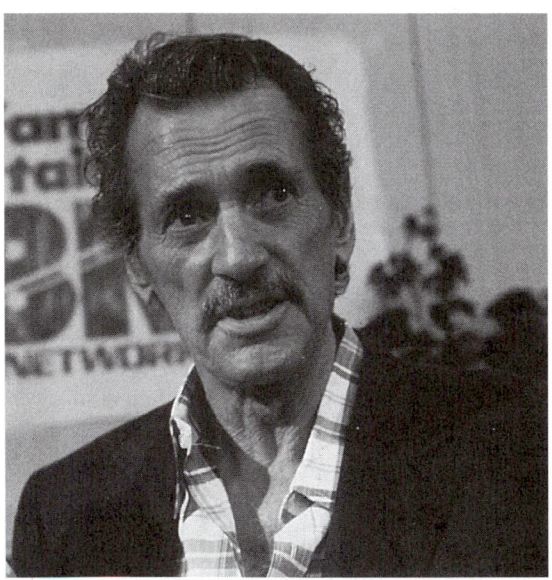

FIGURE 5.1   *As AIDS continues to spread, taking the lives of celebrities such as Rock Hudson as well as ordinary people, psychologists have increased their attention to a variety of intervention strategies to help AIDS victims and prevent the spread of AIDS.*

medical care were vulnerable, so was anyone and everyone. Another piece of the facade was gone. In the meantime, the epidemic was spreading at an alarming rate involving millions across Europe, Africa, India, Haiti and beyond.

As recognition grew that a cure for AIDS would not be ready anytime soon, attention quickly turned to preventive programs. Clinics designed small-group psychoeducational and outreach programs to target known high-risk behaviors (Des Jarlais & Friedman, 1988; Stall, Coates, & Hoff, 1988). As important and successful as individual and small group therapy can be, this effort still could not effectively combat an epidemic involving millions. As more and more information became available, it was apparent that nothing less than a mass public education approach aimed at many strata of society would be necessary to get the message across (Strauss, Corless, Luckey, van der Horst, & Dennis, 1992).

The example of AIDS reflects three basic points about intervention in health and illness. First, health psychologists may need to use a wide variety of intervention strategies, ranging from classic one-on-one psychotherapy to small-group interventions to mass public education campaigns. Training in a single treatment modality, then, is unlikely to be adequate preparation for most health psychologists. Second, many interventions occur only after serious symptoms of the disorder have already appeared. But health psychologists may try to intervene early to minimize potential damage, or they may try to prevent the appearance of a disorder. Finally, producing a change in behavior by the end of an intervention is of little use if the change does not have a long-term benefit—especially when addictive and other high-risk behaviors are involved. Thus generalization and maintenance of change is important to most intervention strategies.

This chapter provides a brief overview of the therapies and interventions commonly used by health psychologists. The chapter begins by discussing the timing of interventions: the difference between tertiary prevention, which occurs largely after the damage is done, and primary prevention, which seeks to prevent the disorder from occurring. Then the chapter turns to variables common to most therapies regardless of theoretical stance or method. Next the chapter highlights the essential features of and current uses for major therapies used by health psychologists. I have chosen to group the therapies into four broad classes: short-term psychodynamic psychotherapy, cognitive therapy, behavior therapy, and pharmacotherapy.

The Timing of Intervention: An Ounce of Prevention

Earlier, we noted the continuing concern about the growing cost of health care and efficient use of the health care dollar. Currently, about 85% of the health care dollar is devoted to direct hospital or physician care, which is typically after the appearance of a malady (Levit, Lazenby, Cowan, & Letsch, 1991). Of the nearly $752 billion currently spent on health care, the federal government devotes only about $600 million to prevention, about 1% of the health budget (U.S. Public Health Service, 1992). Similarly, less than 2% of the total health care dollar is allocated for

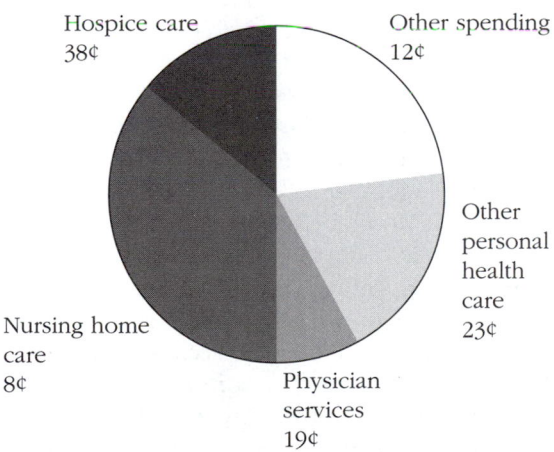

Hospice care
38¢

Other spending
12¢

Other personal health care
23¢

Physician services
19¢

Nursing home care
8¢

FIGURE 5.2 The vast majority of the health care dollar is spent on direct patient services; very little—no more than about 2% total—is spent on research; and only about 1% is spent on preventive research (from Levit et al., 1990).

research of any type. Even of this amount, little is spent on preventive research. Most is used to develop treatments for currently existing disease, including what Pollack (1991) called the medical technology arms race, wherein providers purchase the latest diagnostic and treatment technology, sometimes at costs in the millions for a single instrument, just to stay ahead of the competition.

Beginning around 1962, attention in the mental health field focused on issues of late versus early treatment, and a concerted effort emerged to translate thought into action with practical, community-based programs. But, the concept of prevention applies to physical as well as mental health. Gerald Caplan (1964), one of the principle players in this arena, defined three major types of prevention: primary, secondary, and tertiary prevention.

In broad terms, **primary prevention** is any effort to reduce the incidence of a disease in a population. It seeks ultimately to eradicate a disorder through empirically validated interventions.[1] Many examples of primary prevention are visible in health psychology based on the recognition that high-risk behaviors contribute significantly to diseases such as cardiovascular disease (Perry, Klepp, & Shultz, 1988), addiction, lung cancer (Henderson, Ross, & Pike, 1991), and AIDS (Coates, 1990).

Secondary prevention is treatment of an existing disorder in its early stages, before symptoms become severe and cause irreversible damage. The overall goal is to reduce subsequent problems by intervening in the early stages of a disorder. Secondary prevention depends on early detection of symptoms or markers that identify potential problems. Kivlahan, Marlatt, Fromme, Coppel, and Williams (1990) used this approach in an effort to reduce problem drinking in college students. Their goal was to increase students' ability to control their intake as opposed to total abstinence. The skills training program was partly successful, but

---

[1] A discussion of epidemiology, the science of the distribution and causes of disease, will come in Chapter 6.

there were still reports of occasional heavy drinking bouts after treatment.

Another example is the Swedish Aspirin Low-Dose Trial (SALT) (1991). The subjects were 1360 patients who had suffered but were recovering from a minor stroke or transient ischemic attack. 676 patients were randomly assigned to receive low doses of aspirin. After 32 months, 18% fewer deaths were reported among this group as compared to the remaining group that received conventional medical treatment. Other examples of secondary prevention include exercise for coronary patients and routine testing to detect cervical, breast, or prostate cancer in their early stages.

Tertiary prevention is an attempt to reduce the residual effects of a disorder by containing the severity and shortening the duration of symptoms. Tertiary prevention also attempts to restore people to functional capacity insofar as possible. Many addiction support groups are examples of tertiary rehabilitation efforts. Tertiary care is by far the most common form of practice, whether in medicine, psychiatry, or clinical psychology.

A Surplus of Therapies: Common Themes and Variations

Most people are aware that various psychological therapies have evolved to meet different needs. But they would probably be surprised to find that there are now nearly 400 distinct therapies. In this mass are perhaps 255 psychotherapies with many theoretical orientations representing psychoanalytic, psychodynamic, and existential traditions, among others (Herink, 1980). Also included in this mass are scores of therapies with behavioral or cognitive orientations or both. The four categories of therapies outlined here are primarily for organizational convenience, but they are based on commonly accepted distinctions in therapeutic rationales and techniques.

First, **short-term psychodynamic psychotherapy** (STPP) is generally viewed as a descen-

dant of the Freudian tradition with an emphasis on insight and understanding, even though it is time-limited and more action-oriented than traditional psychoanalysis. The therapist-client relationship and transference is important to therapeutic success (Piper, Joyce, McCallum, & Azim, 1993). The object of the interaction is for the client to confront the self.

Second, cognitive therapies, which are sometimes called **cognitive-behavioral therapies** (CBT), represent an integration of themes from both traditional behavior therapy and dynamic insight therapy. Like short-term psychotherapy and behavior therapy, cognitive therapies are action-oriented and time-limited. Unlike most behavior therapies, cognitive therapies consider the client-therapist relationship important. The focus is on uncovering self-defeating and maladaptive cognitions and then altering perceptions, attitudes, and thought processes.

Behavior therapy is a descendant of learning theory with an emphasis on classical, operant, and modeling processes. Behavior therapies minimize the importance of the therapist-client relationship although they recognize the necessity for a good working relationship. They prefer to focus on direct, quick, and methodical changes in behavior as the primary treatment goal. The goal of the interaction is to help the client confront a problem behavior and change it. Clients are actively involved in the therapy, often contracting about the target behavior to be changed as well as the method of change. BT was at the forefront of the movement to require objective data to show that the specific therapy in question, not some hidden nonspecific factor, produced the desired results.

Health psychologists are not licensed to prescribe and dispense medicines, although debate about whether they should have the privilege is ongoing (DeLeon, Fox, & Graham, 1991; Kingsbury, 1992; May & Belsky, 1992). Still, health psychologists cannot afford to ignore the role that modern **pharmacotherapy** plays in treating both physical and mental disturbance. Health psychologists often work in interdisciplinary teams where multimodal treatment is the norm. Interactions between treatment components can prove problematic, even detrimental to treatment. Without knowledge of how a drug treatment changes mood, cognitive processes, or behavior, the psychologist might overlook signs of progress or come to erroneous conclusions about what components contributed to treatment success.

To aid in standardization of training and the operational specificity of treatment manipulations for outcome research, clinicians have written treatment manuals (Lambert et al., 1988). Training manuals facilitate clinical training and allow researchers to develop rating scales that can assist in outcome research. Training manuals also aid researchers in separating the common factors from the unique factors associated with specific treatment approaches.

Common Denominators: Finding Therapy's Active Ingredient

A perennial problem in comparing the efficacy of various therapies is to determine precisely what caused change in clients and what is unrelated to change. An all too familiar scenario occurs when a therapy has been judged successful, but its success was due to some process that many other therapies also contain. While therapy is in process, any number of factors unrelated to the treatment could produce change in a patient's clinical symptoms. **Spontaneous remission,** for example, is the tendency for certain disorders to remit their symptoms even without outside intervention, with what Schatzberg and Cole (1991) called "the elixir of time" (p. 288).

As a result of extensive research over the past quarter-century, clinicians know much more about these common factors and how they influence the outcome of therapy.[2] Three groups of

common variables are frequently noted: therapist characteristics, therapeutic processes including the therapist-client relationship, and client characteristics.

First, several traits and activities of the therapist exist independently of theoretical orientation. Among the most important are warmth, empathy, positive regard, and support. Others include listening carefully, reflecting, and showing understanding of the client's situation and problem. Most therapists engage in some type of confrontation, but confrontation need not involve hostility or emotionality. Confrontation means only that the therapist will not allow some deceit to interfere with the patient's confronting the problem. Therapists, regardless of their theoretical orientation, also provide many forms of advice, suggestion, encouragement, and persuasion in the course of therapy (Garfield, 1989). Even though many therapists do not subscribe to behaviorist theory, they still give many reinforcements, social and verbal, that move the client in the direction of improvement. Finally, there is a widespread belief that the more experienced the therapist is, the more successful the treatment will be. But data on this subject are far from conclusive, and research is hindered by many problems.

During the therapeutic process, early success and feedback that personal control of symptoms is possible tends to increase the client's perception of personal efficacy. The cognitive changes that are part of this perception occur in a wide variety of therapies and are no longer viewed as unique to a specific therapy.

Another perennial problem in evaluating the therapeutic process is the fact that clients quite often obtain folk therapy from family, friends, clergy—even barbers and bartenders. One study (Cross, Sheehan, & Khan, 1980) showed that people sought advice and counsel outside of therapy to a surprising degree. This behavior occurred more frequently among treated groups than among the untreated control group and was more prevalent among the behaviorally treated group than among the insight treated group. In such a situation, it is difficult to know how much the professionally directed therapy

---

[2] Several excellent comprehensive summaries of common factors in therapy are available including one by Lambert, Shapiro, and Bergin (1988).

contributed to success compared to the nonprofessional counsel.

On the client side, the expectation that improvement will come from the effort of therapy is important. The client may hope for change, but the therapist places on the client a more or less explicit demand for change. The therapist, through a variety of expressed statements, innuendo, and behaviors, may communicate a positive or less than positive belief in the efficacy of the treatment. When the client perceives that the treatment is likely to be successful, the likelihood that treatment will indeed be successful increases. Patients also differ in their motivation for therapy, some coming on their own and others being coerced by family or judicial system to accept an unwanted therapy (Keithly, Samples, & Strupp, 1980). Finally, clients differ in IQ and verbal ability, in their talkativeness and openness, and in the ease with which they establish a trusting relationship with the therapist.

This review of common variables, brief as it is, should serve as a reminder that attributions of success require more than showing that person A was not well before therapy X and was judged healthy afterward. With this background in place, it is now time to look at four intervention techniques.

Short-Term Psychodynamic Psychotherapy: Focus on Feelings

Over the past 25 years, psychotherapy[3] has had to survive several external challenges even as it has gone through a type of identity crisis. The external challenges began with a famous though controversial study in which Eysenck (1952) suggested there was no proof that psychotherapy was effective. Eysenck assembled data showing that psychotherapy was no better than placebo therapy or spontaneous remission.[4]

Nearly 25 years later, several authors used a new quantitative review technique, meta-analysis, to show that various types of psychotherapy were substantially better than placebo therapy (Bergin & Lambert, 1978; Beutler, 1979; Rachman & Wilson, 1980). This position was epitomized in Luborsky, Singer, and Luborsky's (1975) work, a study that contained the much celebrated Dodo Bird conclusion (from Lewis Carroll's *Alice in Wonderland*): "Everyone has won and all [the therapies] must have prizes." Since then, questions of outcome efficacy have been less concerned with establishing the supremacy of one therapy over another (probably a myopic and misdirected effort in the first place) and more concerned with answering the classic question of the best therapy for a particular client with a particular condition. This question rightly assumes that many therapies (though not necessarily all) may be effective, but not equally effective in all circumstances for all people.

A crucial issue, raised in a recent review of psychotherapy with children and adolescents, is as important to the development of critical thinking as it is to the practice of psychology (Weisz, Weiss, & Donenberg, 1992). That is, many of the meta-analyses use so-called research therapy with college student samples as compared to clinical therapy with referred clients. **Research therapy** is often done by people who have been specially trained in the specific therapy using a detailed treatment manual immediately prior to applying the therapy to a well-defined problem with a homogeneous sample of recruited clients. **Clinical**

---

[3] I am using the term *psychotherapy* here in its broadest sense to refer to therapies that focus on changes in the structure of personality—the organization of self—without regard to finer theoretical issues that distinguish the various psychotherapies from each other.

[4] Placebo treatment is typically some form of attention or talk without the direction or focus of the contrast therapy. Eysenck used a figure of 67% for spontaneous remission, a figure that is now regarded as inflated. Lambert's (1976) more recent and better controlled study showed that 40% of clients spontaneously remit their symptoms.

therapy is done by people who have been in practice for varying periods of time with an ongoing, heterogeneous caseload. They often use several different methods because their clients are referred for serious and multiple problems. The problem then is how results obtained in a laboratory clinic can be generalized to a real-world clinical practice. Weisz's group found the problem more critical than some would believe. When they compared laboratory findings with real-world findings, the clinical results were substantially less optimistic than the lab findings would suggest. These results are shown in Figure 5.3.

Psychotherapy's identity crisis, alluded to earlier, stems from the fact that psychotherapy is by no means a unified method nor is it based on a single theoretical perspective. Psychotherapy is practiced by many different professional groups, including psychiatrists, psychologists, social workers, pastoral counselors, and nurses, among others (Strupp, Butler, & Rosser, 1988). Recently, classical long-term psychoanalysis has given way to numerous short-term

psychotherapies—some that still adhere to the psychodynamic tradition, and others that do not. These brief therapies will be the focus of this discussion.

The Background of STPP

Short-term psychodynamic psychotherapy (STPP), sometimes called time-limited therapy, has its roots in Freudian psychoanalysis. STPP is set apart from experiential therapies (Greenberg & Goldman, 1988), which derive from the humanistic client-centered approach of Rogers (1951), and the phenomenological or Gestalt therapy of Perls, Hefferline, and Goodman (1951).[5]

The theory behind long-term psychoanalytic psychotherapy gave a central role to the

---

[5] The article by Greenberg and Goldman contains a review of current training issues in experiential therapy. This article also takes up the issue of empathy as a therapist trait.

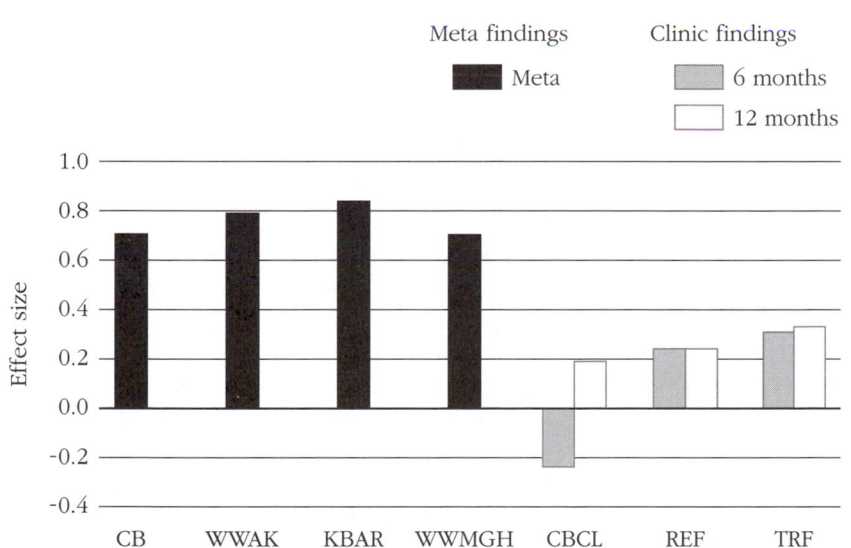

FIGURE 5.3 *Laboratory studies of clinical process may give a distorted impression of therapeutic efficacy, as this figure shows; the effect size from laboratory studies is substantially higher than from real-world clinical studies (from Weisz, Weiss & Donenberg, 1992).*

unconscious, and it emphasized psychic conflicts rooted in distortions in development associated with the psychosexual stages. The predominant treatment techniques were free association and dream analysis. The goal was to facilitate growth of the fixated personality, a type of psychic reconstruction project. The process could take from six months to a year, sometimes even longer. Garfield (1989) cited data showing that the longer psychoanalysis was around, the longer it took to treat patients. In extreme cases, therapy could last as long as 15 years, creating staggering financial burdens. The resulting drawback of long-term therapy is often noted: There is a high drop-out rate, with most clients completing no more than 6 to 8 sessions (Garfield, 1986). Ferenczi and Rank were among the early advocates of brief therapy. There are also tidbits of evidence that Freud was aware of the value of short-term therapy in certain cases. Nonetheless, Freud generally took a negative view of efforts to shorten therapy.

In contrast to the strong theoretical bias of Freudian psychoanalysis, STPP has largely abandoned notions of psychosexual trauma and makes no assumption that one has to "strive for a mythical state of personality transformation" (Garfield, 1989, p. 11). Indeed, the goal of therapy may be simply to develop skills that will carry the person through hard times in the future. STPP focuses on the here and now and is specifically time-limited. Therapy is limited generally to about 20 to 25 sessions, which in practical terms means that therapy should be finished in less than six months. Both therapist and client are pressured to get to the root of the problem quickly and obtain a satisfactory resolution. Finally, dropout problems are reduced and costs contained.

The Practice of STPP

The practice of STPP can be summarized as follows:

1. The therapist focuses efforts directly and quickly on a specific therapeutic goal.

2. The therapist is active and directive.
3. The client also takes an active, participative role.
4. The client has to carry out various active tasks important to the therapeutic process, including homework assignments.
5. Therapy is time-limited with an expectation that both therapist and client understand the criteria for termination (Wells & Phelps, 1990).

In common with most therapies, STPP uses an intake interview to establish the basis of a therapeutic relationship (Garfield, 1989). At the conclusion of the first session, the therapist should have formulated a plan of action for the course of therapy. The therapist continually evaluates the progress of therapy, however, and modifies the approach as necessary. Interpretations of current problems may be derived from everyday circumstances, experiences, and feelings; common sense and logic are as important as theoretical sophistication.

A form of STPP is used in the treatment of depression (Cornes, 1990), and crisis intervention is often modelled on STPP (Ewing, 1990). STPP has been adapted as well to family, marital, and small-group treatment programs.

Applications of STPP in Health Psychology

One example of the use of STPP comes from the work of Christopher Fairburn and his colleagues (Fairburn, Kirk, O'Connor, & Cooper, 1986). They were concerned about the lack of information on the effectiveness of various psychological interventions for use with bulimic patients. Previous research had shown that short-term psychotherapy and behavioral treatments were roughly comparable at short follow-ups, even when the behavioral method had been judged superior at post-treatment. The team used criteria for bulimia preferred in Britain rather than the DSM-III criteria preferred at that time in the United States.

Following detailed manuals, either STPP or cognitive-behavioral therapy (CBT) treatments were provided, lasting for a fixed period of 18 weeks, with 19 total sessions. The STPP sessions were based on the work of Rosen (1979), Bruch (1973), and Stunkard (1976), who all addressed the use of STPP with bulimic, anorexic, and overweight people. A team member who did not know what treatment condition patients belonged to carried out assessments to measure change in clinical symptoms.

One interesting control procedure was used: Clients contracted to not use other therapies during the study, especially during the follow-up period. Thus the maintenance strength of the therapies presumably could be assessed without fear of contamination from competing therapies. The study is also noteworthy because it was a true clinical study, not an analogue study. In other words, the patients were bulimic patients referred from within the hospital catchment area and thus were more representative of real clinical clientele.

Four aspects of the short-term therapy were important. First, the client was directed to pay attention to events and feelings that provoked episodes of overeating. Second, a fact-finding, noninterpretative style was used to help clients recognize and develop confidence in their personal opinions and feelings. Third, clients received information on regulating body weight, dieting, and the potential negative effects of binge eating and purging cycles. Finally, the team attempted to make STPP roughly comparable to CBT in duration and intensity while avoiding intruding specific elements from CBT.

The results showed that both STPP and CBT produced favorable changes in global clinical scores as well as specific indicators related to symptoms of bulimia such as bulimic episodes, vomiting, and weight change. Statistical evaluation of change in these global scores showed that both groups changed significantly over time. The same pattern emerged when general psychopathology and depression indices were analyzed. These changes suggest that both therapies were successful in improving clinical

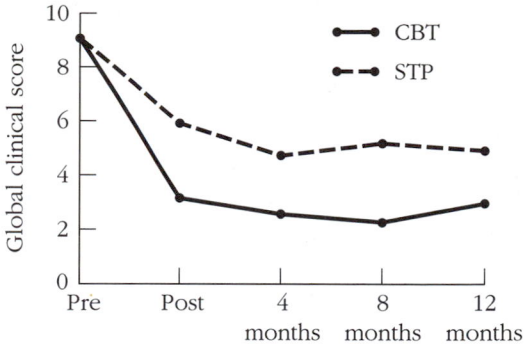

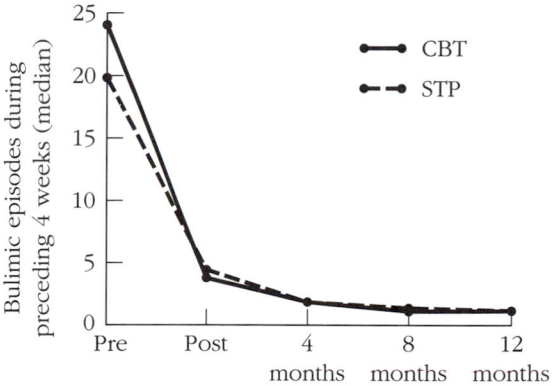

FIGURE 5.4 Changes in global clinical score and bulimic episodes during treatment and follow-up in patients treated with STPP and CBT (from Fairburn, et al., 1986).

symptoms. Throughout the one-year follow-up period, however, the CBT group improved more on global clinical scores and showed lower levels of general psychopathology and lower levels of depression compared to the STPP group. On other specific indices, there was little to choose between the two forms of therapy. Both types of therapy had favorable effects on bulimic episodes, vomiting, eating attitudes (assessed with the EAT scale), and weight gain. Although CBT was usually slightly better, the differences were significant on only one measure, and that was episodes of vomiting at eight-month follow-up.

Cognitive Therapies: Focus on Thoughts

Historically, cognitive therapy (CT) did not evolve until after both psychotherapy and behavior therapy were well advanced. Still, I have chosen to describe CT before behavior therapy because CT represents a link between the internalism of dynamic psychotherapy and the externalism of behavior therapy.

The cognitive therapies have diverse origins and rationales, but they share certain common themes (Mahoney, 1993; Dobson & Shaw, 1988). Hollon and Beck (1986) captured this family resemblance when they defined **cognitive therapy** as "those approaches that attempt to modify existing or anticipated disorders by virtue of altering cognitions or cognitive processes" (p. 443). Cognitive therapists believe that humans actively direct their behavior through internal representations and personal interpretations of external reality. CTs also assume that the cognitive system provides for a wide range of problem-solving strategies. Coping responses reflect how flexible a person is in selecting a strategy to deal with a situation. Another working assumption of most cognitive procedures is that humans have the capacity for self-control. Thus, the methods used in CT often are directed to developing or refining clients' self-control. Finally, cognitive processes (not psychic conflicts) are viewed as interacting causally with learning experiences to affect feelings and behaviors.

Masters, Burish, Hollon, and Rimm (1987) suggested that cognitive methods share common processes that are more or less emphasized. These include rationality, empiricism, repetition, and distraction. **Rationality** uses appeals to logic or reason to bring about changes in people's beliefs or attitudes. **Empiricism** is concerned with a type of personal hypothesis testing. It seeks to confirm or refute beliefs by structuring personal-social situations so one can see the truth or falsity of one's beliefs.

Repetition is founded on the notion that mediating cognitions can be rehearsed and that they will function positively when needed. Finally, **distraction** is a method of redirecting a thought process that is dysfunctional but is not either irrational or inaccurate. Thought-stopping and various cognitive stress coping techniques use distraction.

Just as CTs share common themes, they also share certain fundamental objections to psychodynamic and behavior therapies. CTs generally reject the emphasis on early psychosexual trauma, personality structures, and psychic conflict that is the mark of psychodynamic thinking. CTs also hold that cognitive constructs are more amenable than psychic constructs to operational definition, allowing investigators to directly test the truth or falsity of hypotheses about therapeutic process as opposed to outcome. Finally, CTs tend to resist the mechanistic constructs of the radical behaviorists believing that human behavior is more creative, constructive and interactive than reactive. Here, we review two cognitive therapies: Beck's cognitive therapy and Meichenbaum's self-instructional training (SIT).

Beck's Cognitive Therapy: Testing Faulty Beliefs

Beck's cognitive therapy rejects the primacy of the unconscious in feeling and behavior. It uses logic and persuasion to effect changes, with primary emphasis on empirical testing of belief systems. Beck believes that people carry on internal dialogues that become virtually reflexive and impossible to turn off.

Three negative cognitions play a major role in depression, according to Beck. These are a negative view of self, a negative view of the world, and a negative view of the future. Depressed people may think that they are worthless, unloved, a burden to others, and incapable of making positive contributions to society or others. At the extreme, they may think

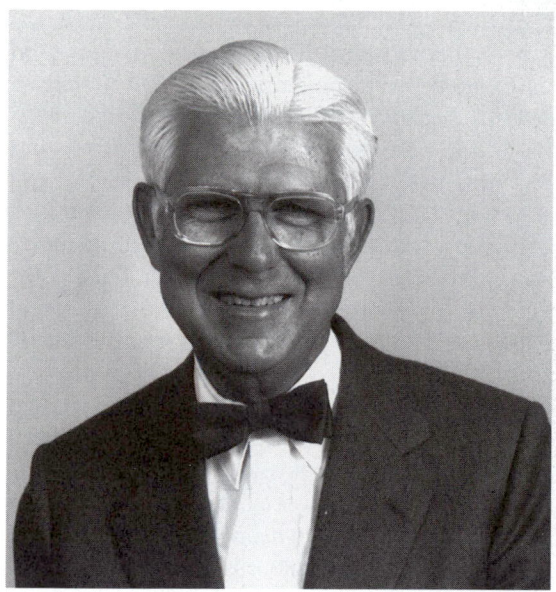

FIGURE 5.5 *Aaron Beck has devoted most of his professional life to the study of depression and development of a cognitive therapy to those suffering from its effects.*

they are so worthless, there is no point in going on, and suicide is a justifiable escape.

Beck teaches clients to examine their thought processes critically and to observe the connection between erroneous beliefs and inappropriate emotional reactions. The therapeutic process includes language techniques to replace reflexive self-defeating labels, homework assignments to test belief systems, and behavioral experiments designed to provide the client with self-correcting information about themselves and their beliefs. The behavioral experiments are graded to control difficulty and increase the likelihood of success. Clients are taught to use three core questions or prompts for self-control: What is the *evidence* for or against this belief? What *alternative explanations* may be reasonable in this situation? Even if true, is it as bad as it seems *(implication)*?

Beck's cognitive therapy was developed as part of his long-standing interest in depression. His treatment method has often been compared to standard medical interventions for depression.[6] After reviewing various studies, Hollon and Beck (1986) concluded that cognitive therapy is as effective, but not necessarily more effective, than pharmacotherapy for acute depressive episodes. One of the potential strengths is that treatment with cognitive therapy has a **prophylactic effect:** In other words, it appears to prevent the recurrence of depressive episodes in the future. There is disagreement on whether this preventive effect is found with pharmacotherapy. Schatzberg and Cole (1991) maintained that prophylactic effects occur with pharmacotherapy, but pharmacotherapy studies reviewed by Hollon and Beck showed no such effect.

Self-Instructional Training: Mediating Cognitions

Donald Meichenbaum (1977, 1985) is known for a number of innovations in cognitive behavior therapy (CBT) including self-instructional training (SIT) and stress inoculation training. Meichenbaum believes, as Beck does, that self-talk directly influences what people do. Self-talk is a form of self-instruction that, for some people, can lead to such problem behaviors as impulsiveness, explosive anger discharges, and anxiety about situations such as taking tests or public performances.

SIT involves five steps. First, the therapist models how to carry out a given task and at the same time verbalizes the sequence of steps used. Then, the client carries out the task while the therapist verbalizes the sequence. Third, the client carries out the task while saying the sequence out loud. Next, the client carries out the

---

[6] The most common medical interventions used tricyclics (TCAs) such as imipramine, or MAOIs (mono-amine oxidase inhibitors) when TCAs proved ineffective. More recently, new antidepressive medications have appeared, such as Paxil, which comes from a class of agents that are selective serotonin reuptake inhibitors. We will discuss this type of medication later.

task while inaudibly whispering the sequence. Finally, the client carries out the task while thinking through the sequence with no external verbal cues. This procedure is highly structured, and it provides for significant practice and repetition. Because behavioral sequences play a prominent role, and forms of differential reinforcement are used, the approach is viewed as a cognitive-behavior strategy.

SIT has been used to treat anxiety disorders (Woodward & Jones, 1980), agoraphobia (Emmelkamp & Mersch, 1982), and obesity (Dunkel & Glaros, 1978). One major criticism of research on SIT is that it is often conducted as an analogue study on trivial problems with nonclinical populations. Thus the external validity of the procedure for use with a true clinical population is often questionable. Studies using SIT with clinical populations of agoraphobics, for example, do not show SIT to be as effective as purely behavioral approaches.

Applications of CBT: The Multimodal Approach

Although there are numerous independent cognitive and behavior therapies, the more common practice is to use a combination of intervention strategies, a practice called **multimodal treatment.** One research team headed by Matthew Sanders (1989) used this approach to treat recurrent abdominal pain (RAP) in school children. RAP occurs in about 10 to 15% of school-aged children. Only about 5 to 10% of these cases have an organic etiology, although subtle physiological dysfunctions may explain some cases. In addition, pharmacological treatments have not proved effective. This leaves a vast majority of the cases with unknown etiology and no viable treatment. Researchers speculate that psychosocial forces may play some etiological role. Both social learning and operant learning theory have been invoked as psychological explanations of RAP. Cognitive-behavior therapies then provide treatments that are consistent with this theoretical point of view.

In the Sanders project, the behavioral component combined self-monitoring of pain with differential reinforcement of other behavior (DRO) for longer pain-free periods. Self-monitoring is widely used as a means to alter high-risk behaviors such as eating, exercise, and smoking rate. The cognitive component also combined several components. These included self-instruction, self-efficacy statements, self-delivered rewards, relaxation training, and imaginal (distractor) techniques for pain control. Generalization procedures and relapse prevention also were part of the treatment package.

Half the 16 subjects were randomly assigned to receive the eight-session multimodal treatment; the other half were assigned to a wait-list control. The wait-list group received the same treatment later. Multiple assessments from the children, their parents, and their teachers were obtained pretreatment, at two interim test times, posttreatment, and at a three-month follow-up. The results, shown in Figure 5.6, provided convincing evidence that the treatment package lowered both the report of pain and the frequency of pain behavior. Note that the control group improved somewhat over the course of the treatment, but the treated group improved more rapidly and eliminated pain more completely. The results on self-reports of pain were significant by Phase 2. More of the treated group maintained their gains at a three-month follow-up: 87.5% of the treated group were completely pain-free, while only 37% of the untreated group were completely pain-free.

Another example of multimodal treatment comes from the work of Susan Jay (Jay, Elliott, Woody, & Siegel, 1991). Jay's team was concerned about the distress, fear, and pain experienced by children undergoing repeated bone marrow aspirations (BMA) or lumbar punctures (LP). The repeated procedures typically lead to high anticipatory anxiety that makes completing the next procedure even more difficult.

Jay's group had found earlier that Valium was effective for anticipatory anxiety, but CBT provided coping skills that were useful during the entire BMA procedure. Based on these findings,

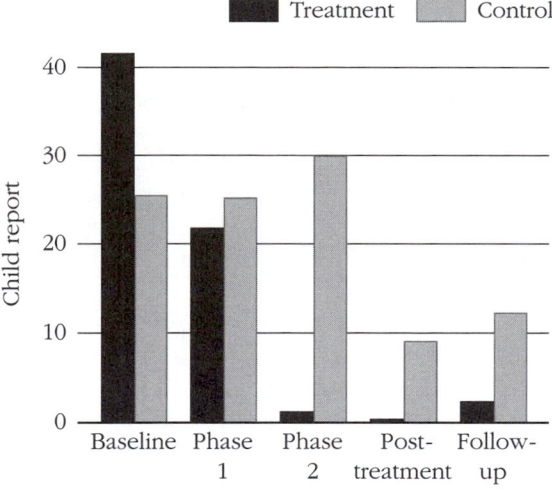

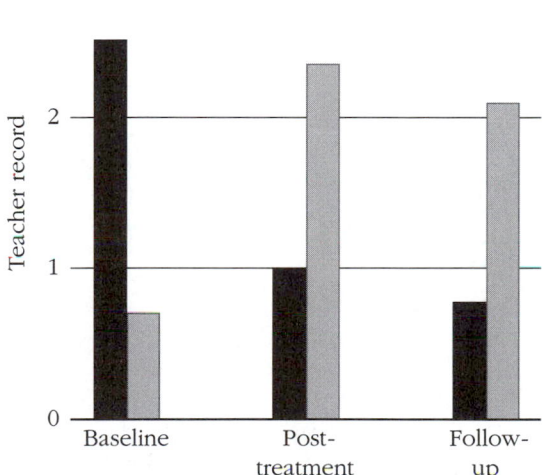

FIGURE 5.6 Mean intensity of child-reported pain across treatment phases, and mean frequency of pain behavior (adapted from Sanders et al., 1989).

the group believed that combining Valium and CBT would have a synergistic effect on distress measures. A **synergistic effect** occurs when the combined effect of two or more treatments is much better than would be predicted by simply adding together the effects of the separate treatments (Schatzberg & Cole, 1991).

More than half the children (45) received the multimodal CBT package by itself, while the remaining children (38) received the CBT package plus the oral Valium. The CBT package consisted of filmed modeling (following the work of Melamed, 1978), breathing exercises, imagery distraction, positive incentive, and behavioral rehearsal. Filmed modeling used peer models to show children what to expect when confronting a particular medical procedure. Breathing exercises involved children's taking a deep breath and letting it out slowly with a hissing sound.[7] In the imagery distraction technique, children heard a story about the medical procedure with a personal hero playing the lead role. They were also taught how to form a pleasant mental image (a trip to Disneyland, for example). Each child then had the choice of which imagery distraction to use. Children could also earn a trophy (positive incentive) for doing the best they could, an effort the team described as trying to transform the medical procedure into a challenge.[8] In the behavioral rehearsal procedure, younger children used the real medical instruments to administer a BMA or LP to a doll while older children carried out a guided demonstration of the procedure. Finally, all children in the Valium group got the same CBT sequence immediately after taking an oral dose of Valium. Administration of Valium was timed so that the peak effect of the drug would occur just after the CBT sequence but at the beginning of the BMA or LP procedure. This might be considered a flaw in the design since the drug could alter the effect of CBT.

The results showed a significant reduction from baseline to posttreatment in behavioral distress, heart rate, and self-reported pain. There was no change in self-reported fear. Further, Valium did not enhance the treatment effect as

---

[7] Some argue that there is an active attention distraction element in deep breathing, qualifying it as a cognitive technique.

[8] The situation was structured so that all children were successful in earning the trophy, making it a noncontingent incentive as opposed to a positive reward.

expected, suggesting that the major effect came from the cognitive-behavioral treatment alone. There was evidence that Valium did interfere with learning coping skills, since the Valium group experienced only about one-third the reduction in distress compared to the CBT group. The authors speculated that since Valium is a benzodiazepam and an arousal-reducing drug, it could have interfered with the children's ability to focus on the instructions in CBT and to confront the medical procedure in a masterful fashion. In conclusion, note that although CBT had a statistically positive effect, the clinical significance is equivocal since distress levels remained at an unacceptably high level in some children.

Before leaving this section, it is instructive to look at a meta-analysis comparing STPP to alternative therapies—here, primarily cognitive therapies. Svartberg and Stiles (1991) found that STPP was slightly superior to no treatment at the end of therapy but not at follow-up. Further, they found that STPP was inferior to the cognitive or cognitive-behavioral therapies at the end of treatment as well as at 12 months' follow-up. The results suggested that the cognitive therapies may provide coping skills that continue to mature and endure.

Behavior Therapies: Focus on Observable Actions

It is likely that behavioral principles have been used to influence human behavior since the beginning of social systems. Pliny the Elder described an aversive counterconditioning procedure used to treat alcoholism (Franks, 1969). In 1798, Itard used systematic reinforcement to teach a feral child basic social skills and the rudiments of speech (DuBois, 1970). Yet the backbone of current behavioral treatments came from the work of people like Pavlov, Watson, Skinner, and Wolpe (Pichot, 1989).

Pavlov's (1927) work in classical conditioning quickly led to a method called **experimental**

psychopathology, producing laboratory analogues of clinical conditions such as phobias. A woman associate of Pavlov's, Schenger-Krestovikova, published an early study on experimental neurosis in dogs. Studies of this nature had implications for treatment based on the logic that if a conditioning process could produce pathology, that same pathology could be remedied by reversing the conditioning process.

Watson built on the Pavlovian legacy even as he tried to make the fledgling discipline a more scientific enterprise. His published report of conditioned emotions in 11-month-old Albert is a clinical analogue of experimental neurosis in humans (Watson & Rayner, 1920). Later, Mary Cover Jones (1924) used a counterconditioning procedure to reverse emotional conditioning in a child named Peter. Although the clinical community probably did not fully appreciate the importance of what Watson and Jones did at the

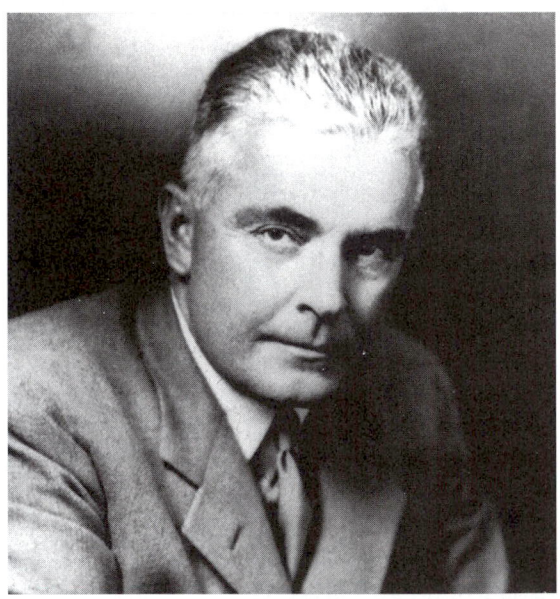

FIGURE 5.7 *John Watson, the founding father of modern behaviorism, carried out early research on the conditioning of emotions, work that also led to one of the early attempts to modify a psychiatric symptom through behavior therapy.*

time, it was the beginning of behavioral therapy for clinical symptoms.

Skinner proposed that behavior changes because of consequences. A protege of Skinner's, Ogden Lindsley, was hard at work by the early 1950s using principles of reinforcement in the mental health arena. He was able to get severely disturbed schizophrenics to engage in cooperative behavior that depended on speaking to one another (Lindsley, Skinner, & Solomon, 1953). It was apparently this group that first used the term *behavior therapy,* a term that was narrowly defined as the application of operant conditioning to psychological problems. Most people now use **behavior modification** to refer to procedures that are operant based, and **behavior therapy** as a general term for any therapy based on learning principles.

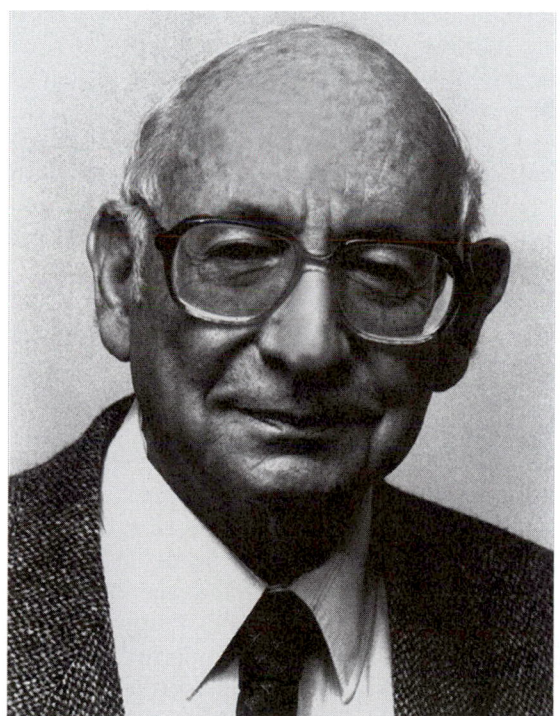

FIGURE 5.8 After becoming disappointed with the success of traditional psychotherapy, Joseph Wolpe developed a behavioral method now called systematic desensitization.

Joseph Wolpe, a South African psychiatrist, became dissatisfied because traditional psychotherapy seemed to produce no lasting effects. He came across contemporary work on experimental neurosis (Masserman, 1943) that served as a model for his own laboratory studies of experimental neurosis. Wolpe synthesized his insights in a classic method, systematic desensitization, which he detailed in his classic work, *Psychotherapy by Reciprocal Inhibition* (1958).

The Rationale of Behavior Therapy

Behavior therapy rests on certain assumptions about human nature and the environmental stimuli presumed to control behavior. A fundamental tenet is that all behavior is learned—whether it is good or bad, safe or risky, whether it occurs at home, school, church, or doctor's office. The sequel to this tenet, indeed the logical foundation for behavioral treatment, is equally important: If a behavior is learned, it can be unlearned. Thus, even maladaptive, high-risk behaviors can be changed by identifying and altering the stimuli that control the problem behavior.

In this system, a person's history of conditioning and reinforcement is most important, whereas intrapsychic conflicts are like the proverbial ghost in the machine. BT views the emphasis on personality categories and diagnostic criteria as unnecessary since maladaptive behavior is only a matter of faulty conditioning, ill-timed reinforcements, or lack of learning. Another hallmark of the behavioral approach is this maxim: If something goes wrong in treatment, look at the program before blaming the client. BT continually evaluates and adjusts treatment based on data collected in process.

Although behavior therapies share many common beliefs, there is still no single unifying theory. There are signs that BTs are becoming more eclectic, including the recognition that treatment success may stem from altered cognitive processes as much as from direct behavior changes.

The Varieties of Behavior Therapy

We noted earlier that scores of behavior therapies have emerged over the years. Among the BTs identified by Masters and his colleagues (1987) are biofeedback, relaxation training, systematic desensitization, assertion training, modeling, contingency management, punishment, and aversive conditioning. Efforts are under way to codify the procedures of specific therapies and to standardize training at the graduate level (Bootzin & Ruggill, 1988). I will describe only applications of biofeedback, relaxation training, systematic desensitization, and stimulus control in health psychology.

Three Faces of Biofeedback: Testing, Education, and Treatment

In principle, **biofeedback** is a well-defined and fairly simple procedure that feeds back information about an internal physical state. It is based on the science of communication and control, **cybernetics,** which assumes that organisms regulate themselves using information fed back to the system from the environment. A simple example of using biofeedback occurs when we step on a scale and use that data to help regulate our weight. In clinical and research setups, biofeedback takes a physiological signal from the body, amplifies it, and then feeds it back, usually in auditory or visual form, to the person who provided the signal in the first place.

To illustrate, consider the procedure of electroencephalography and the brain wave alpha (8–12 Hz). **Electroencephalography** (EEG) measures activity from the brain's neurons. The alpha brain wave received great attention in the 1960s because of its observed link to meditative trance and ecstasy. In its normal state, the brain wave is really a mixture of signals. Further, it is too weak to detect directly. To correct these two problems, the signal first has to be filtered to eliminate noise and competing signals. Filtering eliminates signals faster than alpha (for example, alert signals in the 30 Hz range) as well as signals slower than alpha (drowsy signals below 8 Hz, such as delta and theta waves). Second, the brain signal must be amplified, in some cases as much as a million-fold. Once the signal is strong enough, it can be used to activate an alerting stimulus, such as a tone or a light to tell the person when the desired brain wave is present. EEG biofeedback has been widely used as a means to test hypotheses about brain function and to detect brain pathology. EEG biofeedback may be useful in the treatment of insomnia and epilepsy, but its overall efficacy is not demonstrated. Kamiya (1969) did demonstrate that alpha waves could be produced through EEG biofeedback, but the hoped-for correlate of alpha waves, a state of transcendent ecstasy, never did materialize.

Electromyography (EMG) uses information from the muscles to detect activity (tension) in the muscle fiber membrane (Sturgis & Gramling, 1988). EMG might be used to teach a client to recognize tension that accompanies stress, or to aid a patient in learning relaxation as part of treatment—examples of the teaching aspect of biofeedback.

In clinical treatment programs, EMG biofeedback is often used to treat muscle contraction (tension) headaches, chronic low back pain, and neuromuscular rehabilitation of stroke victims (Agras, 1984). In a neuromuscular reeducation program, a patient would receive information about low-level muscle activation in the form of a visible or auditory signal. The patient might not be able to sense that attempts to move the right arm did produce some muscle activation. Yet the EMG could detect even slight changes in activation. The clinician selects a threshold value for the feedback signal to come on that is initially well within the patient's reach. As the program progresses, the patient is challenged to increase the level of muscle activation. To provide this challenge, the biofeedback equipment is set so that the feedback signal comes on at a slightly higher level than before. Gradually, the patient may regain some control of overt muscle movement. Then, conventional muscular rehabilitation programs may take over to further aid recovery of motor control.

Assessment of cardiovascular activity usually depends on the electrocardiogram, sphygmomanometer, or vasomotor activity. These indicators of heart function have been used in several biofeedback applications. The **electrocardiogram** (ECG) traces electrical impulses from the heart reflecting the activation pattern at the sinoatrial node, which is the heart's primary pacemaker. Abnormal ECGs may indicate the presence of defects such as myocardial infarcts (scar tissue), myocardial ischemia, or arrhythmias. ECG biofeedback has been used in attempts to control arrhythmias.

The sphygmomanometer is the instrument commonly used to measure blood pressure. Blood pressure readings are taken at two points: when the heart is pumping out with force (the **systolic** pressure) and when the heart is at rest (the **diastolic** pressure) (Malasanos, Barkauskas, & Stoltenberg-Allen, 1990). Diastolic pressure is significant because it reflects residual pressure in the system, or pressure that is always there. Blood pressure biofeedback has been used to try to reduce high blood pressure. Often, this procedure produces statistically significant but clinically meaningless change. Stated in other terms, blood pressure may go down enough to be a reliable statistical finding, but the change often is so small from a clinical point of view that it does not change the client's health risk. Further, the changes produced through blood pressure biofeedback often could be brought about just as well by less expensive methods, such as relaxation training (Lustman & Sowa, 1983). In later chapters, we will look at biofeedback techniques and consider how useful they may be in treating a variety of health problems.

Relaxation Training: The Aspirin of Tension Therapy

Relaxation training is the brainchild of Edmund Jacobson, who first wrote about it in 1938. The classic method is progressive muscle relaxation (PMR) or deep muscular relaxation, but there are other relaxation training methods such as autogenics (Schultz & Luthe, 1959) and Benson's (1975) secular meditation. For modern clinicians, the definitive relaxation manual probably is still the one by Bernstein and Borkovec (1978). The major principles and procedures of PMR have become very accessible, even to the extent that PMR is included in some self-help programs. Thus, just as aspirin is inexpensive and readily available, yet powerful in a wide range of applications, so relaxation training has become one of the most economical, widely used, and powerful methods for coping with tension.

Learning progressive muscle relaxation requires the client to work through a sequence of active tension-relaxation exercises for 16 major muscle groups. The sequence typically begins with the preferred arm since tensing a bicep is a

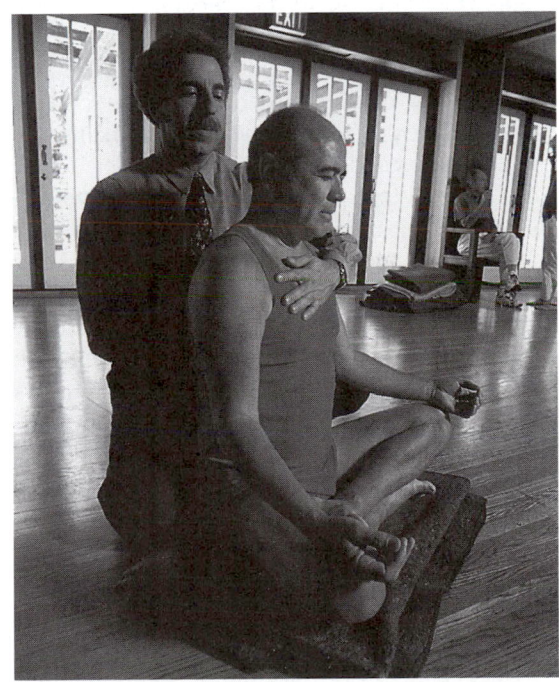

FIGURE 5.9 Patients may learn relaxation with professional help as this person is doing, under the guidance of Dr. Dean Ornish, or with the aid of self-help manuals and tapes.

quick and effective way to experience the difference between tension and relaxation. Then, individual muscle groups are alternately tensed and relaxed from the head to the feet. The tension phase lasts for about 10–15 seconds and the relaxation phase for about 15–20 seconds. Each muscle group is tensed and relaxed 2–3 times before moving to the next muscle group. Early sessions may take as long as 45–75 minutes, but once the skill is acquired, relaxation may be induced in as little as 5–15 minutes.

Clinical applications of PMR are extensive, including treatment of migraine (Sorbi, Tellegen, & du Long, 1989), sleep onset insomnia (Friedman, Bliwise, Yesavage, & Salom, 1991), tension headaches, hypertension, test anxiety, performance anxiety, flight phobias, and Raynaud's disease (Pinkerton, Hughes, & Wenrich, 1982). PMR is used with children suffering from stress-related symptoms (Smith & Womack, 1987) and with cancer patients undergoing various treatments (Burish et al., 1988; Decker, Cline-Elsen, & Gallagher, 1992).

Walsh, Dale, and Anderson (1977), working with a group of clients with essential hypertension, provided evidence that either relaxation or biofeedback can be used effectively to lower blood pressure up to a year after treatment. Blanchard's group (1986, 1989) also studied hypertensive patients on medications. They obtained a significant result, however, showing that thermal biofeedback was successful in 65% of the cases as compared to a 35% success rate with relaxation training. Finally, Blanchard's group also compared relaxation and biofeedback in three headache groups: migraine, tension, and combined migraine-tension. Relaxation alone led to significant improvement in all three groups, but biofeedback led to significant additive gains. In the tension headache group, 73% improved greatly; 52% in the migraine group improved greatly.

The combined results suggest that a number of clinical symptoms can be treated successfully with relaxation training, but caution must be exercised against overgeneralizing. In addition, although relaxation training is generally viewed as a behavioral procedure, there is a distinct possibility that it leads to changes in cognitions and to improved perceptions of self-efficacy (Smith, 1988). Thus, even theoretical issues of what is changed in the process of relaxation training are not resolved.

Systematic Desensitization: Counterconditioning Fears

Assume for a moment that you have a deep-seated fear of going to the doctor's office and getting a shot. The fear is not just a minor fear; it is paralyzing. How can you get rid of it? The preferred standard treatment is systematic desensitization. Presumably, desensitization is based on classical conditioning, but there is still a controversy over the real mechanism behind it, and alternative theories have been offered.[9] Wolpe (1958) called his procedure psychotherapy by reciprocal inhibition, and he explained the logic of it in depth; here, this rationale is necessarily only briefly sketched.

First, fear is a multifaceted response, with behavioral, cognitive, and physiological components. The physiological components include such things as altered heart rate, breathing, perspiration, and stomach and muscle tension. In the process of conditioning, similar stimuli (recall Albert's fear of white furry objects) become conditioned and will also trigger a fear reaction. When arousal does occur, the cognitive system tends to attach the associated fear label, and operant escape behavior will follow closely.

Second, Wolpe was aware of the principle of reciprocal inhibition in the autonomic nervous system (ANS), which is that when the sympathetic system is aroused, the parasympathetic system must be relatively quiet, and vice versa. One correlate of sympathetic arousal is high muscular tension.

The next part of Wolpe's reasoning involves several elements but can be summarized this

---

[9] Alternative explanations usually invoke extinction, habituation, or shaping and modeling.

way. Since conditioned internal arousal triggers the full-blown fear response, it should be possible to countercondition these internal cues thereby preventing the fear response from occurring. Relaxation is a behavioral switch that controls (turns off) sympathetic arousal. Further, Wolpe reasoned that the power of a stimulus to induce fear could be controlled by manipulating the intensity of the stimulus. To do so, he used hierarchies of feared stimuli, which is to say stimuli ranked from low fear arousal to high fear arousal. Then, he asked clients to imagine items from the fear hierarchy, a process called **emotive imagery.**[10]

In its complete form, **systematic desensitization** depends on training in deep muscle relaxation, constructing a hierarchy of feared objects, and imagining the objects while in a state of relaxation. While the rationale may seem complex, it is remarkably simple: If a person relaxes while imagining a feared object, the object will become associated with relaxation, and the person will be counterconditioned to not fear the object. Reducing fear to a low-fear stimulus spreads (generalizes) upward in the hierarchy by reducing fear to higher-fear stimuli even though these higher-fear stimuli have not yet been paired with relaxation. As the client pairs more intense images with relaxation, fear is gradually eliminated even from the most feared object. The term **desensitization,** then, means to remove the sensitizing power of a feared object.

Systematic desensitization has been used widely to treat simple phobias and sexual dysfunction (see Emmelkamp, 1986, for a review). It has also been used to treat so-called blood phobics, people who need to be able to tolerate medical procedures. Morrow and Morrell (1982) used desensitization to treat cancer patients who had developed conditioned aversion responses, including nausea, to chemotherapy.

Stimulus Control: Altering the Environment

Operant techniques assume that behavior changes because of the consequences of behavior and that various stimuli in the environment become associated with the behavior as well. These stimuli may then become powerful cues that trigger the same behavior later. For example, watching television may become a stimulus for snacking, making it difficult to control weight. Reading in bed may be a nice relaxing way to go to sleep; but if done routinely, reading may become a stimulus to become sleepy even when one is reading material that is demanding and important. Stimulus control has been adapted to a wide range of problem behaviors including smoking reduction, weight control, study habits, and sleep disturbance.

There are compelling reasons to attempt to develop a behavioral method for treating insomnia. Insomnia occurs in more than 25% of people aged 60 and older, and it becomes more prevalent with age. Insomnia customarily has been treated through pharmacotherapy. In the 1960s and 1970s, the drugs of choice were typically barbiturates (Gillin, 1991). Now, the treatment of choice is a sedative-hypnotic benzodiazepine (Schatzberg & Cole, 1991).[11] Unfortunately, drug treatment becomes more problematic and risky with age due to altered metabolic function and sleep-related respiratory impairments that may be exaggerated with sedative medication.

Morin and Azrin (1988) wanted to provide a method to treat geriatric insomnia patients, and they decided to compare a traditional stimulus control method against a cognitive imagery treatment. Both these active interventions were compared against a wait-list control group who were promised treatment six weeks later. This project did not use a pharmacotherapy group, though all subjects were screened with regard to

[10] Besides emotive imagery, stimuli can be presented with pictures. Also, desensitization can be carried out *in vivo*—in other words, in the real world with real objects.

[11] The use of barbiturates is declining now that more effective drugs are available with fewer negative side effects.

current medications. Also, subjects were selected only if they complained of **sleep-maintenance insomnia,** the inability to stay asleep, as distinguished from **sleep-onset insomnia,** the inability to get to sleep. Still, the technique described here is effective for both sleep-maintenance or sleep-onset insomniacs (Engle-Friedman, Bootzin, Hazlewood, & Tsao, 1992).

Morin and Azrin used a variation of a stimulus control procedure introduced by Bootzin, Engle-Friedman, and Hazelwood (1983). The procedure consists of instructing the client to implement a set of behaviors designed to control the major stimuli involved in sleep onset and maintenance. Six behaviors are identified.

1. Go to bed at night only when sleepy.
2. Use the bed for sleep and sex only. Do not use the bed for reading, TV watching, work, or worry.
3. If sleep does not come within 15–20 minutes, or sleep does not return after waking in 15–20 minutes, get out of bed, and return only when sleepy again.
4. Repeat step 3 as often as necessary through the night.
5. Get up in the morning at the same time regardless of the amount of sleep the previous night.
6. Do not nap during the day.

The imagery training procedure, a variation of the counting sheep technique, required the client to imagine a sequence of six common objects, a candle, a lightbulb, an hourglass, a kite, a stairway, and a palm tree on a beach. Guided instruction and practice was provided before clients used the procedure in the nightly routine. The rationale of the technique is that the mind will become quiescent if it is focused on neutral as opposed to arousing objects or events.

Analysis of the data showed that both the stimulus control and imagery groups improved significantly compared to the control group. These differences are shown in Figure 5.10. Although the stimulus control group made greater gains than the imagery group—gains that

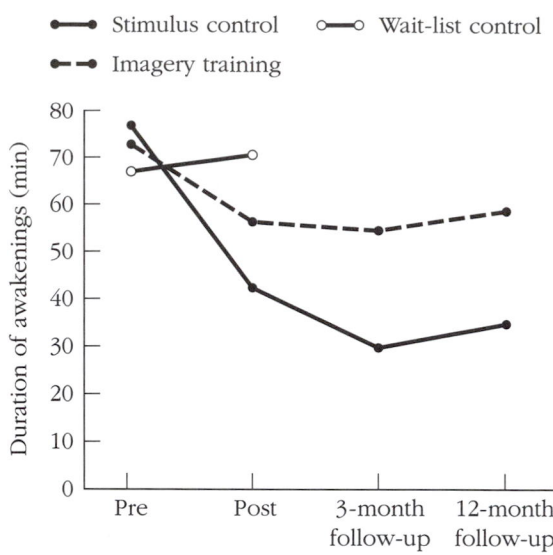

FIGURE 5.10   *These data show the effectiveness of stimulus control compared to imagery training and a wait-list control group at the end of treatment and at 12 months' follow-up (from Morin & Azrin, 1988).*

were maintained at 3 months' and 12 months' follow-up, the differences were not significant. On a subjective measure of satisfaction, the stimulus group was significantly more satisfied with the progress of their treatment than the imagery group. Sleep partners were also more satisfied with the stimulus control procedure.

In sum, the procedures described here suggest that behavioral methods may be used effectively to intervene in a variety of health conditions (headaches and pain, for example), to alter high-risk behaviors (overeating, for example), or to alter a psychological state (fear or anxiety, for example). Note, however, that the intervention's success or failure is often related to a complex set of interactive factors (patient, condition, context, therapist, and so forth). Further, clinicians have to be wary of claiming success for an intervention that has only statistical, not clinical, importance. Finally, in current practice, behavioral techniques are often combined with other methods, such as cognitive and pharmacological interventions, in a type of multimodal therapy. We turn now to the last category of health interventions, those involving medications.

Clinical Pharmacology: Focus on Neurochemistry

Probably the most commonly used biomedical intervention is **pharmacotherapy,** the use of drugs to alter physical or mental symptoms in patients. Pharmacological agents have become not only the socially preferred means of treatment, but sometimes the overused and abused means of treatment (Avorn et al., 1992). There are more than 70,000 prescription drugs and more than 200,000 over-the-counter preparations on the market. In 1990, U.S. expenditures reached $32.3 billion for prescription drugs and $22.3 billion for nonprescription drugs (Levit et al., 1991).

Still, many health care professionals do not share the medical establishment's enthusiasm for drug therapy. The division of opinion tends to break down along disciplinary lines. The medical profession, including psychiatrists, tends to overvalue drugs, whereas psychologists and other nonmedical clinicians tend to be skeptical or devalue drugs (Klerman, 1988). Further, the value judgment is usually based on discrepant views of etiology: The medical profession is prone to suspect biological etiology, which justifies drug treatment. Nonmedical health care providers are more likely to suspect psychosocial etiology and often express the view that drugs mask psychological symptoms and interfere with therapy rather than aid it.

Klerman (1988) noted three reasons psychologists, psychiatrists, and mental health professionals need to be aware of issues in psychopharmacology. First, large numbers of clients probably use recreational drugs or are receiving drugs for medical purposes. Treatment decisions may be misguided and judgments of success or failure erroneous if the therapist does not know the client's drug history. Second, treatment decisions are based on outcome studies that compare psychotherapy to drug therapy or some combination of therapies. Finally, a continued significant thrust in research and theory is to explain how chemical substances affect various aspects of cognitive processing and behavior.

Basic Terminology in Pharmacology

The science of **pharmacology** is concerned with drugs and their physiological effects, including drugs' ability to alter cell function. **Psychopharmacology** is concerned with how drugs influence the brain, change mood, alter cognitive processes, and modify behavior. The term **drug** refers to any substance that alters bodily functions, changes mental processes, and influences behavior. The term **medication** refers to drugs used specifically for the purpose of preventing illness or restoring health. Drugs that produce psychological changes are **psychotropic** (or psychoactive) drugs. The changes they bring about result from interactions with brain **neurotransmitters,** or chemicals that permit neurons to communicate with each other.

Problematic Issues in Pharmacology

Whatever the type of medication, drugs can and often do have **side effects,** outcomes separate from the intended change in body function or symptom. Not all side effects are undesirable, but when negative effects are known to occur, they are called **contraindications.** A commonly cited example is the appearance of tardive dyskinesia from prolonged use of antipsychotic drugs. **Tardive dyskinesia** is marked by involuntary, irregular muscle movements, including tongue rolling, hand clenching, grimacing, and pelvic thrusts.

Three potentially negative effects occur from prolonged use of prescription drugs: substance dependence, substance tolerance, and substance withdrawal. In **substance dependence,** the person loses control over the use of a substance. **Substance tolerance** occurs when the drug does not produce the same effect as it first did, and the person has to increase the dose to get the same effect. Finally, **substance withdrawal** consists of unpleasant physical and emotional symptoms that occur when the person quits using a drug after using it for a long period of time.[12]

Two other problems in pharmacotherapy should be noted. First, there is a problem with **polypharmacy,** prescribing multiple medicines for patients. Drug interactions can produce unpredictable problems, exaggerate negative side effects, or lead to physical crises (such as hypertensive crisis) or even death (Schatzberg & Cole, 1991). Second, prescribing drugs for a **nonapproved use** is a widespread practice. In such cases, the drug is used to treat symptoms on the basis of informal clinical experience or preliminary data from clinical trials but prior to approval of the use by the Food and Drug Administration (FDA). One example is the use of imipramine to treat agoraphobia.

Drugs are classified in various ways: by chemical structure, by mode of neurochemical action, by mode of psychological action, or by clinical use. Classifying drugs by structure, we might speak of the phenothiazines, the tricyclics, or the benzodiazepines. Classifying drugs by neurochemical action, we might speak of the monoamine oxidase inhibitors or neuroleptics. Psychomotor stimulants or hallucinogens are examples of drugs classified by psychological effect. To refer to a drug as an antipsychotic, antidepressant, or antianxiety agent is to use a clinical form of classification. Here, we use the clinical classification scheme.

The Antidepressants: Tricyclics and Inhibitors

Pharmacotherapy for depression is as old as written history. The ancient medical literature of the Hindus reveals that they used a ruwolfia extract, called the medicine of sad men, to treat depressed people. Modern drug therapy has used three major drugs: tricyclic antidepressants (TCAs), monoamine oxidase inhibitors (MAOIs), and selective serotonin reuptake inhibitors (SSRIs). The TCAs and the MAOIs were discovered accidentally while looking for treatments for schizophrenia and tuberculosis, respectively. Two common TCAs are amitriptyline (Elavil) and imipramine (Tofranil).[13] Phenelzine (Nardil) and isocarboxazid (Marplan) are among the MAOIs (Potter, Rudorfer, & Manji, 1991).

TCAs were originally thought to work through blocking the neuronal reuptake of norepinephrine or serotonin. It is now known that their operation is more complex, including effects on both pre- and postsynaptic receptors and other neurotransmitter systems. Although TCAs are approved for treatment of depression, certain aspects of the drug action are important to understand. TCAs are slow acting, typically taking between two and four weeks to show any effect. In clinical practice, treatment may last as long as 6 to 12 months. There are also problematic side effects, including dry mouth and eyes, heartburn, urinary hesitance (with prolonged use), memory problems, speech blockage, confusion, and, infrequently, visual hallucinations. Nicotine and barbiturates are known to cause TCAs to break down, thus reducing their effect. TCAs have found their way into nonapproved but frequent clinical use. Nonapproved uses include treatment of insomnia, headache, agoraphobia with panic attacks, chronic pain, and bulimia.

MAOIs were typically prescribed for depression when the TCAs had not proved effective. Long-term use has the potential to bring about acute hypertensive crises, depending on the patient's other medications and diet. Because of the numerous negative side effects, MAOIs are now infrequently prescribed.

The preferred medication for depression has shifted to the SSRIs. SSRIs include sertraline HCl

---

[12] More detail on addictions is presented in Chapters 8 and 9.

[13] The names of the drugs in text are in so-called generic form with the brand name in parentheses.

TABLE 5.1 *Major psychotherapeutic drugs with structure, generic name, and trade name (adapted from Klerman, 1988).*

THERAPEUTIC USE	CHEMICAL STRUCTURE OR PSYCHOPHARMACOLOGIC ACTION	GENERIC NAME	TRADE NAME
Antipsychotics (also called "major tranquilizers" or "neuroleptics")	Phenothiazines		
	Aliphatic	Chlorpromazine	Thorazine
	Piperidine	Thioridazine	Mellaril
	Piperazine	Trifluoperazine	Stelazine
	Thioxanthenes		
	Aliphatic	Chlorprothixene	Taractan
	Piperazine	Thiothixene	Navane
	Butyrophenones	Haloperidol	Haldol
	Dibenzoxazepines	Loxapine	Loxitane
	Dihydroindolines	Molindone	Moban
	Rauwolfia alkaloids	Reserpine	Sandril
	Benzoquinolines	Tetrabenazine	
Antidepressants	Tricyclic antidepressants (TCAs) Tertiary amines	Amitriptyline	Elavil
		Imipramine	Tofranil
		Doxepin	Sinequan
	Secondary amines	Desipramine	Norpramin
		Nortriptyline	Pamelor
		Protriptyline	Vivactil
	Monoamine oxidase inhibitors (MAOIs)	Phenelzine	Nardil
		Tranylcypromine	Parnate
		Pargyline	Eutonyl
		Isocarboxazid	Marplan
Psychomotor Stimulants	Amephetamines	Amphetamine	Benzedrine
		Dextroamphetamine	Dexedrine
	Other	Methylphenidate	Ritalin
Antimanic		Lithium	Eskalith
		Carbamazapine	Tegretol
Antianxiety (also called "anxiolytic" or "minor tranquilizers")	Benzodiazepines	Chlordiazepoxide	Librium
		Diazepam	Valium
		Chlorazepate	Tranxene
		Oxazepam	Serax
		Lorazepam	Activan
	Triazolobenzodiazepine	Alprazolam	Xanax
	Triazolam	Halcion	
	Propanediol carbamates	Meprobamate	Miltown
	Barbiturates	Phenobarbital	Luminal

(Zoloft), fluoxetine HCl (Prozac), and paroxetine HCl (Paxil). A substantial body of literature suggests that depressed people have lower serotonin function. The SSRIs act selectively at presynaptic receptors to prevent reuptake. The result is improved serotonergic activity at the synapse.

One clinical trial compared paroxetine to imipramine and placebo for treatment of depressed outpatients (Dunbar et al., 1991). The groups were randomly established and consisted of about 240 patients in each of the three treatment conditions. Compared to placebo, both paroxetine and imipramine produced significant improvement in depression as measured by the Hamilton Rating Scale for Depression. Improvements appeared earlier for paroxetine, however, and fewer subjects dropped out because of side effects compared to imipramine. Analysis of data from nearly 7000 patients suggested that paroxetine has no significant effects on cardiovascular or EEG function (Boyer & Blumhardt, 1992). The primary side effect that occurs with the SSRIs is nausea.

The antidepressant fluoxetine HCl (Prozac), released in 1988, has been featured prominently in the news. Several cases suggested Prozac might cause some people to have adverse reactions and commit suicide. The anecdotal nature of the case reports, however, does not provide conclusive evidence that Prozac is at fault or that other factors may not have played a role. Prozac does appear to be very effective against major depression, with fewer negative side effects than the TCAs or MAOIs. Prozac is being studied as a possible therapy for bulimia and obsessive-compulsive disorders, as well as for obesity, since it appears to promote weight loss.

Anti-Anxiety Agents: Controlling Anxiety, Panic, and Stress

Most people probably would not know what benzodiazepines are. Still, mention some common trade names—Librium, Valium, and Ativan—and recognition will probably be instant.[14] These anti-anxiety drugs may be the social class status drugs of the era. They are often prescribed by primary care physicians on the basis of patient complaints that they feel upset or anxious. The benzodiazepines, introduced in the 1960s, and the barbiturates, developed in the early 1900s, are the most common anti-anxiety medications. Benzodiazepines account for 90% of the market. Barbiturates now account for only about 7% of the market.

Benzodiazepines are known to have a wide safety margin for dosage. Still, both animal and human studies suggest that dependence will occur with prolonged use (Salzman, 1991; Schatzberg & Cole, 1991); one of these medications—alprazolam (Xanax)—is highly addictive. One study showed that patients may continue to experience withdrawal symptoms six to eight months after discontinuing the medication (Rickels, Schweizer, Csanalosi, Case, & Chung, 1988).

The benzodiazepines are routinely prescribed for acute symptomatic relief of anxiety, muscle tension, insomnia, and epilepsy; they are also prescribed for preoperative anesthesia. One benzodiazepine, oxazepam (Serax), has been used to help patients withdrawing from alcohol abuse.[15] Susan Jay's group used Valium for children facing painful medical procedures. Patients with panic disorders, with or without depression, have been found to improve on either alprazolam or imipramine (TCA) (Deltito, Argyle, Psych, & Klerman, 1991).

Phenobarbital is probably the most widely used barbiturate. It is used as a daytime sedative. As a long-acting sedative, it is sometimes called the "methadone" of the barbiturate group, because it is used to withdraw patients from short-acting sedatives and occasionally from alcohol (Schatzberg & Cole, 1991).

While the benzodiazepines and barbiturates are the most commonly used drugs to combat anxiety, other drug groups may be used, including buspirone, antihistamines, phenothiazines, and meprobamate (Miltown). Another group of drugs, called beta-blockers (propranolol), typically act to reduce the somatic symptoms of anxiety. They are prescribed for hypertension and to prevent the recurrence of angina, arrhythmias, and migraine headaches. The side effects

---

[14] The generic names are chlordiazepoxide (Librium), diazepam (Valium), and lorazepam (Ativan).

[15] See Chapter 9 for more detail on this use.

include hypotension, fatigue, impotence, and gastrointestinal upset, among others.

Hypnotic Agents: Pharmacologic Treatment for Insomnia

Sleep disturbances can be defined as any deviation from a normal sleep pattern that interferes with daily functions (Williamson, Davis, & Prather, 1988). Sleep disturbances are of special significance for a variety of reasons. First, they may indicate emotional distress caused by acute or chronic stressors. Sleep disturbances may interfere with the feeling of physical well-being because of the accompanying loss of energy and general fatigue. Finally, sleep disturbances may interfere with recovery from serious illness or surgery.

The benzodiazepines, notably first flurazepam (Dalmane) and later triazolam (Halcion), were routinely used for treating sleep disturbances (Gillin, 1991). Triazolam is a short-acting benzodiazepine hypnotic. One group compared triazolam to stimulus control for sleep-onset insomnia (McClusky, Milby, Switzer, Williams, & Wooten, 1991). Although triazolam produced superior immediate results, behavioral treatments were more successful for the long term. These results suggest that triazolam may be used for a short time for a quick relief, but then phased out as behavioral control is established. Further, excessive reliance on triazolam has the potential to produce so-called **rebound insomnia,** a quick return of insomnia after a brief period of relief. This effect may lead to even more anxiety and confusion, and it has the potential to lead to escalating dosages, abuse, and dependence.

Pharmacologic Treatment of Substance Abuse

It is common knowledge that certain drugs have been used to treat drug addiction, even drugs that produce their own form of addiction. Methadone, for example, is a long-acting opiate, so withdrawal symptoms will not appear as quickly as if one had taken a short-acting drug such as morphine. Disulfiram has been used to treat alcoholism, though its operation is very different from methadone. Disulfiram interacts with the presence of alcohol in the stomach to produce physical symptoms of discomfort, such as nausea. The benzodiazepines are also used to counter symptoms of alcohol withdrawal. Clonidine, another beta-blocking drug, is widely used to block physiological symptoms of opioid withdrawal.

Rounsaville, Weissman, Crits-Christoph, Wilber, and Kleber (1982) compared elements of a multimodal drug treatment program in the treatment of opiate addicts. The treatment facility used drug-free treatments such as interpersonal psychotherapy, supportive-expressive therapy, and cognitive-behavioral therapy. The facility also used antidepressant pharmacotherapy, and a methadone maintenance program. About 66% of the clients were on a methadone maintenance program, but all treatment groups, including the methadone group, received intensive individual or small-group therapy. Controls were clients who had presented themselves for assessment and screening but who did not enter active treatment. The team did not observe any symptomatic improvement resulting from either antidepressant pharmacotherapy or from the drug-free treatments. The only factor that seemed important was length of treatment: The longer clients stayed in treatment, the more symptoms were reduced. A recent review of various medications used to treat cocaine, cannabinoid, sedative, or hallucinogen abuse also found no evidence of superiority for one medication over another (O'Brien, 1996).

Summary

As health psychology becomes increasingly involved in clinical services and research on intervention efficacy, health psychologists will need to be aware of the range and utility of various intervention strategies available. This chapter, while not a comprehensive treatment of this area, summarizes current common treatments and applications. Other treatments will be encountered in the remaining pages of the book, but this background will serve to refresh, update, and speed assimilation of treatment concepts introduced later.

1. A central theme of this chapter is that treatment is often multimodal and theoretically eclectic. Single treatment strategies rooted in a narrow theoretical context are becoming less frequent in current practice.

2. Health psychology has important reasons to be concerned about primary prevention—that is structuring environments and lifestyles to prevent the appearance of illness.

3. Secondary prevention strategies are those efforts that seek to reduce risk and minimize damage after symptoms have already appeared. One example is intervention in the early stages of drug use to prevent the appearance of habitual addictive behaviors.

4. Tertiary prevention, which constitutes the majority of clinical work, includes those strategies that seek to reduce impact, shorten the duration of symptoms, and rehabilitate the client. Tertiary prevention occurs after some damage has usually already been done.

5. The number of psychological therapies has increased dramatically to possibly as many as 400 therapies, including 255 psychotherapies and scores of behavioral therapies.

6. Despite their different approaches, therapies share numerous common factors that may influence outcome. These include therapists' characteristics, the nature of the therapeutic process including the therapist-client relationship, and client characteristics.

7. The most important therapists' variables include warmth and empathy, positive regard and support, and ability to listen and understand the client's situation and problems.

8. In terms of process, many therapies, whatever they are called, expose and desensitize clients to various fears and insecurities. The particular process may not be as important as the exposure. Many therapies also provide useful information, instruction, and advice that may be helpful.

9. Clients vary in motivation, type of disorder, degree of disturbance, and expectations for therapeutic success.

10. Brief psychodynamic therapies have become more widely accepted and commonly used in the recent past. Cost containment, better client motivation, and greater client satisfaction help to explain the popularity of this approach.

11. The brief therapies share with long-term psychotherapies a concern for insight and understanding, but they are more directive and goal-oriented. By definition, they are also time-limited, to about 20–25 sessions maximum.

12. Cognitive therapies focus on changing attitudes, beliefs, expectations, and personal representations and interpretations of reality.

13. Cognitive therapies appear to share certain common processes, such as rationality, empiricism, repetition, and distraction. The emphasis varies, however, from one cognitive approach to another.

14. Beck's cognitive therapy and Meichenbaum's self-instructional training are frequently used cognitive interventions.

15. Behavior therapies focus on overt behavior. They use conditioning, reinforcement, and modeling approaches, among others, to change behavior.

16. Behavior therapies are often used to reduce high-risk behavior, increase compliance with medical regimens, increase healthy behaviors such as exercise, or reduce tension and fear.

17. Commonly used behavior therapies include relaxation training, desensitization, and stimulus control.

18. Pharmacotherapy is the use of drugs to alter physical or mental symptoms. It is often more favored by professionals in the medical establishment and less favored by professionals in psychology.

19. Health psychologists often serve on interdisciplinary treatment teams and work on research projects that require knowledge of the relationship between drugs and behavior. Psychological therapies are often compared to drug therapies to determine the most effective intervention strategies.

20. The use of drugs for therapeutic purposes is not without danger. Prescribed drugs may produce unwanted and sometimes dangerous side effects. Drugs may also lead to tolerance and, in some cases, abuse and dependence.

21. The most common pharmacotherapies revolve around antidepressants, anti-anxiety agents, hypnotics and sedatives, and drugs to facilitate withdrawal from addictions.

22. Multimodal therapy uses a combination of intervention strategies dependent on the client's situation. Brief dynamic therapy might be used for depression, cognitive therapy to restructure faulty belief patterns, behavioral therapy to increase compliance with a medical regimen, and pharmacotherapy for specific symptoms.

Key Words

behavior modification
behavior therapy
clinical therapy
cognitive therapy
contraindications
desensitization
distraction (CT)
drug
drug withdrawal
emotive imagery
empiricism (CT)
experimental psychopathology
medication
multimodal treatment
neurotransmitter
nonapproved use (drug)
pharmacology
pharmacotherapy
polypharmacy
primary prevention
prophylactic effect
psychopharmacology
psychotropic

rationality (CT)
rebound insomnia
repetition (CT)
research therapy
secondary prevention
short-term psychotherapy
side-effects
sleep-maintenance insomnia
sleep-onset insomnia
spontaneous remission
substance dependence
substance tolerance
substance withdrawal
synergistic effect
systematic desensitization
tardive dyskinesia
tertiary prevention

Study Questions

1. What is the difference between primary, secondary, and tertiary prevention, and how may health psychologists be helping to shift the focus to primary prevention?

2. What are the core common ingredients of therapy, and why are they important to understanding when a therapy is effective or not?

3. Describe the essential characteristics of short-term psychodynamic therapy. How does it differ from the other three therapies discussed in this chapter?

4. What are the customary uses for short-term psychodynamic psychotherapy in the health psychology arena?

5. Describe the major characteristics of cognitive therapy. How does it differ from the other therapies discussed in this chapter?

6. How is cognitive therapy most often used in health psychology?

7. Describe the basic characteristics of behavior therapy, and indicate how it differs from the other three therapies discussed in this chapter.

8. What are the most common applications of behavior therapy?

9. Describe the basic characteristics of behavior therapy, and indicate how it differs from the other three therapies discussed.

10. What is pharmacotherapy, and how does it enter into the work of health psychologists?

11. What are the major classes of drugs used in treating medical and psychiatric patients?

12. What is multimodal therapy, and why is it important to the practice of health psychology?

Class Projects/Activities

1. Invite health psychologists, clinical psychologists, behavior therapists, and psychiatrists to present descriptions of their practice to class. If possible, select the participants to represent the different therapies described in this chapter.

2. Have a panel discussion on the relationship between psychological therapies and pharmacotherapy. Present the strengths and weaknesses of each approach fairly, and suggest how the two approaches might work well together.

3. Find recent literature on the controversy about whether psychologists should or should not be allowed to prescribe drugs. Have a debate on the issue with one team taking the pro side and one team taking the con side. (If you have access to currently practicing psychologists who are on opposite sides of the issue, invite them to class to present the two views.)

4. Find recent examples (case studies or research projects) of multimodal therapy in health psychology and present them to the class to show how different therapeutic interventions are used simultaneously.

Suggested Readings

Dobson, K. S. (Ed.) (1988). *Handbook of cognitive-behavioral therapies*. New York: Guilford Press.

Journal of Consulting and Clinical Psychology, April 1993, 61. Special section: Recent developments in cognitive and constructivist psychotherapies. (Includes contributions by Aaron Beck, Albert Ellis, Don Meichenbaum, and others.)

Journal of Consulting and Clinical Psychology, August 1993, 61. Special section: Curative factors in dynamic psychotherapy.

Klerman, G. L. (1988). Drugs and psychotherapy. In S. L. Garfield & A. E. Bergin (Eds.). *Handbook of psychotherapy and behavior change* (pp. 777–818). New York: Wiley.

Wells, R. A., & Giannetti, V. J. (Eds.) (1990). *Handbook of the brief psychotherapies*. New York: Plenum.

WEBSITES   *Information and Innovation in Therapy*

ADDRESS	DESCRIPTION
http://www.cmhc.com	☆ Mental Health Net—Psychotherapy
http://www.behavior.net/	☆ Behavior On-Line
http://www.nacbt.org	☆ National Association of Cognitive-Behavioral Therapists
http://www.wwnorton.com/blurbs/npb/ psylinks.htm	Psychology/Psychotherapy Resources—links to top five sites
http://www.pharminfo.com/pin hp.html	☆ Pharmaceutical Information Network—great data source for the layperson as well as the professional
http://www.lycaeum.org	The Lycaeum—with drug information archives
http://www.coedu.usf.edu/behavior/	Behavior Analysis Homepage
http://www.cwru.edu/orgs/div29/div29.htm	APA Division 29—Psychotherapy

CHAPTER **6**

Biobehavioral Research: Experimental, Clinical, and Epidemiological Strategies

The death of A. Bartlett Giamatti on 1 September 1989 sent shock waves through the academic and sports communities. These two seemingly disparate groups had become strange bedfellows, wedded by the personality of Giamatti and his indomitable love of America's game—baseball. He was a man who was just as much at home in the classroom teaching Renaissance literature as he was being a fan at his beloved Fenway Park in Boston. He was just as comfortable reciting poetry as he was the records of baseball's legends. He became president of Yale at the age of only 40, and in this capacity, he walked its halls for a decade. He loved literature, it is true, but baseball's allure proved irresistible. When asked to become the National League's president, he did. And because his service to the league was as illustrious as his work in academia, he was asked to serve as baseball's commissioner.

For those who were close to him, the problem was how to deal with the grief of sudden loss. For others, Giamatti's death at 51 prompted a predictable round of speculation about causes. He was overweight, though we have no information about his diet. He was a chain smoker, smoking three to four packs a day. For at least the five months preceding his death, he apparently worked 22 hours a day, getting only 2 hours' sleep a night. He also had to deal with an immense pressure: confronting one of the great sports legends of all time, Pete Rose, who had

This chapter is a modified version of the methods chapter appearing in the author's publication *Stress and Health* (1992). It is used here with permission of Brooks/Cole.

just been charged with betting on baseball, possibly betting on his own team. There were even rumors of threats against Giamatti's life if he went through with sanctions against Rose. Some speculated that this monumental stress killed him. Some suggested that whatever stress he felt was only the last straw, the final load added to several other physical risk factors. Others said that stress had nothing to do with it at all.

For a group of scientists whose profession is epidemiology, their job is to untangle the web of causes: the etiology or origins of disease. How does one go about untangling such complex webs as risk factors for cardiovascular disease? How do we go about tracing the complex links between psychosocial stress and immune system suppression? This chapter is concerned with the process of theory building and research methods used to investigate just such issues. Space limitations once again dictate brevity. Those who want to pursue more in depth reading will find specialized discussions in Kasl and Cooper (1987) and Karoly (1985).

Modes of Thinking in Science

We should not assume that science approaches theory building with uniformity. Our theories of health and illness show great diversity. Gary Schwartz discussed four ways of thinking about nature: formistic, mechanistic, contextual, and organistic (Schwartz, 1982).[1] **Formistic thinking** is categorical, either-or thinking. It does not admit middle categories or series of categories. In this way of thinking, you are either sick or well; Type A or Type B; alcoholic or nonalcoholic. There is no middle ground. In one sense, formistic thinking is a necessary prelude to scientific inquiry because science must first categorize relevant events before it can establish causal connection. Formistic thinking, though, can only lead to overly simplistic, if not primitive, models of environment-behavior relations.

Mechanistic thinking assumes that cause-effect chains are singly determined; that is, there is one cause linked to one effect. To the mechanistic mind, a specific germ causes a certain disease. A specific stressor has one and only one effect. A lifestyle choice produces one fixed outcome. The notions that multiple causes may contribute to an effect and that multiple outcomes may derive from a single cause are foreign to this way of thinking.

Contextual thinking takes the view that any effect depends on context. Contextual thinking is relational and multicausal thinking. In addition, the context of the observer may provide alternative, equally plausible explanations of an event. Stress may be good or bad depending on how you view it. Disease may be caused by a set of interconnected factors including decisions to engage in high-risk behaviors that lead to exposure or lowered resistance. Disease may be related as well to attitudes toward preventive behavior and compliance with medical regimens.

Finally, **organistic thinking** is systems thinking. The healthy functioning of an organism results from the interplay of numerous components, both within the organism and between the organism and its environmental context. The interactions are complex, resulting in interactive multicausal, multieffect models. Contextual thinking and organistic thinking are clearly compatible and provide, according to numerous authors, the framework within which satisfactory models may be developed that explain how psychosocial forces contribute to maintaining health or increasing risk for illness.

Health research also distinguishes between proximal and distal causes. **Proximal causes** are events hypothesized to operate in the recent past. Acute infections, respiratory disorders, injuries, and serious accidents (acute stressors), among other things, are typically treated as proximal causes. **Distal causes** are those presumed to act from some remote time past. Rheumatic fever in childhood may be the cause of heart problems in adulthood. It is all the more difficult to untangle the causal web when the complex matrix of biopsychosocial variables must be considered across long time spans.

---

[1] Schwartz credits these to Pepper's (1942) notion of world hypotheses.

Further, we distinguish between precipitating factors and predisposing factors. **Precipitating factors** are insults, physical or psychosocial, that immediately precede the onset of a breakdown. These are similar to proximal causes, but the terminology is introduced for reasons that will become clear momentarily. **Predisposing factors** are biological-genetic factors that influence organic or constitutional weakness and probably also determine stable personality traits.

These two sets of variables have been integrated in the diathesis-stress theory. This theory suggests that there is an interplay between predisposing factors and precipitating factors. The predisposing factors set a threshold, low or high, for breakdown through constitutional strengths and weaknesses. Whether a weakness ever appears depends on the amount of stress—the precipitating force—that the person experiences. In a sheltered environment, free of germs and risks of exposure, even a very weak person might never show signs of illness. Conversely, a person under severe, continuous assault might break down even though genetic predispositions are strong. Theory and method in health science research have increasingly sought to incorporate this intermix of variables to provide more powerful explanatory models of health and illness.

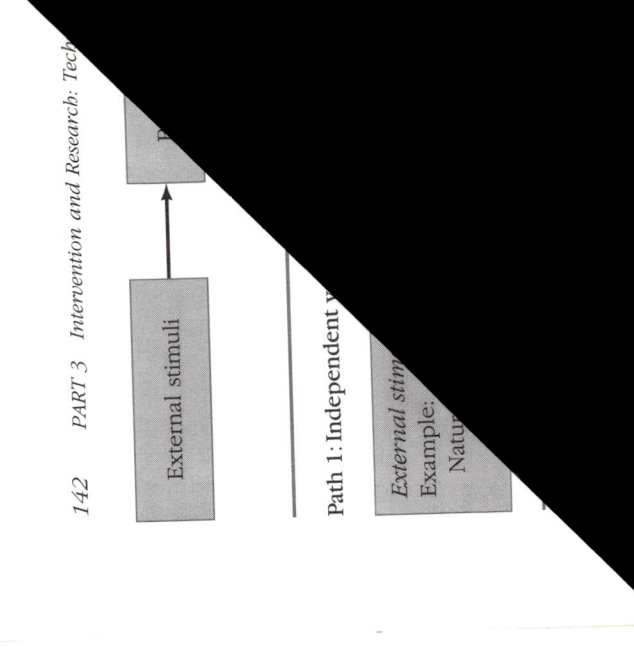

The Logic of Scientific Method

Scientific method is a serial process that seeks to establish cause and effect relationships. The cause is the independent variable (IV), whereas the effect (or outcome) is the dependent variable (DV). In the social-behavioral sciences, the independent variable is usually an environmental stimulus, and the dependent variable is some behavior. In design terms, the **independent variable** is the treatment condition manipulated by the investigator, whereas the **dependent variable** is the behavior that is measured. For example, it is widely assumed that chronic stress causes a decline in health. Stress is the independent variable, and decline in health is the dependent variable.

Independent Variables: Biomedical Versus Psychosocial Stimuli

A social psychologist might study variations in the type of social support systems (perhaps intimate and extended networks versus impersonal and limited networks) that people have and how these systems protect against the effects of stress. Environmental psychologists might compare reactions to different physical stressors (such as natural versus technological disasters). Clinical health care personnel might be concerned about how different therapies (for example, relaxation versus cognitive restructuring) alter subjective reports of stress or feelings of tension. In each case, the independent variable is some aspect of the external environment.

Alternatively, we might focus on internal differences in the host organism. For example, we might categorize people with regard to their autonomic reactivity (hyperreactive versus hyporeactive) and its influence on stress reactions. We could test for differences in levels of trait anxiety and categorize people from high to low on this personality variable. Then we could assess differences in stress reactions related to this trait. In each of these examples, an internal personal trait is used as the independent variable. In the first case, we selected a biological characteristic; in the second, a psychological trait.

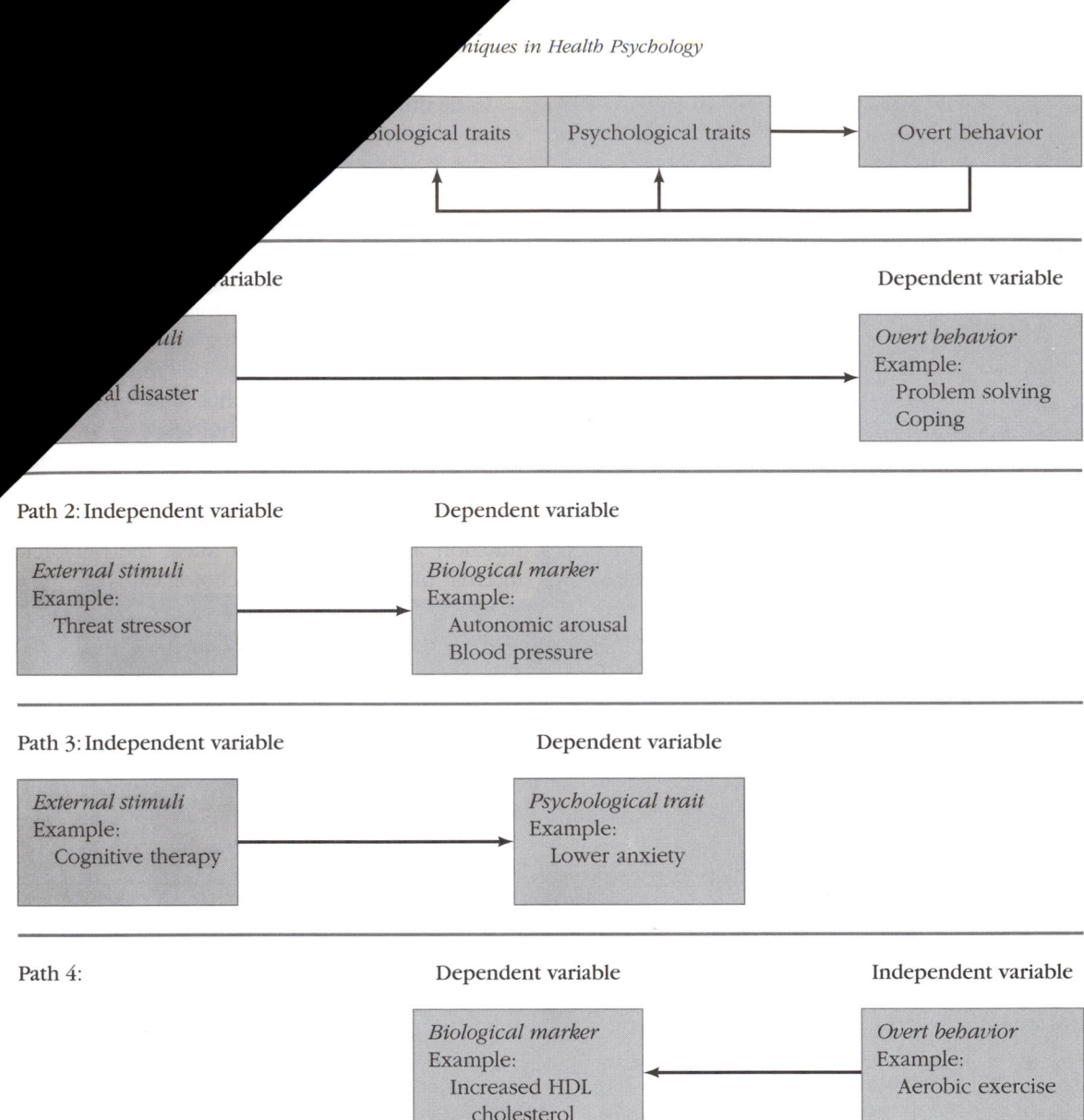

Biological traits → Psychological traits → Overt behavior

variable | Dependent variable

...li |
...al disaster | → | *Overt behavior* Example: Problem solving Coping

Path 2: Independent variable | Dependent variable

External stimuli Example: Threat stressor | → | *Biological marker* Example: Autonomic arousal Blood pressure

Path 3: Independent variable | Dependent variable

External stimuli Example: Cognitive therapy | → | *Psychological trait* Example: Lower anxiety

Path 4: | Dependent variable | Independent variable

Biological marker Example: Increased HDL cholesterol | ← | *Overt behavior* Example: Aerobic exercise

FIGURE 6.1 *Possible stimulus-response sequences that structure stress and health research (from Rice, 1992).*

Finally, we might take differences in behavior patterns as the stimulus event. For example, we might classify people in terms of the frequency and intensity of exercise. We could then look at several different dependent measures such as changes in cardiovascular systems, alterations in physical fitness, improvements in level of depression, or differences in subjective reports of stress.

Dependent Variables: Measuring Outcomes

Dependent variables are also defined primarily by their point in the chain. Recall the study by Kiecolt-Glaser's group discussed in Chapter 3. These researchers wanted to know whether immune competence changes following relaxation training as compared to social support or no contact (Kiecolt-Glaser et al., 1985). Their dependent variable was change in natural killer cell activity. Others are concerned about the origins of the Type A personality. Does it result from genetic factors, or does it result from familial patterns of discipline? Here, Type A is measured as an outcome variable. In another context, it might be a stimulus variable similar to trait anxiety. Finally, we might be concerned that coronary risk relates to a mood state such as chronic intense hostility. In this case, the dependent variable is a cardiovascular measure such as blood pressure or serum cholesterol, and the independent variable is an internal psychological mood.

A variety of dependent measures focus on internal biological changes. This focus reflects the notion that biomedical measures somehow are more real than psychosocial or behavioral measures. Robert Kaplan (1990) made a compelling argument for behavior as the central outcome of health research. He noted that numerous interventions result in clinical improvement, such as reducing blood pressure, but quality of life indicators are unchanged. Further, Kaplan cited the highly touted study showing that aspirin reduced deaths from myocardial infarction. The rest of the story was not publicized: Total coronary deaths did not decrease. Aspirin changed only the distribution of deaths among the categories. As Kaplan noted, though, families are rarely as much concerned with how their loved ones die as they are with the fact of their loss.

Taking the Measure of Health: Issues in Assessment

It is clear from the foregoing that health psychologists frequently use assessment methods to establish levels of an independent variable or to measure dependent variables. Assessment issues thus have become so important that entire books are devoted to assessment techniques (biomedical, psychosocial, or behavioral), to assessment in special populations (women and minorities, for example), and to assessment for different health conditions (heart health, cancer,

or pain, for example) (Bellack & Hersen, 1988; Blechman & Brownell, 1988; Karoly, 1985, 1988).

When health psychologists need a psychosocial test, they usually have two choices: either find a currently available standardized test that has been developed for the target situation and clientele, or develop the test from scratch. If they must develop the measure, they must also test it before basing clinical or research judgments on it. Testing the test basically means determining how reliable and valid it is.

Testing the Tests: Norms, Reliability, and Validity

When we say a test is standardized, we mean that it was built with specific rules so that it can be—indeed, must be—administered the same way every time (Anastasi, 1988). This standardization may include verbatim instructions and precise timing of test segments, among other things. Any variation in scores on the test, then, can be more logically attributed to real variations in the trait and not to differences in the conditions of taking the test.

Standardized tests also provide norms—in other words, group means, percentiles, and standardized scores for selected representative reference groups. Raw scores are generally meaningless by themselves, but norms provide a way for the clinician to compare groups or individuals to a standard. It is customary to provide normative data for common demographic traits such as age and sex, but many other demographic variables may be included for specific purposes.

The Reliability Criterion: Issues of Accuracy

Since so much rides on the outcome of tests, the instruments must themselves be subjected to careful scrutiny to ensure that they yield accurate results. Such scrutiny is no less important when the test in question is biomedical than when it is psychosocial. The technical sophistication and the appearance of quantitative precision that accompanies most biomedical tests may lead to a premature judgment that the tests are both reliable and valid, when in fact the tests have not been thoroughly tested (Kaplan, 1990). The same is true of computerized clinical psychological tests and interpretations (Matarazzo, 1986). Psychology has developed extensive procedures for testing the tests—procedures that we can discuss only briefly.

Good tests must meet two fundamental criteria: that is, they must have reliability and validity. Reliability means that the test measures consistently. Validity means that the test measures what it is supposed to measure.

Professional test designers recognize four major types of reliability: test-retest, alternate forms, split-half (also called internal consistency), and Kuder-Richardson reliability. Which type of reliability is most important depends on the way you intend to use the test. In test-retest reliability, a test is administered at one time and then later at a second time. If it gives approximately the same scores both times, it has test-retest reliability. Reliability is measured as the correlation (Pearson r) between the two scores obtained from the same people on the two test days. Alternate forms reliability requires two separate tests that are nearly equivalent in content. The reliability measure is the correlation between two scores taken from the same people on two distinct but equivalent forms of the test.

Perhaps the most common measures of consistency are so-called internal consistency measures, such as the split-half and the Kuder-Richardson reliability. Split-half reliability is similar to obtaining alternate forms reliability from a single administration. Each person receives two scores from a single test—for example, one score from the odd-numbered items and one score from the even-numbered items. Reliability is the correlation between the two halves of the test. Kuder-Richardson reliability is an inter-item consistency measure based on the person's performance on each item obtained from a single test. A well-known alternative to the Kuder-Richardson procedure is Cronbach's alpha. These internal consistency measures are used often because they are the quickest and simplest to compute.

The Validity Criterion: Issues of Credibility

Reliability is of little value if a test does not measure what it is supposed to measure. Suppose that I set out to construct a personality test that measures as many meaningful facets of personality as possible. Further, suppose that the test yields precisely the same score for the same person every time it is given. Still, a colleague points out that my test is measuring only one very narrow facet of personality—say, dominance-submission. In this case, no matter how reliable my test is, it is not a valid general measure of personality. At the same time, it is impossible to determine the validity of a test unless it is also reliable. In this sense, reliability sets the upper limit for validity.

There are three major types of validity: content validity, criterion-related validity, and construct validity. Content validity requires that the test content fairly represents the behavior domain to be measured. Ensuring content validity does not entail a statistical analysis, but an exercise in expertise and logic resulting in the systematic selection of items for inclusion in the test. Content validity is often confused with face validity, which involves a simple intuitive judgment that test items look like they tap what the scale claims to measure. Criterion-related validity is assessed by checking the test against a relevant performance-based measure. For example, we might check a graduate entrance exam against a composite academic performance index near the end of the person's graduate program.

One of the most important forms of validity is construct validity, which is concerned with whether the test measures the specific trait or theoretical construct of concern. To illustrate this notion, consider the construct of trait anxiety. When we say that a test measures anxiety, we should provide evidence that this trait is precisely what the test measures. We may do so by checking the test against other tests of anxiety with a known track record. Further, we may use physiological measures of anxiety obtained in the laboratory under different conditions designed to induce varying degrees of anxiety. Under conditions of high threat, a high-anxiety person should show a high score on the test as well as a strong physiological response. If these cross-checks are all positive, we may conclude that the anxiety test is a valid measure of the anxiety construct. This procedure is what Campbell (1960; Campbell & Fiske, 1959) called convergent validation.

Donna Lamping (1985) reviewed several problems that occur when health psychologists apply traditional assessment strategies and instruments to current clinical problems and research issues in health psychology. These can be summarized as follows:

1. *Conventional tests often have inadequate content validity for medical problems* because they were developed for use with a physically normal population.

2. *Conventional tests are often used with inappropriate norms for medical populations* because they were developed for psychiatric or normal populations.

3. *Most tests have been developed with a unidimensional conceptualization of behavior* and were not meant to apply to behavior when one is ill.

4. *Most conventional tests lack contextual specificity,* being developed for use as general trait measures and not for use in specific contexts such as being in a hospital with a life-threatening illness.

5. *Most tests are insensitive to the rapid changes* that can take place when a patient is confronting serious health problems.

Testing Causal Connections: Educated Guesses

To return to the steps in the scientific method, the common strategy is to test the truth value of a hypothesis by directly manipulating the causal

variables presumed to influence behavior. A **hypothesis** is a tentative answer to a research question—a prediction of what behavior we expect under specified conditions.

A prototypic experiment illustrates the process. Suppose a research group wants to know whether relaxation training will reduce migraine headaches. As a first step, the researchers inspect the methods and results of previous research. The goal is to become familiar with migraine and its treatment. Based on this review, the researchers state a plausible hypothesis: Relaxation training (IV) will be effective in reducing both the frequency (DV_1) and severity (DV_2) of migraine attacks.

The team then obtains a volunteer group of migraine sufferers. The researchers review medical records (with client permission, of course) to ensure that each subject fits the definition of migraine. Including nonmigraine pain patients (for example, chronic low-back pain patients) would confuse interpretation of results.

Then, the investigators randomly assign subjects to one of two groups, the experimental group or the control group. **Random assignment** permits the assumption that no differences exist between the groups except that introduced by the independent variable. Unfortunately, random assignment is not always possible. People cannot be randomly assigned to disease categories, such as coronary heart disease. They cannot be assigned randomly to behavioral or personality profiles, such as the Type A behavior pattern (Friedman & Booth-Kewley, 1987). Because of this, the investigator must use a quasi-experimental design (Cook & Campbell, 1979). *Quasi* literally means resembling. A **quasi-experimental design** resembles a true experiment in most respects but still falls short. The resemblance is that both true and quasi-experiments have treatments, outcome measures, and sampling units (Rosenthal & Rosnow, 1991). The difference is that quasi-experimental designs cannot assign subjects completely at random to the treatment conditions.

The **experimental group** receives training in relaxation, while the **control group** receives no training. This difference between the two groups constitutes manipulation of the independent variable. In reality, the control group very seldom receives nothing. More often than not, the control group receives an **attention placebo.** An attention placebo may be given by having a series of nonspecific informational meetings. These meetings would be roughly equal to the contact time the experimental group receives but would not provide training in relaxation.

Over time, subjects provide data on the frequency and intensity of their headaches. These measures are the dependent variables. **Baseline measures,** or pretreatment data, tell the experimenters where the behavior was before treatment and whether the experimental and control groups were equivalent at the outset. After treatment, the data will allow the investigator either to refute or to confirm the hypothesis that relaxation changed frequency and intensity of headaches. If the groups were not equivalent in headache measures at the beginning, then any favorable change in the dependent variable could not be assigned reliably to the relaxation treatment. Similarly, if the treatment and control groups were still equal in headache measures at the end of the experiment, even if they were both significantly lower, the investigators could not be confident that relaxation provided an effective treatment.

We should take steps to protect against the chance that subjects know or guess the research hypothesis. This possibility could bias the results (Rosenthal, 1966). To control for this possibility, a special group of collaborators may collect and tabulate the data. They are special because they do not know the purpose of the experiment nor do they know to which group the subjects belong. Technically, this technique is a **double-blind control.** If these collaborators are blind to group membership but know the hypothesis of the experiment, then it is a **single-blind control.** A recent meta-analysis of modeling procedures to prepare children for surgical operations revealed the importance of this control: Treatment effects all but disappeared in experiments using adequate blind procedures, but remained quite strong (almost three times the effect size) in experiments not using blind control procedures (Saile, Burgmeier, & Schmidt, 1988).

Using Subjects for Research: Ethical Dilemmas

An important criterion for conducting responsible research is that subjects receive information about the basic procedures and any personal risks involved from their participation. Researchers provide this information in an **informed consent** form. Subjects read and sign the informed consent form to show they understand the procedures and risks and agree to participate.

Ethical issues in research can be very complicated. Any agency that uses federal moneys must form an **Institutional Research Board** (IRB) to review projects and ensure that investigators comply with ethical guidelines. When deception is involved, the investigator must be certain that such deception is necessary to test the hypothesis. If deception is used, then subjects must receive a **debriefing** to explain what the deception was and to remedy any ill effects that might result. A serious dilemma (exemplified in our prototype experiment) occurs when a possibly helpful treatment is given to one group but is withheld from the control group. In these circumstances, some investigators ask their subjects to give their informed consent to possible assignment to the control group. Kiecolt-Glaser's group used this procedure in the study of relaxation versus social support mentioned earlier. Still, investigators typically offer the treatment to the control group after completing the study.

Making Sense of the Numbers

When the project is complete, investigators must try to make sense of the numbers. In order to reduce the chance that personal bias will influence interpretation, scientists use numerous statistical tools. In our hypothetical project, the team would compute the average number of headaches and the mean intensity ratings for the experimental and control groups. If the relaxation group showed a sizable decrease in headaches or greatly reduced pain, the hypothesis is confirmed. The problem is to know what makes a sizable decrease or change in severity of pain. It is possible that decreases reflect nothing more than uncontrolled chance factors.

We use **inferential statistics** to enable us to state with mathematical precision how confident we can be that results are attributable to the experimental treatment. To be safe, the team sets a confidence level (or level of significance) before the project begins. The **confidence level** defines a statistically significant result by reference to a probability so rare that the results are not likely to have occurred by mere chance. Conventionally, scientists use confidence levels around p = .05 or p = .01. A confidence level of .05 states that the results could occur by chance no more than 5 times in 100. A confidence level of .01 states that the results could occur by chance no more than 1 time in 100. Chance factors usually refer to a combination of sampling error, measurement error, or experimental error. If the decrease in frequency or severity of headaches is reliable by a statistical test, then the investigators say that the hypothesis is true.

There is, of course, always a small chance that when we say the experimental hypothesis is true, it is in fact false. This chance exists because the decision itself depends on the statistics of chance. Stated in other terms, when we say the results could not occur by chance more than 5 times in 100, we have no way of knowing whether this result is one of the 5 chance outcomes that could occur, or one of the non-chance outcomes that means our experimental hypothesis is confirmed.

Two types of decision errors may occur. One is the Type I error just described, which occurs when we say that our experimental manipulation is responsible for the observed changes in behavior, but in reality, the result is due to chance. The likelihood of making a Type I error is exactly the confidence level we have set. The second decision error is a Type II error, which occurs when we overlook a meaningful experi-

mental outcome. In this case, we say that chance was operating when in fact our experimental manipulation did have an effect. The second type of error occurs more often when we have set a more restrictive confidence level.

Typically, investigators especially want to avoid Type I errors when they are deep into a program of research, and particularly when they are refining a theory. Conversely, they do not want to make a Type II error when they are just beginning a new research program of discovery, or they are working in more applied areas where overlooking a potentially useful treatment may be particularly undesirable.

Operational Definitions and Repeatability

Scientists take steps to ensure that the procedures used to test hypotheses are explicit and repeatable. Researchers must make certain that special constructs and terms are stated clearly and precisely. A research project may appear elegant in design, but if its central constructs are fuzzy, interpretation of results will be an exercise in futility. Some terms are concrete and have well-defined referents, such as *heart rate*. Other terms are more abstract or theoretical, such as *stress* or *ego* (Clark & Paivio, 1989).

When ambiguity exists because a term has several connotations (for example *pain, stress, anxiety,* or *headache),* then scientists use an operational definition. An operational definition is a statement about the procedures the researcher used to establish levels of an independent variable or to measure a dependent variable. To illustrate, pain might be defined qualitatively as a particular type of pain—low-back pain as opposed to headache pain. Then the pain might be quantified as a score on a standardized pain scale. The investigator may want to look at differences in cognitions and attitudes between high pain and low pain groups. The high pain group might be defined as the top 40% on the pain scale and the low pain group the bottom 40%. This provides an operational definition of pain.

TABLE 6.1   Comparison of key features of research designs (from Rice, 1992).

TYPE OF DESIGN	DEGREE OF CONTROL	METHOD OF ANALYSIS
Case-study method	No control over any variables, whether experimental or extraneous	Subjective (clinical) interpretation Possible comparison to normative data when using standard psychometric exams
Reversal designs	Direct control over experimental or treatment variables Limited or no control over extraneous variables	Graphical—comparison of treatment period to baseline May include some statistical analysis with multiple groups or baselines
Field studies	No direct control over most variables Statistical control over demographic variables	Statistical—yields descriptive values such as means and normative data Comparisons between subgroups with inferences about differences
Correlational studies	Statistical control over demographic variables	Statistical—results in correlation coefficient and estimate of variance
Pre-post designs	Direct control over experimental or treatment variables Added levels of control depend on type of control group(s) used	Statistical—comparison of target behavior after treatment to pretreatment levels Comparison to control groups to eliminate competing explanations for change
Experimental designs	Direct control over hypothesized causal variables Potential to control most important extraneous variables	Statistical—descriptive and inferential Comparison between groups
Epidemiological studies	Varies with specific type of design but potentially very good control Many variables must be controlled by selection rather than by direct manipulation	Statistical—both descriptive and inferential Comparisons between treatment conditions Comparisons between groups exposed to different risk factors
Meta-analysis	Only decisional control over how to select and combine studies	Statistical—aggregate effect size Comparison of effect sizes in subsets of studies

Finally, the end of data analysis does not necessarily mean the end of responsibility for subjects. If the results support the contention that relaxation was effective, the team would provide relaxation training to the control group. Typically, this action would satisfy the investigator's ethical obligations to subjects in the experiment. We are reminded that various ethi-

DESIGN STRENGTHS	DESIGN WEAKNESSES
Extensive data about the individual	Subject to bias of the observer
May be of heuristic value when it leads to testable hypothesis	Cannot test causal hypotheses
	Cannot be repeated
May be the only way to document rare cases/ disorders	Limited generality
Weak causal connections may be inferred	Usually carried out with very small n
Study is repeatable	Limited generality
Especially useful in early development of clinical treatments	Cannot eliminate many sources of contamination
Potential to obtain quantitative data on many variables from many subjects	Cannot test causal hypotheses
Establish norms and/or trends	May be subject to reporting biases such as selective memory, failures in memory, or expectancies about the nature of the study
May be of heuristic value	
May provide data on social/ecological phenomena that cannot be studied in the laboratory	Not repeatable with disaster events
Can be repeated with most survey studies	
Identify relations between any number of variables	Cannot determine causal connections
Identify potentially interesting causal variables for controlled study	Significance of the coefficient does not reveal the amount of variance explained
Stronger inferences of causal link as controls become better	Limited causal inferences with no control group or weak controls
More generality than reversal designs (this depends on sampling and n	Potential ethical questions with untreated controls
Repeatable	
Most powerful design to establish causal links	Criticized for using artificial tasks
Multicausal links	Can be difficult to interpret with large number of variables
Interactions can be established with extended (factorial) designs	Cannot manipulate some variables for ethical reasons
Repeatable	Ethical issues with untreated controls
Generality good but related to sampling and task demands	
Usually conducted in natural environment	Difficult to obtain good control over many variables
Useful for issues of disease etiology and lifestyle disease links	Costly in terms of time and effort
Repeatable	Outcomes are often still subject to more than one interpretation
Generality good	Ethical issues with untreated controls
Resolves issues from conflicting results	Must work with existing data no matter how clean or dirty the data are
Resolves disputes due to disparate methodologies	Potential bias of using only published studies
Resolves disputes between competing theoretical models	
Repeatable	

cal issues confront investigators involved in this type of research (O'Leary & Borkovec, 1978).

This discussion represents the bare essentials of the logic of experimental design. We now turn to research strategies used in health psychology research. Table 6.1 summarizes the more common strategies. You may find it helpful to refer to this table as you read about each design.

Case Studies: The Intensive Analysis of One

The case study has a long and venerable history in clinical circles. Originally, it signified an intensive examination of a single client. Any and all facets of the client's medical, psychological, familial, educational, and social background could provide information crucial to treatment. The case study method also proved useful in opening new areas of inquiry, such as behavior modification research. The case study method led to formal methods for single-subject designs and the experimental analysis of behavior, a technique that will be described later. The major limitation of the case study method is that it cannot directly test hypotheses.

A recent example of the case study comes from the work of Norman Cousins. This example is unique in that the subject and observer were the same person. Cousins first gained national recognition as editor of the *Saturday Review.* Later, he took a senior lecturer position at the UCLA School of Medicine. When Cousins suffered from a serious collagen disease, he found traditional medical treatment unsatisfactory and left the hospital against medical advice. He documented these experiences in *Anatomy of an Illness* (1979).

Cousins generated a great amount of interest because of what he did after leaving the hospital. He checked into a hotel where he spent several hours a day watching classic comedy movies. He reported that ten minutes of laughter had an anesthetic effect enabling him to sleep for two hours without the aid of other medications. He also observed a drop in sedimentation rate, an indicator of the severity of the inflammation, during laughter. In a short while, he felt that he was significantly improved, and he resumed normal activities. Cousins noted later, though, that the press had made much more of the humor issue than was merited. Humor is not a cure for illness, but a practice that arouses the spirit and positively conditions the mind. Humor, then, is a metaphor for positive emotions like hope and cheerfulness, emotions that can be powerful allies on the road to recovery (Cousins, 1983, p. 50). Numerous studies followed up on Cousins's hypothesis, testing whether laughter is indeed the best medicine and whether humor is an effective coping strategy (Martin & Lefcourt, 1983). These studies confirmed that although laughter may be healthy, the issue is far too complex to be summed up in simplistic statements.

Field Studies: Constructing Plausible Explanations

Think for a moment about how you might try to find answers to the following questions. What are the mental and physical health outcomes for victims of a natural catastrophe, such as Hurricane Andrew, which ravaged Florida and Louisiana in August 1992? Can we provide any information to patients waiting for painful medical procedures that will minimize their anguish and promote recovery? Are air traffic controllers at increased risk for nervous breakdowns and physical health problems? Does high caffeine consumption increase coronary risk? What is the relationship between physical fitness and coronary risk?

Each of these questions is important and deserves to be answered. Each situation presents a problem, though, concerning where and how to observe whatever stress-health connection may be present. Hurricanes are natural disasters. Surgery takes place in hospitals, not in research labs. Air traffic controllers may face very different work conditions depending on the size of the city and the amount of airport traffic. Those conditions cannot be re-created in a laboratory. Caffeine consumption and physical fitness are behaviors whose effects on coronary condition may not show up for years. These situations, then, require research strategies that differ from the laboratory experiment.

For these questions, investigators often turn to a family of designs called field studies. Included in this group are survey research, ex post facto designs, and correlational designs.

Survey Research: Sampling at Large

Survey research is a widely used procedure that seeks to discover typical attitudes or behaviors in large representative samples. Surveys require extensive time for face-to-face interviews or require respondents to fill out lengthy questionnaires. The most elaborate survey research is the U.S. census, which occurs every ten years. Other visible examples are Gallup polls and Roper polls, which tap attitudes on social and political issues. These polls assess changes in behavior tendencies such as religious affiliation, sexual mores and conduct, and health behaviors. A Gallup (1984) poll on fitness, for example, showed that about 59% of the adult population engaged in daily exercise, more than twice the number as in 1961.

Surveys are helpful to indicate trends in attitudes and behaviors, but they also suffer from several limitations. Since survey data are self-reported, we must be concerned with the credibility of those reports. Most surveys expend little effort to verify data. Surveys often ask people to report blood pressure or other biomedical statistics without cross-checks. The investigator also must hope that respondents interpret questions in a consistent way. Surveys also may suffer a reactivity effect: The respondent's answers may change as a result of being a subject. Respondents may have no opinion before the interview but form an opinion on the spot to satisfy the social demand characteristics of the interview. Finally, surveys do not allow the investigator to manipulate causal variables or to control for confounding variables.

Ex Post Facto Studies: Looking Back

One special type of field study is the **ex post facto study.** This design is unique because the investigator must select variables to study after the event has already happened. Natural and technological disasters call for an ex post facto study. Experimenters cannot manipulate variables to produce suicides, abuse, or rapes, for obvious ethical reasons. The only choice is to wait until the events occur and then try to answer important questions in retrospect.

Shirley Murphy (1984) used an ex post facto design when she studied victims of the Mount St. Helens volcano eruption. She collected data on a variety of physical and emotional symptoms. Catastrophe research might use **archival data** from hospitals or social and governmental agencies. Door-to-door surveys with pre-set questions or face-to-face interviews can provide clues to alterations in physical and mental health status. A descriptive analysis may be possible that summarizes the traumas reported by the group. With careful planning and execution, it is sometimes possible to test hypotheses about likely changes following such an event. It would still be impossible to directly test hypotheses about what precipitated an event such as suicide or abuse.

Correlational Designs: What Is the Relationship?

Correlational research is not experimental in the strict sense of the term. Nonetheless, this type of research can be very useful in tracking down variables that are potentially relevant for more extensive experimental investigations. Correlation is a statistical procedure that assesses the relationship between two or more variables. More precisely, the correlation coefficient is a quantitative index of the extent to which individuals occupy the same relative position on two scales. Correlation coefficients, expressed as r, range from +1.00, a perfect positive association; through 0.00, showing no association; to −1.00, a perfect inverse association. A strong negative relationship is just as informative as a strong positive relationship.

A study by Sorbi and Tellegen (1988) illustrates the correlational approach in stress research. Survey studies suggested that stress events frequently precede the onset of migraine headaches. Since no one had tested the strength of this relationship previously, Sorbi and Tellegen decided to do so. They treated stress as cause (also called the predictor variable) and migraine as effect (also called the criterion variable).

A group of 29 migraine patients responded weekly to an event-specific coping list. This list contained a stress scale based on the notion that everyday life events are stressful. Stress events could be objectively categorized into threat and challenge. Patients used a diary to record migraine attacks hourly. Sorbi and Tellegen found that threat events preceded migraine but challenge events did not. The reported correlation was $r = +0.50$. This was significant beyond the .01 level, a result that would be expected to occur by chance less than once in 100 instances.

Several caveats apply to correlational research. First, correlation does not imply causation. Associations may be produced by the operation of another hidden variable, or the association may be simply a matter of coincidence. There can be no causation unless there is first correlation, however. Thus, correlational research can be very useful to identify patterns of association that may be subjected later to closer scrutiny with experimental techniques.

Second, even when the observed correlation is high, the explained variance (technically r^2) is smaller. Explained variance, a technical term, can be understood without going into the statistics behind the term. Assume for the moment that stress tends to cause migraine headaches. How much of the variability in migraine attacks can be reliably attributed to stress? We would not expect stress to be the only cause of migraine. Biomedical factors (for example cardiovascular factors) probably explain some variability in migraine attacks as well. The correlation observed in the Sorbi and Tellegen study suggests that stress explains no more than 25% $(r^2 = .50^2 = .25)$ of the variability in migraine headaches. About 75% of the variability is unexplained by this relationship and must be due to the operation of other factors.

Scientists still regard the laboratory experiment as the pinnacle of research procedure. Nonetheless, designs implemented in the natural environment or with small groups of clients in a clinical setting are known for their great heuristic value; that is, they are a rich source of new hypotheses that may be tested later in more optimal controlled conditions.

Clinical Research: Pre-Post Intervention Designs

Clinical research usually works with clients who seek help for distressing or painful symptoms. Researchers try to find the best treatment to use with a specific type of client presenting a distinct set of symptoms. They are rarely satisfied with the knowledge that a treatment works; they also want to know *how* it works. They want to identify the effective agent of change in the treatment and the process variables that are crucial to success.

Current clinical research may be thought of as a process of give and take among lab, clinic, and field settings. Hypotheses generated in applied settings may eventually be tested in more controlled settings. On the other side, insights gained from controlled studies may become the rationale for even more effective clinical interventions.

Single-Subject Research: Baseline Reversal Designs

The simplest clinical study is the **single-subject design.** Although many variations are possible, the most general is the so-called **baseline reversal design,** or AB design, in which A is the baseline and B is the treatment phase. During baseline, the clinician obtains data that indicate how frequent or intense the behavior is before treatment. Then, the clinician selects a therapy that presumably should improve the symptoms and begins treatment. Later, the clinician compares treatment data to baseline data. If the symptoms are gone or reduced, there is reason to believe that the treatment will be effective in the future. To be sure that the treatment and not some coincidental outside factor produced the improvement, baseline conditions may be restored. If the symptoms reappear, we have even more confidence that the treatment was the effective agent. This is an ABA design.

Mark Hegel and his colleagues worked with three women who displayed hyperventilation syndrome (Hegel et al., 1989). They taught each patient to use controlled diaphragmatic breathing plus the relaxation response. As Figure 6.2 shows for one patient, episodes of chest pain and shortness of breath declined systematically after this treatment was introduced. The treatment gains were still evident 12 months later. Results were similar for the other two patients.

An interesting example of an ABAB baseline reversal design comes from the work of Roque and Roberts (1989). The ABAB baseline reversal design tracks behavior for a specified period of time prior to treatment. Then the clinician begins treatment and continues to collect data during treatment. Later, treatment is terminated, and the conditions that existed in baseline are reinstated

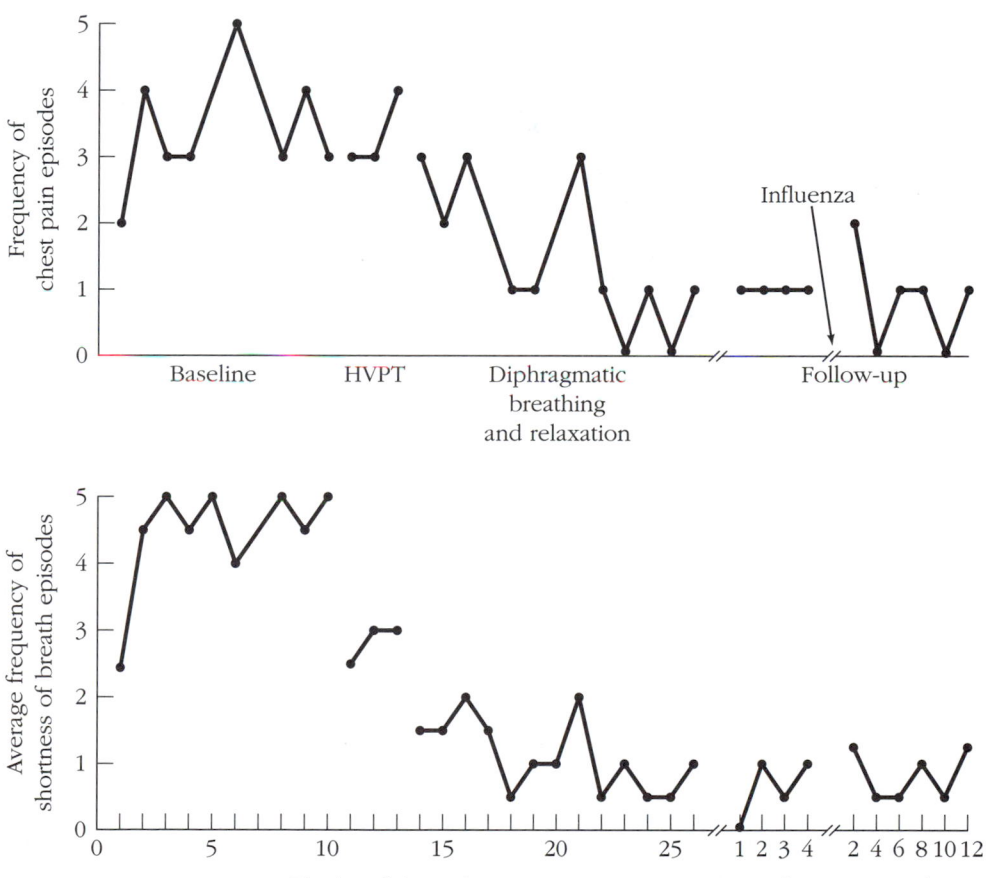

FIGURE 6.2 *Frequency of chest pain episodes and average frequency of shortness of breath episodes for patient G. A. for baseline, treatment, and follow-up (adapted from Hegel et al., 1989).*

as much as possible. Finally, treatment conditions are repeated to ensure that the client is ethically released with maximum therapeutic benefit.

Rogue and Roberts carried out their study in the natural environment with a group of unsuspecting subjects, drivers on the public streets of Tuscaloosa, Alabama. Subjects never gave consent for participation, but they were observed anonymously and without disclosure of their behavior to any authority.

Rogue and Roberts were concerned about high-risk driving behaviors such as speeding and failure to wear seat belts. The researchers wanted to find out whether public posting of compliance with speed limits would help to control speeding. Their subject population consisted of drivers on a defined stretch of urban highway in Tuscaloosa, Alabama. Speed was detected through inductive loop detectors. Feedback on the rate of compliance with the speed limit was provided daily by a roadside sign that read "DRIVERS NOT SPEEDING YESTERDAY, *nn*%" on top and "BEST RECORD, *nn*%" below.

Rogue and Roberts monitored speed for 10 days, 24 hours a day, in order to establish their baseline. The percentage of drivers complying with the speed limit was calculated and used for the subsequent phase of the experiment. As a control, the road sign that would display the percentages was erected so that it was in place during the baseline, but it was covered so that no information was conveyed to the drivers. In the treatment phase, the sign was uncovered, and the percentage of drivers who were in compliance with the speed limit was posted. The daily posted rates were accurate reflections of prior data. The results showed that posting compliance rates led to even more compliance among low and middle range speeders. Unfortunately, high speeders did not seem to reduce their speed at all. But additional interesting results confirmed the speed-reducing effect of posting.

After the posting period was finished, another baseline was established. This second baseline

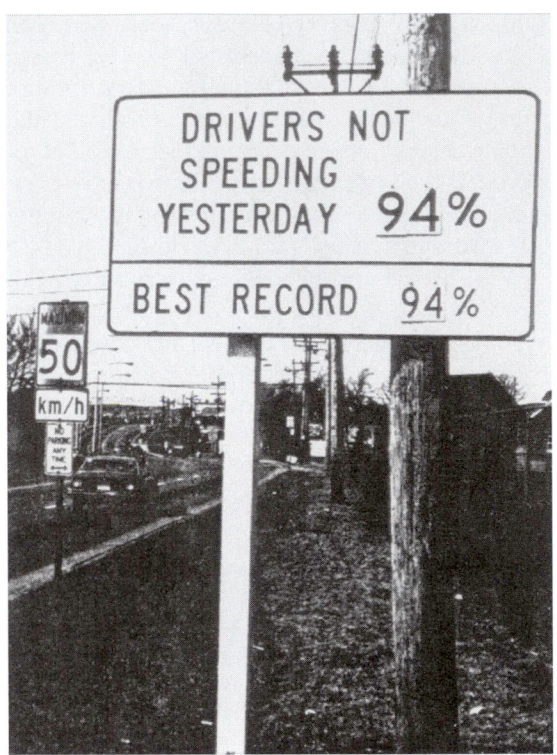

FIGURE 6.3   *An environmental sign of the type used by Rogue and Roberts to reduce speeding (from van Houten, Nau, & Marini, 1980).*

showed an increased speeding level in all groups of drivers, almost like a rebound effect. But this return to the baseline level is convincing data that the posting treatment was effective. Finally, the research team used a fourth treatment period in which inaccurate and inflated compliance rates were posted. When this occurred, more high speeders were likely to reduce their speed. In fact, the higher the posted rate of compliance, the greater the effect on the high speeder. Still, the overall effect on the high speeder was not significant.

These reversal designs can be very helpful. Yet they lack control, and use of a single subject limits generalizability. Of course, nothing prevents using multiple subjects as well as multiple baselines in a baseline reversal design. When an AB design uses a large number of subjects, it is usually called a pre-post design.

Pre-Post Designs: The Workhorse of Therapy Research

In a **pre-post design,** a group of clients with common symptoms responds (pretesting) to a standard scale (or set of scales). This step shows how severe the symptoms are before treatment. Then all clients receive treatment for a set time. In a posttest, clients respond to the same scale (usually an equivalent form of the same scale). The clinician then compares scores on the pretest to scores on the posttest to find out whether the treatment was effective.

This design seems elegantly simple on the surface, but it is also subject to problems of control. Factors external to the intervention may have produced the change. Clients may obtain helpful informal therapy from family, friends, or clergy. Clients with acute stress reactions may improve because the stressor retreats as quickly as it entered. In the absence of a control group, we cannot tell.

Pre-post design with untreated control

To solve this problem, the clinician may use an untreated control group having the same clinical symptoms as the treatment group. One way of managing this procedure is to use the **wait-list control,** diagrammed in Table 6.2. Volunteers may be solicited through local advertising. After the pretest, the clinician randomly assigns about half the volunteers to a wait list. To facilitate this process, volunteers are given a convincing cover story—that the clinic can provide treatment to only a few people at a time, and treatment will be provided as soon as space is available.

TABLE 6.2   *A pre-post design with wait-list control group (from Rice, 1992).*

NONFACTORIAL DESIGN WITH WAIT-LIST (UNTREATED) CONTROLS

Treatment group	Pretest (T1)	Treatment phase	Posttest (T2)
Wait-list control	Pretest (T1)	Waiting period	Posttest (T2)

When the treatment group completes therapy, we treat the wait-list group. Before beginning treatment, though, subjects on the wait list again fill out the scales that were used in pre-testing. The logic is straightforward. If the treatment group improved while the wait-list group did not, then the treatment must be responsible, not external factors. This design is superior to both the baseline-reversal and the pre-post design, but it still has flaws. For example, we know that clients' belief in a therapy alone creates a greater chance for cure. This is the **placebo effect.** To solve this problem, we use an attention-placebo control group.

Pre-post design with attention control

A study at the Sloan-Kettering Cancer center led by Sharon Manne illustrates this approach (Manne et al., 1990).[2] Manne and her associates were concerned about the extreme distress experienced by children undergoing invasive and painful chemotherapy. Children often must be physically restrained for venipuncture procedures. Manne cited evidence that these children receive as many as 300 venipunctures in the course of treatment. The procedure usually becomes more aversive as the veins become less accessible.

Manne's team designed a behavioral-cognitive treatment program with four components. First, children could divert attention by using a party whistle during venipuncture. Second, paced breathing substituted for undesirable behaviors such as struggle and refusal to sit still. Third, children could earn cartoon or celebrity stickers as positive reinforcement for cooperation. Finally, parents received instruction to encourage use of the party whistle and paced breathing.

---

[2] The procedures and analysis of this study are simplified to highlight the main design features and outcomes. The researchers also used sophisticated statistical analyses that are beyond the scope of this text.

Participating were 23 children, 13 in the treatment group and 10 in the attention-placebo group. All subjects provided baseline data during a scheduled venipuncture procedure plus three data sets following intervention. Parents in the attention-placebo group received instructions to use whatever procedures had been successful in previous sessions. For both treatment and control dyads, psychologists were present during venipuncture sessions. One flaw existed in the design: The researchers could not use blind control. The treatment team, including medical personnel, knew whether the children belonged to the treatment group or the attention group.

Manne's team rated children's distress over three trials. The results of the experiment were clear. The behavioral-cognitive treatment significantly reduced the amount of observed child distress. Children in the treatment group required less physical restraint after intervention than before and significantly less than the control group. The control group did improve but not as much. This result illustrates the role of attention that would be obscured by an untreated control design. (See Figure 6.4.) Parents also rated their children's pain as much lower

following intervention. The intervention was just as successful with young children (three years old) as with older children (nine years old), and with both boys and girls. Children in the treatment group did not report lower subjective pain, however, suggesting that behavioral control under distress and subjective experience of distress are not necessarily linked.

Factorial Designs: Combining Independent Variables

The previous designs manipulated only one independent variable. They are easy to interpret, but of doubtful generality. Events in the real world are rarely if ever determined by just one factor. Factorial designs combine two or more independent variables in a single experiment. We gain significant information with this strategy. Each independent variable can be tested as though a single-variable experiment is under way. At the same time, the interactions of variables also can be tested. Interactions reflect the way multiple factors combine to produce outcomes not predicted by the operation of variables studied in isolation. No single-variable experiment, no matter how well designed, can

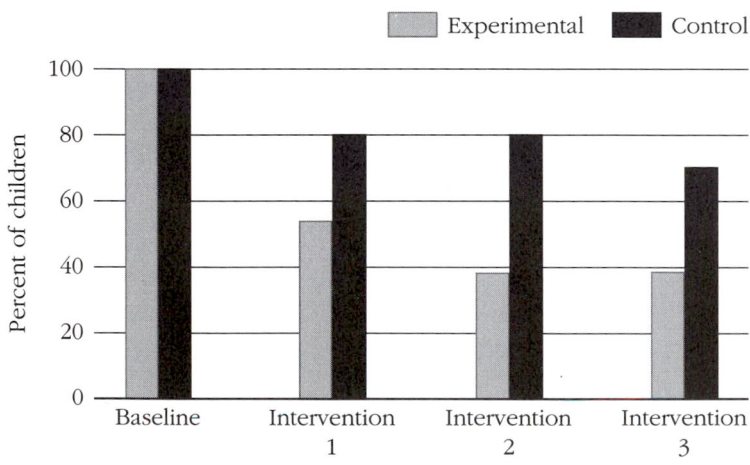

FIGURE 6.4   Mean frequency of use of restraint across baseline and three intervention trials (percentage of children) (from Manne et al., 1990).

ever provide information about interactions. Neither can we link a group of single-variable experiments to obtain information about interactions. The only way to study interactions is to combine the influence of suspect variables in one experiment.

A study conducted by Kenneth Allred and Timothy Smith (1989) illustrates the factorial design. Allred and Smith were following a line of inquiry begun by Suzanne Kobasa (1979a, 1979b) on the hardy personality. Numerous studies suggested that people who display a hardy personality are resistant to stress-induced illness. Investigators usually credited this to an adaptive cognitive style and reduced physiological arousal. To test this idea, Allred and Smith assessed both cognitive and physiological responses of males who were high and low on measures of hardiness under conditions of a laboratory-manipulated threat.

This study used two independent variables: personality hardiness and threat as a stressor. First, Allred and Smith used the Abridged Hardiness Scale and the Revised Hardiness Scale. They divided subjects into groups of high and low hardiness by taking the combined median split of the two scales.[3]

Second, Allred and Smith randomly assigned subjects to receive either a high evaluative threat condition or a low threat condition. Subjects in the high threat condition believed that they would take a test that could predict academic and vocational success. Subjects in the low threat condition believed that they would provide physiological measures while doing a cognitive task where answers were unimportant. Each independent variable had two levels, resulting in a typical 2×2 factorial design, shown in Table 6.3. The dependent variables were systolic and diastolic blood pressure plus a

TABLE 6.3   *A schematic representation of the* 2×2 *factorial design used by Allred and Smith (1989) and the expected outcome for the dependent variables (from Rice, 1992).*

	High threat	Low threat
High hardiness	Low arousal positive thoughts	No change compared to low hardy
Low hardiness	High arousal negative thoughts	No change compared to high hardy

self-statement inventory to assess positive and negative thoughts.

Analysis of the data showed that hardy subjects had only marginally lower arousal when they were waiting for the task to begin. Hardy subjects had higher systolic blood pressure, perhaps because of more active coping efforts. High hardy subjects in the high threat condition also had more positive thoughts than low hardy subjects in the same condition. The results supported the hardy cognitive style on the one hand, but suggested that the physiological links between hardiness and health status are by no means simple.

Indeed, Dienstbier (1989) has shown that organisms subjected to intermittent stressors develop a type of physiological toughness and resilience that allows for a more efficient response to stress. The base rate for sympathetic operations is reduced, which translates to a lower level of chronic arousal. At the same time, the sympathetic-adrenal-medullary complex can react more swiftly and strongly to challenge or threat. Further, brain catecholamines (neurotransmitters) are not depleted as rapidly as when sympathetic nervous system activity is high. This fact is significant because depletion of catecholamines undermines mental and physical performance. The resulting deficits could have a critical effect on ability to cope successfully with stress. Finally, experience with

---

[3] A median split divides the group into two equal halves. If the subject scored in the same half on each median split, they stayed in the study. Otherwise, they were dropped from the study.

intermittent stressors suppresses the pituitary adrenal-cortical response, which appears to translate as enhanced immune system function.

Mixed Designs: Comparing Between Groups Across Time

Quite often, clinical research and field trials require that the investigator examine the effectiveness of a treatment across time. Typically, the dependent measures are taken pre- and posttreatment, but other measures may be taken at different times during treatment and at several follow-up times. It is not uncommon for such work to collect observations years after the original intervention. In the parlance of experimental design, these are repeated measures on the same subjects.

In addition, there may be differences in client traits that are considered theoretically important, or different potentially useful treatments that are still unproved. Indeed, it may be that one treatment is most useful with one type of client, whereas another treatment is most useful with a different type of client. To test hypotheses of this nature, the investigator must use separate groups. The first approach, involving repeated observations on the same subjects, is a **within subjects design.** The second approach, assigning different subjects to different treatments, is a classic **between groups design.** When the project requires both the within subjects and between groups approaches, it is a **mixed design.**

Friedman, Bliwise, Yesavage, and Salom (1991) used a mixed design to compare two different treatments, sleep restriction therapy (SRT) and relaxation training (RLT), for sleep insomnia in adults. Sleep restriction therapy limits the time in bed when sleep is disturbed and increases time in bed as sleep becomes more efficient (Spielman, Saskin, & Thorpy, 1987). Subjects were obtained from the community, carefully screened for inclusion in the study, and alternately assigned to either SRT ($n = 10$) or RLT ($n = 12$).

Multiple dependent measures were used, including total sleep time, time in bed, sleep efficiency (defined as the ratio of total sleep time to time in bed multiplied by 100), and time to sleep onset, among others. Each measure was obtained for two-week observation periods and converted to three period means: The first mean was for a two-week baseline; the second mean was for the last two weeks (weeks 3 and 4) of treatment; and the third mean was for a two-week follow-up scheduled three months after treatment. Total sleep time did not improve for either group during therapy, but it rose significantly in both groups by follow-up. RLT subjects were spending more time in bed after treatment, but were significantly less efficient than SRT subjects. By this criteria, SRT seemed to have the more salutary effect on sleep. The authors

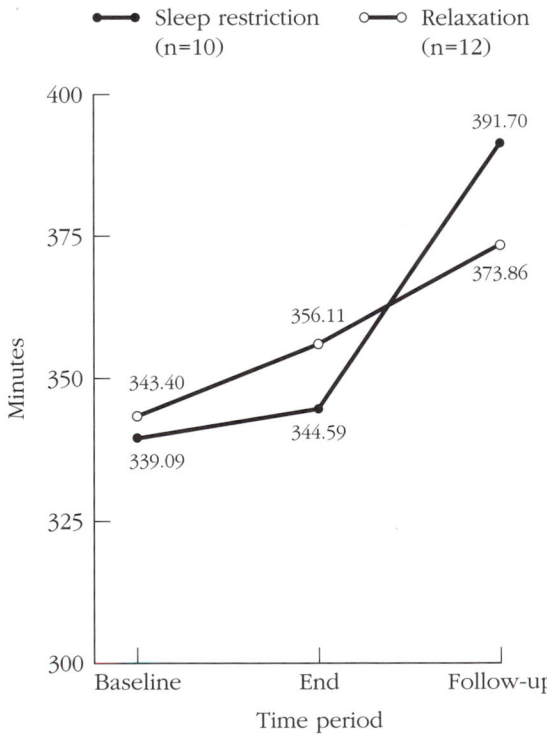

FIGURE 6.5   A comparison of sleep restriction therapy to a relaxation procedure with three months' follow-up (from Friedman et al., 1991).

noted, however, that there were subjects in both groups for whom the treatment did not seem to be effective. This result suggests that it is necessary to know more about how client traits interact with the qualities of specific treatments before better matches can be made.

Quasi-Experimental Designs: Comparing Assessed or Static Groups

We saw earlier that a quasi-experimental design is a design that has a family resemblance to a true experiment but is different in crucial ways. The primary difference is that in a quasi-experimental design, the investigator cannot assign subjects completely randomly to the different treatments. This limitation may occur because a trait being used for grouping cannot be directly manipulated. For example, sex of subjects is used very often as a grouping variable, but the investigator must use the presence of the variable as it already exists in the subjects. Trait anxiety, depression, coping style, and preexisting medical condition are just a few examples of subject traits that must be assessed by inventory or selected for based on documented diagnosis. In each case, the degree of a trait or the presence versus absence of a trait, rather than random assignment, determines group membership. Many of the so-called experimental designs technically may be quasi-experimental designs by this criteria. For example, the Allred and Smith (1989) study described earlier technically is a quasi-experimental design because the researchers used an assessment procedure to assign subjects to high hardiness or low hardiness groups.

Epidemiology: The Science of Epidemics

Epidemiology, the science of epidemics, seeks to understand the distribution and etiology of disease (Lilienfeld & Lilienfeld, 1980). The historical origins of this science are ancient and venerable, but the modern era may be traced to the work of John Snow around 1850. Snow, a founding member of the London Epidemiological Society, noted that death rates were eight to nine times higher than normal in a London district south of the Thames. Snow discovered that one particular company supplied water to this region and that this was the only company to draw its water from a highly polluted area of the Thames. Snow inferred from these facts that cholera came from "poison" transmitted by the polluted water.

Epidemiologists use many dependent measures not typically encountered in psychosocial research. The most common are mortality, morbidity, incidence, prevalence, and relative risk. **Mortality** is a period death rate per base of the population. For example, the annual death rate from cardiovascular disease is approximately 326 cases per 100,000 people. **Morbidity** measures the presence of disabling symptoms in a population. Heart patients may experience severe fatigue, require corrective surgery, or suffer nonfatal strokes.

The rate at which new cases of a disease appear in a given period is **incidence. Prevalence** is the number of cases of a disease that exist at a given time; thus prevalence is the total number of cases, whether old or new. The rapid change in AIDS during the middle 1980s illustrates these two measures. Early in 1986, the total number of cases—prevalence—was about 18,907. At that time, new cases began to appear at an alarming rate—incidence. In this case, the incidence statistic was much more important than the prevalence statistic. Finally, **relative risk** (RR) is the measure of association between a marker trait and the disease. It is expressed as a ratio:

$$RR = \frac{\text{Incidence of disease in exposed group}}{\text{Incidence of disease in nonexposed group}}$$

Grobbee and his colleagues used this measure in their report on caffeine and cardiovascular disease in men (Grobbee et al., 1990). Men who drank four or more cups of coffee per day (whether caffeinated or decaffeinated) had a relative risk of 1.04. In concrete numbers, 589 non–coffee drinkers suffered some cardio-vascular disorder compared to 613 men who drank four or more cups of coffee per day ($613 \div 589 = 1.04$). This difference was so small that it could be explained by sampling differences or measurement error. One interesting result was that men who drank decaffeinated coffee had a relative risk of 1.67 (572 nonexposed compared to 1002 exposed). This difference was statistically significant. The authors concluded that there is no support for the notion that coffee consumption increases risk for coronary disease.[4]

The logic of epidemiology follows the usual scientific progression from description, to explanation, to prediction and control (Kleinbaum, Kupper, & Morgenstern, 1982). In general, epidemiology first tries to describe the health status of a population. Researchers count current cases of illness (prevalence) or measure the rate at which new cases of an illness appear in a given period (incidence). Using these measures, comparisons can be made between subgroups of the population, as Snow did for people living below the Thames as opposed to those living above. Differences between subgroups may lead to useful and testable hypotheses (pollution of the water caused the illness).

The second step is to explain the **etiology,** or origins, of a disease. Etiology constructs a coherent picture of the factors that contribute to an illness. Numerous markers may be identified, including demographic characteristics (sex, age, ethnic group), biological and genetic factors, environmental variables, socioeconomic variables, and personal health habits and lifestyle (such as coffee consumption). The emphasis is on groups at risk. There is no attempt to predict illness in individuals (Cockerham, 1982).

Epidemiologists may test models developed in the second stage by trying to predict prevalence and distribution of diseases. If predictions are accurate, confidence that the etiological

model is correct increases. Finally, epidemiologists may use the knowledge gained in prior studies to control diseases. Outcomes could include implementation of preventive steps, eradication, prolongation of life, or improvement in the health status of afflicted persons.

There are many variations to epidemiological studies, more than we can discuss here. We can use a very common procedure, the clinical trial, to illustrate. A **clinical trial** is a field experiment to verify that a therapeutic agent is effective. The study presented also illustrates a **prospective design;** that is, it followed subjects through the natural history of a disorder. In contrast, a **retrospective design** attempts to reconstruct probable causes by looking back on a disorder after it has already occurred.

Recently, medical nutrition research suggested that beta-carotene may act as a dietary anticarcinogen. Animal models (discussed in more detail later) suggested that carotenoids slow down development of tumors but do not reduce the number of tumors (Krinsky, 1989). Case-control studies showed that increased consumption of fruits and vegetables with high levels of beta-carotene reduced the risk for cancer. Unfortunately, case-control studies do not allow us to eliminate competing explanations, since we cannot control for many other variables.

Greenberg's group reported the results of a large-scale randomized double-blind clinical trial in people with a prior history of nonmelanoma skin cancer (Greenberg et al., 1990). The researchers randomly assigned 1805 patients to one of two groups. The treatment (exposed) group (913 patients) received 50 mg of beta-carotene daily. The placebo (nonexposed) group (892 patients) received capsules identical in appearance to the beta-carotene capsules.

The team monitored compliance with the therapy through regularly scheduled questionnaires. If subjects did not take the pills, or there was a substantial difference in compliance between the groups, no firm conclusions could be made. Greenberg's group anticipated another potential problem, that the nonexposed group might obtain black market supplies of beta-carotene. To check on compliance, the

---

[4] Note, however, that the results across many studies are mixed, so the jury is still out on the exact role of caffeine in coronary risk.

researchers tested subjects' blood samples for levels of beta-carotene. This is a **manipulation check.** Patients in the exposed group had an eight-fold increase in beta-carotene while patients in the placebo group showed no change from prestudy levels.

Patients received routine medical examinations at yearly intervals over a five-year study period. There were two dependent measures: time to the occurrence of new skin cancer and number of new skin cancers. The results clearly conflicted with earlier case-control studies: Beta-carotene did not protect the exposed group against recurrence of skin cancer. The exposed group had an average of .29 new cancers per study year whereas the placebo group had an average of .25 new cancers. The rates also did not differ at checkpoints during the five-year period of the study. The authors pointed out that their study used subjects with a particular type of cancer. From this sample, then, it would be unwise to conclude that beta-carotene offers no protection for all cancers.

Meta-Analysis: Analyzing the Analyses

Meta-analysis is the new kid on the block when it comes to analysis of experiments. Richard Light, a Harvard statistician, and David Pillemer, a Wellesley College psychologist, developed the technique in the early 1970s (Light & Pillemer, 1984), but it was Gene Glass (1976) who coined the term. Meta-analysis is observational, not experimental. It generates new data, but only through use of old data, not through manipulation of causal variables. It is a statistical technique that sums up the results of studies concerned with similar hypotheses.

Historically, science has progressed by contributing a volume of studies that probe the breadth and depth of an issue. In the process, a group of studies might seem to converge to a common solution only to be upset by another group of studies showing discrepant results. When a critical mass accumulated, some un-daunted soul would pore over the results and try to extract order from the jaws of chaos. The written record of this effort is a **qualitative literature review** (or a narrative review). Entire journals are devoted to these reviews (*Psychological Bulletin* and *Psychological Review*), and they play an invaluable role in helping interested parties keep up with a research topic.

Still, qualitative reviews suffer from the bias of expert opinion. No matter how expert the reviewer is, the review still involves subjective judgment. Further, qualitative reviews lack methodological rigor, and they place undue emphasis on the level of significance of studies under review (Johnson, 1989).

In contrast, meta-analysis provides an objective tool to conduct a **quantitative literature review.** Presumably, the results of a meta-analysis can be placed in the public domain for scrutiny, whereas expert opinion cannot. Also, the process is subject to replication and should lead to the same outcomes and interpretations.

In brief, meta-analysis accounts for the magnitude of effect, which is defined as the absolute size of the difference between experimental and control conditions. Magnitude of effect is not based solely on statistical significance. By pooling the results of many studies, the effect of certain stimulus variables can be seen more clearly. In several situations, meta-analysis led to much different conclusions than those obtained from a narrative review.

An example of this approach is found in the work of Fernandez and Turk (1989). Their research revolved around issues of pain management and the efficacy of behavioral and cognitive therapies to reduce pain. Fernandez and Turk used a pool of 46 articles with a composite sample of 2000 subjects. They showed that previous qualitative and quasi-statistical studies led to confusion about the potency of cognitive coping strategies. Earlier reviews suggested that acknowledging pain was the most effective method of altering pain perception, whereas neutral imagery was the least effective. Meta-analysis showed the opposite result. On one matter, though, all the analyses agreed: Cognitive strategies produce substantive improvement over untreated or placebo controls.

Although meta-analysis has had remarkable success, it is not a panacea. It has its pitfalls and critics. The investigator must make many decisions about which studies to include and exclude, how to group studies when definitions vary, how to treat missing data, and so on. Also, studies with significant effects are overrepresented in the published literature, whereas studies with nonsignificant findings are much less likely to be published. In their meta-analysis of the disease-prone personality, Friedman and Booth-Kewley (1987) criticized the excessive speculation that has often resulted from meta-analyses. The authors pointed out that the most valuable product of meta-analysis should be more refined empirical work to resolve discrepancies. Finally, there is concern that meta-analysis distances us even further from the client, whose well-being is the primary concern of much of the research.

Program Evaluation: Assessing the System

Health psychologists do not just evaluate people. They also evaluate agencies, large and small, and the various services these agencies provide. This effort is commonly called program evaluation. Sechrest and Figueredo (1993) defined evaluation in general as an activity aimed at deciding the worth of various activities. Program evaluation is very different from the standard research process, and it often entails very different statistical procedures. Indeed, the recent trend in program evaluation has been toward qualitative methods and away from the traditional rigorous quantitative methods that marked the inception of the enterprise. Further, far from being an objective and detached scientific inquiry, program evaluation now is often committed to furthering certain social values.

Traditionally program evaluation has focused on structure, process, or outcome (Miller, 1981). Structural features include the physical and psychosocial environment of the service agency: facilities, staff, and equipment. As recent work suggests, evaluating structure may also require sensitivity to the sociopolitical context of the agency. Health care agencies are subject to many pressures, including federal, state, and regional funding biases that can shift radically with the winds of politics and taxpayer demands.

Health care agencies must meet external accreditation criteria as well. Evaluations may be conducted using these criteria to determine whether the agency is in compliance. A subcomponent of this type of evaluation includes determining staff competency. Program evaluators do not establish the criteria of professional competency any more than they would actually test a professional's competency. Using the criteria from accrediting agencies and professional licensure groups, however, it is possible to determine whether the agency is staffed with people properly trained to provide services the agency expects to deliver.

Process evaluation refers to how frequently and how effectively specific services are supplied to specific populations. Outcome evaluations determine to what extent the agency has met its goals and provided successful treatment to its clients.

Shadish, Cook, and Leviton (1991) identified five key issues in program evaluation (p. 32):

1. Social programming: how social programs and policies develop, improve, and change, especially in regard to social problems
2. Knowledge construction: how researchers learn about social action
3. Valuing: how value can be attached to program descriptions
4. Knowledge use: how social science information is used to modify programs and policies
5. Evaluation practice: the tactics and strategies evaluators follow in their professional work, especially given their constraints

Social programming is the hallmark of progressive government, but as we are all too often painfully reminded, social programming may not have the intended positive effect. Quite often, a social program fails because few legislators take the time to think about how the program may be expected to have the desired effect. One trend in program evaluation is to depend more on theory-based evaluation. Simply put, a carefully thought out theory should help focus evaluation on the specific process and outcomes that will show whether the program is serving its intended purpose.

Knowledge construction concerns how researchers discover vital information about a given social program. The dispute between the quantitative and qualitative camps is often based on disagreements about what data are most relevant to this purpose. To illustrate, quantitative data may show that a drug rehabilitation program has had limited success in treatment but fail to show why. Qualitative data may show that the program did not adhere to its treatment model, but still miss the crucial fact that disagreement between management and staff on how to implement the program led to different practices that undermined the program.

The value issue appears to be more vital today than ever. Sechrest and Figueredo (1993) use the PUSH/Excel program as an example of this situation. The Push to Excellence program to help disadvantaged youths was the brainchild of Jesse Jackson. The first evaluation of PUSH/ Excel used traditional quantitative methods and reached distinctly negative conclusions. These conclusions were drawn because the evaluation team could find no consistent program at the many different sites. Arguments in support of continuing the program, though, never provided data to refute the outcomes. In fact, the arguments suggested that data were irrelevant and that the program should be valued in its own right since it was to help disadvantaged, largely minority populations.

Knowledge use is concerned with how the information feeds back to the program or policymakers monitoring the program. The original idea was that policy or program elements could be changed by making evaluation data available. As Sechrest and Figueredo

pointed out, that view seems hopelessly naive. Evaluation research has advanced very little in terms of how to make use of its knowledge. In part, this failure may be due to the fact that programs are embedded in complex extended social networks. Unless evaluation research includes the entire social network in the evaluation scheme—a step that may be wholly impracticable—inadequate use of knowledge is not likely to improve.

Finally, evaluation practice is concerned with the merits of different methods of assessment. One core issue already discussed is the relative merit of quantitative versus qualitative evaluation. Another issue is the distinction between formative and summative evaluation. Formative evaluation is generally nonpunitive evaluation that tries to help correct weaknesses before an end point and potentially punitive evaluation occurs. Summative evaluation is the end point or outcome assessment. It is intended to determine whether the program has met its objectives, what degree of success the program enjoys, and what the program's cost-benefit ratio is. In a general sense, evaluation research must turn a critical eye to its own methods, just as traditional research and statistical practice has inspected its methods over the years.

Animals in Health Research: Models of Obesity, Addiction, and Aging

Most of the research designs we have discussed used human subjects, but animal studies are not irrelevant to health research. In fact, a substantial amount of research on health variables and methods of intervention began with animal models before the work moved on to human populations.

To begin, several arguments have been made in support of animal research (Johnson, 1990). First, the need to provide therapeutic assistance to the physically and mentally ill has always seemed a compelling reason to pursue research with animals. This need is based on the demand, indeed the public clamor, for treatments to meet catastrophic health needs. Second, animal research has proved historically to be nearly invaluable in providing information about numerous crucial issues including brain-behavior relations; genetic substrates of stress, addictions, obesity, and aging; and development of treatments (both behavioral and pharmacologic) for depression and anxiety, among other maladies. Third, animal models enable researchers to control and manipulate certain factors that could not be controlled so easily with human subjects. Fourth, although animal rights activists recommend simulations and culture experiments, these techniques cannot begin to provide the information that is needed where the complexities of human behavior and health needs are concerned. Fifth, the evolution of the comparative sciences (comparative psychology, for example) has produced more detailed knowledge of parallels between animals and humans in biological and psychological systems. When a scientist selects a particular animal subject, the selection is typically directed by that same knowledge. In turn, generalizations to humans can be made with increased confidence, although final confirmation with a human population is still important. Finally, though not an argument for animal research, it has been noted that the number of animals used in psychological research is in actuality relatively small, and that experiments inflicting severe pain are rare even though their frequency has been highly exaggerated (Coile & Miller, 1984; Miller, 1985).

I will touch on just a few of the more noteworthy examples of animal research. At the biological end of the continuum, psychological research has used animals for a wide range of neuroanatomy, neurophysiology, and neurotransmitter studies. This work has been important to understanding brain-behavior connections, many of which are important to health psychology. As one example, understanding the role of the hypothalamus in regulating food intake depends largely on animal models. Overall regulation of hunger and food intake is now known to be a complex system that involves brain centers and feedback of information (both neural and chemical) from the digestive system. Further, knowledge of obesity and fat storage mechanisms has benefited greatly from animal research. In turn, all this knowledge has led to more focused research and better understanding of eating disorders in general, including obesity, anorexia nervosa, and bulimia.[5]

A second important research area involving animals attempts to answer questions about the genetic basis of high-risk behaviors. For example, the past 25 years have seen much research on the genetic basis of drug addiction (George, 1988, 1990) and alcoholism (George, 1987; Geer, McKechnie, Heinstra, & Pyka, 1991). Among the more important issues explored via the genetic animal model are (1) sensitivity to drug effects; (2) tolerance, dependence, and withdrawal; (3) and the rewarding (or aversive) effects of drug use. (See the review by Crabbe, Belknap, & Buck, 1995.) Animal models of genetic influence enable an investigator to look at the transmission of a trait over several generations (five to seven generations is not uncommon) in a matter of only a few years, when the same research with humans would require 100 to 120 years. Animals from the lowly fly, to rodents, to primates have served for this type of work.

Hans Selye's (1956, 1976) research on stress was conducted largely with rats as subjects.[6] Thus, much of what we know about the body's emergency response system (the physiology of stress) comes from this type of work. Over the past 20 years, we have seen the emergence of the field of psychoneuroimmunology (Ader, Cohen, & Felten, 1987). The basic notions of immunology and connections between the immune system and the brain and endocrine system have been based on animal models. Investi-

---

[5] See Chapter 10 for more detail on eating disorders.
[6] Research on stress and health, including Selye's work, is discussed in Chapter 7.

gators also have provided evidence that the immune system can be classically conditioned. Finally, dose-response links for newly designed medicines or for high-risk toxins like sidestream smoke and carcinogens are based largely on animal research.

Of course, sensitive ethical issues beyond the scope of this chapter have sparked lively debates on both sides of this issue. Perhaps the most intense debates ensued following revelations from Edward Taub's laboratory that involved neglect, if not abuse, of animal subjects. Despite the negative press surrounding this situation, the research program itself is an example of the analogue approach applied to closed-head injury and rehabilitation methods (Pons et al., 1991). Later chapters will frequently refer to studies based on animal models.

Summary

In this chapter, we have discussed several methodologies used to study psychosocial factors related to health and illness. The coverage has been selective to provide a background for studies introduced later in the text.

1. Case studies look in great depth at a single individual, but do not establish cause and effect relations. Case studies can be of heuristic value in generating hypotheses for further clinical testing.

2. Field studies observe many behaviors that occur in natural settings. Most do not control for extraneous variables and thus cannot provide information about cause and effect. Yet they have more ecological validity than laboratory studies, and like the case study, they are of heuristic value.

3. At the most primitive level, clinical experiments use single-subject designs and compare baseline data to data following treatment. Extensions of this basic design include the single-group pre-post design, the pre-post design with untreated control group, and the pre-post design with an attention-placebo control group. Each design improves on the preceding one by increasing the control that eliminates alternate explanations for the success of the treatment.

4. Factorial designs are the first step to multicausal hypotheses. Factorial designs combine two or more independent variables and allow us to test how these variables interact to produce outcomes not predicted from study of the variables in isolation.

5. Epidemiological research assesses the distribution of diseases in a population. It also seeks to discover the etiology or causes of disease. When changes in mortality (deaths) and morbidity (disabling symptoms) occur with different rates in subgroups of a population, important clues may appear to guide further research.

6. One of the most common research designs in epidemiology is the clinical trial. This method randomly assigns subjects to different therapies and then tests the success of the therapy for a certain disease. Psychosocial epidemiology is now extending these methods to study relations between psychosocial factors and health status.

7. Meta-analysis is a newcomer to the quantitative analysis of data. It works on data from already completed studies. The technique analyzes effect size—the size of the difference between the experimental and the control group. This information enables investigators to evaluate the consistency of findings, assess the importance of either demographic or situational variables used by previous investigators, and resolve contradictions among existing studies.

8. Health psychologists may also be called upon to do program evaluations, which assess the structure, process, and outcomes of an agency. The overall purpose is to determine the extent to which an agency is meeting its goals in providing effective client services.

9. Animals are used in various projects to obtain information on disease and health processes that may not be as readily obtained with human subjects. Genetic processes, for example, can be much more easily observed in a rodent sample than in a human sample.

Key Words

archival data
attention placebo
baseline measures
baseline reversal
    design
between groups
    design
case study method
clinical trial
confidence level
contextual thinking
control group
correlational research
criterion variable
debriefing
dependent variable
distal cause
double-blind control
epidemiology
etiology
ex post facto study
experimental group
factorial designs
formistic thinking
hypothesis
incidence
independent variable
inferential statistics
informed consent
Institutional Research
    Board

manipulation check
mechanistic thinking
meta-analysis
mixed design
morbidity
mortality
operational definition
organistic thinking
placebo effect
precipitating factors
pre-post design
predictor variable
predisposing factors
prevalence
prospective design
proximal cause
qualitative literature
    review
quantitative literature
    review
quasi-experimental
    design
random assignment
relative risk (RR)
retrospective design
single-blind control
single-subject design
survey research
wait-list control
within subjects design

Study Questions

1. What is the significance of the distinction between unicausal and multicausal models for health psychology?
2. How might single-subject case studies be useful to the health psychologist?
3. What are the strengths and weaknesses of the correlational design?
4. When an investigator decides to use a control group, what factors must be considered?
5. What is epidemiological research, and how does it differ from classical laboratory research?
6. What is meta-analysis? How is it being used today to add to our knowledge base in health psychology?

Class Projects

1. If the department has current active projects that can use students as subjects, consider volunteering to get an inside view of the research process.

Suggested Readings

Engel, G. L. (1977). The need for a new medical model: A challenge for biomedicine. *Science, 196,* 129–136.

Evans, A. S. (1978). Causation and disease: A chronological journey. *American Journal of Epidemiology, 108,* 249–258.

WEBSITES   *Research and Methods in Health Behavior*

ADDRESS	DESCRIPTION
http://www.carleton.ca/~cmckie/research.html	Research Engines for the Social Sciences
http://www.cdc.gov	☆ Center for Disease Control—provides latest data on epidemiology of disease
http://tin.ssc.plym.ac.uk/	Social Science Meta-Index to social science resources
http://www.essex.ac.uk/social-science-methodology-school	Social Science Methodology School Home Page—Data Analysis and Collection
http://www.apa.org/science/lib.html	☆ APA's Introduction to Library Resarch—for students and non-psychologists
http://sci.psychology.research	Newsgroup for research issues in psychology

Stress, High-Risk Behaviors, and Health

Health psychology has gradually built a base of information revealing a vital connection between psychosocial events and health. The psychosocial events include environmental events that trigger stress reactions and high-risk lifestyle choices. Lifestyle choices encompass many things from diet and exercise, to drug use or abuse, to high-risk sexual behavior.

Early Canadian and U.S. studies revealed that about 50% of premature mortality could be attributed to lifestyle (Lalonde, 1974; Institute of Medicine, 1979). Seven of the ten leading causes of death involve important behavioral components. Four behaviors in particular seem crucial to changing health risk: managing stress; changing diet to reduce fats, salts, and sugars and to increase carbohydrates; increasing exercise; and reducing the use of drugs, especially tobacco and alcohol. Given the rapid spread of AIDS, it seems prudent to add a fifth behavior to this list; avoiding high-risk sexual behavior.

The importance of the stress-health connection is reinforced by a research legacy, spanning nearly 40 years, showing that cognitive-behavioral reactions to stress can change the way the body operates. In some cases, the body's protective systems may work at a higher level of efficiency than normal, thus providing even more resistance to illness. In other cases, such as prolonged and unremitting stress, protective mechanisms may begin to weaken, thus making the person more vulnerable to illness than under normal conditions. You first glimpsed this important connection in Chapter 3 where we discussed the new field of psychology, psychoneuroimmunology. While many questions remain, the breakthroughs in this area provide some of the strongest evidence to date of the connection between mental processes and body functions.

The focus of Chapter 7 will be a more thorough study of how stress works to alter body functions and thus to influence health for better or for worse. In the course of this discussion, we will describe definitional issues in stress research. In order to complete the details of a stress model, we must go over several theoretical issues, including the currently most influential theory of stress, Lazarus's transactional model. Later, we will take a focused excursion into the brain and neuroendocrinology. This discussion will provide the background necessary to understand more intricate facets of the immunocompetence model, which posits that stress alters the ability of the body to protect itself from disease. Just as cognitive-behavioral

reactions to stress may tip the scale in the direction of lowered resistance and poorer health, they may also be allies. The techniques used to defend against stress or to transform potentially negative stress into positive challenge are called coping skills. A growing body of research shows that coping techniques can be learned and then brought into play to preserve health or to help in the battle against an illness in progress.

In Chapters 8 and 9, we will take up the issue of substance abuse, a very serious high-risk behavior in our society. Current theory and research is concerned with definitional issues, because physical and psychological models of craving and dependence have not always been consistent with each other. General theories of addiction have emerged that try to address the common features that link addictions. Later in Chapter 8, we will look at the epidemiology, etiology, and treatment of smoking. Smoking is regarded as the single most modifiable high-risk health behavior, because it contributes to more than 400,000 deaths each year yet is largely voluntary. Chapter 9 considers the epidemiology, etiology, and treatment of alcohol addiction.

Chapter 10 deals with nutrition, diet, and eating disorders that influence health. Obesity is a significant problem for many people worldwide. The physiology and psychology of obesity will be discussed. Several biomedical and psychosocial treatment models will also be described. Finally, many young women struggle with the eating disorders of anorexia nervosa and bulimia. We will briefly describe these disorders and some of the programs developed to help treat these problems.

In the last chapter in this section, Chapter 11, we will look at how high-risk sexual behavior contributes to the origin and spread of AIDS.

Stress Models: Symptoms, Sources, and Coping

When Hurricane Andrew approached the heavily populated east Florida coast, everyone knew it had the potential to be a killer storm. Fortunately, early warnings and precautions by area residents served to prevent heavy loss of life. Still, no one could be fully prepared for the magnitude of the physical loss suffered by those in its wake. Even as the storm left to continue its devastation in Louisiana, and another hurricane, Iniki, ravaged Hawaii, survivors could do little more than look on with a mixture of shock, grief, and awe at what took place in so short a time. We may never have a completely accurate account of the loss, but estimates suggest that it will take years and cost more than $20 billion for homeowners, businesses, and government to rebuild.

Beyond the physical loss, though, such natural disasters have both direct and hidden psychological effects. We do not know yet what the mental health fallout may be, but many studies carried out worldwide over the past 25 years provide insights about what can be expected from such catastrophes. The experience of shock and grief is nearly universal, and survival guilt also occurs. Other aspects of the psychological aftermath include anxiety, phobic fear, an increased sense of vulnerability, helplessness, frustration, depression, and anger. Sleep disturbances are common, as is loss of appetite. Disaster victims tend to increase use of alcohol, cigarettes, sleeping pills, antidepressants, and tranquilizers (Joseph, Yule, Williams, & Hodgkinson, 1993).

Many disaster victims are forced to relocate for either short- or long-term stays in unfamiliar,

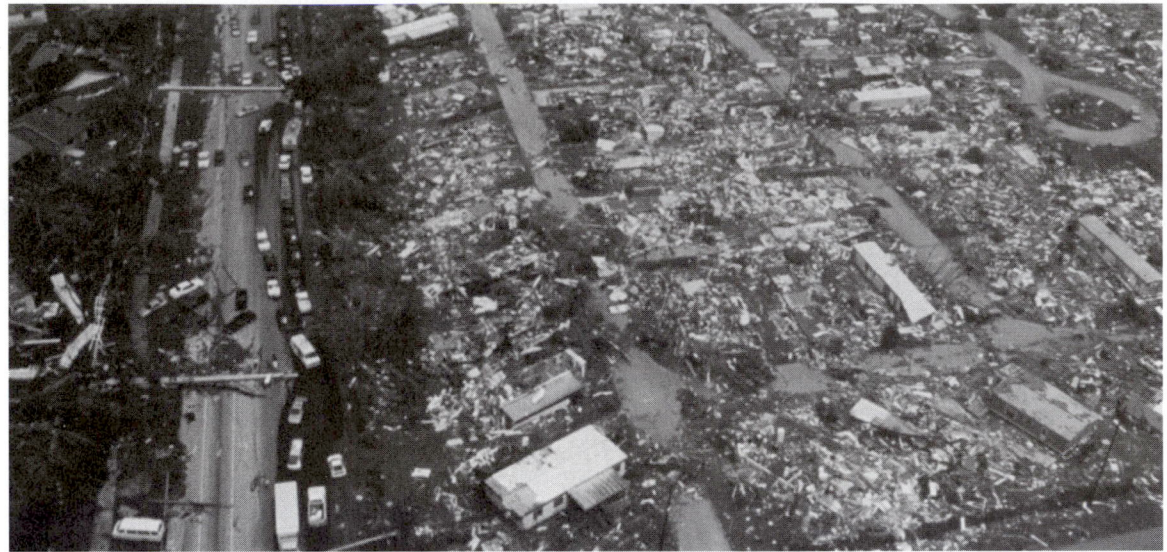

FIGURE 7.1   The devastation of Hurricane Andrew surveyed from the air.

crowded, and often substandard conditions (Riad & Norris, 1996). The pervasive disruption in daily routine and diminished sense of well-being contaminate personal relationships, including placing intolerable strains on already fragile marriages (McLeod, 1984). Clinically, these symptoms are part of the syndrome called post-traumatic stress disorder (PTSD). One south Florida resident survived Hurricane Andrew but lost everything including the furniture business he had worked years to build. When he took his life later that October, the tragedy was attributed to PTSD.

Still, health psychologists and stress researchers want to answer another important question: Can stress feed back information to the physical system that changes how the body functions? In turn, do these physical changes expose the person to even greater risk of illness? If the answer to both these questions is yes, then we must ask what specific mechanisms and communication pathways provide for this dialogue between mental events and body processes. On the positive side, what steps can people take to combat the insidious effects of stress? The

answers to these questions are the subject matter of this chapter.

To begin, we will look at epidemiological data that tells how pervasive stress is, and we will set about the difficult task of defining stress. We will then discuss the logic and research suggesting that stress does have important consequences for health and illness. In this context, we will examine information on the physiological systems involved in translating psychosocial stress to physical outcomes. Finally, we will consider several coping strategies that people can use to combat the negative effects of stress.

Stress Takes Its Toll: Demographics and Distribution

In 1985, a National Health Interview Survey asked people to respond to a stress questionnaire (Silverman, Eichler, & Williams, 1987). The sample was a nationwide group of civilian citizens 18 years of age and older. The survey reported results in percentages and used a weighted procedure so that the total number of people reporting stress and coping behaviors could be estimated. Roughly 41%, or 34 million people, reported a lot of stress in the preceding two weeks. Less than 2% reported they did not know what stress was.

Women were more likely than men to report stress (23% versus 18%), an effect that was even more pronounced in those over 65 years of age. Both higher levels of income and education were associated with more stress than middle levels of income and education, but lower income levels (poverty levels) were also associated with greater stress. About 17% of the sample thought about getting help for stress, and about 69% of those considering help actually sought it. Finally, those reporting the greatest amount of stress also reported that they rarely ate breakfast, usually slept six or fewer hours per night, and were less physically active. These findings are consistent with research suggesting that diet, exercise, and rest are important stress-related behaviors.

These statistics only scratch the surface of the wide range of stress effects. To fully appreciate what stress can do, it is necessary to consider how stress influences the family, the workplace, and ultimately the individual's health status. Holmes and Rahe's (1967) work on life-event stress suggested the three most potent sources of stress are death, divorce, and separation. Although divorce and separation do not invariably lead to negative outcomes (Barber & Eccles, 1992), disruption to the family still remains one of the single greatest sources of stress. Single-parent homes generally suffer more pressure from financial strain and scheduling than two-parent homes. Most members of the family suffer some decline in both emotional and physical health as a result of divorce or separation, and children often encounter additional adjustment problems (Grych & Fincham, 1990). Unfortunately, life-change stress and abuse in families are also linked (Smith, 1984). At the extreme end, about 20% of homicides are the direct result of family violence that itself appears to result from stress (Emery, 1989).

There are gender differences in the experience of stress due to differences in acculturation and role definition. Marjorie Fiske (1993) summarized some long-term research on this issue carried out by the Institute for Social Research. This work showed that single women experienced more stress than single men. Young married women without children appeared to experience less stress than men, however. On the other hand, divorced women appear to experience more stress than men, typically because of uncertain finances and difficulties in managing time constraints stemming from child care, housework, employment, and social life. Later in the life span, widowed women were less likely to experience stress than widowers. Some speculate—and speculation it is—that this discrepancy results from the traditional expectation that the woman will be the principal home manager and caregiver. Presumably in the process of carrying out these duties, she has become more adept at self-care and self-management, while presumably the man has become more dependent on the woman. When the man is widowed, then, he may have more difficulty readjusting his life to a spouse's absence than a woman does.

In the workplace, occupational stress became a category in the DSM-III-R and continues in the DSM-IV (American Psychiatric Association, 1987; 1994; Sauter, Murphy, & Hurrell, 1990). One estimate suggests that about one in every three days of absenteeism is related to stress (Veniga & Spradley, 1981). The federal government estimates that 100,000 workers die each year from job-related diseases, and another 390,000 develop some type of job-related illness. In addition, 14,000 workers die each year from accidents on the job. Another 2.2 million suffer some type of disabling injury (Institute of Medicine, 1979). It is likely that acute reactive stress contributes to some of these job accidents (Green, 1985).

Issues in Defining Stress: Three Faces of Stress

It is easy enough to find commonsense definitions of stress. It has been called simply "that great confusion of mind." Stress also has been defined by example: Stress is your boss asking if you ever thought about a different career. It is your spouse asking if you know a good divorce lawyer. The poet Bukowski described it as "the shoelace that breaks with no time left."

Still, scientists look for formal, precise definitions that they can submit to direct scientific scrutiny and around which they can build a general theory. In the course of his long career, Hans Selye, the founder of modern stress research, came to understand that the task of defining stress involved serious problems. He wrote that "stress, like relativity, is a scientific concept which has suffered from the mixed blessing of being too well known and too little understood" (Selye, 1980, p. 127). In recent years, three definitions of stress have been used: stress as a physical force, stress as subjective emotional tension, and stress as body arousal. Each provides a partial view of stress, but each can be integrated in a fourth definition that is part of the cognitive-transactional model of stress.

Stress as External Pressure: The Physical Force Approach

The external pressure view is the most simplistic. It suggests that stress exists as a property of an external event. In the world of physical objects and events, stress is like a strong wind against a bridge or a skyscraper. Engineers presumably only have to calculate the load or force a structure must endure and then build it to be strong enough to resist that force. In regard to psychosocial events, stress is typically illustrated by an unpredictable and uncontrollable event. For example, in October 1991, a gunman drove through the front window of a Killeen, Texas,

restaurant during the noon lunch rush and began randomly shooting anybody in sight. The gunman's timing was unpredictable and the forces unleashed were largely uncontrollable for most of the people present. In this instance, then, stress could be attributed to the external savage force present in the gunman's actions. The view of stress as external pressure suggests that all the person can do is try to withstand that pressure. This approach suggests that external stress is something that places severe pressure on a person, and all the person can do is to try to survive.

Stress as Internal Tension: The Psychological Approach

The subjective tension view suggests that stress is an internal state of psychic struggle, tension, anxiety, perhaps even panic, that involves a perception of threat or harm. Stress is the internal war that goes on inside when we try to cope with something that seems overwhelming. We may use psychic processes such as denial or rationalization, which are generally considered negative defenses. We may also struggle with stress in very positive ways, perhaps by generating creative solutions to solve difficult problems. In any case, psychic struggle takes time and energy. If the struggle goes on over a long time and there seems to be no end in sight, stress drains energy and stymies motivation.

Stress as Body Arousal: The Physiological Approach

The third view, originally propounded by Selye in 1956, suggested that stress is "the nonspecific response of the body to any demand made upon it." (1974, p. 27). Selye used the term **distress** for unpleasant, bad, and damaging stress and the term **eustress** for positive, satisfying, or good stress. In his model, stress is dependent on some demand, but it makes no difference whether the demand is bad or good. Stress is not defined in terms of the demand itself, however. To meet the demand, the body reacts with a higher arousal level and expends more energy; and it is this body arousal and energy expenditure that constitute stress.

The theoretical context of Selye's system came from his own profession, physiology, and the notion of homeostasis, taken from the work of his predecessor, Walter Cannon (1932). **Homeostasis** is the tendency for any biological organism to maintain a steady state, or stable internal environment. The simplest example of a homeostatic mechanism is hunger. Being deprived of food leads to depletion of blood sugar, a condition that is monitored by regulatory centers in the brain. When deprivation reaches a threshold level, the organism senses it and takes action to find food. Consuming food restores the internal balance, and food-seeking activity ceases. In Selye's view, stress alters body equilibrium, which requires compensatory action to restore balance.

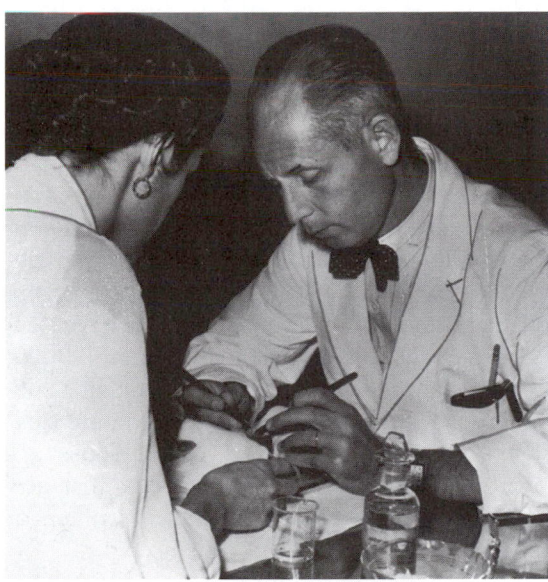

FIGURE 7.2   Hans Selye is regarded almost universally as the founder of modern stress research (Source: UPI/Bettmann).

Linking Stress Terms: Stressors, Strain, and Stress

Investigators now use alternative terms to get around the definitional problems just described. External forces are called stressors. **Stressors** are stimuli or environmental demands that trigger coping responses. Stressors need not exist in any strictly objective sense, however. They have to exist only in the mind of the beholder as mental constructs of external reality. Next, both internal subjective tension and body arousal are called strain. **Strain** can be either the mental or the physical wear and tear that follow attempts to cope with a stressor, or both. In these terms, **stress** is a process, not a state.

An Integrative Approach: Refining and Connecting Models

As you read about each of the views just described, you may have thought about ways the model could be modified to make it more complete. An external force interacts with organic traits of physical structures. In the same way, people are not passive recipients of external pressure, but organisms whose personality traits and physical strengths or weaknesses influence the way they react to stress. Psychological tension does not occur in a vacuum. Such tension is usually the result of some external reality, even if that reality has been distorted. Emotional upheaval is accompanied by physiological arousal and energy expenditure. The easiest way to look at the three views is that each has emphasized one part of the stress equation at the others' expense. Each facet is necessary, but no one component is sufficient in and of itself to encompass all that stress involves. Richard Lazarus has attempted to provide a more complete definition of stress in the context of his transactional model of stress. This view is the single most influential model of stress at this time. As such, it is the core context within which the other information on stress discussed here is interpreted.

Stress as a Transaction: The Cognitive Approach

The model of stress formulated by Richard Lazarus and his colleagues (Lazarus & Launier, 1978) is referred to as a cognitive-transactional model. The model was first formulated in the 1970s, but it continues to be a very influential theory even as it continues to evolve (Lazarus, 1991b, 1993). One of the more concise definitions from this model states that stress is "neither an environmental stimulus, a characteristic of the person, nor a response but a relationship between demands and the power to deal with them without unreasonable or destructive costs" (Coyne & Holroyd, 1982, p. 108).

Stated in other terms, stress exists only when environmental demands exceed the person's ability to cope. If the person's coping resources are adequate, no stress occurs, even if an outsider might view the demand as extreme. Conversely, if the person's coping skills are weak and ineffective, stress may occur, even though to an outsider, the demand may appear slight. Table 7.1 is a mnemonic device that is useful to remember the various stress terms introduced up to this point.[1]

Lazarus believes that the transaction between a person and the environment is based on three separate appraisals: a primary appraisal, a secondary appraisal, and a reappraisal. In a **primary appraisal,** the person considers the personal stakes involved in an encounter (Lazarus, 1991b). The primary appraisal is equivalent to asking the question, "Am I in trouble or not?" The outcome is that an event may be interpreted as irrelevant, benign-positive, or stressful. (Figure 7.3 provides a schematic view of the Lazarus theory.)

An appraisal of irrelevance may occur as follows. Say you get up feeling a little irritable one morning. You leave for class or work a tad late. While waiting anxiously at a stoplight, you hear a horn honk behind you, and your first thought is that the person is honking at you to get going. You may even have a momentary flare of anger. Then you see in the rearview mirror that the person is waving to an acquaintance in the next lane. Immediately, you realize that the honking had nothing to do with you—it was, in other words, irrelevant.

As for the other possible primary appraisals, benign-positive events are usually desirable events that do not place undue demands on the person. Lazarus described three stressful appraisals: challenge, threat, and harm-loss. **Challenge** exists when a situation is demanding, but the person feels capable of meeting the demand, and the emotional tone is one of excitement and positive anticipation. **Threat** exists when the situation demands more coping ability than is available. The distinction between challenge and threat is not entirely clear in the writings of Lazarus. A **harm-loss** appraisal occurs when the person feels that personal harm may result from the encounter, or

TABLE 7.1 *The components of stress: A Mnemonic Device.*

S = **Stressor:** a stimulus event or mental construction of an event that triggers internal tension

T = **Transaction:** ongoing negotiations between the person and the environment

R = **Resistance:** the private struggle that goes on while trying to cope with the stressor

E = **Energy spent:** both mental and physical energy that are part of the cost of coping

S = **Strain:** the wear and tear that results from coping efforts

S = **Solution or slide:** coping efforts may yield a solution, but continued stress may lead to a gradual decline in energy and motivation

---

[1] Note that stress as a process involves many feedback loops. This mnemonic is only intended to help organize the basic components of stress and not to suggest an inevitable linear progression.

The Stress Process

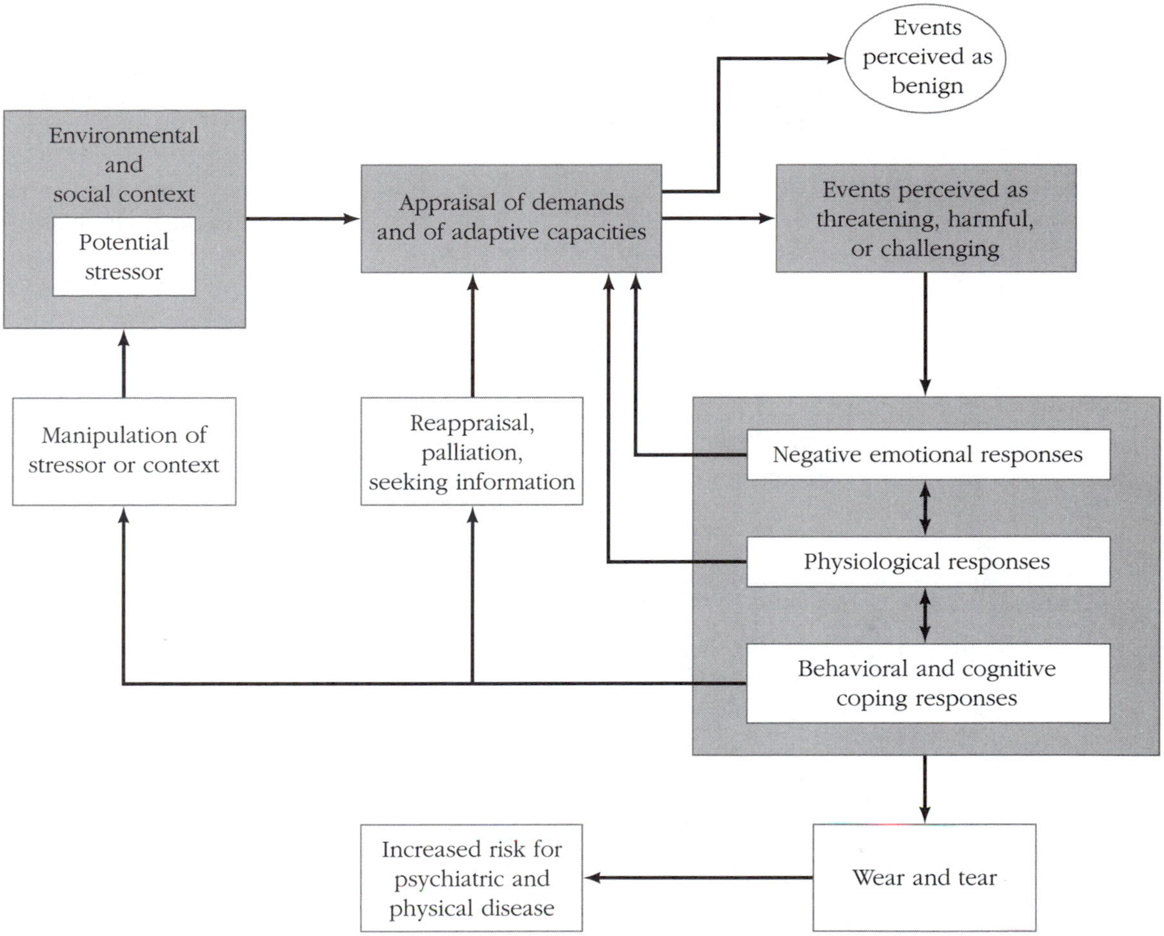

FIGURE 7.3   *A schematic diagram of the transactional model of stress. Note that appraisal processes may suggest no stressor is present (irrelevant or benign events). In this model, the physiological stress response is expected to occur only after an appraisal that something harmful is present, but it may feed back to influence the perceptual and interpretive process. Finally, note that increased risk for mental or physical illness typically occurs after some efforts have been made to cope and some wear and tear has occurred. (Used by permission of Jeffrey Ratliff-Crain.)*

that something personally very important may be taken away. Receiving news of an inoperable tumor would be an example of a harm appraisal. Finding that one's entire life's savings had been wiped out by a corrupt investment counselor would be a loss appraisal.

Next, a **secondary appraisal** answers the question, "What can I do about it?" At this point,

the person compares skills (adaptive capacities) with demands. If skills are adequate to the demand, there is little or no stress. If skills are lacking, stress is likely to occur. Finally, in the **reappraisal** process, the person uses feedback of new information or results of prior coping efforts to check the accuracy of both primary and secondary appraisals.

Lazarus's approach has several important implications. First, any given event may be interpreted as stressful by one person but not by someone else. Assume that someone in southeast Florida was unhappy with her lifestyle and home. Hurricane Andrew might be interpreted as a welcome chance to change location, build a new home, switch jobs, and begin a new life. Others might find the prospect of weathering such a vicious storm a challenge, like skyboarding and bungee-jumping thrill-seekers who find encounters with danger the ultimate uplifting experience (Zuckerman, 1971). Most external stimuli cannot be defined as stressful in any absolute sense. Instead, cognitive appraisals that compare demands to coping skills determine whether events are stressful or not.

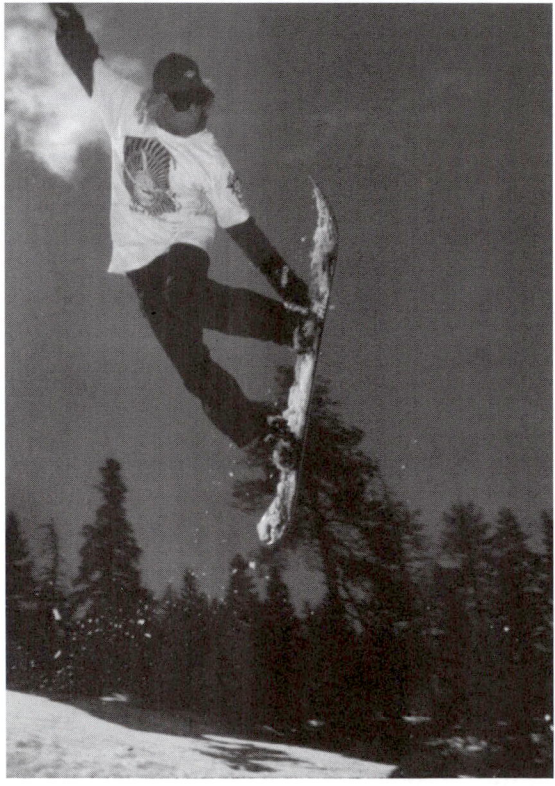

FIGURE 7.4   A snowboarder with nothing between him and the ground but his ability to control his board.

Second, the same person could interpret equivalent events as stressful at one time but not another. Wrecking a new car may be interpreted as catastrophic when one is already dealing with serious financial pressures. The same event may be only a minor setback when finances are on a firm footing, or the person was unhappy with his car and sees an opportunity to get a new, more desirable car. Changes in physical condition—being physically tired, tense, or ill—can influence, perhaps even distort, cognitive interpretations. In a similar vein, changes in psychological states can affect appraisals. Emotional moods and motivational states differ across time and are powerfully connected to the interpretive process (Lazarus, 1991b).

Third, personal constructs of reality do not have to be veridical; in other words, they do not have to be consistent with some external standard of reality. Misperceptions, even distorted perceptions, may trigger an emotional upheaval, physiological arousal, and a full stress reaction. In support of this notion, there is evidence that the brain does not distinguish between its thought of an event and the actual event (John, 1967). In other words, the body responds in the same way whether you are in reality being chewed out by a supervisor, or you are just mentally reliving the experience of being chewed out, or you are just imagining that the reason you have been summoned to the boss's office is to be chewed out for some imagined flaw in your work. The bottom line is that the mind at times creates its own fictions, some gentle, some not so gentle. When the fictions are not so gentle, stress may result.

Is Stress Always Big? Stress Boulders and Stress Pebbles

It is probably most common to think of stress as something that results from major calamities such as the death of a loved one or a natural disaster that wipes out an entire life's work. A useful visual mnemonic may be to think of this as the boulder model of stress. Still, an alternative view suggests that stress may be linked to minor events. A visual mnemonic may be to think of this as the pebble model of stress, like a small stone in the shoe. Not being able to find your keys when you are late for an appointment or finding that you have no money for lunch can cause a stress reaction just as much as a major calamity can. Two classic lines of research have been carried out to compare the boulder and pebble models of stress. Later, we will review evidence from each model linking stress to health or illness.

The Boulder Model: Death, Divorce, and Bankruptcy

The first line of research, begun by Holmes and Rahe (1967), went to great lengths to test the notion that major stress is linked to an increased rate of illness. Holmes and Rahe accepted the notion that both good and bad stress require efforts to readjust and thus put demands on the physical body. Their research program included building a scale to quantify the amount of stress a person had experienced in the recent past. This scale, the Social Readjustment Rating Scale

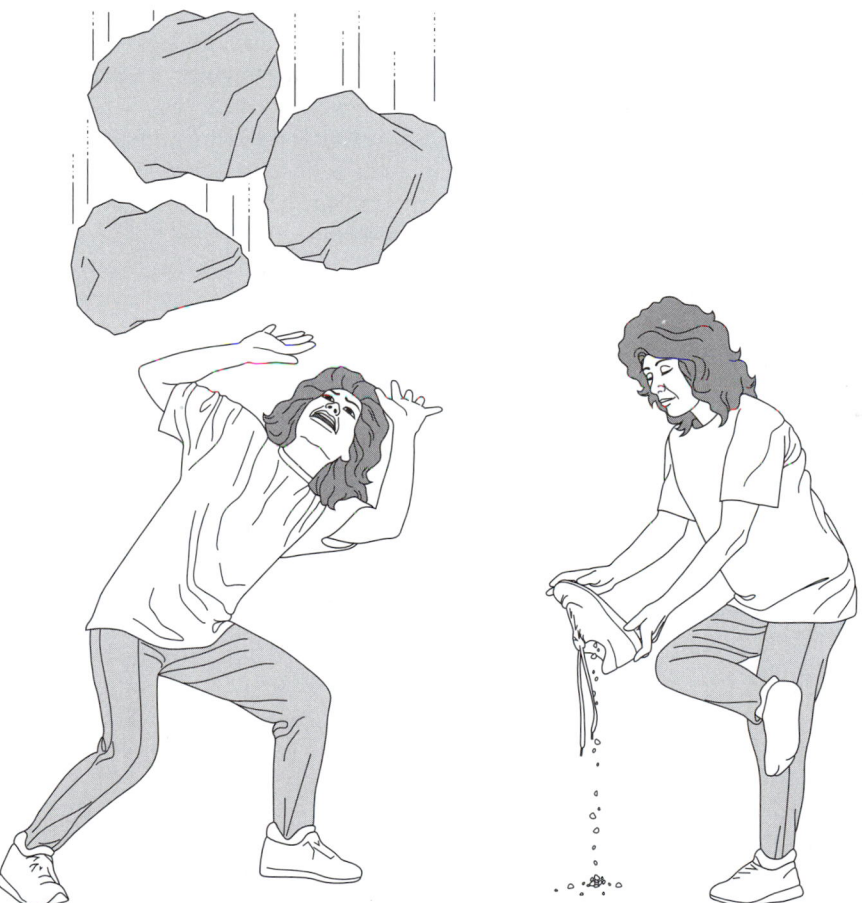

FIGURE 7.5   One view of stress suggests that the real problem is with boulders—infrequent but huge problems that cannot be dealt with. The other view suggests that the real problem is the little pebbles that get in our shoes or the proverbial straw that breaks the camel's back.

(SRRS), identified 43 items, each with a Life-Change Unit (LCU) score (see Table 7.2). The items and scores were based on ratings from several large samples.

It is apparent that major catastrophes lead the list with high scores and that minor problems (such as a minor law violation) are low on the scale. Note also that the scale has a mixture of negative and positive events. Respondents simply circle the left-hand number for any and all life-change events that have occurred to them in the past six months. Then the associated LCU score (on the right) is circled and added. Total LCU scores over 300 define a major life crisis; scores between 200 and 299 define a moderate life crisis; and scores between 150 and 199 define a mild life crisis. Scores under 150 are regarded as normal. The key point for our purposes is this: People who had a major life crisis in the past six months were more likely to display higher rates of physical illness than those with lower levels of life-change stress. We will have more to say on this later.

Both the rationale and the scale itself are often criticized in hindsight (Schroeder & Costa, 1984; Monroe & Simons, 1991). Development of newer life-event scales during the past decade has not softened the criticism. Still, this was the first major innovation in the effort to quantify life events as stressors. It was also part of the first wide-ranging effort to establish a link between stressors and health status.

The Pebble Model: Lost Keys, No Lunch Money, and Flat Tires

The alternative view, that stress is an accumulation of small irritants, has been advocated most by Richard Lazarus and his group. They developed the Hassles Scale to quantify stress of this nature (Kanner, Coyne, Schaefer, & Lazarus, 1981). They also split bad and good stressors so that they could look at effects based on this distinction. They called the negative events hassles, and the positive events uplifts. **Hassles** are little things such as getting a flat tire on the way to work, breaking a favorite piece of china, or losing a billfold or purse. **Uplifts** are positive events such as news that a baby is expected, finding an error in your bank account in your favor, or scoring higher on a test than expected.[2] Presumably, negative happenings produce a drain on energy and body resources that ultimately could lead to health problems. On the other side, positive events should be associated with better health outcomes. This distinction is a major difference between the boulder (catastrophic) model and the pebble (minor irritant) model.

At the same time, hassles scales have been criticized for using items that reflect psychiatric symptoms rather than objective life events. Items that refer to drug use and sexual difficulty, for example, may tap lowered mental health status that follows stress rather than themselves being stress events. Stated in other terms, the items may only reflect the problems they are intended to predict. This possible difficulty is especially problematic when stress is supposed to predict subsequent health problems. Some use this contamination hypothesis to attack the credibility of the hassles account of stress and illness.

A longitudinal study carried out by Lu (1991), however, found that hassles add to the load of psychological symptoms over time even when prior mental health symptoms and risks are controlled for. This finding tends to refute the criticism that hassles scales are measuring, not stress, but only mental health.

Another research group headed by Paul Kohn attacked the problem differently by developing a decontaminated hassles scale (Kohn, Lafreniere, & Gurevich, 1991). This study found that trait anxiety and hassles both contributed to the

---

[2] It should be apparent that any of these events could also be a major catastrophe under certain circumstances. A flat tire in a very dangerous section of a large city could be life-threatening. A significant error in the bank account could spell financial ruin. Still, the notion is that everyday irritants can pile up and produce as much or more difficulty than the rare catastrophes.

TABLE 7.2 *Rank of life-change events with associated life-change units (LCUs)*
(from Holmes & Rahe, 1967).

RANK	LIFE EVENT	LCU
1	Death of spouse	100
2	Divorce	73
3	Marital separation	65
4	Jail term	63
5	Death of close family member	63
6	Personal injury or illness	53
7	Marriage	50
8	Fired at work	47
9	Marital reconciliation	45
10	Retirement	45
11	Change in health of family member	44
12	Pregnancy	40
13	Sexual difficulties	39
14	Gain of new family member	39
15	Business readjustment	39
16	Change in financial state	38
17	Death of close friend	37
18	Change to different lines of work	36
19	Change in number of arguments with spouse	35
20	Mortgage over $10,000	31
21	Foreclosure of morgage or loan	30
22	Change in responsibilities at work	29
23	Son or daughter leaving home	29
24	Trouble with in-laws	29
25	Outstanding personal achievement	28
26	Wife begins or stops work	26
27	Begin or end school	26
28	Change in living conditions	25
29	Revision of personal habits	24
30	Trouble with boss	23
31	Change in work hours or conditions	20
32	Change in residence	20
33	Change in schools	20
34	Change in recreation	19
35	Change in church activities	19
36	Change in social activities	18
37	Mortgage or loan less than $10,000	17
38	Change in sleeping habits	16
39	Change in number of family get-togethers	15
40	Change in eating habits	13
41	Vacation	13
42	Christmas	12
43	Minor violations of the law	11

TABLE 7.3   Selected items from the Hassles Scale and items from the uplifts potion of the scale (from Kanner, Coyne, Schaefer, & Lazarus, 1981).

HASSLES			SEVERITY
1. Misplacing or losing things	1	2	3
2. Concerns about owing money	1	2	3
3. Trouble relaxing	1	2	3
4. Being lonely	1	2	3
5. Not getting enough sleep	1	2	3

UPLIFTS			HOW OFTEN
1. Feeling healthy	1	2	3
2. Completing a task	1	2	3
3. Quitting or cutting down on smoking	1	2	3
4. Buying clothes	1	2	3
5. Making a friend	1	2	3

perception of stress, but trait anxiety was the stronger of the two. In addition, hassles had a significant impact on minor ailments and on psychiatric symptoms. It appears that as trait anxiety increases, a person is more vulnerable to the impact of hassles and will reflect that impact more in both mental and physical symptoms.[3] The analysis still is consistent with the notion that stable organismic traits interact with environmental events to predict outcome.

Culture also likely enters into the experience of hassles. Black students in southern California, for example, report a higher frequency and severity of hassles than white students in the same area (Jung & Khalsa, 1989). The students also reported a major difference in the type of hassle experienced: black students had more economic hassles, whereas white students had more work hassles. Two additional findings are

noteworthy that did not differ between black and white students. First, as the severity of hassles increased, so did severity of depression. This finding is of interest since depression is one of the negative moods often linked to poor health. Second, the more the person felt that family support was available, the less depression occurred; in other words, the presence of social support appeared to act as a buffer against the appearance of depression, though it did not buffer against stress itself.

The Last Straw: Boulders Make the Load, Pebbles Break the Back

These two views of stress, the boulder and the pebble models, have vied for attention over the past quarter century. A more centrist view is that both types of stress occur sporadically, but that they interact with each other. Thus, no less than three scenarios may exist to explain the origins of stress. The first scenario suggests that catastrophic events may be sufficient to produce stress reactions in some people. The second scenario suggests that an accumulation of small irritants in a short time may lead to stress reactions in some people (people with high trait anxiety, for example). Third, hassles may be like the last straw, the infinitely small piece added to the load that finally breaks the camel's back.

The Diathesis-Stress Model: Setting and Crossing Thresholds

Before discussing the link between psychosocial stressors and physical changes, it may be useful to consider a model that addresses interactions between host (organismic) and environmental factors. This model, first proposed by Paul Meehl (1962; see Fowles, 1992, for a recent review) to explain schizophrenia, is called the diathesis-stress model. The diathesis component reflects inherited strengths and weaknesses, predisposing factors, that set a threshold for risk.

---

[3] One problem with this study is that the scale content is substantially different from the conventional hassles scale, so that it is difficult to compare the results to other hassles studies.

The stress component reflects precipitating factors that present the risk occasion.[4]

Predisposing factors are constitutional traits that set the organism's strengths and weaknesses, influence response sensitivities, and have the net effect of creating a tolerance threshold for environmental pressures. Predisposing factors establish the limits of vulnerability to disease and capacity to resist stressors. The fact that one person may express stress physically as an ulcer whereas another person may express stress as accelerated coronary artery disease could be explained by reference to the diathesis component.

An extreme but rare example of a constitutional weakness is **severe combined immune deficiency** (SCID) (Jones, Ritenbaugh, Spence, & Hayward, 1991). SCID patients may lack either T cells or B cells (or both), which ordinarily help the body fight invading organisms.[5] One of the most widely publicized cases was that of David, who was born in Houston in 1971. He lived most of his 12 years in a germ-free isolation bubble designed to protect him from everyday infections that most people would never even notice (Demaret, 1984a; 1984b). To David, however, even a mild infection could be life-threatening. The night David died was the first and last time his mother could touch him without surgical gloves and mask or through the bubble.

Environmental stressors, called **precipitating factors,** vary in type, severity, and duration. Some stressors are biological, such as bacterial and viral infections or industrial toxins. Other stressors are psychosocial, such as a disagreement with a teacher over grading or a spat with one's spouse over chores. Some stressors are mild and brief, such as finding that one has no money prior to an important lunch date. Others are intense and chronic: Consider the example of a person who is laid off work, who faces continuous financial pressure for months and ongoing threats from the bank to foreclose on the home. Even a strong person might break down under such circumstances.

Most organisms learn how to resist stressors through coping strategies. A quick trip to the automatic teller machine on the way to lunch solves the money problem. Finding part-time work and working out a partial payment schedule with the bank may get through the crisis until work resumes. The point is that whether a person ever reveals a weakness or not depends on whether the stressor presents itself above the threshold of tolerance.

Monroe and Simons (1991) reviewed the diathesis-stress theory in the context of life-stress research. They noted that the problem of defining stress (an issue we discussed earlier) still plagues the model. Further, they argued that we should not assume that stressor events add together in summative fashion to push the organism over the threshold of tolerance. More likely, subtle components of stressors combine in unique ways to produce stress.

It is now time to examine more carefully the issue of stress and health status. In order to do so, we must first examine the body's role in stress. This effort will require excursions into the neuroanatomical, neurochemical, and genetic bases of the stress response. As we proceed, we will discover that stress physiology is indeed complex. Still, our efforts to understand the complex interplay of biomedical and psychosocial forces lead to much richer theoretical notions of stress.

---

[4] I must emphasize that there is no conflict between the diathesis-stress model and the biopsychosocial model. In one sense, the biopsychosocial model simply tries to make explicit the nature of the interactions between predisposing and precipitating factors.

[5] The immune system, including T cells and B cells, was discussed in Chapter 3.

Stress Physiology: Genes, Brain, Glands, and Immune System

Research on biomedical aspects of stress physiology reveals a complex interactive communication network composed of the brain, the glands, and the immune system. Sensitivity within this system is probably set in part by genotypes (diathesis) that are only incompletely known (Goldstein, 1994). In addition, older notions suggesting that certain body systems operate autonomously can no longer be entertained. It is preferable to think of the nervous system as a complex cybernetic system with multiple (redundant) positive and negative feedback loops, and the immune system as a fully integrated member assisting in the task of maintaining homeostasis (Ader, 1983). These feedback loops provide information to other parts of the system on a timely, need-to-know basis. At the same time, these feedback loops may have the effect of amplifying or attenuating responses in different parts of the system. Here, we will discuss only the essential systems and links between elements of the system. This discussion assumes that

the reader has some background in neuro-anatomy.[6]

Brain Regulation in Stress Reactions: A Primer of Neuroanatomy

The brain's role in the stress response involves potentially all of its centers. We can simplify this complexity, though, by focusing on three centers most crucial to the stress response (shown in Figure 7.6). These three are the hindbrain and the visceral brain in the central nervous (CNS) and the autonomic nervous system, a

---

[6] Students who want to refresh their knowledge or obtain more background information may turn to one of several general psychology texts, such as Kalat (1993) or Baron (1992). More advanced information may be found in physiological psychology texts, such as Kalat (1992) or Pinel (1993).

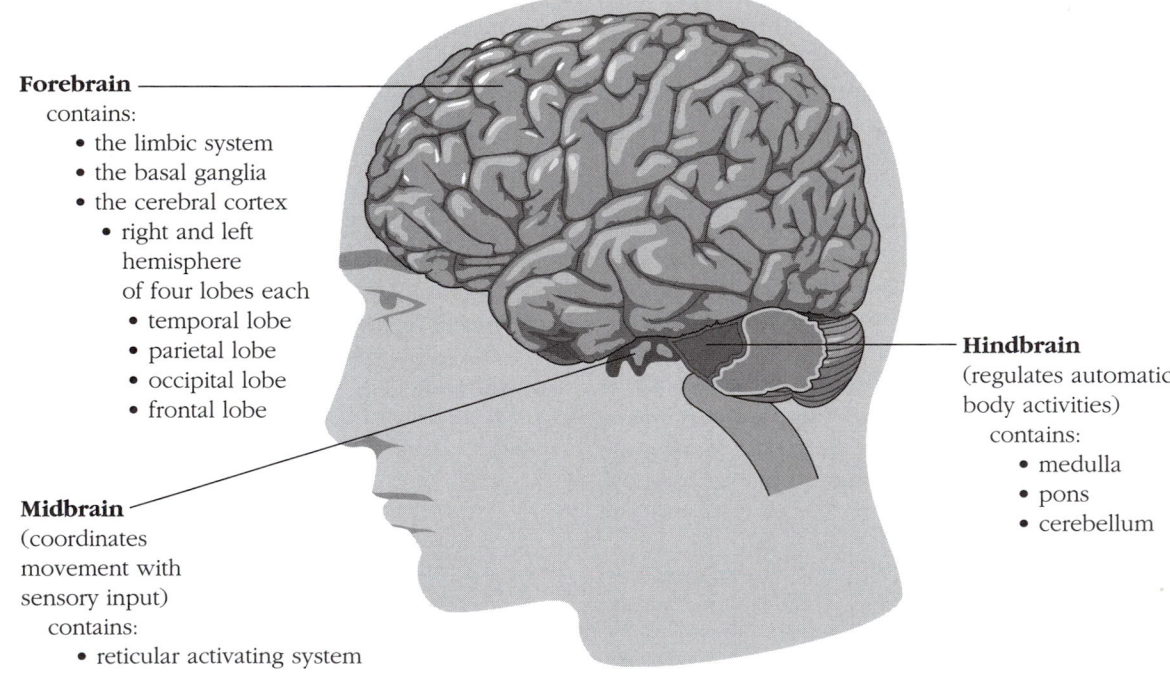

Forebrain
contains:
- the limbic system
- the basal ganglia
- the cerebral cortex
  - right and left hemisphere of four lobes each
    - temporal lobe
    - parietal lobe
    - occipital lobe
    - frontal lobe

Midbrain
(coordinates movement with sensory input)
contains:
- reticular activating system

Hindbrain
(regulates automatic body activities)
contains:
- medulla
- pons
- cerebellum

FIGURE 7.6   General view of the brain showing the hindbrain, midbrain, and forebrain structures (from Durand & Barlow , 1997).

subdivision of the peripheral nervous system (PNS). The **hindbrain,** the first and oldest part of the brain to evolve, controls many life-support functions, such as sleep and arousal, plus cardiovascular and respiratory control. The **visceral brain,** located at the midbrain level, is a complex system in itself. It is responsible for interpretation of stimuli that may arouse emotions, and it then controls the fight or flight response as necessary. The **autonomic nervous system** (ANS) controls three different tissues, cardiac muscle, most of the glands, and all smooth muscle (Liebman, 1979). Later, we will discuss the controlling balance provided by two ANS components, the parasympathetic and the sympathetic nervous systems.

The Hindbrain: The Brain's Grand Central Station

The hindbrain appears as a bulb-like outgrowth at the top of the spinal column. It houses two major control centers, the medulla and the

reticular formation (RF). Figure 7.7 shows these structures in more detail.

The **medulla** can be likened to a neural Grand Central Station. Autonomic and motor nerve fibers arrive from the body and depart from the brain through this concourse. The most important medullary centers are the autonomic nuclei and the reticular formation. The **autonomic nuclei** carry on life-support processes such as respiration, heart action, and digestion. Stress can trigger changes in the usual synchrony of control that originates from these nuclei.

To illustrate, normal breathing occurs at about 12 breaths per minute, with two seconds for inspiration and three seconds for exhalation (Guyton, 1977). But state anxiety can lead to the appearance of being out of breath. Suppose your instructor asks you to come to the front of the class to give an impromptu speech on neuroanatomy, and you have not read the material. You may notice an immediate change in your breathing rate. How did this happen?

In essence, after the midbrain interprets the stimulus as a stressor,[7] the cortex sends a signal to the respiratory nuclei. In response, the respiratory balance is changed so that more inhalation—deeper breathing—occurs. In turn, more oxygen enters the bloodstream than normally would. In true cybernetic fashion, interpreting the deep breathing as a signal of distress, the system may amplify the imbalance even more. This effect is what Figure 7.3 suggested in the feedback loop linking appraisal, threat, physiological response, and feedback to appraisal.

In the extreme, the process just described can result in **anxiety hyperventilation,** when the person feels many symptoms customarily associated with a heart attack. These may include

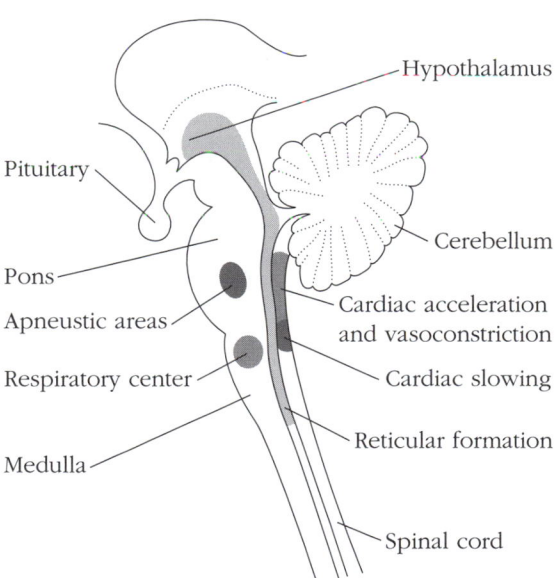

FIGURE 7.7   A view of the brain stem region showing the reticular formation, and the cardiovascular and respiratory control centers (from Rice, 1992).

Pituitary

Pons

Apneustic areas

Respiratory center

Medulla

Hypothalamus

Cerebellum

Cardiac acceleration and vasoconstriction

Cardiac slowing

Reticular formation

Spinal cord

[7] The event might be interpreted as threat if we see our skills as inadequate to meet the demands of the moment. But it might be interpreted as harm-loss if we perceive the potential for acute embarrassment in front of peers, or we have reason to believe that failure to perform well could mean failure in the class and academic probation or suspension from school.

shortness of breath, pounding heart, dizziness to the point of fainting, and perhaps even **paresthesia,** a numbness or tingling in parts of the body. Even though there is a clear physical sequence of control, we still think of hyperventilation as a psychogenic reaction, one that comes from a mixture of psychological traits and social circumstances, not from physical pathology. When hyperventilation occurs so frequently or intensely as to disrupt a person's life, clinical intervention may be called for. Hyperventilation can be relieved, for example, by practiced breathing and relaxation (Hegel et al., 1989).

The **reticular formation** (RF), so named because of its net-like appearance, is a bundle of fibers with about 100 tiny nuclei and many diverse roles to play. The RF runs like a great rope through the middle of the brain stem, upward into the hypothalamus and thalamus. One important RF function is brain-body communication. Through the descending pathway, the RF relays signals, including signals of distress, from the hypothalamic-pituitary complex to organs controlled by the autonomic system (Figure 7.8 shows these connections). Psychosocial stressors thus have a direct path to

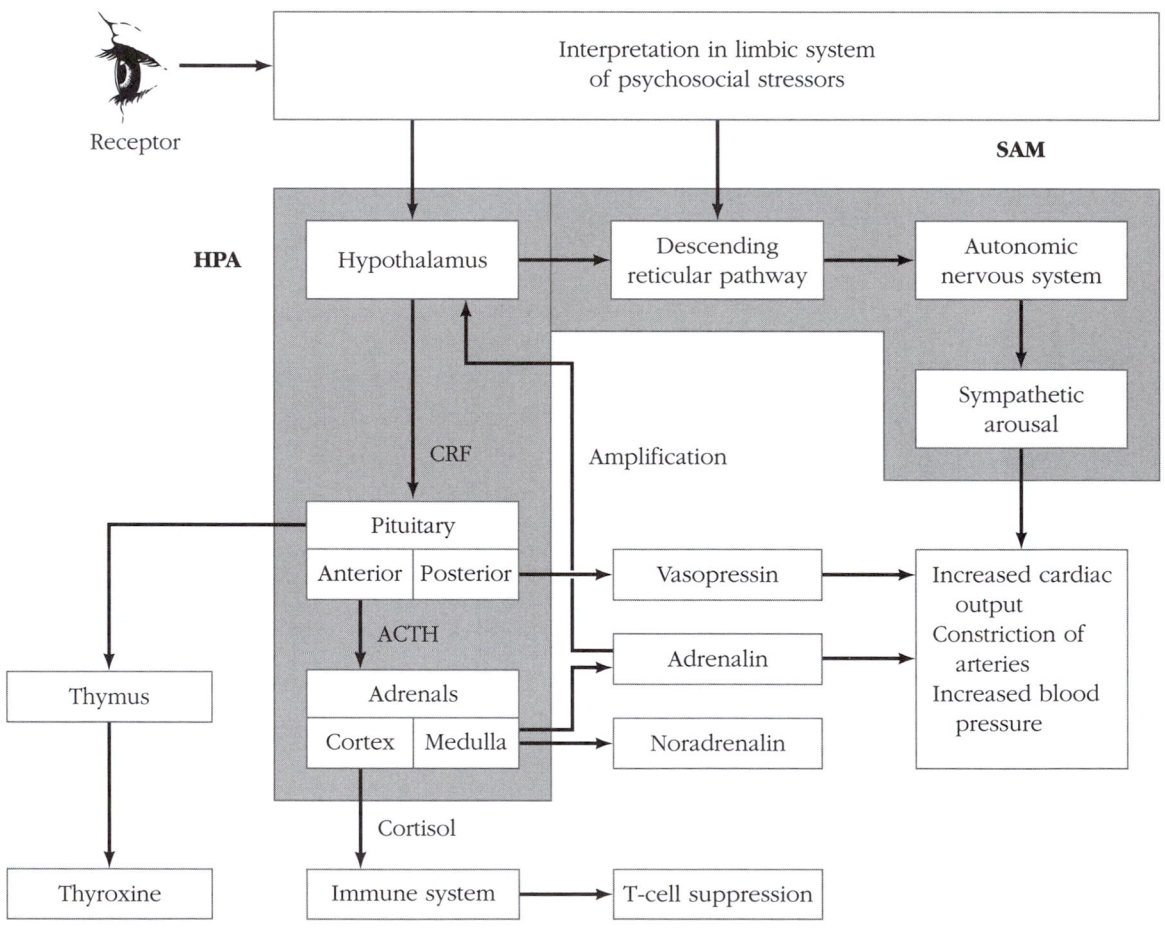

FIGURE 7.8   *A conceptual model of the HPA and SAM complexes with feedback circuits. These components of the neuroendocrine system regulate much of the physiological response to stress (from Rice, 1992).*

change the operation of such important systems as the cardiovascular, glandular, and immune systems.

Through the second, ascending pathway, the RF signals the brain of the existence of a physical stressor, such as an injury to the body. Such stressors may be translated into a variety of emotional states that produce psychological discomfort and tension. The reticular formation and thalamic centers are involved in the awareness of pain. Because pain usually produces negative emotions, an amplification effect may occur that increases sensitivity to the pain itself. Under normal circumstances, though, this signal system leads to activation of the body's natural healing processes.

The Visceral Brain: Preparing for Fight or Flight

The visceral brain, a cluster of structures that owes its name to extensive connections with the **hypothalamus,** is the center that controls visceral (gut level) systems involved in fight or flight reactions. The cluster includes the **thalamus,** the hypothalamus-pituitary complex, and parts of the **limbic system.** These structures are illustrated in Figure 7.9. Because the visceral brain plays a crucial interpretive role with potential stressors, it is vital to any explanation of how the brain responds to stress. We will start with the thalamus and limbic system and return to the hypothalamus later.

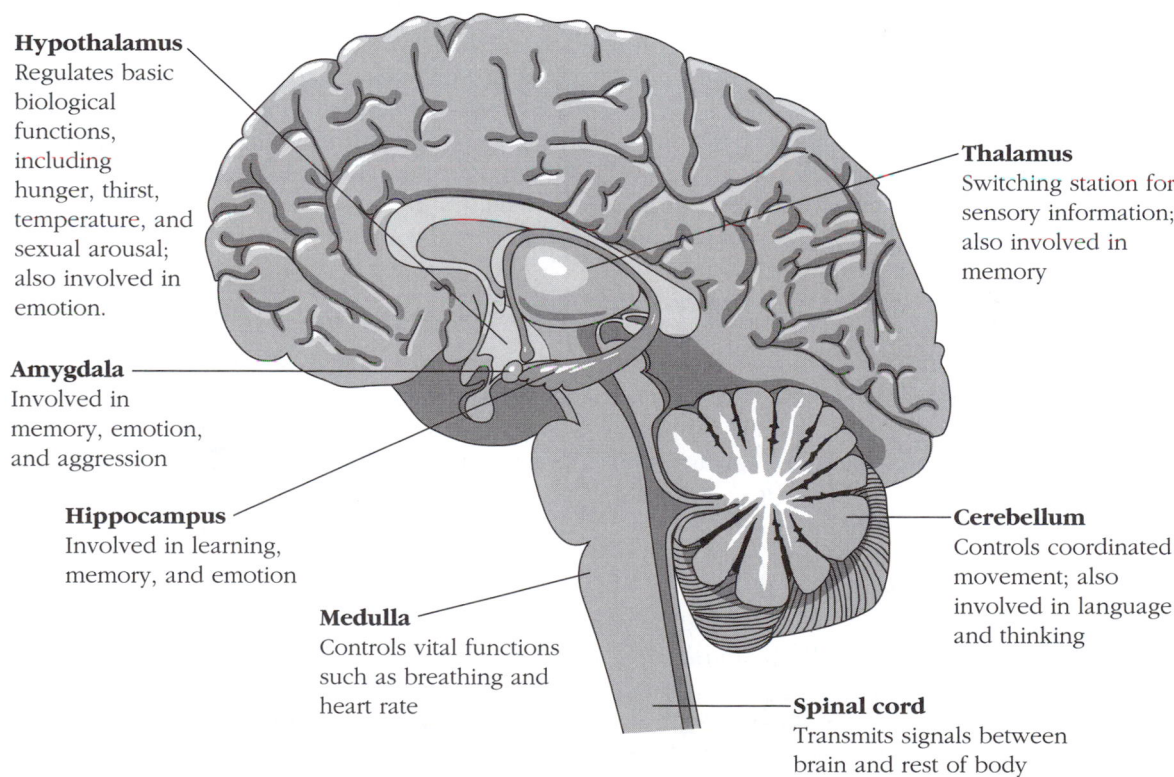

Hypothalamus
Regulates basic biological functions, including hunger, thirst, temperature, and sexual arousal; also involved in emotion.

Amygdala
Involved in memory, emotion, and aggression

Hippocampus
Involved in learning, memory, and emotion

Medulla
Controls vital functions such as breathing and heart rate

Thalamus
Switching station for sensory information; also involved in memory

Cerebellum
Controls coordinated movement; also involved in language and thinking

Spinal cord
Transmits signals between brain and rest of body

FIGURE 7.9   *A cross-section of the brain exposing the major components of the visceral brain (from Goldstein, 1994).*

The thalamus contains relay nuclei for every sensory system except the sense of smell. It is strategically positioned to evaluate emotional content in sensory information. Another thalamic function is pain perception. Pain researchers identify three types of pain: pricking pain, burning pain, and aching pain (Guyton, 1977). Each specialized pain pathway terminates in the thalamus. We will discuss pain in more detail in Chapter 13.

The limbic system is part of the primitive brain concerned with survival. It includes the thalamus, hypothalamus, amygdala, hippocampus, and septum (see Figure 7.9). The functions most often associated with the limbic system include anger, aggression, punishment, reward, sexual arousal, and pain. Damage to the septum may result in extreme irritability or even rage responses with unprovoked aggression. Damage to the amygdala produces the opposite type of reaction, suggesting that these two centers balance aggressive tendencies, with the amygdala starting and the septum moderating aggression.

Damage to the hippocampus results in a failure to form new memories and may slow down or block several types of learning (Milner, Corkin, & Teuber, 1968). The hippocampus also plays an important role in regulating the pituitary-adrenal stress response, as we shall see later (McEwen & Mendelson, 1993).

The hypothalamus is located just above the roof of the mouth, toward the back. Nearly every brain area interacts with the hypothalamus in some way. Because of this intricate linkage, the hypothalamus can respond to psychosocial stimuli ranging from external events to associative memories, obsessional ruminations, or even imaginary stressors. Most important, the hypothalamus connects directly to the **pituitary gland,** the master gland of the body, and then to the adrenal cortex. The hypothalamus also monitors concentrations of hormones originating in other parts of the body. By this means, the hypothalamus powerfully affects nearly every visceral system in the body. This hypothalamus-pituitary-adrenal cortex (HPA) complex is one of two major axes involved in control of the stress response. The second major axis is the sympathetic-adrenal medulla (SAM) complex.

The role of the hypothalamus in stress is clearly revealed in the following four functions.

1. The hypothalamus initiates activity in the autonomic nervous system.
2. The hypothalamus stimulates secretion of **adrenocorticotropic hormone** (ACTH) from the anterior pituitary.
3. The hypothalamus stimulates production of antidiuretic hormone (ADH), or **vasopressin,** which is then stored in the posterior pituitary.
4. The hypothalamus stimulates the anterior pituitary to release thyrotropin, which tells the thyroid glands to produce **thyroxine.**

To perform these tasks, the hypothalamus has two dedicated centers. One center stimulates sympathetic activity and the production of pituitary stress hormones. The other center slows down sympathetic activity and inhibits the production of pituitary stress hormones. These functions will be further clarified as we turn our attention to the autonomic nervous system and the master gland.

The Autonomic System: Balancing Tension and Calmness

If the RF is the great sentry system, then the autonomic nervous system is the great balancer, working to keep an equilibrium between tension and tranquility. The ANS is not autonomous or involuntary, as was earlier thought. Controlled by the brain stem, hypothalamus, and spinal cord, the ANS in turn controls heart activity, blood pressure, digestion, urinary and bowel elimination, and other bodily functions. The ANS has two parts, the **parasympathetic nervous system** and the **sympathetic nervous system.** Most of the time, these two work in dynamic but antagonistic tension. When one is active, the other is relatively quiet or passive, and vice versa. Although this coinhibition is the most often discussed mode of operation, the systems may be coactivated as well, and at times the two may be uncoupled to operate independently (Berntson, Cacioppo, & Quigley, 1991). Two brief examples may be cited. Cannon (1932) noted that extreme fear responses display coactivation: Increases in heart rate and blood pressure indicate sympathetic control, but emptying of bowel and bladder indicate parasympathetic control. Second, the male sexual response requires support from both systems, the parasympathetic system for erectile response and the sympathetic system for the ejaculatory response.

The parasympathetic nervous system is dominant when we are quiet and relaxed. This promotes positive rest and reconstruction of the body after higher levels of energy expenditure. At this time, blood collects in central organs for digestion and storage of energy reserves. Breathing is balanced and slow, heart rate idles, blood pressure drops as does body temperature, and muscle tension relaxes.

The sympathetic nervous system is the fight or flight system. It serves to mobilize the body for defensive action during emergencies or during states of heightened emotionality. The alarm signal itself originates in the hypothalamus. In consort with activation of the adrenal medulla (secretion of adrenalin), the body quickly mobilizes itself for action. The effect of sympathetic arousal is to increase blood pressure, blood flow to large muscles and muscle strength, overall energy expenditure, blood glucose concentration, mental activity, and rate of blood coagulation (Guyton, 1977). When the emergency is past, the hypothalamus typically recalls the parasympathetic system, and then the body begins to repair destructive effects from the emergency. Undesirable effects of prolonged sympathetic arousal include elevated blood pressure and ulcers.

The emergency system response is, in itself, a highly functional, adaptive, and positive feature. When large muscle responses are possible, the body effectively discharges its tension and everything returns to normal. A major problem encountered in modern society, though, is that arousal of the emergency response often occurs without allowing for discharge of the tension. Large-scale responses must be inhibited and feelings masked with a facade of politeness and civility. The result may be one of chronic activation with consequent long-term alterations in physiological systems linked to the emergency response. For this reason, stress and stress-related illnesses are often referred to as diseases of civilization.

Hormonal Processes in Stress: The Master and Adrenal Glands

Early in his research program, Selye noted that stressors activate a response in the HPA complex described earlier. The adrenal cortex secretes **glucocorticoids,** which are steroid hormones that mobilize energy resources, combat inflammation, and promote healing (Pinel, 1993). Selye found that after chronic stress the adrenal cortex in rats was enlarged, the thymus gland was atrophied, and lymphatic response became impaired.

The full process begins when the hypothalamus uses its own hormone, **corticotropin-releasing factor** (CRF) to stimulate release of B-endorphin, prolactin, and adrenocorticotropic hormone (ACTH) from the anterior pituitary. In turn, ACTH activates the adrenal cortex to release glucocorticoids (such as cortisol) (Kant, Meyerhoff, Bunnell, & Lenox, 1982). Information then feeds back to the hypothalamus to continue the regulatory process. The presence of almost any stressor leads to a swift rise in the level of ACTH and the glucocorticoids. For example, one psychosocial stressor, the death of a spouse or child, typically triggers ACTH release. The overall response is, again, an adaptive response in the service of homeostasis. As long as the stress remits or adaptive behaviors manage the stress, no harm is done.

One glucocorticoid, **cortisol,** provides more energy to the body through conversion of body stores into glucose, but it can also have negative effects on the immune system. Hypersecretions of cortisol are seen in major depression (Gold,

Goodwin, & Chrousos, 1988), and cortisol also may act to suppress the **immune system** (O'Leary, 1990). Immune suppression reduces the number and effectiveness of lymphocytes and thus impairs the body's resistance to infections and disease (Dantzer & Kelley, 1989; Jemmott & Locke, 1984) and possibly cancer (Riley, 1981). Figure 7.10 shows interactions within this system and provides an example of a biological negative feedback system enmeshed in a complex hierarchical system.

Selye's ideas have been revised and extended in the years since his research. It is known that the pituitary secretes several hormones besides

ACTH. Specifically, the anterior pituitary secretes five stress hormones in addition to ACTH, and the posterior pituitary secretes two stress hormones, vasopressin and oxytocin.

Further, we now know that the second axis, the sympathetic-adrenal-medullary axis (SAM), is actually the primary or first response to stress (Antoni, 1987) Stress activates the sympathetic system and increases the release of **epinephrine** (also called **adrenaline**) and **norepinephrine** (also called **noradrenaline**). These hormones appear to be released rapidly following stress, whereas the glucocorticoids appear to be delayed in an attempt to restore balance in the system. McEwen and Mendelson (1993) refer to this as glucoid counter regulation of the primary stress response.

Under conditions of severe stress and heightened activation of the sympathetic system, the body can be flooded with epinephrine and norepinephrine. In fact, norepinephrine can remain elevated for some time after the stress terminates (Aslan, Nelson, Carruthers, & Lader, 1981). Most important, these hormones may feed back to amplify the effect of sympathetic arousal. For example, parallel to the sympathetic system, epinephrine has a powerful effect on the heart. Epinephrine increases both the rate and strength of the heart's contractions and raises blood pressure. Through feedback to the hypothalamus, epinephrine can increase secretions of ACTH to higher levels, thus serving to keep the HPA complex aroused. This arousal amplifies the effect of changes in other visceral systems and increases the level of activity in the HPA loop. Thus, activation of these two complexes, HPA and SAM, can have powerful effects during chronic stress.

In the brain, the distribution of adrenaline and noradrenaline differs across brain regions depending on the type and timing of stressors (Ward et al., 1983). Noradrenaline is detectable in the hypothalamus, amygdala, and thalamus of rats within an hour after immobilization stress, in the hippocampus and cerebral cortex during the second hour, and later in other centers (Tanaka, et al., 1983). The brain is also extremely sensitive

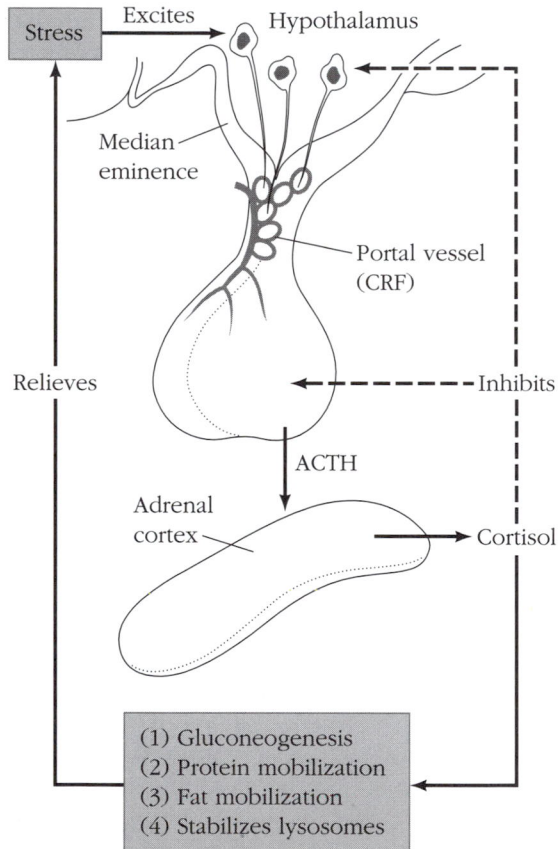

FIGURE 7.10   This shows how cortisol may alter the system to help combat stress, but may also work to change the immune system (from Guyton, 1977).

to the presence of adrenocorticosteroids. These hormones can produce changes in mental function, which in turn raise adrenocorticosteroid levels even higher. Under these conditions, people become more vulnerable to stress, because they cannot deal effectively with daily problems (Riscalla, 1983).

Genetic Contributions to Stress: The Tip of the Iceberg

Evidence for genetic contributions to stress reactivity may be gleaned from information on genetic influences in the development and operation of physiological systems in general and stress response systems in particular. The strategy has been to test for genetic influences by assessing sensitivity in the neuroendocrine (HPA and SAM, for example), cardiovascular, and autonomic nervous systems.

Goldstein (1994) summarized a number of results from animal studies. Certain strains of rats show major differences in activity within major stress systems. One hypertensive strain shows excessive renal sympathetic nervous activity in response to challenge from several different stressors. Strain differences in production of vasopressin and strain differences in levels of catecholamines have also been observed. Numerous investigators have used these same strains because of genetic differences in neurochemical and behavioral reactivity to stressors (Irwin & Livnat, 1987). These results suggest that reactivity of the major stress response systems is subject to a genetic influence.

Many investigators have come to believe that dopamine exerts a powerful influence in the brain with effects that touch on humans' mental health, internal reward (pleasure) mechanisms, and drug addiction and tolerance. It should not be surprising, then, that the role of dopamine in stress has also been considered. In a recent study, European investigators considered this issue in the context of a genotype that affects the adaptation of the brain dopamine system to stress (Puglisi-Allegra, Kempf, & Cabib, 1990).

Many details of this study are beyond the scope and space limitations of this work, but the major conclusions are still important and meaningful.

This research team used two different inbred strains of mice; inbreeding ensures more genetic similarity within strains and heterogeneity between strains.[8] In Puglisi-Allegra's work, the different strains of rats were placed in conditions of chronic stress, and measures were taken to determine dopamine receptor sensitivity. One strain showed a markedly increased sensitivity of dopamine receptors in the brain and marked lowering, if not outright elimination, of a typical climbing response used to escape from aversive situations. The other strain showed hyposensitivity of the dopamine receptors and no interference with the typical climbing response. Puglisi-Allegra argued that this result shows a genetic influence in the adaptation of the dopamine receptor in response to chronic stress.

Richard Rose and Margaret Chesney (1986) reviewed the literature on cardiovascular stress reactivity and found evidence of a genetic contribution as well. Stress researchers have been aware of subjects who show exaggerated cardiovascular responses to stressors. A tendency to such responses now is generally accepted as a familial trait since this tendency runs in families. Classic twin studies support this notion as well. In addition, Rose and Chesney provide evidence that the heightened cardiovascular response to stress is a precursor of hypertension and thus may be a marker that could be used to intervene before a medical condition results.

These findings taken in total suggest that specific mechanisms are built into the brain and endocrine system that provide a pathway for psychosocial stressors to introduce changes in the physical system. The cardiovascular system, digestive system, muscles, and immune system

---

[8] A parallel from years past was Tryon's (1940) breeding of maze-bright and maze-dull animals. After seven generations, the variability within each group fit a normal curve, but the brightest of the dull strain was far below the lowest of the bright strain.

all may be affected by stressors. These changes are largely positive, adaptive features of a system that seeks to maintain overall equilibrium. It appears that only when the stress is unremitting or unmanaged is there potential for the physiological changes to translate into increased risk for mental or physical illness. We turn our attention now to this specific issue: under what conditions stress may have unfavorable results for health status.

Are Stress and Health Related? Searching for Links

The notion that stress may affect health status is also connected with the work of Hans Selye. As noted at the outset, Selye defined stress as the body's nonspecific efforts to meet demands placed on it. Recall that in Selye's view, it made no difference whether stress was bad or good: There was demand on the body and resulting physiological arousal.

Early in his research program, Selye observed extensive biochemical changes following stress. He also observed that an organism's functional integrity may be threatened with unremitting stress. To integrate this data and attempt to explain how stress changes the body over time, he formulated a classic theoretical model, the **General Adaptation Syndrome** (GAS). Since then, several lines of research have refined the idea so that today, a clearer picture can be presented of the relationship between stress and physiological function.

The General Adaptation Syndrome: Alarm, Resistance, Exhaustion

Maintaining an internal state of equilibrium is a lifelong task that requires energy expenditure on a daily basis. Stress is just one type of environmental demand that disturbs internal balance. Adjustment to stress demands, though, occurs in stages. The time course and progress through these stages depends, first, on the severity and

duration of the stressor and, second, on how successful the organism's coping reactions are. Since each organism has a finite reserve of energy, the more severe and chronic a stressor is, the more likely it is that the energy reserve will be depleted. If and when that occurs, the organism may reach a survival crisis point. These ideas are formally described in the three stages of the General Adaptation Syndrome: the alarm reaction, the stage of resistance, and the stage of exhaustion.

The **alarm reaction** is the first response to a stressor. It makes no difference to the organism whether the stressor is acute (short-term) or chronic (long-term), since this judgment can be made only in hindsight. To the organism, any event that is judged to be a stressor requires immediate defensive reactions. During this stage, the sympathetic-adrenal medulla (SAM) complex initiates the arousal that serves to mobilize body resources to counter the demands. For a short time, the organism may be at increased risk, because the body's defenses may operate at lower efficiency than normal. Metabolic processes are catabolic or destructive, and weight may drop as a result. If the stressor passes quickly or the person's coping skills are

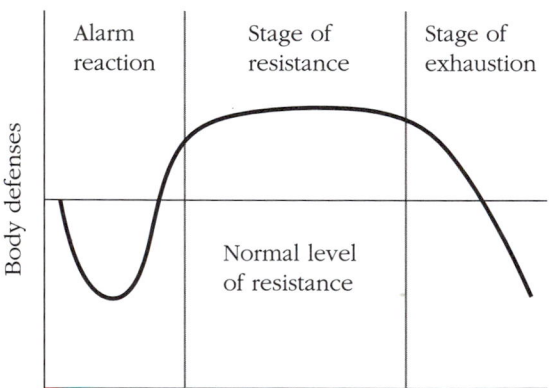

Time course of general adaptation syndrome

FIGURE 7.11   The three stages of Selye's GAS are associated with changes in body arousal and ability to defend against stress (adapted from Selye, 1956).

adequate to meet the demands, however, the crisis subsides and the body returns to normal with no ill effects.

The **stage of resistance** occurs when a stressor persists over a long time (by definition, such a stressor is usually a chronic one), or the person's coping skills are not adequate. Then, the body mobilizes its defenses above normal operational level, an action that is under the control of the HPA complex, including introduction of the glucocorticoids. During this time, the body may put up greater than normal resistance to illness. Metabolic processes are anabolic or restorative, and the organism may return to normal weight. Still, the body cannot sustain high energy expenditure indefinitely. Continued defensive arousal taxes the body's resources and ultimately leads to the last stage.

If the stressor does not abate or the organism has not found an effective coping strategy, the **stage of exhaustion** will follow. In this stage, the neuroendocrine system has reduced capacity to release defensive hormones. The body may be unable to produce lymphocytes to protect against disease (Keller, Weiss, Schleifer, Miller, & Stein, 1981), and thus the immune system functions at lower efficiency (Vaernes, Ursin, Darragh, & Lambe, 1982). The organism then experiences increased vulnerability to functional illnesses (colds or flu, for example) or structural illnesses (ulcers for example). In some rare cases, death may occur. These diseases of adaptation, as Selye (1976) called them, include disorders such as ulcers and hypertension.

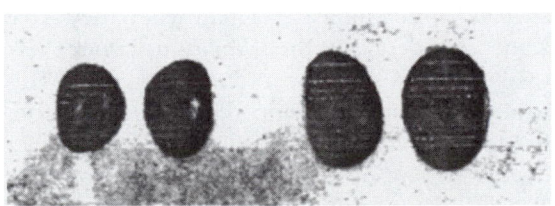

FIGURE 7.12 *This picture shows an abnormally enlarged adrenal compared to a normal adrenal gland.*

Two points about this stage are important. First, in most cases, stressors will cease before the organism reaches this stage, or the organism will use effective coping strategies that reduce or eliminate the stressor. Thus, the stage of exhaustion is neither an inevitable nor common outcome of stress. Second, the physical disorders most likely to develop depend on biological predispositions to weakness in the afflicted system. This fact is consistent with a diathesis-stress notion.

The Executive Monkey Study: Is it Responsibility or Error?

One of the first studies to demonstrate that stress might be linked to biological insult was the famous executive monkey study conducted by Joe Brady and his colleagues (Brady, Porter, Conrad, & Mason, 1958). In this study, four pairs of monkeys were placed in an avoidance learning situation. One monkey was the responsible monkey, always required to make the lever presses that would avoid shock for both members of the pair. The second monkey had no control: It could only wait passively, its comfort depending solely on the actions of the other monkey. The outcome of this study has been broadcast far and wide: The four executive monkeys died of ulcers while the other four monkeys survived with no apparent ill effects. The public took great interest in these results, perhaps because the experimental situation seemed to parallel the corporate maze in which executives carried extreme responsibility and also suffered from such health problems as ulcers.

Weiss's Rebuttal: Control, Predictability, and Information

Later, though, Stephen Weiss could not replicate Brady's study. It was discovered that Brady and his colleagues had made a fatal experimental error. When Brady's group began the experiment, both monkeys received shock. The first monkey to press the control lever was designated as the executive monkey. Since the four executive monkeys were self-selected, not randomly selected, it is possible that other characteristics of the first responders could explain the outcome better than the popular responsibility explanation. The monkeys could have had higher activity and arousal levels than the control monkeys. This characteristic could be associated with an overreactive gastrointestinal system (diathesis), which could explain the ulcers and death. Although the outcome could not be disputed—the monkeys did die of ulcers—the proposed explanation was open to question.

Weiss's subsequent studies systematically identified crucial factors that determine when physiological insult may result from stressor events. In one experiment, two groups of rats were exposed to a series of shocks (Weiss, 1968). One group could escape the shock with a lever press, while the other group could not. The helpless animals were more likely to develop ulcers than those who had control. In a second experiment, Weiss (1971a) added predictability, a visual signal that told rats when shock would occur. With predictable shock, the rats had fewer ulcers as compared to rats exposed to unpredictable shock. This lower rate of ulcers held true even without a controlling response available. Finally, Weiss (1971b) arranged for feedback to signal animals that their responses were effective in terminating the shock. Again, the animals receiving feedback had fewer ulcers than those who could escape but had no such feedback. Taken together, these studies suggest that the physiological effects of stress may be greatly reduced if the organism can engage in controlling behavior against a stressor that is predictable and also receives feedback about the effectiveness of its behavioral control. Note that these core features—control, predictability, and feedback—may be considered part of the organism's cognitive appraisal system. Even though this line of research originated in the context of Selye's theoretical system, then, the outcomes are fully consistent with Lazarus's transactional model.

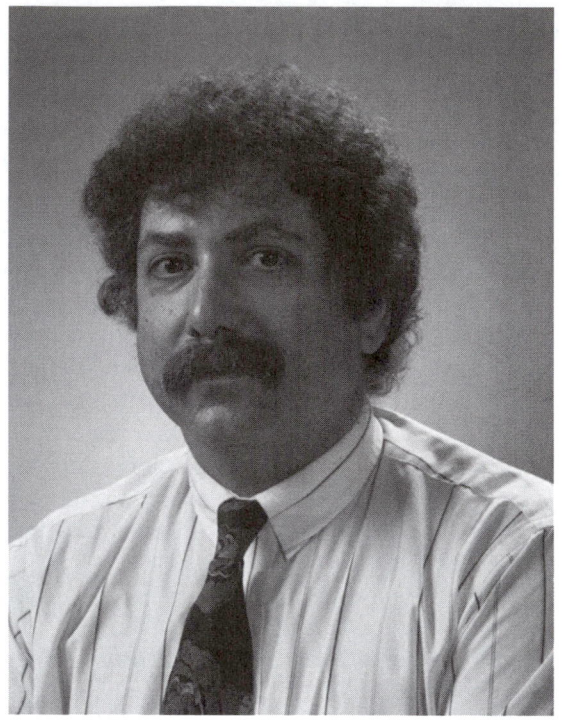

FIGURE 7.13   In the years since the Three Mile Island nuclear accident, Andrew Baum studied the residents of the area and provided especially pertinent data on coping responses in a natural setting.

The effect of controllability is also demonstrated in field studies of natural and technological disasters. Andrew Baum's work (Baum & Fleming, 1993) shows that people experience more stress when there is less predictability and when they feel less confident in their ability to control risk (as in the case of a nuclear disaster such as Three Mile Island) than when they have some confidence in their ability to control risk (as in the case of exposure to radon gas). This result was obtained even though people confronted with toxic radon exposure had a higher degree of perceived risk than those living near TMI or a toxic landfill. The physiological markers used to measure stress (urinary epinephrine, norepinephrine, and cortisol) vary in a way that is consistent with this interpretation.

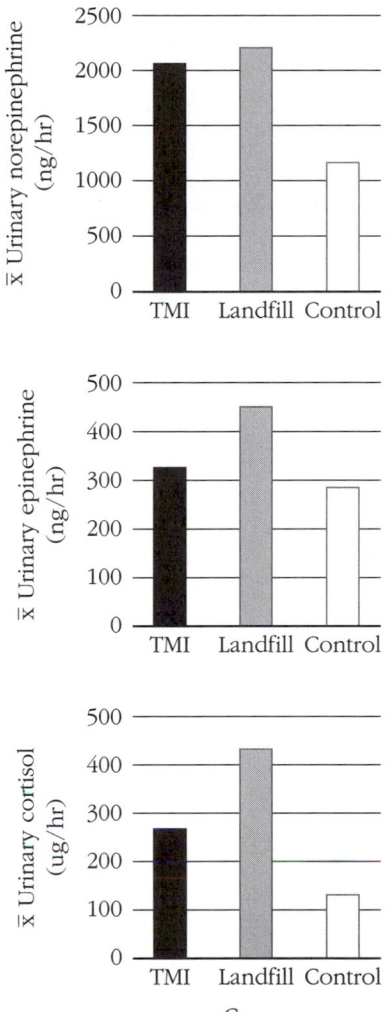

FIGURE 7.14 *From Andrew Baum's work at Three Mile Island, we have come to understand that naturally occurring stressors also cause increases in stress hormones (from Baum & Fleming, 1993).*

Since cortisol has been identified as a stress hormone, it is noteworthy that predictability affects the amount of cortisol in the system. The less predictable the stressor, the more cortisol in the system. As cortisol increases, so do associated negative physical changes (Frankenhaeuser, 1986). Overall, the assembled infor-

mation should make clear that however stress and health are related, the connection is not a simple one.

Stress Boulders: Predicting Illness from Life Events

During the 1970s and 1980s, scores of studies were carried out extending the findings of Brady's group, based on the logic that life change requires adaptive energy expenditure and increases risk for illness. Rubin (1974), working in the real-world environment of aircraft carrier pilot trainees, found a result that paralleled the original Brady study. Pilots, who had full responsibility for their craft and the life of their radar intercept officers (RIOs) in addition to their own safety, showed an elevated adrenocortical response on flying days. Their RIOs, who had no control over the craft, reported more subjective anxiety but showed only a slight but nonsignificant increase in adrenal response. Nelson (1974) reported that among enlisted sailors, only a few men accounted for most of the sick days. A cross-check revealed that these sailors were in routine, menial jobs, some of which were either hazardous or uncomfortable or both.

Holmes and Masuda (1974), in an early review of this literature, found an impressive array of supporting evidence. The early studies, though flawed by reliance on retrospective reports, suggested that increased rates of myocardial infarction, fractures, diabetes, tuberculosis, and leukemia occurred following increases in life-change stressors (Rabkin & Struening, 1976; Rahe & Arthur, 1978). These findings held across age groups, occupational groups, and cultures.

One of the best recent examples comes from Sheldon Cohen's laboratory and his research on stress, colds, and the immune system (Cohen, Tyrrell, & Smith, 1991). This project is exemplary for three reasons. First, it was a true experimental design that used a controlled virus challenge. Second, it collected medical and serological data on infections and colds over time using a prospective method while subjects were under direct control of the investigators. Third, it used meticulous controls to eliminate alternative explanations for the relationship between stress and immune response to cold viruses.

These controls warrant some comment. Cohen and his colleagues were aware of many sources of confounds in studies on stress, the immune system, and health. For example, people can differ in immune system reactivity, which might explain the appearance of illness. Further, subjects who have been exposed to a virus naturally could be more vulnerable independent of the laboratory virus challenge. Also, the presence of real-world stressors might lead to a negative change in dietary behavior, loss of sleep and increased fatigue, increased reliance on smoking to allay anxiety, or any combination of these. It is possible that these health behavior changes could predict the illness better than the stress. Finally, many theorists resort to some personality explanation to explain health risks. The link between negative affect and illness may be one of the most common connections discovered to date (Friedman & Booth-Kewley, 1987).

Cohen's group wanted to control for as many of these other explanations as possible. First, they used three measures of stress: a life-events scale (List of Recent Experiences), the subject's perceived coping ability, and an index of negative affect. Then, all subjects received extensive medical and health behavior tests prior to exposure. They provided blood samples to measure preexperimental serologic status relative to the viruses to be used, and the level of cotinine in the blood. Cotinine is commonly used to determine whether the subject is currently smoking.[9] After participants completed these measures, Cohen's team exposed each of the 420 subjects to one of five respiratory viruses and quarantined them for seven days, either singly or in pairs.

The outcome of Cohen's study showed that the rates of infection and clinical colds increased in a dose-response manner with increases in the stress-index score. This relationship did not change even when the control variables were entered in the regression model. Stress levels were not related to increases in clinical colds among the infected, however. Thus, in Cohen's view, the link between stress and colds is primarily due to increased rates of infection among subjects with higher stress-index scores, not to increased frequency of cold symptoms following infection. This distinction is important, since it indicates that the alteration in the immune system occurs in response to stress even when the full-blown symptoms of a cold do not appear.

The criticisms of life-events scales mentioned earlier also present a dilemma for those attempting to confirm a connection between stress and illness. Brett and her colleagues provided evidence that life-stress scales are

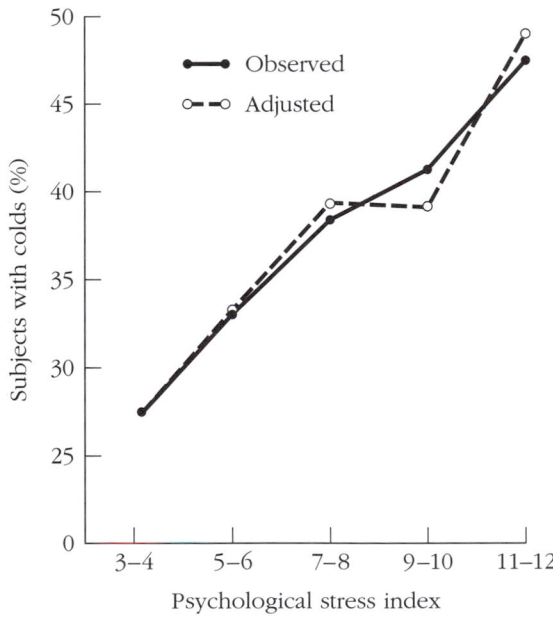

FIGURE 7.15   *Exposure to cold virus challenge showed a relationship between stress and the rate of colds (from Cohen, 1991).*

---

[9] See Chapter 8 for more on cotinine and smoking.

contaminated with items that tap mood and disposition. They also presented evidence that cautions us to accept the stress-illness link with some skepticism (Brett, Brief, Burke, George, & Webster, 1990). The rationale is that ratings of life stress may reflect a pessimistic cognitive style and negative emotional set more than they reflect inherent stressful features of the life event.

When Brett's group used measures of life change free of negative affect bias, the relationship to physical symptoms mostly disappeared. When the researchers constructed scales with extreme negative affect, the relationship to physical symptoms was even stronger than to total life-events scores. Brett's group also showed that negative affect correlated very strongly with depression. Thus, negative affect may be a general mood-dispositional tendency that carries the burden of depression and lower quality of health. In sum, Brett's research provided an argument that negative affect is the major contributing factor linking life change and illness. This result is all the more interesting when we consider that negative affect has played a major role in coronary-risk research.

Stress Pebbles: Predicting Illness from Hassles

Given the difficult task of connecting major life stressors to health and illness, we should not expect any easier task in confirming a link between hassles and health. Lazarus and his colleagues claimed that hassles predict illness better than life-change stress does (Coyne, & Holroyd, 1982), and there is some support for this notion. For example, in the study discussed earlier, Kohn and his colleagues (1991) found that hassles were positively and significantly linked to minor ailments and to psychiatric symptoms. Further, a study among the Navajo Indians in New Mexico found that both hassles and life events related to increased risk of hospital admission two years later (Williams, Zyzanski, & Wright, 1992). Nakano (1989) could

not replicate these findings working with a Japanese sample, however, suggesting that the hassles-illness link may have limited cross-cultural generality.

A study conducted in India, though, adds an interesting dimension to this debate. Lepore's research team compared hassles to major life-events stress among the urban poor in India (Lepore, Evans, & Palsane, 1991; Lepore, Palsane, & Evans, 1991). In the incredibly crowded conditions encountered by the urban poor, major life events (the crowding itself and inadequate housing and water supply, for example) were strongly associated with higher levels of psychosomatic symptoms, but hassles were unrelated to such symptoms. Lepore's team argued that major life events may be the more valid measure of stress among poor, urban groups in developing countries.

What Can We Do About Stress? Stress Coping Strategies

The details just presented may make it appear that once stress hits, some negative change in the physical system inevitably follows. The truth, though, is very different. Even genetic influences in reactivity leave much room for intervention to prevent potential ill effects from ever materializing. Two additional points are noteworthy. First, since stress is a relation between the person and the context of an event, many events that appear to be stressors may be reappraised quickly and given reduced psychic significance. In such cases, the initial arousal quickly passes, the body returns to normal, and no ill effects occur. Second, we can improve stress coping skills already available and add new skills as needed to help combat the effects of stress. Quite often, the role of a health psychologist is to help clients develop coping skills. In this section, then, we will discuss the major coping strategies. More details on coping techniques will be provided in later chapters in the context of specific disorders.

How Shall We Define Coping? Efforts to Minimize Stress

Folkman and Lazarus (1980) attempted to provide an inclusive definition of coping as part of the cognitive-transactional theory of stress. They defined coping as all the cognitive and behavioral efforts to master, reduce, or tolerate external or internal demands. Internal demands typically reflect the outcome of cognitive appraisals or emotional conflict. Further, coping usually aims at one of two outcomes: It seeks to alter the relationship between self and environment, or it seeks to reduce emotional pain and distress.

A more recent effort to define coping sought to integrate the work of various stress theorists. In this definition, **coping** is "any effort, healthy or unhealthy, conscious or unconscious, to prevent, eliminate, or weaken stressors, or to tolerate their effects in the least hurtful manner" (Matheny, Aycock, Pugh, Curlette, & Silva-Cannella, 1986, p. 509). This definition highlights several crucial elements of coping. First, people do not always use the most healthy coping strategies. People may deny the facts to the point of completely distorting their reality. They may eat to excess while hiding from threatening social situations. They may use violence to resolve power struggles in personal relationships. Second, a person does not have to be consciously aware of a strategy the person is using to cope in order for that strategy to be considered a coping method. Third, coping strategies do not have to eliminate a stressor altogether. They may also work to prevent the appearance of or simply to weaken the stressor. Fourth, coping strategies are used to reduce emotional or physical hurt, even though typically some cost is involved whenever dealing with a stressor.

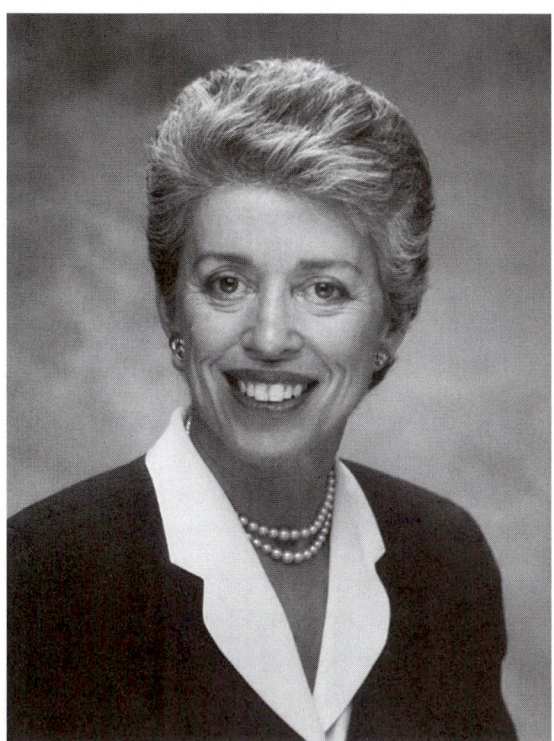

FIGURE 7.16   Susan Folkman has worked extensively in the area of stress and coping.

A Taxonomy of Coping: Combative and Preventive Coping

Just as various definitions of coping have been proposed, several ways to classify coping efforts have been offered. Consistent with the notion that coping seeks to change the relationship between self and environment or to reduce emotional pain, the cognitive-transactional model proposed two types of coping. In the first, emotionally focused coping, the person tries to control and release negative feelings (such as anger, frustration, and fear) provoked by the stressor event. In the second, problem-focused coping, the person tries to develop concrete plans of action and exerts as much direct control as possible. A cognitive reappraisal that changes the meaning of an event is one way to change the relationship between self and environment.

Andrew Baum and his coworkers looked at these coping styles in the context of a technological disaster (Baum, Fleming, & Singer, 1983).

Baum's group asked a small sample of local residents to describe the personal coping strategies they used after the Three Mile Island nuclear accident. The scale used for this purpose measured the extent to which people used an emotion control coping style designed to control their emotions as opposed to the problem control coping style.

Next, Baum's group classified each person as high or low in emotionally focused coping and high or low in problem coping. Then, they counted the number of symptoms reported for each coping style. The results were very revealing. People who were low in emotionally focused coping reported nearly three times the number of symptoms compared to those who were high on this dimension. People who were high in problem coping reported nearly three times the number of symptoms compared to those who were low on this dimension. How can this outcome be explained?

Baum's group believes that the most effective strategy in disaster situations is to focus first on getting rid of the negative emotions. In addition, victims probably should not be concerned about trying to control the problem through direct confrontation. The team reasoned that a disaster such as Three Mile Island confronts people with a situation that is inherently uncontrollable for anyone without technical training. Attempts to assert direct control, then, seem to add stress by increasing personal feelings of frustration at not being able to do anything about the problem. In other stressful situations, though, a problem-solving approach may be the most effective means of coping with stress. Personal control may be both possible and effective for resolving interpersonal conflict, for example.

Perhaps the most inclusive view of coping strategies comes from the work of Matheny and his associates (1986), who provided the definition of coping set out earlier. A summary of this approach appears in Table 7.4. In their view, there are two main categories of coping efforts, preventive coping and combative coping. From a learning perspective, preventive coping is

TABLE 7.4   *Preventive and combative coping methods (adapted from Matheny et al., 1986).*

PREVENTIVE STRATEGIES	COMBATIVE STRATEGIES

1. Avoiding stressors through life adjustment
2. Adjusting demand levels
3. Altering stress-inducing behavior patterns
4. Developing coping resources
  a. physiological assets
  b. psychological assets
    confidence
    sense of control
    self-esteem
  c. cognitive assets
    functional beliefs
    time management skills
    academic competence
  d. social assets
    social support
    friendship skills
  e. financial asssets
	1. Monitoring stressors and symptoms
	2. Marshaling resources
	3. Attacking stressors
	  a. problem solving
	  b. assertiveness
	  c. desensitization
	4. Tolerating stressors
	  a. cognitive restructuring
	  b. denial
	  c. sensation focusing
	5. Lowering arousal
	  a. relaxation
	  b. disclosure
	  c. catharsis
	  d. self-medication

avoidance learning, and combative coping is escape learning.

In **preventive coping,** we try to prevent stressors from appearing through cognitive restructuring that alters the perception of demand, or through increasing resistance to the effects of stress. The skills involved in preventive coping, because of their proactive nature, may take the most time and effort to develop. Building these skills may involve changing habitual behavior patterns, such as a sedentary lifestyle, that are often very difficult to alter, requiring constant attention over long periods. Developing these skills also may involve working on stable personal traits that resist change but can be altered to some degree nonetheless. For example, increasing optimism and self-efficacy may require long-term efforts with outside support or counseling plus incremental successes before these qualities become part of the person's habitual coping style.

In **combative coping,** a stressor triggers a defensive counterstrike, in which we attempt to subdue or defeat the stressor in some fashion. This strategy is essentially reactive. Combative strategies include skills that can often be learned through relatively short-term programs. One of the most common tension reduction methods, for example, is progressive muscle relaxation. This technique can be acquired quickly either with professional instruction or can be self-taught through reading and tapes. Another skill, **stress monitoring,** involves the person's attention to the signs and symptoms of stress. Before one can apply stress management techniques effectively, we must have some personal awareness of what stress is doing to us mentally and physically. Stress monitoring also enables us to identify the sources of stress more readily. Other techniques included in this category are problem solving, assertiveness training, and desensitizing disabling fears.

Note that a taxonomy is descriptive, an abstraction from behaviors displayed by many people over many situations and time frames. A taxonomy is not prescriptive: There is no reason to believe that everyone should use all these strategies. Instead, we each have coping strategies we have learned over the course of time, which we may use more or less by force of habit. There is evidence, though, that the choice of coping strategies varies by the type of person.

A research team headed by Peter Vitaliano at the University of Washington suggested that coping profiles can be constructed for different problem groups (Vitaliano et al., 1990). The coping categories used in this study included problem-focused coping, wishful thinking, social support, avoidance coping, and self-blame. Vitaliano's group compared four groups: psychiatric patients, physical health problem patients, medical students, and spousal caregivers. Within each of these groups, they also compared subjects with anxiety and depression to subjects with no anxiety or depression. Psychiatric patients used less problem-focused coping and sought less social support while using more wishful thinking and avoidant coping. The groups with physical health problems used more problem-focused coping and sought more social support than any other group besides the spousal caregivers. The reader can find other interesting comparisons with a more careful study of the graphs. Still, the study suggests that a study of coping styles may be useful in distinguishing different groups, and it may provide clues on where coping strengths and weaknesses exist.

Further support for this notion comes from research showing that one coping style—the self-focused coping style—may contribute to higher blood pressure in real-life stress situations. This coping style, defined by Richard Lazarus's group, is a pattern of coping with stress using self-blame, restrained emotions, and social isolation (Folkman & Lazarus, 1980). Carol Dolan and her research team studied male college students with the aid of ambulatory blood pressure monitoring (Dolan, Sherwood, & Light, 1992). Subjects first were classified as either high or low on the Self-Focused Coping Scale (SFCS). Then, they were tracked over two days: one a regular class day, the other an exam day. Dolan's group found that the high self-focused coping group had both higher systolic and diastolic blood pressure not only during tests, but also for the remainder of the day including rest periods. Most important, this difference between high and low self-focused copers was significant on test days but not on regular class days. Based on other related work, the authors suggest that affiliation, rather than isolation, on high stress days may help to ease the physiological effects of stress.

What Can I Do About Stress? The Practical Side of Coping

These principles have been presented largely in the context of the theory and research on stress and coping. On a practical level, the motivated learner can strengthen and develop personal coping skills fairly easily. In addition, several coping techniques mentioned here will be discussed in detail in subsequent chapters. The following represents a thumbnail sketch of advice on coping with stress.

First, using the information presented above, analyze your coping strengths and weaknesses. Then, concentrate some period of time to developing coping skills that reduce or minimize weaknesses. Third, develop hobbies and distractions that provide downtime from the pressures of studies and work. Even exercise can be viewed as a hobby, a very healthy hobby. Fourth, develop, maintain, and strengthen social networks that can buffer stress. These include family, friends, colleagues at work, and local social groups or agencies. Fifth, recognize that religious belief systems can function as effective cognitive structures to combat stress and that church groups can function as helpful support agencies. Sixth, consider the power of humor to diffuse and reduce stress. In other words, treat humor as one type of coping skill. Seventh, a healthy sense of optimism, tempered always by some degree of hard-nosed realism,

appears to be helpful both in warding off the impact of stress and in preventing the insidious effects of chronic arousal in undermining health (Scheier & Carver, 1987). Finally, successful encounters with stress tend to engender more success. Repeated success in coping with stress also tends to generate psychological resilience, reinforce self-efficacy, and may breed physiological toughness (Dienstbier, 1989)—the ability of the system to roll with the punches, so to speak, and to be less reactive when stress hits.

Summary

This chapter looked at the complex relationship between stress and health. A crucial part of this relationship is the way psychosocial stressors may be translated into physical processes with potential to damage the body. In later chapters, we will have occasion to look at stress in relationship to cardiovascular disease, cancer, pain, AIDS, and chronic disorders. This background should dispel any notion that the stress-health link is only speculative. On the contrary, the information accumulated goes a long way to describe what sequence of events follows the organism's efforts to ward off threats from either acute or chronic stressors.

1. The effects of stress can be seen almost everywhere—in mental conflict, physical fatigue and illness, disrupted family dynamics, disturbed social relations, lowered job satisfaction, and economic loss. About 41% of the population may suffer from moderate to severe stress at any one time.

2. The diathesis-stress model proposes that disorder depends on the interaction between predisposing factors and precipitating factors. Genetic predisposing factors influence the person's constitutional strengths and weaknesses, setting a threshold for vulnerability to stress. Environmental precipitating stressors, given an opportunity to emerge, determine whether the threshold of vulnerability is crossed or not.

3. Over the years, the definition of stress has ranged from an external force, to internal psychic struggle, to internal physical arousal. The transactional view of stress combines most of these features, and suggests that stress is the result of cognitive appraisals that match demand to coping resources. If demand is great while coping resources are weak, the result is stress.

4. A common mistake in talking about stress is to view it as always bad. In technical terms, bad stress is distress. It usually carries some threat of substantial loss or harm to the person if allowed to go unchecked. On the other side, good stress is called eustress. It is challenging and growth-promoting stress.

5. Early views of stress also focused largely on catastrophic stress, the huge boulders of life that crash down once in a while. An alternative view is that the little pebbles are what matter: hassles that occur every day throughout the day, like a stone in your shoe. Possibly the two types of stress combine—boulders make the load, but pebbles, like the proverbial straw, break the back.

6. Both life-events stress and hassles are related to an increased prevalence of illness. Though hassles may be more strongly related than life events, the issue is far from clear at this time.

7. Further research has determined that predictability, control, and feedback are important in determining whether stress will occur. In most situations, the ability to control a predictable event with feedback about the effect of exerting control greatly reduces the chances of stress.

8. Hans Selye was among the first to observe the link between stress and changes in the body system. His research identified the HPA complex and revealed that stress outcomes include enlarged adrenals, a system flooded with adrenalin and noradrenaline when stress is chronic, and gastric ulcers.

9. Selye proposed the General Adaptation Syndrome to account for the long-term effects of stress. This syndrome includes the alarm reac-

tion, the stage of resistance, and the stage of exhaustion.

10. Evidence compiled from both animal and human studies indicates that genetic factors contribute to stress reactivity.

11. The HPA complex, the hypothalamic-pituitary-adrenal complex, is one of the major links between brain and glands that results in potentially damaging effects and ultimately illness. Flooding with cortisol from the adrenals may then impair immune function.

12. The SAM complex, the sympathetic-adrenal-medullary complex, is another major component in active stress coping. Activation of the SAM axis leads to increased blood pressure, more blood flow to large muscles, more muscle strength, higher energy use, and better mental alertness.

13. The visceral brain includes the hypothalamus, thalamus, and parts of the limbic system. It controls visceral (gut-level) systems involved in fight or flight reactions.

14. The autonomic system acts in part to preserve homeostasis, the balance or equilibrium between resource conserving and resource expending forces. The parasympathetic system is the resource-conserving side, while the sympathetic is the resource-expending side.

15. Coping efforts are directed to reduction or prevention of the harm that may come from unmanaged stress. Coping strategies may be reactive and combative or else proactive and preventive.

16. Common combative coping strategies include stress monitoring, relaxation, problem solving, assertiveness, desensitization, and cognitive restructuring.

17. Common preventive coping strategies include adjusting one's lifestyle, behavioral risks, and building psychological and social resources.

18. Development of coping strategies is one of the clinical teaching activities often carried out by health psychologists, but coping skills may be acquired on a self-taught basis as well.

Key Words

adrenocorticotropic hormone (ACTH)
alarm reaction
anxiety hyper-ventilation
autonomic nervous system
autonomic nuclei
challenge
combative coping
coping
corticotropin releasing factor (CRF)
cortisol
distress
epinephrine (adrenaline)
eustress
General Adaptation Syndrome (GAS)
glucocorticoids
harm-loss
hassles
hindbrain
homeostasis
hydrocortisone
hypothalamus
immune system
limbic system
medulla

norepinephrine (noradrenaline)
parasympathetic nervous system
paresthesia
pituitary gland
precipitating factors
predisposing factors
preventive coping
primary appraisal
reappraisal
reticular formation (RF)
secondary appraisal
severe combined immune deficiency (SCID)
stage of exhaustion
stage of resistance
strain
stress
stress monitoring
stressor
sympathetic nervous system
thalamus
threat
thyroxine
uplifts
vasopressin
visceral brain

Study Questions

1. What is the diathesis-stress model? How is it consistent with the biopsychosocial model?
2. How may the three older definitions of stress be reformulated to provide more consistent use?
3. How does Lazarus integrate environmental with cognitive elements in his transactional view of stress?
4. What evidence is there for a genetic contri-bution to stress reactivity? How does this information fit with the diathesis-stress view?
5. What are the key neural elements that control the stress response? What is the role of the HPA and the SAM complexes in stress reactivity?
6. How might coping strategies operate to reduce physical arousal and negative effects from stressors?

Class Projects

1. Find additional information on different cop-ing strategies. Use a small group discussion format to learn how to implement a strategy, what the range of applications may be, and what the degree of success is for the strategy.
2. Ask your instructor whether the class may fill out and discuss group results from one or more standard stress scales.
3. If possible, invite a specialist in stress man-agement to speak to the class.

Suggested Readings

Ader, R. (1983). Developmental psychoneuroimmu-nology. *Developmental Psychobiology, 16,* 251–267.

Brady, J. V., Porter, R. W., Conrad, D. G., & Mason, J. W. (1958). Avoidance behavior and the develop-ment of gastroduodenal ulcers. *Journal of the Experimental Analysis of Behavior, 1,* 69–72.

Matheny, K. B., Aycock, D. W., Pugh, J. L., Curlette, W. L., & Silva-Cannella, K. A. (1986). Stress coping: A qualitative and quantitative synthesis with impli-cations for treatment. *Counseling Psychologist, 14,* 499–549.

Monroe, S. M., & Simons, A. D. (1991). Diathesis-stress theories in the context of life stress research: Implications for the depressive disorders. *Psycho-logical Bulletin, 110,* 406–425.

O'Leary, A. (1990). Stress, emotion, and human immune function. *Psychological Bulletin, 108,* 363–382.

Rice, P. L. (1992). *Stress and health* (2nd ed.). Pacific Grove, CA: Brooks/Cole.

WEBSITES   *Stress and Health*

ADDRESS	DESCRIPTION
http://www.gasou.edu/psychweb/mtsite/index.html	☆ Mind Tools—includes stress and time management information, plus shareware and many useful links
http://www.health-net.com/stress.htm	Health Net Managing Stress Home Page
http://www.stressfree.com	Stress Free Net—personal and occupational stress solutions
http://gladstone.uoregon.edu/~dvb/trauma.htm	Trauma Information Pages for PTSD and major disaster support
http://www.dartmouth.edu/dms/ptsd/	National Center for PTSD—includes index and access to the PTSD Research Quarterly
http://www.ssnr.com	☆ Society for the Study of Neuronal Regulation—biofeedback resources and applications
http://www.stress-o-s.org.uk/	Stress On-line Support from Great Britain

CHAPTER **8**

Substance Abuse I: Kicking Harmful Habits

Hardly a day goes by that we are not reminded of the frightening power of drugs to alter human potential. Drugs may, almost instantly, twist hope and joy into despair and sadness. Drugs have no respect for wealth, power, or position. Drugs care nothing of careers or occupations, and they contaminate the work, destroy the careers—sometimes take the lives—of philosophers, doctors, lawyers, writers, musicians, laborers, and sports celebrities alike. Many centuries ago, the poet Horace wrote: "Pale Death kicks his way equally into the cottages of the poor and the castles of kings." The brief sketch that follows serves to illustrate some of these points.

A Ledger of Drug Abuse: Freud, Cocaine, and Tobacco

It is now widely known that Sigmund Freud used cocaine during his early career. Beyond this bare fact, Freud's long-term habit of smoking cigars led to even more serious health problems and apparently a painful death.

Freud believed that cocaine could cure heroin addiction, a mistake in judgment that was to cost him dearly. Although Freud later changed his mind about cocaine, he first reported that it was pleasant to use with none of alcohol's negative effects (Freud, 1885/1974). Freud prescribed cocaine for a friend, to be taken by injection, a prescription that had disastrous consequences for the friend and left Freud with a deep sense of guilt for years. Before learning how risky cocaine could be, he sent periodic doses, with instructions for its use, to Martha Bernays, his fiance. Freud's own dependence grew presumably out of his attempt to fight fatigue, depression, and boredom. He even took cocaine prior to a social function at Charcot's residence because he was afraid that his fragile command of the French language would let him down. Peter Gay described Freud's early position as a blend of "scientific reporting and strenuous advocacy." [1988, p. 43]

Later, in 1917, through self-examination, Freud found a growth on his palate. Perhaps Freud believed that he, the physician, could heal himself, because he did not seek help for six years. At this time, it became apparent that Freud's cigar addiction had resulted in cancer. Still, his doctors tried to shield him from the truth: His condition was extremely serious. After a botched surgery and severe bleeding nearly killed him, he was fitted with an oral prosthesis

only to live with severe pain for his remaining 16 years. Near the end of his life, the ulcerated cancerous tissue in his mouth was so foul smelling that even his pet chow cringed from Freud's breath. When he died in 1939, it was from multiple large doses of morphine given by his doctor at Freud's personal request (Gay, 1988).

Our goal in this and the next chapter is to understand the biopsychosocial factors that contribute to initiation and maintenance of drug abuse. We will begin with definitional issues and consider the multicausal matrix of drug use. Later, we will consider both the epidemiology (distribution) and etiology (origins) of drug use. We will discuss the health and economic costs of abuse. Then, we will consider two drugs that are frequently abused: nicotine in this chapter and alcohol in the next. We will review the most promising intervention methods, but we must consider serious limitations that still exist. Along the way, it should become clear that health psychologists have many different roles to play in understanding, preventing, and treating drug abuse.

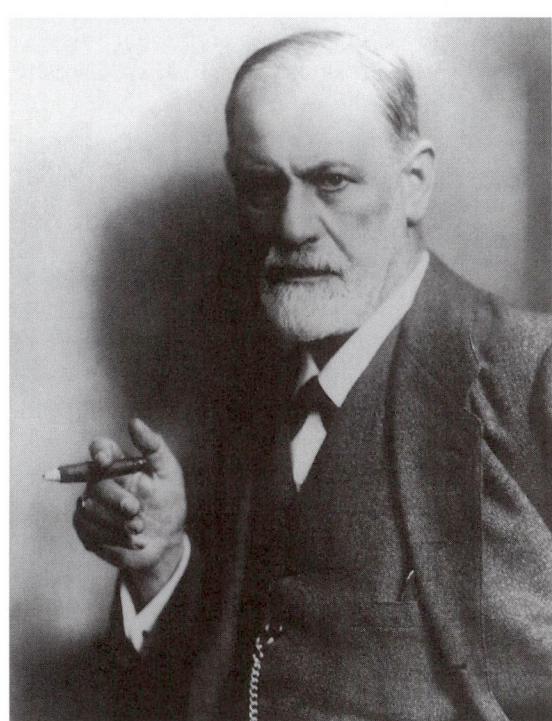

FIGURE 8.1   Freud, who fought an addiction to cocaine, also was a lifelong cigar smoker, a habit that resulted in mouth cancer.

Chaos in Definitions: Abuse, Dependence, and Tolerance

Defining drug abuse and dependence should be straightforward. Yet, there is new concern about the accuracy and clarity of terms we use to talk about drug abuse in general and the criteria we use to classify specific drug dependencies in particular. This concern has emerged as a result of difficulties encountered in clinical practice, and from laboratory research that challenges traditional views of craving and dependence (Wise, 1988). We will come back to some issues in the controversy later.

To begin, I will use the clinical standard, DSM-IV, which prefers to use the terms *substance abuse, dependence, craving, tolerance,* and *withdrawal* (American Psychiatric Association, 1994). **Substance abuse** is a maladaptive pattern of substance use that leads to clinically significant impairment or distress and continues or recurs periodically over a long period of time (American Psychiatric Association, 1994). Substance abuse is more inclusive than drug abuse, since people abuse substances other than drugs. People sniff glues, paints, or other chemicals to get high. Substance abuse also covers medications and over-the-counter drugs. (Later, when I refer to drug abuse, it is because our concerns in this and the next chapter revolve around a few specific drugs—nicotine, alcohol, and cocaine—and not all substances of abuse in general.)

The first marker of substance abuse, *maladaptive pattern of use,* is a behavior pattern in which the person continues to use the substance in spite of signs that it is causing social, work, or psychological or physical problems, or the person continues to use the substance in situations where its use is dangerous, such as while driving. Other behavioral effects include substantial time and effort involved in obtaining the drug and noticeable changes in mood, thinking, and perception. National health statistics may include other categories when reporting drug abuse, such as drug psychoses, dependence, and abuse with harmful effects for a fetus (Rice, Kelman, & Miller, 1991).[1] This custom primarily serves to make reporting more convenient, but it may contribute to unfortunate confusion when diagnostic and theoretical clarity is preferred.

The term **substance dependence** is used when there is evidence of tolerance, withdrawal when trying to quit, persistent craving or unsuccessful efforts to cut down. Further, social and occupational pursuits may be impaired, but the person continues to use the drug knowing that it is causing problems. Numerous biomedical studies have called into question traditional views of drug action, what defines craving, and the relation between dependence and patterns of use (Wise, 1988). Simply stated, a person can be dependent on a drug but not abuse it. One oft-cited example is of cancer patients who depend on morphine but still do not abuse

morphine. Smokers depend on nicotine but typically show no impairment in social or work relationships.

In contrast, people may also abuse a drug without being dependent on it. This may be the case among people who use a preferred drug for recreational purposes but do not demonstrate the other behaviors associated with dependence (Barnes, 1988). For example, a 1991 survey of high-school students showed that LSD has been making something of a comeback with more than 9% of white males and 5% of white females using it. LSD had become the recreational drug of affluent teenagers, the 1990s' suburban equivalent of the keg party (Seligmann, 1992, February 3). Timothy Leary, the guru of LSD in the 1960s, openly advocated drug use as a mind-expanding experience, and throughout his life he seemed to have escaped the expected negative effects of drug use. Based on recent research, this situation is not too surprising, since hallucinogenic drugs do not always lead to physical dependence.

Craving is an intense desire for the drug despite repeated attempts to cut down or quit. There are frequent periods of intoxication from the drug, and the person gives up other important activities in order to consume it. In addition, substantial periods of time and effort may be spent in trying to obtain the drug, even through illicit channels. *Tolerance* occurs when the drug does not produce the same effect it first did. Then, to achieve the same effect, the dose has to be markedly increased. Tolerance varies greatly with the person and the drug, making tolerance difficult to identify.

Finally, **substance withdrawal** refers to unpleasant physical and emotional symptoms that occur when the person quits using a drug he or she has used for a long time. Withdrawal has some features common to most types of drug dependencies, but some reactions are specific to the drug being used. Withdrawal from amphetamine dependence, for example, leads to depression, fatigue, hyperphagia, and hypersomnia. Withdrawal from barbiturates or benzodiazepines usually includes tremors, disorientation, tachycardia, and hypotension (Schatzberg

---

[1] For more information on how drugs may harm the fetus, including fetal alcohol syndrome, see Chapter 9.

& Cole, 1991). The problem of withdrawal also complicates the issue of defining dependence: It is never entirely clear whether people use a drug because of the high it gives—an *approach* response; because of psychosocial stress they are trying to elude—an *escape* response; or because they cannot endure the pain that withdrawal brings—an *avoidance* response. It is also likely that which response is more important changes with the history (time line) of drug use. The approach response is more likely important in the early stages of drug use, whereas the avoidance response is probably more important in the later stages of drug use.

The Tangled Web of Addiction: On Cause and Effect

Researchers are trying to untangle the complex web that accounts for both the initiation and maintenance of drug use and abuse. To this point in time, though, we have suffered more from a confusion of riches than a shortage of models. At the most general level, we can identify three views of drug use. The **medical model,** also called the **disease model,** tries to explain drug abuse largely in terms of physical properties of the drug itself and the effect of the drug on biological systems. Although drug addiction does not fit the classic notion of a disease, the medical model suggests that physiological and neurological reactivity to drugs may provide clues to vulnerability to addiction. One strong line of evidence is based on the genetic component in addiction, which influences sensitivity to drugs, tolerance for drugs, and rewarding versus aversive effects of drugs (Crabbe, Belknap, & Buck, 1995).

The **psychological model** examines everything from needs, drives, motives, modeling and vicarious reinforcement, to self-concept, self-efficacy, personality types, and pathological personalities (Shedler & Block, 1990). Although strong arguments can be made that psychological variables are crucial to the initiation and maintenance of drug use, most drugs undeniably change the way the physical system works and may do physical harm. Thus, the psychological model may not adequately explain the powerful physical factors involved in dependence, tolerance and withdrawal.

The **social model** has considered variables such as peer group pressure (van Roosmalen & McDaniel, 1989), dysfunctional families or weak family ties (Ellickson & Hays, 1992), differential association, advertising, social control, and public policy (Agnew & White, 1992; Tayman & Pennell, 1992). In the final analysis, though, no one model is adequate to explain both initiation and maintenance of drug use.

Far from deciding which model is correct, the problem now seems to be to determine how the three models may be integrated to form a comprehensive view of drug use. The problem is made more difficult because the three interacting variables—biological, psychological, and social—can be viewed at any given time as either cause or effect.

For example, we often talk about how drugs change physical functions such as altering metabolic or CNS function, treating drugs as cause and change in the biological system as effect. But it is possible that biological predispositions set thresholds for risk. Genetic endowment may bless one person with a metabolic system that sheds alcohol with little or no recognition of its existence in the system, and may curse another with a system that absorbs alcohol quickly with powerful consequences for body, brain, and behavior. In this case, the biological system (genetics) is cause, and addiction is an effect (Miller & Giannini, 1990).

Psychological variables may be related to both initiation and maintenance of drug use. One line of inquiry tries to discover personal traits that distinguish between abstainers, experimenters, and abusers (Shedler & Block, 1990). In this approach, the psychological variable is causal, and drug abuse is a symptom of personal maladjustment. But we are also concerned that drug abuse may change cognitive and personality functions. At this point, drug abuse is cause, and change in psychological function is effect.

Finally, many teenagers, especially females, face tremendous peer pressure to use drugs to be part of the group (Evans, Smith, & Raines, 1984; van Roosmalen & McDaniel, 1989). In this case, social process is cause, and drug abuse is effect. Conversely, drug abuse often disrupts interpersonal relations, both intimate and work related. When the analysis focuses on this relation, drug abuse is cause, and disturbed social relationship is effect.

Theoretical Views of Addiction: Chemistry, Cognitions, and Social Strain

As researchers pursue clues to the mystery of drug abuse, several people have attempted to integrate the fruits of this research in omnibus theories—in other words, broad-scale theories explaining all types of drug abuse. These theories are not at the same level as the Grand Unifying Theories (GUTs) of physics (Hawking, 1988), but they do offer interesting possibilities for higher order descriptions of drug abuse. In the next few pages, I will review the most prominent general theories. As you read each one, consider how each theory fits into the causal matrix discussed earlier.

The Biomedical View: Addiction as Genetics

One biomedical view suggests that the causes of addiction are buried in the genetic code (Miller & Giannini, 1990). Animal models are in use to study the genetics of risk, especially for alcoholism (George, 1988; 1990). Still, the first and most widely used method to demonstrate a genetic link was the concordance study. A concordance study looks for a trait in monozygotic twins (MZ) and computes a **concordance index,** which is the percentage of pairs of twins with the same trait. The same rate is then computed for dizygotic twins (DZ). A higher concordance rate in MZ twins compared to DZ twins supports the

notion that a genetic contribution exists for that trait, since monozygotic twins have the same genetic code.

Numerous studies of concordance have been carried out in the context of addictions such as smoking, alcoholism, and cocaine. Still, the extent to which genetics plays a role is unclear. One problem researchers face is the influence of other factors that may covary with genetics, such as familial and environmental variables. To get around the problem of covariation, researchers may look for adopted monozygotic twins. If the concordance rates are high, even when the pair of twins have been reared in different environments by adoptive parents who do not show the trait, then there is stronger evidence for a genetic contribution. Even if the concordance rate is very high and other variables have been well controlled, concordance studies do not identify the chromosome or gene that actually controls the process. To do so requires additional, often painstaking, research.

The Biomedical View: Addiction as Altered Neurochemistry

Another biomedical theory views all addictions as a single class of behaviors (Sunderwirth & Milkman, 1991). In this view, altered neurochemistry may explain the effects of addiction as well as the physiological basis of craving.

For example, Giannini and Miller (1989) pointed to six different neurotransmitters that research has implicated in addiction. These include gamma aminobutyric acid (GABA), acetylcholine, norepinephrine, dopamine, serotonin, and β-endorphin. These neurotransmitters are shown in Figure 8.2 with their central action, the drugs that alter their action, and the brain locations where their activity can be detected. Giannini and Miller proposed a biopsychiatric model and argued that "drugs of abuse do not interact uniquely with the brain to produce highly specific symptoms" (p. 173). Instead, they suggested that the effect of drugs is to increase or decrease the availability of a limited number of neurotransmitters.

Neurotransmitter/ central action	Drugs of abuse that affect neurotransmitter action	Central location
γ-Aminobutyric acid (GABA) General inhibition of other neurotransmitters	Alcohol Barbiturates Benzodiazepines Chloral hydrate Ethchlorvynol Meprobamate Methaqualone (?) Phencyclidine	Throughout brain 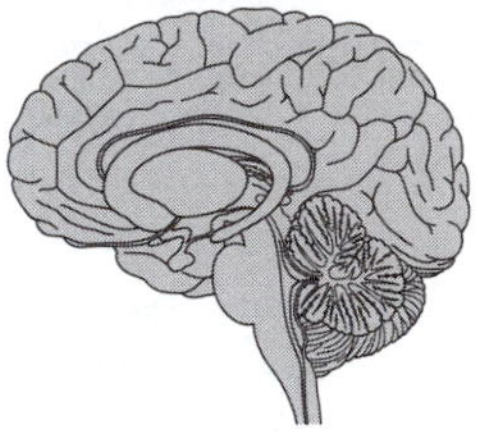
Acetylcholine Counterbalances dopamine Maintains memory Initiates short-term memory	Phencyclidine	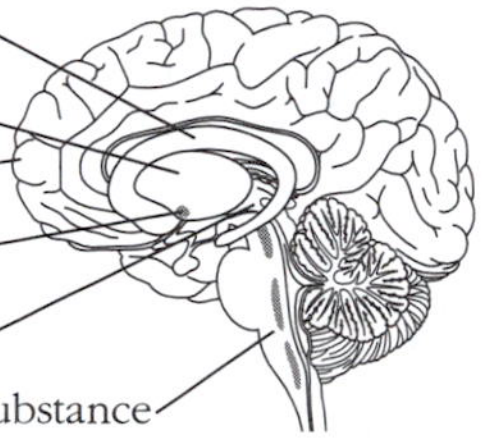 Caudate nucleus Lentiform nucleus Cerebral cortex Nucleus basalis of Meynert Nigrostriatal tract Reticular activating substance
Norepinephrine Modulates mood Maintains sleeping state	Amphetamines Cocaine Opiates Phencyclidine	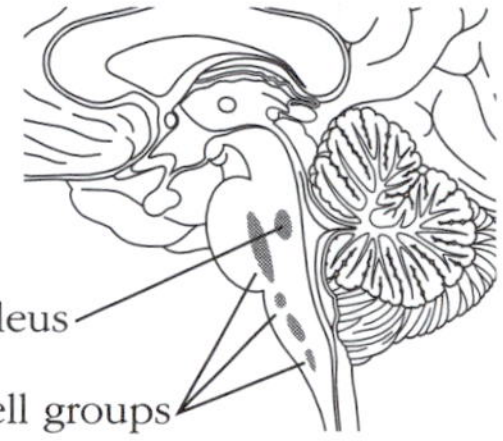 Nucleus locus ceruleus Pontine and medullary cell groups
Dopamine Counterbalances acetylcholine Stimulates pleasure center Modulates mood Affects intellectual processes Inhibits prolactin release	Amphetamines Cocaine Phencyclidine	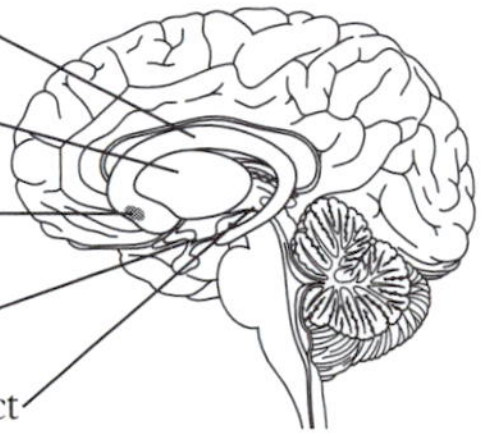 Caudate nucleus Lentiform nucleus Nucleus accumbens Tuberoinfundibular pathway Nigrostriatal tract
Serotonin Modulates mood Initiates sleep Involved in REM sleep	Psychedelic agents Phencyclidine	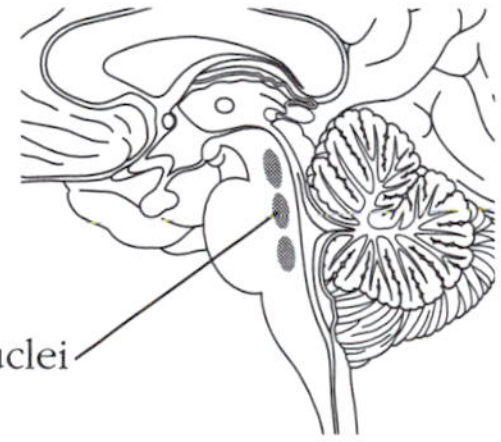 Pontine raphe nuclei
β-Endorphin Modulates mood Modulates pain perception Inhibits norepinephrine release	Opiates Phencyclidine	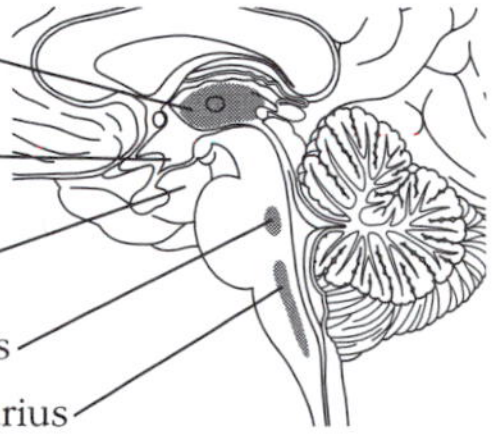 Thalamus Arcuate and premamillary nuclei Hippocampus Nucleus locus ceruleus Nucleus solitarius

FIGURE 8.2   The major neurotransmitters thought to be the neurochemical substrate of drug abuse (from Giannini & Miller, 1989).

According to the most frequently cited neurochemistry model, ingestion of any one of several drugs depletes dopamine (Dackis, Gold, & Pottash, 1986). Amphetamines and cocaine, for example, first elevate the release of stored dopamine from presynaptic vesicles into the synaptic cleft, but then block reuptake. Next, the dopamine in the synaptic cleft is degraded so that it cannot be recycled, resulting in an overall loss of available dopamine (Giannini and Miller, 1989). In addition, negative mood states—including depression, loss of a sense of well-being, and an increase in anxiety—appear related to abnormal dopamine levels. Addiction behaviors are carried out presumably to restore dopamine neurotransmission, alleviate feelings of anxiety, and renew a sense of pleasure. Even though psychological states, including self-controlled behaviors, are involved, the primary explanatory power is accorded to the dopamine depletion process.

Pleasure Centers in the Brain: Addiction as Self-Reward

Many years ago, two McGill University psychologists reported on a study that used electrical stimulation as the method to deliver reinforcement to rats' brains while the rats learned an operant response (Olds & Milner, 1954). This study is another one of science's stories of serendipity, an accident that proved interesting in its own right. James Olds, a social psychologist, and Peter Milner, a graduate student in physiological psychology, intended to implant electrodes in a rat's brain stem reticular region. But, because of a small error in calculating brain coordinates, the researchers hit the septal region instead. After the surgery, they found that this rat would work frenetically just to deliver stimulation to itself. At one point, the rat's response rate reached 100 bar presses per minute, and, in contrast to its response rate for food reinforcement, the rat could not be satisfied by any amount of stimulation.

Olds and Milner, along with many other

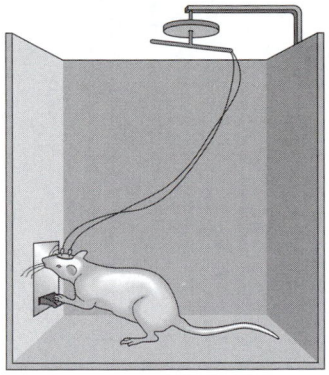

FIGURE 8.3   *A typical operant arrangement for studying rewarding self-stimulation (from Kalat, 1995).*

investigators, replicated this discovery in several different situations, with many other subjects, and with many additional interesting observations (Gallistel, Shizgal, & Yeomans, 1981). This brain center soon became known as the reward or pleasure center (see Figure 8.4). The customary account given for the behavioral effects of rewarding self-stimulation was that the animals were working to restore or maintain the same level of pleasure.

It is only a short step from here to the position that drugs operate on the brain's reward center: Drugs induce a pleasurable high that the user then tries to reinstate. Wise and Bozarth (1987) and Wise (1988) integrated evidence from research on the brain reward center and on dopamine depletion to argue that all addictive substances share psychomotor stimulant properties that activate a common neural reward mechanism. These authors believe that this neurophysiology, rather than withdrawal distress or psychosocial conflict, is the biological basis of psychological dependence and craving. Finally, these researchers argued that the operation of the brain's reward center may explain why treatment of addictions is so difficult. According to Wise (1988), these internal reward mechanisms exert a controlling influence over addiction that is far more powerful than any environmental stimulus.

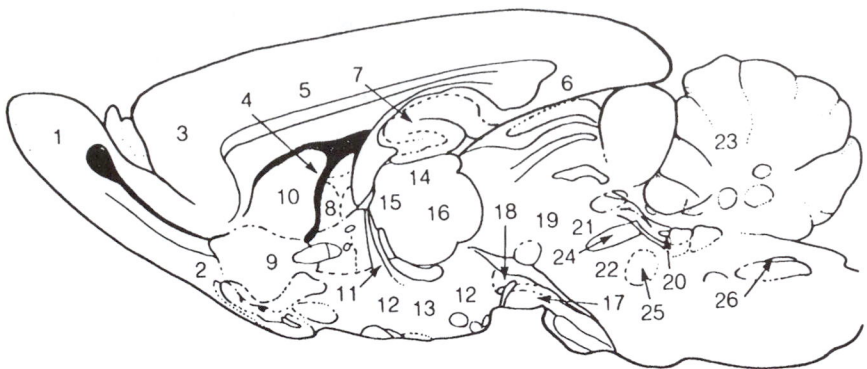

TELENCEPHALON

1. Olfactory Bulb
2. Prepyriform Cortex
3. Prefrontal Cortex
4. Subfornical organ
5. Cingulate Cortex
6. Entorhinal Cortex
7. Hippocampus
8. Septum
9. Nucleus Accumbens
10. Striatum

DIENCEPHALON

11. Fornix
12. Lateral Hypothalamus
13. Ventromedial
    Hypothalamus
14. Mediodorsal Nucleus
    of Thalamus
15. Nucleus Paratenialis
    of Thalamus
16. Central Nucleus
    of Thalamus

MESENCEPHALON

17. Substantia Nigra
18. Ventral Tegmental Area
19. Periaqueductal Grey
20. Mesencephalic Nucleus
    of Trigeminal Nerve
21. Dorsal Raphe
22. Median Raphe

METENCEPHALON

23. Cerebellum
24. Superior Cerebellar
    Peduncle
25. Motor Nucleus of
    Trigeminal Nerve

MYELENCEPHALON

26. Nucleus Tractus
    Solitarius

STRUCTURES NOT SHOWN

Globus Pallidus
Amygdala
Habenula

FIGURE 8.4   A diagram of major reward centers in the brain. The septum, site of Olds
and Milner's rewarding self-stimulation study, is just below the point numbered 8 (based
on Pinel, 1993).

The Opponent Process View: Habits, Habituation, and Addiction

Solomon (1977; Solomon & Corbit, 1974) proposed a general homeostatic motivational model of drug addiction based on the view that emotion-arousing stimuli follow a standard pattern of affective dynamics. This pattern is shown in Figure 8.5. The model is homeostatic because it assumes the body works to keep emotions stable as much as possible. The model is

motivational because it assumes people are driven to maintain or restore pleasant affect and to terminate or avoid unpleasant affect.

Solomon and Corbit called their view **opponent process theory,** a label derived from their core argument: A primary peak emotion is opposed by a secondary affective after-reaction. The **primary process,** also called the *a process,* reaches a peak quickly and then levels off due to the rising influence of the slower **opponent process.** This opposing *b process* tries to restore the balance disturbed by the strong primary process. The adaptation phase reflects the net effect during the time when both primary and opponent processes are maximal. But the primary process also stops quickly when the stimulus ceases, while the opposing influence, always a step behind, continues to work. This causes a type of rebound effect when the emotion displayed by the person is the opposite of the prior peak emotion. The overall effect can be likened to depression following intense excitement and happiness.

One additional assumption in the theory is crucial to our purpose. After repeated exposure to a stimulus, the peak emotional response *habituates* (diminishes) but the after-reaction becomes much stronger. This finding is supported by observations that, after repeated exposure, the b process kicks in faster, reaches its peak sooner, and persists longer. Thus, emotional highs are not as intense, but emotional lows are much stronger.

How does this process relate to drug abuse? Solomon (1977) says that the use of most drugs leads at first to strong emotional reactions, called **affective pleasure.** With alcohol, the feeling may be described as being relaxed or mellowed out. With amphetamines, the feeling may be described as a high or euphoria with great energy. In either case, the drug induced emotional state is associated with the primary process. When the drug has worn off, though, a strong after-reaction occurs called **affective withdrawal.** With alcohol, there may be headaches, nausea, and a feeling of being down or blue. With amphetamines, there may be mild depression and fatigue. In either case, the response is the biphasic one that opponent process theory predicts.

Opponent process theory suggests that drug tolerance is a result of the habituation of the a process. The emotional reaction is not as strong after repeated presentations, so the person has to increase the dose to achieve the same high as before. At the same time, long-term use may be associated with diminished pleasure in taking the drug because of the amount that has to be

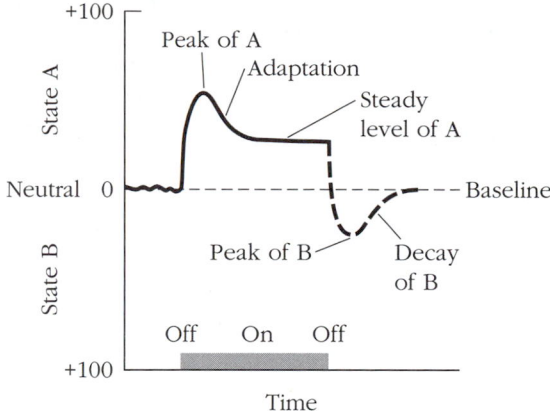

I. The standard pattern of affective dynamics produced by a relatively novel unconditioned stimulus

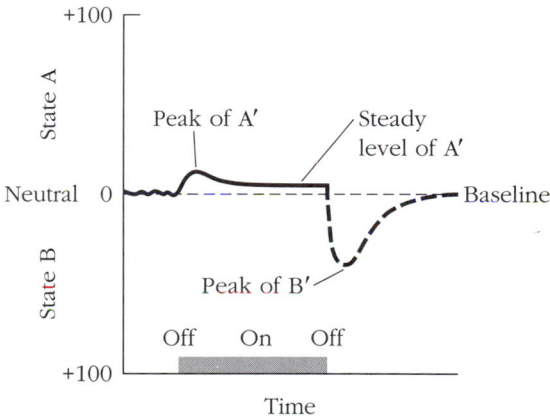

II. The standard pattern of affective dynamics produced by a familiar, frequently repeated unconditioned stimulus

FIGURE 8.5   *Solomon's opponent process theory suggests that emotional reactions that accompany drug use plus drug tolerance can be explained by differences in adaptation of A' and B' (from Solomon, 1980).*

taken to restore the primary emotion. This diminished pleasure is called **affective tolerance.** Still, the after-reaction continues to strengthen, so that withdrawal effects are even more aversive. At this point, regardless of diminished pleasure, the person often feels compelled to go on taking the drug to remove the extreme low. This is one logic behind the notion that, whatever one's reasons for beginning drug use were, continued drug use is primarily an avoidance response.

Finally, any attempt to quit may be frustrated because although withdrawal symptoms can persist for a long time and be very painful, merely taking the drug again will immediately remove the symptoms. From a learning point of view, this competition between short-term and long-term rewards is a stacked deck that is almost always cut in favor of the short-term reward. This model makes it easy to predict, as Rosenhan and Seligman (1989) pointed out, that drugs with short half-lives and intense withdrawal symptoms will be the most likely to produce drug dependence.

The Learning View: Pavlov's Dogs and Drugs

Mention Pavlov's dogs and most people will think of a dog in harness salivating to a tone that has been repeatedly paired with food. But Pavlov (1927) also had some intriguing ideas on drugs and conditioning. Two aspects of the conditioning model of addiction are important for our purposes. The first relates to the process of habituation, and the second relates to conditioning of contextual cues. We have already encountered the notion of habituation in discussing the opponent process theory. Drug tolerance is assumed to result from habituation: In other words, response to a drug is reduced due to repeated arousal with the same stimulus. The opponent process theory and the classical conditioning model are thus compatible. Ramsay and Woods (1997) note that central mediating responses to drug use are also learned and

these mediating responses may be activated by appropriate conditioned stimuli without the drug being present. The model proposed by Ramsay and Woods shows that biological and conditioning models of drug dependence and tolerance may also be highly compatible.

The issue of conditioned contextual cues goes back at least to the work of Pavlov himself. Pavlov believed that drug ingestion rituals can be viewed as classical conditioning trials (O'Brien, Childress, McLellan, Ehrman, & Ternes, 1988). The logic behind this is fairly simple. A drug addict usually has a ritual that includes a place, a method, and a set of basic tools needed to administer the drug. The drug itself results in powerful systemic effects. The environmental stimuli that are part of the ritual form a compound CS, while the systemic effect is treated as a powerful UCS.[2] With repeated pairings, the cues associated with the ritual may trigger reactions like those that occur with the drug itself. This is just the relationship that Pavlov and his colleagues noticed. One of Pavlov's dogs was repeatedly injected with morphine by the same experimenter. Later, when the dog merely saw the experimenter with a syringe (a CS), the dog acted just as though it had received a morphine injection. It began to salivate, vomit, and appeared to be sedated (a complex CR) even though no morphine had actually been given.

The effect of contextual cues on drug consumption is illustrated by the work of Hinson and his associates (Hinson, Poulos, Thomas, & Cappell, 1986). They gave rats a series of morphine injections in a distinctive room (DR) environment, and a series of saline injections in a home room (HR) environment. Later, when the rats had the opportunity to drink a morphine solution in both environments, they ingested significantly more morphine in the morphine-associated DR environment than in the saline-associated HR environment.

---

[2] The classical conditioning model was presented in Chapter 3.

This effect helps explain a finding from the Vietnam war. The extent of drug use and abuse in Vietnam has been widely reported. Studies of veterans returning to the states turned up some startling results, however. In one study, veterans were compared to addicts of comparable age treated at federal facilities in Lexington, Kentucky, and Fort Worth, Texas (Robins, Helzer, & Davis, 1975). Those addicted in Vietnam, of course, returned to a very different stateside environment. Those addicted in the states, though, often returned to virtually the same environment where they had acquired their addiction. The surprising result was that only about 7% of the veterans became readdicted when they returned, whereas significantly higher percentages of stateside addicts relapsed. This finding suggests that addiction may be environment specific.

Environment specificity can be extended to other aspects of the addict's experience, including the potential for overdose. This line of reasoning is based on Shephard Siegel's work (1988), probably the most notable proponent of the conditioning model of drug dependence. Siegel's group (Siegel et al., 1982) provided two groups of rats with identical heroin use histories in the same environment. Then, some of the rats were given a high dose of heroin in their old familiar drug setting, while another group received the same high dose but in a different setting. Rats injected in the new environment were much more likely to perish than those injected in the old one. To understand how this result can explain classic overdose deaths among hard-core users, though, we must add one more bit of information.

The conditioning model of addiction assumes that the body reacts in a compensatory fashion to counteract the strong effects of the drug. The cues normally present when shooting up also become linked with this compensatory action, and the protective response becomes a type of conditioned response. It protects the body against wild fluctuations that could be life threatening. In fact, the addict's drug tolerance may depend in part on these cues (Poulos &

Cappell, 1991). When an addict shoots up in a new environment, though, the cues for the compensatory response are weaker, if not completely absent. Thus, it is as though the addict is taking that same high dose as a first-time user, and the result can be lethal (Siegel, Hinson, Krank, & McCully, 1982). As appealing as this theory is, and despite the clinical case observations that support it, it remains unverified with human subjects.

Although much research has revolved around the opiates, a substantial body of evidence shows that tolerance also is context specific with nonopiate drugs such as ethanol, pentobarbital, amphetamine, scopolamine, haloperidol, and several benzodiazepines (Hinson & Siegel, 1986; Siegel & Sdao-Jarvie, 1986).

A Cognitive Model: Abuse as Automated Action Schemata

Stephen Tiffany (1990) contended that the resurgent interest in urges and cravings has not led to adequate models of addiction. Most urge theories explicitly or implicitly point to three components of the drug urge: the subjective experience of the person who feels the need for the drug; the emotional states tinged with a hedonic quality that accompany drug seeking and anticipation of drug ingestion; and the motivational forces derived from subjective experience that presumably activate drug-seeking behavior. Unfortunately, neither physiological variables nor psychological processes are closely related to the self-report measures used to confirm urge models. Indeed, much of the data reviewed by Tiffany suggests that psychological processes supporting drug-use behavior function independently of urges.

Tiffany proposes that drug abuse is controlled by automatized action schemata stored in long-term memory. The basic propositions are supported by a variety of indirect and direct laboratory work on the nature of voluntary (controlled) and involuntary (automatized) cognitive processes and skills. As a simple example, we may think of the first time we went out to learn how to drive a car. For most of us, it was a time of some strain as we struggled to learn the rules of the road while also trying to coordinate complex perceptual-motor actions to keep the car moving smoothly between the lines. After a few months of practice, however, driving became so automatic that we could do it with little or no conscious effort; the end result, in other words, was an automatized action schemata for driving cars.

According to Tiffany, automatized action schemata have five important features. The first three are more or less self-explanatory: Because of the numerous repetitions and practice in carrying them out, automatized action schemata are fast, effortless, and to a large degree unconscious. The last two features require added explanation. Action schemata are carried out without intention (autonomy) and show a tendency to ballistic completion. The feature of intention suggests that behaviors may be initiated without intent if the contextual cues are suitable and strong. This notion is reminiscent of the Biblical maxim: "When I want to do good, I don't; and when I try not to do wrong, I do it anyway" (Romans 7:19). The term ballistic completion means that once the behavior begins, it runs its course. Indeed, it may be very difficult, if not impossible, to stop the behavior once it has begun. Both of these points are thought to be crucial to understanding drug abuse.

Tiffany argued that drug seeking and drug consumption are behaviors that have been practiced over and over, and thus take on an automatized action schemata. These actions are fast and efficient, carried out often without specific intent, and difficult to impede. The physiological components of drug abuse may result from a combination of contextual cues, effortful processing, and somatovisceral adjustments that anticipate the motor sequences.

Still, two important questions must be asked: How does drug use get started, and how is it sustained to the level of an automated procedure? Here, Tiffany fell back on the notion that

many of the drugs of abuse have powerful rewarding properties that sustain a high rate of self-administration in the early stages. The theory seems to tie together a substantial body of data from dopamine depletion, brain reward center, and conditioning phenomena. At the same time, it has not received the critical and detailed inspection, both logically and empirically, that is needed to determine whether it can lead where other theories have failed.

Comparing Social Models: Association, Control, and Strain

Agnew and White (1992) used data from 1380 New Jersey adolescents to compare the relative contributions made by several social variables to delinquency and drug abuse. The authors designed their study to compare three social theories of drug abuse: differential association, social control, and general strain theory (GST). **Differential association theory** suggests that positive relationships with powerful but deviant peer models influences the adolescent to engage in a variety of antisocial behavior including drug use. **Social control theory** believes that it is the absence of positive relationships with significant others, such as parents, teachers, and other conventional embodiments of social value and control that leads to a failure in social control.

General strain theory tries to identify the conditions that influence the type of response that may occur under strain. GST suggests that strain occurs (1) when attempts to achieve positively valued goals are frustrated; (2) when previously achieved positively valued possessions are removed or threatened; and (3) when aversive consequences are applied or threatened. The two most important variables considered to mediate the effect of strain are association with delinquent peers and self-efficacy. Agnew and White showed that strain had a greater effect on delinquency and drug use when adolescents had many delinquent friends. Self-efficacy was related to delinquency but not drug use, perhaps because people low in self-efficacy react with anger, aggression, and theft. Their responses, in other words, are relevant to delinquent antisocial behavior but less relevant to drug use.

Taking a different tack, Shedler and Block (1990) constructed in-depth personality profiles of family units beginning when the child was 3 and continuing to age 18. The parents of frequent users and abstainers were described as cold, unresponsive, and pressuring. Abstaining children were described as overcontrolled, timid, fearful, immobilized by stress, and morose. Frequent user children were described as maladjusted, insecure, interpersonally alienated, emotionally withdrawn and unhappy. On the other hand, the parents of experimenters (children who experiment with but do not regularly use drugs) were described as responsive, spontaneous, supportive, protective, and able to find fun in situations. Their children were described as warm, responsive, active, curious, open to new experience, and cheerful. Based on a comparison of personality profiles and interactions at age 7 and again at 18, Shedler and Block conclude that the psychological differences between abstainers, users, and experimenters can be traced to quality of parenting in early childhood.

With this definitional and theoretical background in place, it is time to turn to specific addictions. We begin with a most pervasive addiction, smoking.

Nicotine Dependence: Risks, Origins, and Quitting

Tobacco is the generic name of the plant species *Nicotiana*. The name reveals the active ingredient, the alkaloid nicotine, which gives the smoker a kick and ultimately leads to physical dependence. A tobacco leaf may contain from 2% to 10% nicotine, depending on the strain and the method of processing.

Use of tobacco is undeniably a part of Americana. Tobacco was unknown in Europe and probably most of the eastern regions of the world until Spain's explorations and conquests in the late 15th and early 16th century. At that time, tobacco was in use among Indian groups of both North and South America, largely for ceremonial and social activities. It was believed, though, that tobacco had medicinal value, and on this basis, it was exported first to Europe and then, in less than 100 years, to the rest of the world. Sir Arthur Helps (1859, *Worry*), perhaps speaking sarcastically, wrote: "What a blessing this smoking is! Perhaps the greatest that we owe to the discovery of America." It is one gift of that era that might have been better left unbestowed.

But tobacco was, for the settlers, the main staple with which they could obtain manufactured goods from Europe, a fact that entrenched tobacco in the commerce and economy of America. From the middle of the 19th century on, tobacco was mass produced for a populace whose appetite seemed insatiable. By 1990, the tobacco industry manufactured and sold 534 varieties of cigarettes plus numerous smokeless tobaccos. To get the word out, the industry multiplied its advertising budget sevenfold between 1974 and 1984 (Davis, 1987). It now spends over $3.25 billion trying to convince consumers that smoking is chic or macho (FDA Consumer, 1995).

By 1955, the prevalence of tobacco use was estimated at nearly 53% of the population, a figure that remained more or less constant through about 1963. Although the data now show a gradual decline, tobacco use in 1990 still occurred among more than 25% of the population (28% males and 23% females) (MMWR, May 22, 1992). A 1991 Youth Risk Behavior Survey reported that, among high school students, a median 12% reported smoking on 20 of the preceding 30 days (MMWR, Sep. 18, 1992). It is estimated that every day nearly 3000 adolescents take their first steps toward a lifelong habit of smoking (Jason, Ji, Anes, & Birkhead, 1991). Thus, although the trend had been gradually declining, that decline may be leveling off. There are concerns about increased use among

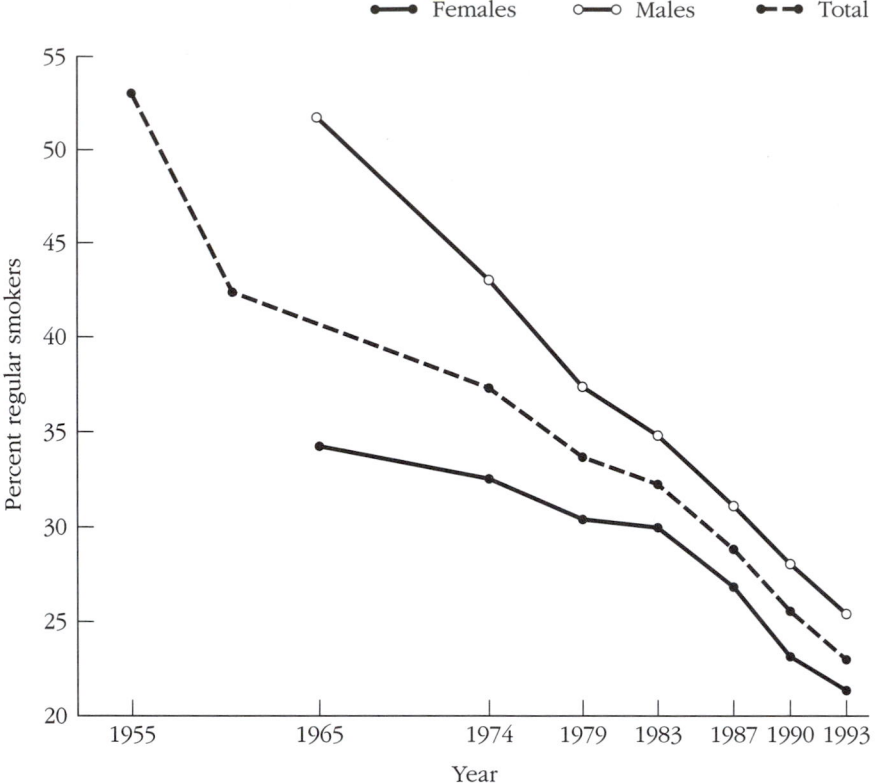

FIGURE 8.6   *This shows the decline in smoking that has occurred among the population 18 years and older since use peaked between 1955 and 1963 (data from National Center for Health Statistics, 1996).*

some segments of the population (youth and women) that may offset if not reverse the trend. Tobacco is second only to alcohol in rate of use, but it ranks first in association with morbidity and mortality, as Table 8.1 shows.

According to one study, prevalence of smoking differs by ethnic group. This study, Monitoring the Future, is under the direction of the University of Michigan's Institute for Social Research (Bachman et al., 1991). It began in 1975 and continues to sample nearly 17,000 high school students each year. The research team provided data showing that the 12% overall prevalence is fairly typical for white males (12.5%) and white females (13.3%) smoking a half-pack or more per day. Among black males and females, however, the prevalence rate is

much lower: 3.3% and 2.2% respectively. Prevalence is lower among Mexican Americans (5.2% and 2.5%) and Asian Americans (4.4% and 4.5%) as well. Among Native Americans, though, the prevalence is 18.4% for males and 23.4% for females. The encouraging note is that, regardless of ethnic group, the trend in prevalence is largely toward lower use.

The authors point to one discrepancy from national data on drug use: that black adults are highly visible in morbidity and mortality data related to drug use and abuse. Bachman's group argued that this disproportionate visibility can be explained by the two worlds of drug use in the black community. On the one hand, a small minority abuse drugs to the extreme and pay for it dearly with various health problems. On the

TABLE 8.1   Drug use and its results.

DRUG	EVER USED[a]	CURRENT USER[a,b]	MORBIDITY	MORTALITY
Alcohol	85.0[b]	53.4	cirrhosis of liver	129,000[c]
			pancreatitis	
			gastritis	
			hypertension/stroke	
			cancer	
			organic brain damage	
			seizures	
			delirium tremens	
			birth defects	
			fetal alcohol syndrome	40/100,000
			auto accidents:	
			injuries	
			deaths	19,777
Caffeine[d]	85.0	85.0	hypertension	
			headache	
			tremors	
			anxiety	
			depression	
Cigarettes	75.1	28.8	cardiovascular disease	426,000
			gastritis	
			peptic ulcer	
			lung cancer	
			impaired fetal growth	
			spontaneous abortion	
Smokeless tobacco	14.9	3.4	oral cancer	
			gum recession	
Marijuana/hashish	33.1	5.9	accidents	75
			respiratory illness	
			lung cancer	
			impaired immune response	
			impaired memory	

[a]All values for "ever used" and "current user" are given as percentages.
[b]A current user is defined as one who has used the drug sometime in the past month.
[c]This figure includes 4000 deaths annually due to mixing alcohol with other drugs.
[d]This category is not included in the household survey but is added to show comparison of a widely used stimulant.

continued

other hand, a large majority is abstinent to the extreme.

Risk Statistics: Smoking's Terrible Tale

Information compiled by several health agencies shows that smoking is anything but a benign recreational activity. A 25-year-old who smokes one pack to two packs per day has a life expectancy that is eight years less than a nonsmoker (Horovitz, 1988). Recent estimates indicate that smoking causes at minimum 426,000 deaths per year, or about 1 in 6 deaths from all causes (Davis, 1987; MMWR, 1992, March 13). It is interesting to compare reactions to this fact and the emotions that continue to run at a high level for those killed in Vietnam. We built a wall in memory of the 58,022 soldiers who died dur-

TABLE 8.1   Drug use and its results (continued).

DRUG	EVER USED[a]	CURRENT USER[a,b]	MORBIDITY	MORTALITY
Cocaine	10.7	1.5	chronic rhinitis	2000
Crack	1.3	0.2	perforation of nasal septum	
			seizures	
			depression	
			unpleasant tactile sensations	
Hallucinogens	7.4	0.4	agitation	
LSD	5.5	0.4[e]	hyperactivity	
PCP (phencyclidine)	3.1	0.2[f]	flashbacks	
			depression	
			psychosis	
Inhalants	5.7	0.6	CNS damage	
			depression	
			heart failure	
			suffocation	
Stimulants/	7.1	0.9	sleep disturbance	
Amphetamines[g]			depression	
			hypertension	
			headaches	
			malnutrition	
			cardiac arrest	
Depressants/	3.5	0.4	accidents	
Sedatives				
Tranquilizers	4.8	0.6		
Analgesics/	5.2	0.6	pulmonary edema	4000
Narcotics			respiratory arrest	
Heroin	1.0	0.3	convulsions	
			premature birth	
			fetal addiction	

[a]All values for "ever used" and "current user" are given as percentages.
[b]A current user is defined as one who has used the drug sometime in the past month.
[e]The statistical basis for reporting use in the past month was of such low precision that NIDA did not give an estimate. The value reported here is for use in the past year.
[f]The statistical basis for reporting use in the past month was of such low precision that NIDA did not give an estimate. The value reported here is for use in the past year.
[g]All percentages listed for psychotherapeutic agents, whether stimulants, sedatives, tranquilizers, or analgesics, are for nonmedical use.

ing more than 16 years of U.S. involvement in Vietnam. Yet eight times as many deaths occur *each year* due to smoking, and many still act as though there is no great urgency.

Manson's group (1992) estimates that smoking is directly responsible for 21% of mortality from heart disease, or about 115,000 deaths annually. One prospective study using female nurses compared smokers to nonsmokers for fatal coronary disease. It revealed a relative risk that was 11 times higher for those smoking more than 45 cigarettes per day, 5.5 times higher for those smoking more than 25 cigarettes per day, and 2 to 3 times higher for those smoking between 1 and 14 cigarettes per day (Willett, et al., 1987). Smoking also contributes directly to about 150,000 deaths from various types of cancer, most notably lung cancer: About 80% of lung cancer mortality is attributed to smoking (Lopez, 1992; Jaret, 1986).

There is a suggestion that smoking does not predict morbidity or mortality among the elderly. But two studies paint a very different picture. First, smoking is a risk factor in 7 of the 14 major causes of death among those over 65 years of age (Orleans, Rimer, Cristinzio, Keintz, & Fleisher, 1991). Second, among elderly current smokers, the total mortality rate is twice that among cohorts who have never smoked (LaCroix et al., 1991).

The preceding statistics focus on mortality, but data on morbidity reveal a similar harmful effect from smoking. Smoking-related diseases may result in $43 billion in lost productivity and $22 billion in health care costs (Davis, 1987). Male smokers suffer from short-term illnesses at a rate that is about 14% higher than nonsmokers. For women, the morbidity rate is 21% higher than nonsmokers. Male smokers lose about 33% more workdays than their nonsmoking colleagues, and women smokers lose about 45% more workdays (Tucker, 1985). One puzzling but as yet unexplained finding is that former smokers have a higher risk for ulcerative colitis than current smokers (Boyko, Koepsell, Perera, & Inui, 1987). Smokers have more respiratory problems, including reduced lung function and both acute and chronic bronchitis. Reduced lung function is present in both male and female adolescents smoking as few as five cigarettes per day. Girls appear to be more vulnerable than boys (Gold et al., 1996).

Even the fetus is vulnerable to the side effects of smoking. Smoking during pregnancy lowers birth weights, retards brain growth, and increases risk for sudden infant death syndrome (SIDS). Despite ample warnings about hazards to the unborn, many women continue to smoke during pregnancy, and male partners release sidestream smoke that also exposes the fetus.

Toxic By-Products of Smoking: Carbon Monoxide and Fat

In addition to altering metabolism and destroying phagocytes, nicotine produces the deadly by-product carbon monoxide. Marijuana has the same effect, but at a rate per cigarette that is five times greater (Wu et al., 1988). Figure 8.7 shows the complex set of events that transforms tobacco into new by-products. Carbon monoxide has a 200 times stronger attraction to red blood cells than oxygen. It infuses the blood through the lungs displacing oxygen and interfering with oxygen distribution throughout the body. The end result is that the heart has a heavier load, both because its own supply is reduced and because it now has to work harder to supply the rest of the body. As a result, smokers can feel fatigue sooner, especially during attempts to exercise. This could contribute in part to the lower rate of compliance with exercise routines noted among smokers as a group.

Carbon monoxide has yet another insidious side effect: It appears to increase the rate of fatty deposits in the cardiovascular system. To complete the double-barreled assault, inhaling nicotine stimulates the release of adrenaline. Adrenaline causes fat cells all over the body to change so that they dump their fatty acids into the bloodstream, increasing the risk for atherosclerosis (Horovitz, 1988).

Assessment Issues: Biochemical, Behavioral, and Self-Report

Before we talk about issues in smoking research and interventions, we must discuss one major methodological problem researchers confront. This problem can be phrased as a question: How do you reliably measure how much a person is smoking?

Investigators often depend on self-report measures that estimate the frequency (days per week) and intensity (number of cigarettes or packs per day) of smoking. These reports are often done retrospectively, so that both fallibility of memory and self-serving biases may enter in. Behavioral measures may include both self-monitoring (possibly subject to faking), and informant counting of cigarettes smoked using a

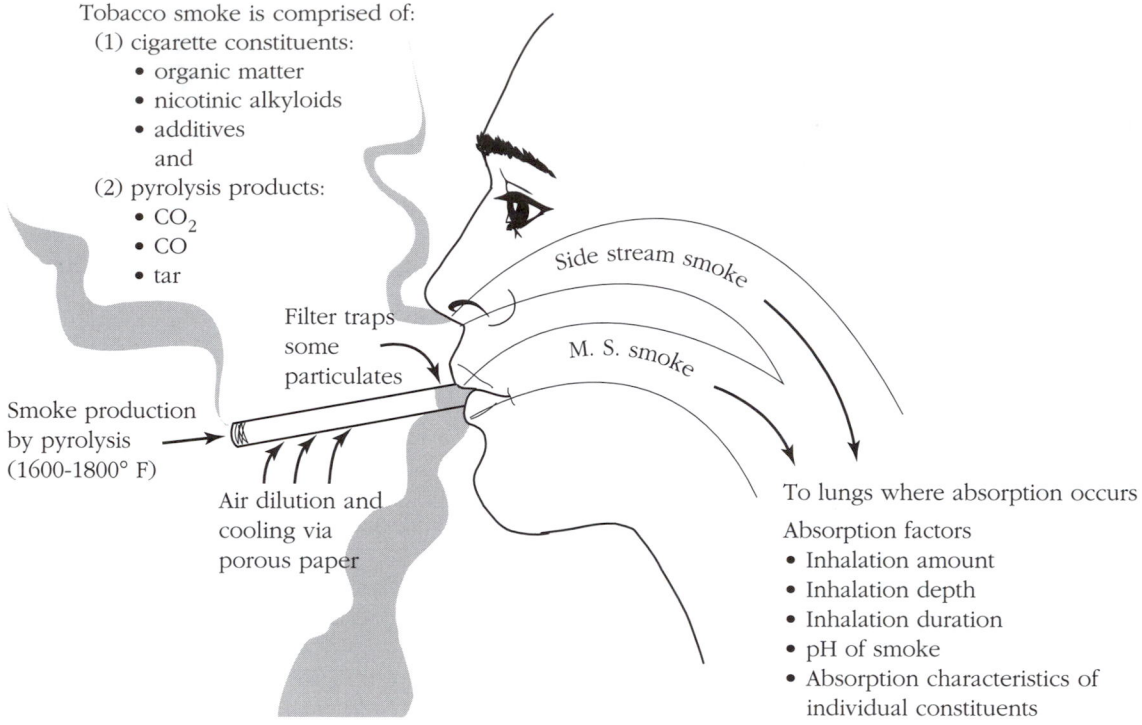

Tobacco smoke is comprised of:
  (1) cigarette constituents:
    • organic matter
    • nicotinic alkyloids
    • additives
      and
  (2) pyrolysis products:
    • CO_2
    • CO
    • tar

Filter traps
some
particulates

Smoke production
by pyrolysis
(1600-1800° F)

Air dilution and
cooling via
porous paper

Side stream smoke

M. S. smoke

To lungs where absorption occurs

Absorption factors
  • Inhalation amount
  • Inhalation depth
  • Inhalation duration
  • pH of smoke
  • Absorption characteristics of
    individual constituents

FIGURE 8.7   *The sequence of events involved in converting nicotine to deadly by-products (from Henningfield & Woodson, 1989).*

mechanical counter, a charting method, or even a miniature computer.

Three biochemical measures have been frequently used to assess active smoking behavior and to evaluate the success of intervention programs (Velicer, Prochaska, Rossi, & Snow, 1992). These are thiocyanate (SCN), carbon monoxide (CO), and cotinine. On the surface, nicotine seems the most obvious marker for smoking. Unfortunately, nicotine has a half-life of no more than two hours and thus is not a very useful measure. Tests for SCN, moreover, are not very sensitive for light smokers and are easily contaminated by certain foods (cauliflower and beer, for example). Velicer and his colleagues have suggested that SCN should no longer be regarded as a valid test.

CO can be assessed in the bloodstream, but it is also insensitive for light smokers, and it is easily contaminated because of air pollution (environmental plus secondhand smoke) and

lactose intolerance. Still, it is regarded as a useful test because it is easy to obtain and relatively inexpensive.

Cotinine is a by-product of nicotine. Tests based on either saliva or blood samples provide very sensitive tests of recent smoking even in light smokers. Since nicotine is unique to tobacco, cotinine provides a very specific test of recent smoking. There are racial differences in absorption, but the false negative rate is still less than 2% overall. In spite of the fact that it is more complex and expensive than SCN or CO, cotinine has become the method of choice.

Physical Dependence: Tolerance, Withdrawal, and Dose-Response

Although virtually everyone recognized long ago that various drugs—alcohol, heroin, and cocaine, among others—have the potential for physical dependence, nicotine has been often treated with more or less benign neglect. Yet professionals in addiction research have known for nearly a century how dangerous nicotine can be. The dose-response relationship, a reasonably reliable sign of physical dependence, was the subject of study already at the turn of the century (Henningfield & Woodson, 1989).

In addition, research showed that when low-tar cigarettes were introduced to the market, smokers offset the lower nicotine content by increasing the number of cigarettes smoked per day, by smoking closer to the tip, or both (Benowitz, Jacob, Kozlowski, & Yu, 1986).[3] Smokers' behavior changed because they suffered withdrawal symptoms from reduced nicotine intake if they stuck to their previous smoking habits. By the 1970s, a solid base of information unequivocally showed that nicotine is a powerful drug with the capacity to produce physical dependence, although with wide individual differences (Shiffman, 1989). The commonly reported withdrawal symptoms include anxiety, concentration problems, sleep disturbance, depression, hunger, irritability, and restlessness. John Hughes (1992) found that withdrawal symptoms fit into three clusters defined by mood, appetite, and insomnia.

In low to moderate doses, nicotine is a stimulant that arouses the central nervous and cardiovascular systems. After a short initiation period, users report that smoking reduces anxiety and restrictions on smoking increase anxiety. With high doses, nicotine actually can have depressant effects on the system. The body metabolizes the smoke fumes rapidly so that nicotine crosses the blood-brain barrier in a mere ten seconds from the first inhalation (Horovitz, 1988). In the brain, nicotine stimulates release of catecholamines, adrenaline-like substances that accelerate heart rate and raise blood pressure. Effects in the cardiovascular system are amplified under conditions of stress (MacDougall, Dembroski, Slaats, Herd, & Eliot,

1983). These physical changes are part of the lift that smokers experience and crave.

Nicotine use is also subject to partial tolerance effects since subjective feelings, EEG, and cardiovascular responses diminish greatly with repeated doses. Increased doses generally restore these responses up to a point. Note the two qualifications made in these statements. First, partial tolerance points to the fact that even with repeated doses, some responsiveness still remains. Second, it is possible, though not certain, that a ceiling for tolerance occurs because large doses of nicotine become aversive and may serve to control further intake.

Although most of the evidence on physical dependence seems clear and convincing, there is one contradictory line of evidence. Saul Shiffman (1989) studied a group of smokers, called tobacco chippers, who constitute no more than 5 to 10% of smokers. Chippers smoke at most five cigarettes a day about four days each week. When compared to a group of dependent smokers, chippers inhaled the same as dependent smokers, but they showed no signs of withdrawal when abstinent. Shiffman noted that chippers report less stress, have better stress coping skills and better social supports than the dependent smokers.

Genetic-Familial Origins of Smoking

As the difficulty of quitting smoking continues to frustrate smokers and clinicians alike, some research has turned to the issue of a genotype for smoking. The rationale of this approach is that there may be genetically determined differences in responsivity to nicotine. Previous research using an animal model showed that nicotine does not affect the physiological system and behaviors the same way in all mice strains (Marks, Burch, & Collins, 1983).

A recent study on genetic influences in smoking adds to the body of evidence that a genotype may influence lifetime smoking practices (Carmelli, Swan, Robinette, & Fabsitz, 1992). According to Carmelli's group, earlier twin, family, and adoption studies showed an overall smoking heritability index of 0.53. The

---

[3] The practice of smoking closer to the tip is particularly dangerous because toxic particles increase their concentration as the cigarette is smoked down to the tip.

heritability index expresses the proportion of phenotypic variation (smoking behavior) attributed to genetic variation. The Carmelli team analyzed data from 4774 twin pairs. They found that three components of smoking behavior—never having smoked, being a current smoker, and quitting smoking—were moderately influenced by genetic factors. Note that the results of this study were immediately challenged because Carmelli's group failed to distinguish genetic variation from familial variation (Austin & Newman, 1993; Levy, 1993). Further, although animal models suggest genetic strain differences in binding to nicotine receptors, Carmelli's study once again only points in the direction of a genetic influence without identifying a specific mechanism.

Psychological Origins of Smoking

Psychological models of smoking focus on aspects of social learning, personality process, or both.[4] Learning models may include simple conditioning constructs as well as the powerful effects of parental and peer modeling. Simple conditioning suggests that smoking behavior may increase because it is followed by a pleasurable high. This explanation must, of course, use other constructs to explain how smokers become entrapped given the initial aversive effects—nausea and headache—that occur after the first smoking experience. In addition, learning models suggest that environmental stimuli become classically conditioned cues that support smoking behavior.

Social learning theory suggests that, no matter what physiological and conditioning processes maintain the addiction, initiation of smoking is due to modeling and vicarious reinforcement, combined with cognitive expectancies and values. Perhaps the clearest expression of the expectancy element is provided by Ajzen and Fishbein's (1970, 1980) theory of reasoned action. These researchers argued that a person forms the intention to carry out an act (behavioral intention) based on attitudes toward the act and normative expectations of how others would react. Behavioral intent is a significant predictor of actual later smoking behavior (Norman & Tedeschi, 1989).

Attitudes toward smoking are formed in the crucible of life, where the person sees the consequences and desirability of smoking. Parents and peers make smoking appear mature, if not glamorous or macho. In addition, failure to conform to a salient peer group's standards (normative expectations) may have negative psychosocial consequences, including a sense of rejection and feelings of loneliness. In this view, the initial aversive effect is not at all problematic; the power of peer modeling is so strong that it easily overcomes any short-term aversive affect.

This analysis is consistent with the six major risk factors for beginning smoking (Camp, Klesges, & Relyea, 1993):

1. Presence of smoking friends or family members
2. Overestimation of peer smoking by a factor of 2
3. Perception of maturity, independence, or toughness as a value of smoking
4. Perception that personal support is lacking or lower expectation for academic success (Ellickson & Hays, 1992)
5. Being a risk taker or being rebellious
6. Enjoyment of emotional and/or pharmacological effects of smoking

To this list, Camp's group would also add the perception that smoking serves to control weight. We will discuss this issue in more detail later.

According to the health belief model (reviewed in Chapter 4), we must perceive a threat to personal health (vulnerability) before we are motivated to take action. Cigarette ads present models who are the picture of health and vitality: They are models of invulnerability. Peers

---

[4] I am using the term *social learning* here to subsume a wide range of conditioning, reinforcement, modeling, and expectancy variables that can influence both initiation and maintenance of smoking.

also normally endorse the invulnerability myth, encouraging one another to believe that ill health happens only to the old, and even then always to someone else. Still, Riche and Thelen (1989, May) presented evidence suggesting that smokers are aware of their increased health risks and rate their own chances of developing health problems more highly than nonsmokers'.

Mass media education campaigns now are trying to counteract the image presented by tobacco industry ads. These education campaigns show the ugly side of smoking, and they emphasize both the immediate and long-term negative effects that can occur. In addition,

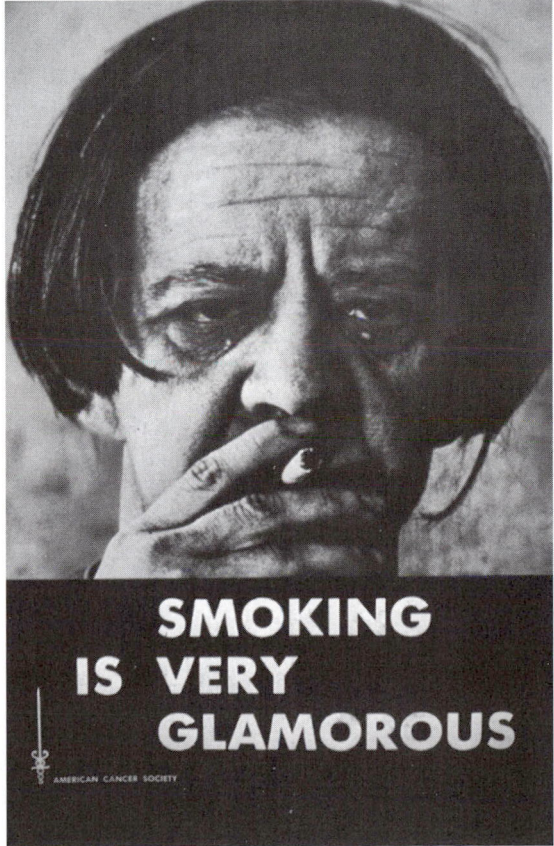

FIGURE 8.8 *Psychosocial factors in smoking can be used to help deter youths from beginning smoking, as by getting them to focus on negative social consequences of smoking.*

antismoking campaigns may try to build both self-efficacy and self-esteem by suggesting that people who resist the pressure to smoke or quit smoking are capable and determined people, part of a growing peer group that devalues smoking.

To this point, only a small amount of research has been done relating personality traits to smoking. Such research usually focuses on how smoking serves to reduce the impact of negative emotions, such as anxiety and distress, that result from intrapsychic conflict and interpersonal or environmental stressors. In general, the smoker is described as extraverted, somewhat neurotic, and tense. There is a sex difference, however, in that higher anxiety is found in female smokers than in male smokers. These findings relate to the factors causing people to begin smoking, though, not those that keep people smoking (Spielberger & Jacobs, 1982). Heavy smokers show more psychological disturbance than light smokers, and they show less tolerance for stress when not allowed to smoke than when allowed to smoke. In addition, people with psychosocial assets—feelings of self-efficacy, internal control, and good social networks—are able both to resist pressure to begin smoking (Stacy, Sussman, Dent, Burton, & Flay, 1992) and to quit smoking more readily than those lacking such assets.

Social Origins of Smoking: *Alive with Pleasure?*

Many social, political, and economic forces interact in the marketplace. Nowhere is the complexity of this equation more evident than when government and the tobacco industry confront each other on issues of public versus business interest. On the one hand, the government still works to prop up the industry, while trying all it can to persuade people not to smoke. Among the most cynical of government actions was to supply millions of dollars to developing countries to open new tobacco markets for U.S. producers, knowing all the while that it was promoting a habit that could have few positive and mostly negative outcomes.

On the other hand, the tobacco industry ignores most data on health while they try to persuade people to take up smoking, reassuring them all the while that they have come a long way or that they can feel alive with pleasure. In a move that some regard as callous, the industry has also specifically targeted women, youth, minority groups, and blue-collar workers (Davis, 1987).

The government's efforts to curtail smoking include increased taxes, stepped-up enforcement of minimum age limits for access to tobacco products, antismoking ad campaigns, legislated controls on broadcast advertising, and a requirement that tobacco products carry the now famous warning that smoking may be hazardous to health. More recently, the federal government has threatened to have nicotine declared a drug and thus ban public over-the-counter sales (FDA chief urges curbs; 1995, March 16). The federal government has also threatened to require the tobacco industry to fund antismoking ads aimed at teenage smokers, primarily based on the notion that the tobacco industry is targeting vulnerable groups to increase profit margins. Finally, the Clinton Administration proposed a ban on sale of tobacco products through vending machines and a ban on distribution of free samples ("Tobacco," 1995, August 17). Such efforts face opposition from the tobacco industry and consumer groups that want freedom of choice no matter what the consequences. Some efforts to regulate drug use may be counterproductive (MacCoun, 1993), but some studies suggest that social policy interventions can be useful.

In a study that focused on enforcement, Jason's group found that using a compliance check procedure on local merchants reduced sales to minors from 70% to less than 5% (Jason et al., 1991). In California, an additional 25¢ tax was imposed on each pack of cigarettes beginning in 1989. Of the money from this tax, 20% was used to fund a health campaign that began in 1990. Results suggest that cigarette consumption has dropped by 14% overall since the beginning of this program. It is estimated that a tax of two dollars per pack could save as many as two million lives over time. These efforts suggest that enforcement and economic sanctions can have a positive effect on smoking behavior.

Passive Smoking: The Matter of Social Etiquette

Among the most divisive issues in recent years is the conflict between nonsmokers' and smokers' rights. Bans on public smoking are on the increase and now cover most airline flights, restaurants, and public buildings. As recently as 1988, though, more than 40% of employed adults worked at sites where smoking was still permitted in designated or other areas (MMWR, 1992, May 22). More than 43% of nonsmokers reported some or moderate discomfort from secondhand smoke, and nearly 16% reported great discomfort.

Studies in both the home environment with children and in the work environment with adults confirm that passive smoking, or exposure to environmental tobacco smoke (ETS), has the potential for unhealthy outcomes. Even rats

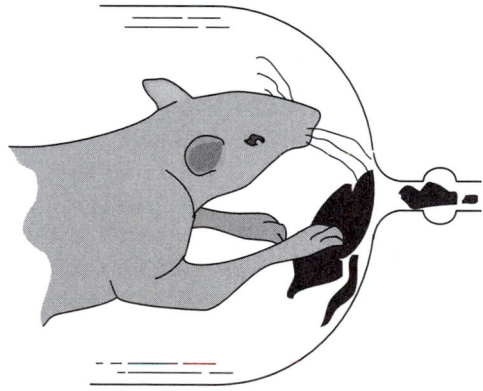

FIGURE 8.9   *In this study on the effects of passive smoke inhalation, Paul Silverman found that rats, hamsters, and mice all developed a simple method of preventing smoke from entering their environment by stuffing feces in the chamber inlet (based on Silverman, 1978).*

seem to find ETS aversive. As a study by Silverman (1978) showed, rats appear to engage in insightful problem-solving behavior to prevent smoke from entering their environment. Irritation of the eyes and nose are common. Breathing rate increases as does heart rate and blood pressure. The Surgeon General and the National Academy of Science both published reports in 1986 stating for the first time that passive smoke inhalation causes disease, most notably lung cancer (Fielding & Phenow, 1988). **Sidestream smoke,** the aerosol given off by the end of a smoldering cigarette, contains more carbon monoxide, toxins, and carcinogens than does **mainstream smoke,** the smoke inhaled by the smoker.

Among the strongest evidence suggesting a direct association between passive smoke inhalation and disease is the dose-response relationship (Celermajer et al., 1996). Even when the active smoker smokes only a few cigarettes or even just *one* cigarette per day, the passive smoker still shows increased risk compared to those who have no such exposure. The short-term urinary marker, cotinine, correlates positively with increased exposure to passive smoke. In addition, there is evidence for respiratory disorder, as measured by reduced expiratory volume and flow and upper respiratory problems, in both adult and child nonsmokers living with smokers, and arterial damage in healthy young adults.

Combining the results of several studies, the best estimate of the relative risk for lung cancer is 1.34. The estimates are even higher, between 1.7 and 1.8, for children with asthmatic conditions (Chilmonczyk et al., 1993). Once again, there is a clear dose-response relationship, as shown in Figure 8.10.

For those concerned about involuntary exposure, it appears that the social custom of common courtesy—asking before smoking—is not an effective control. In an analysis of data from 22,000 adults, 47% of the smokers lit up without asking if others minded. Further, only 4% of nonsmokers reported being able to ask a smoker not to smoke (Davis, Boyd, & Schoenborn, 1990).

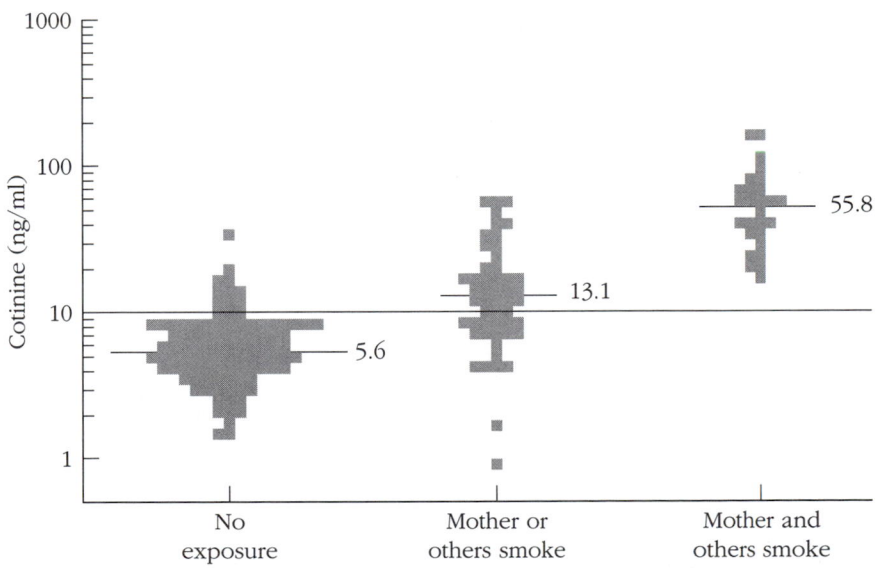

FIGURE 8.10   *This graph shows clearly the dose-response relationship between passive inhalation and presence of urinary cotinine in children: The more people that smoked in the child's environment, the higher the level of cotinine (from Chilmonczyk, 1993).*

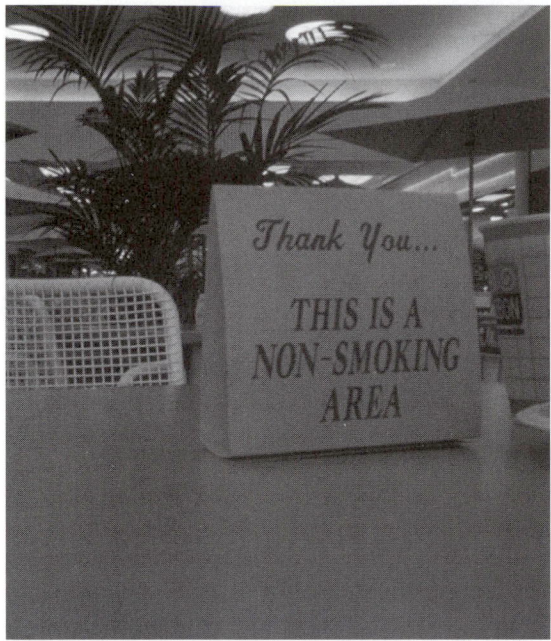

FIGURE 8.11   Signs like this one are increasingly encountered by smokers as the public and politicians become more aware of the hazards of environmental smoke.

Quitting Smoking: The Promise of Perseverance

Mark Twain said: "To cease smoking is the easiest thing I ever did; I ought to know because I've done it a thousand times." Twain was obviously poking fun at his personal weakness. But his was a shortcoming undoubtedly shared by many others. Many contemporary issues in smoking cessation research were reviewed in a special section of the October 1993 *Journal of Consulting and Clinical Psychology.*

Most recent evidence suggests that more people are trying to quit smoking with the encouragement and support of friends and family. Health data also provide clear and compelling evidence that those who quit, whether young or old, will benefit in reduced illness and coronary risk (Hermanson, Omenn, Kronmai, & Gersh, 1988). About 80% of smokers say they would like to quit, but no more than about 14% are able to quit in any given year (Biener & Abrams, 1991). The good news is that nearly 50% of all the people who ever smoked have quit over the past 25 years. Most important, the smoker's increased risk of heart disease decreases rapidly within 2 years of quitting, and by 10 to 15 years after quitting, the smoker's risk is no higher than someone who never smoked (LaCroix et al., 1991). Of those who do quit, though, about 95% quit on their own without the benefit of a professionally directed program. Indeed, an analysis by Cohen's group (Cohen et al., 1989) showed that it made no difference whether people tried to quit on their own or went into a formal program. This conclusion has been challenged recently, as we shall see later.

The good news must be tempered by some bad: Many people quit for a while but quickly fall back into their old habits. Intervention in smoking, or in any drug addiction for that matter, has proved one of the thorniest clinical problems of the past quarter century.

A classic early review by Leventhal and Cleary (1980) led to three ideas about quitting smoking. The first is that many programs may show significant early drops in smoking rate, but that all the methods have failed to produce lasting change. The second idea is that no single therapy has proved more successful than any other therapy over the long run. The third notion is that most cessation programs show a high dropout rate. Over the intervening years, it has also become somewhat of a truism that the single most important predictor of success in quitting smoking is persistence: continuing to try to quit. According to this view, the program may be nothing more than a vehicle used by some people to accomplish what they want to do.

Barriers to Quitting: Craving, Pleasure, and Anxiety

Anyone who wants to quit smoking faces significant obstacles. In one study of older smokers, the most common barriers were concerns about craving cigarettes, loss of subjective pleasure in smoking, and being tense or irritable after trying to quit (Orleans et al., 1991). These concerns, though, were mediated by the personality variable of self-efficacy. Those low in self-efficacy were most concerned about craving, pleasure, and irritability, whereas those high in self-efficacy were more likely to contemplate quitting. In addition, the latter group had more concerns for health and had more carefully calculated the health benefits of quitting.

Smoking Cessation and Weight Gain

An oft-cited motivation for continued smoking is to avoid the weight gain thought to occur with cessation. Even though a substantial percentage of quitters (13%–72%) remain the same weight or even lose weight (Bosse, Garvey, & Costa, 1980), the notion that weight gain follows quitting is now widely accepted. The official voice of Division 38, *Health Psychology,* even devoted an entire issue to the topic of smoking and weight. In this issue, Klesges and Shumaker (1992) summarized information from prior epidemiological studies showing that body weight and smoking are positively connected. First, smokers weigh about 7 pounds less than their age-mates who do not smoke. Second, when people start smoking, they tend to lose weight. Third, when people quit smoking they tend to gain weight. Women gain on average 8.4 pounds, and men gain about 6.2 pounds. Animal research provides consistent findings (Grunberg, Bowen, & Morse, 1984).

Two major hypotheses have been advanced to account for the weight gain. One suggests that smoking alters metabolic processes so that food absorption is less efficient. Equally possible, though, is that smoking alters the rate at which calories are burned. The second hypothesis suggests that food becomes more attractive and flavorful after quitting, which leads to increased food intake. But the ex-smoker does not increase all food consumption in equal degrees. Quitters increase sugar intake more than most

other foods, a fact that may explain part of the weight gain.

To explore these notions more thoroughly, more precise measures were needed. Contemporary research now considers three biological processes in the "quit smoking, gain weight" equation: energy intake, energy expenditure, and energy balance. At first, operational definitions of energy intake amounted to little more than calorie counting, but now, using **macronutrient analysis,** energy intake measures consider the type of calorie as well. This approach recognizes that fats, proteins, and carbohydrates have different effects in the body that cannot be judged on the basis of their calorie content alone (Grunberg et al., 1992). Energy expenditure refers to the calories burned, which changes with type, rate, and intensity of physical activity. Generally, smokers lead a more sedentary life, exercise less often and less strenuously, and abandon new exercise programs more rapidly than nonsmokers do (Morgan & Goldston, 1987). Energy balance refers to the relationship between intake and expenditure.

Using the macronutrient approach, Judith Rodin (1987) followed middle-aged smokers before and after smoking cessation programs. A cotinine test was used to validate abstinence. Rodin observed that smokers who gained weight did so because of sizable increases in calories from sugar, but those who stayed the same or lost weight actually reduced the amount of dietary sugar. Maintaining the same caloric intake as before quitting, though, usually led to weight gain whether sugar was increased or not. Further, those who lost weight or stayed the same engaged in more activity than those who gained weight.

These results suggest that whether or not weight gain follows quitting depends on both diet and exercise. From a prescriptive viewpoint, smokers who want to quit but are afraid of weight gain should first reduce caloric intake moderately but look very critically at sugar content. Second, they should begin a regular exercise program, an action that may itself further help to curb smoking (Taylor, Houston-Miller, Haskell, & Debusk, 1988).

Stages on the Way to Quitting: Intention, Action, and Continuation

Numerous investigators have proposed that recovery from an addiction involves several stages linking motivational and emotional tensions with cognitive-decisional processes. Perhaps the best known of these models is the one proposed by Prochaska and DiClemente (1983; Prochaska, DiClemente, & Norcross, 1992).

In this model, the smoker moves through five stages: precontemplation, contemplation, preparation, action, and maintenance. In the precontemplation stage, the smoker does not actively think about quitting smoking. Precontemplators seem to be least convinced that any health risks are associated with smoking (Owen, Wakefield, Roberts, & Esterman, 1992). Smoking behavior goes on at its normal rate and serves as a type of baseline for later evaluation. During contemplation, the smoker seriously thinks about quitting sometime in the near future (about six months out) but has not made the commitment to do so. During the third stage, preparation, the person not only thinks about quitting, but wants to do so in the next month (intention) and has tried (behavior) some method for quitting in the last year. The action phase is the period up to about six months after the smoker quits. This stage includes overt attempts to modify behavior and environment to overcome smoking. Finally, the maintenance stage extends from six months until the behavior is no longer regarded as a problem. Prochaska's group (1992) also suggested that the type of intervention must be targeted to the smoker's specific cognitive stage in order to be effective.

The stage model has a variety of supporting evidence to its credit, including that it is related to self-efficacy and to the decision process itself (DiClemente et al., 1991). In addition, the stage model has demonstrated cross-cultural generality (Dijkstra, deVries, & Bakker, 1996), and generality across other high-risk behaviors, such as cocaine abuse, weight control, exercise adoption (Marcus, Rakowski, & Rossi, 1992), and HIV risk reduction, among others.

Clinical Interventions: Pharmacological, Behavioral and Cognitive

Clinical interventions for smoking run the gamut from biomedical techniques, including specially formulated nicotine gums and skin patches, to behavioral and cognitive therapies, to social support groups, to mass media TV campaigns (Gruder, et al., 1993). Most interventions are tertiary or secondary treatments at best. At the same time, there is great interest in preventive programs. Saul Shiffman (1993) argued that in spite of this wide range of therapies, few innovations and little progress have followed the period of intense innovation in the 1960s. We will review some of these clinical interventions to conclude this chapter.

Pharmacological interventions: nicotine gum and skin patches   Over the past two decades, several replacement therapy programs have been tried, including nicotine gum, nasal solutions, and the transdermal patch. Nicotine gum may be manufactured to look and feel like a chewing gum. It is formulated to contain an amount of nicotine that presumably will replace the nicotine obtained from smoking and thus reduce the urge to smoke. Nicotine polacrilex (Nicorette), for example, provides for a replacement therapy based on a biomedical model of dependence. After using gum concentrations at two mg and four mg respectively, mean plasma concentrations of nicotine are about 33% and 67% of what would be found after smoking (Tønnesen et al., 1988).

The results of studies on nicotine gum have been mixed at best. The study carried out by Tønnesen's group was one of the better controlled projects, though still flawed. It used a double-blind placebo-control dose-response design to look at the link between degree of dependence, the concentration of nicotine in the gum, and success in quitting. After excluding volunteers with medical or psychiatric disabilities, subjects were classified into high, moderate, and low dependence groups. The high dependent group (Hi-Dep) was subdivided into two groups, one to receive two-mg gum throughout the treatment period, the other to receive four-mg gum for the first six weeks followed by two-mg gum for the balance of the treatment. The moderate and low dependent groups (Ml-Dep) received two-mg gum throughout, or a placebo gum with capsaicin to simulate the taste of nicotine. The placebo was not used with high dependent subjects.

The results, displayed in Figure 8.12, revealed that smoking reduction rates at six weeks ranged between 41.5% for the Ml-Dep placebo group, to 81.5% in the Hi-Dep four-mg group. The Hi-Dep two-mg group had a reduction of 54.5%, and the Ml-Dep two-mg group had a reduction rate of 73.3%. The 41.5% abstinence rate in the placebo group points once again to the powerful effect of expectancy. At two years' follow-up, though, the comparable rates were 9.4% for Ml-Dep placebo, 33.3% for Hi-Dep four-mg, 6.1% for Hi-Dep two-mg, and 28.3% for the Ml-Dep two-mg group. It seems clear from this outcome that dose interacts with dependence to determine the effectiveness of gum intervention, both early and late in the program.

There are numerous problems with nicotine gums, though. A recent meta-analysis suggested that the success of nicotine gum treatment depends on the intensity of therapy (Cepeda-Benito, 1993). Nicotine gum serves well as an adjunct with extended programs but does not seem to help with brief programs, as judged by maintenance at about 12 months. Further, nicotine gum has been judged safe in clinical trials, but it still may produce unpleasant side effects such as palpitations, headaches, mouth blisters or sores, stomach upset, and hiccups.

The nicotine patch is a high-tech solution that appears to avoid some of the aversive properties of nicotine gum. Side effects, though relatively rare, most often include headache, nausea, and vertigo. The patch is worn during the day and releases nicotine through the skin into the bloodstream. Although it produces significantly higher rates of abstinence than placebo patches, abstinence was only 17% after 12 months (Tønnesen, Nørregaard, Simonsen, & Säwe, 1991). John Hughes (1993) calculated the ratios of abstinence, comparing nicotine gum and the patch over several studies. He found the patch produced a likelihood of abstinence more than two times higher than nicotine gum.

Behavior therapies: incentives and stimulus control Among the many behavioral methods used to change smoking behavior are contingent reinforcement, self-monitoring, stimulus control, contracting, and aversive techniques. Contingent reinforcement provides

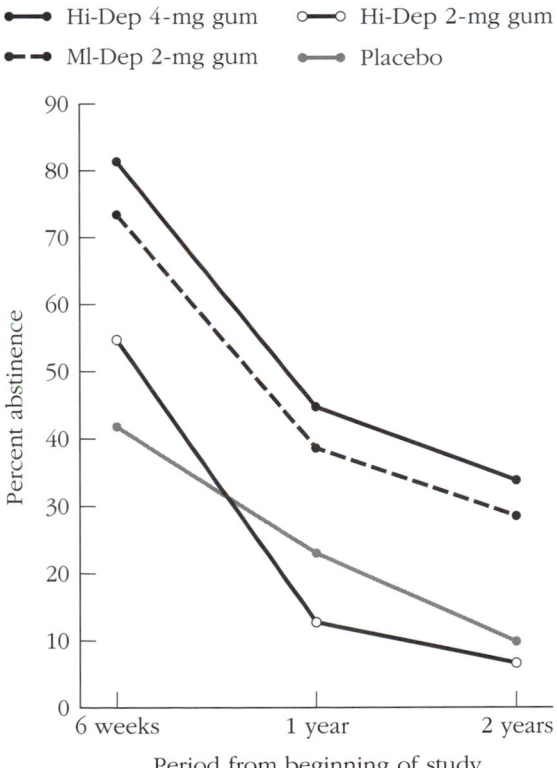

FIGURE 8.12   *In the Tønnesen study, nicotine gum was effective in increasing abstinence, but the effect was tied to the subject's degree of dependence (from Tønnesen et al., 1988).*

monetary or other incentives to quit and may increase rewards for continued abstinence. At Johns Hopkins University, Maxine Stitzer's group used a monetary incentive of $40 to participate and up to $200 for complete compliance (Stitzer, Rand, Bigelow, & Mead, 1986). The investigators reported that 68% initiated quitting, but after three weeks, only 18% were still abstinent, 36% had resumed some smoking, and the remainder had resumed heavy smoking. Self-monitoring requires the smoker to keep track of cigarettes smoked on a continuous basis and then plot the frequency of smoking on a daily basis. This method produces a decline in smoking without further interventions, but it is not generally effective in stopping smoking altogether.

Stimulus control tries to locate and control or eliminate environmental stimuli that may sustain smoking. A timer may be set to go off at irregular intervals, signaling the person that smoking is allowed. Since the timing is random, it should dissociate smoking from regular environmental cues (Shapiro, Tursky, Schwartz, & Shnidman, 1971). Clients may be told to confine their smoking to a certain place. Such methods often reported success rates of up to 75% at program completion, but follow-up usually showed sustained change closer to the 30% to 40% level.

A recent study conducted at the University of Wisconsin under the direction of Diane Zelman found that treatment success depends on smokers' traits (Zelman, Brandon, Jorenby, & Baker, 1992). Zelman's group compared rapid smoking (RS)[5] to nicotine gum (NG) therapy combined with either skills training (ST) or support counseling (SC). They also measured negative affect, craving, and withdrawal. Overall, the skills training program led to higher abstinence at the end of training than did support counseling (98% versus 88%), whereas the nicotine gum and rapid smoking therapies were virtually identical. These results had to be qualified, though, when survival analysis at one year showed no significant differences between the treatment combinations. The one-year survival showed statistically equivalent abstinence rates of 28% (RS + ST), 36% (RS + SC), 40% (NG + ST), and 39% (NG + SC).

When subjects were divided on negative affect, however, a very different picture emerged. Subjects high in negative affect fared better with support counseling, but subjects low in negative affect fared better with skills training. In the low negative-affect group, cessation was 25% to 35% higher even at 3 months' and 12 months' follow-up. High craving produced a less satisfactory response, but here, the nicotine gum therapy was clearly superior to rapid smoking. These results suggest that the type of therapy, whether biomedical, psychosocial, or combined, must be adjusted to the unique traits of the person trying to quit.

Workplace Smoking Bans: The Pitfalls of Legislated Change

Yet another approach to changing smoking habits is to legislate change in the workplace. Many businesses, especially those whose service involves continuous contact with the public, have implemented no-smoking policies. Some policies are established with the employees' advice and consent, either informally or through union negotiations. Other smoking bans have been imposed more or less unilaterally by management, although some have done so only after complaints and pressure from nonsmokers. Overall changes in lifestyle combined with support from the work environment and co-workers appears to predict who the successful quitters and people prone to relapse will be (Lueger & McDonald, 1992).

A study recently completed in Australia provides some insights into what one might expect from such programs (Borland, Owen, Hill, & Schofield, 1991). The investigators collected several different types of information. They tried

---

[5] Rapid smoking requires that the person smoke multiple cigarettes in quick succession.

to ascertain how well workers understood the ban and what beliefs and opinions workers held about smoking in general and the ban in particular. The researchers also asked workers to indicate whether they intended to quit smoking and how soon. Finally, the investigators included a self-efficacy scale and obtained behavioral measures of smoking (duration in years and daily habits, among others). Success in quitting smoking was most strongly predicted by low habit strength, a desire to quit, few previous attempts to quit, educational level, and the existence of social supports to help quit. This study rejected a common article of faith: that the only variable to consistently predict quitting is the attempt to quit. Instead, this study found that the more prior attempts to quit, the more likely the smoker would suffer a relapse.

Public Education and Policy: Smoking Prevention

Given the inconsistent results obtained with tertiary treatment methods, it is not surprising that attention has shifted in part to the development of preventive programs. This trend is encouraged by data on the age of onset for smoking: If people have not started to smoke by the time they are 20 or 21, they are not likely to smoke ever. The school system then becomes a logical setting to implement prevention programs. Several school-based programs designed to prevent smoking have been reported in the literature.

Gregory Botvin and his colleagues (1980) worked with a junior high group in grades 8 to 10. Their work was based on a social-psychological model attacking three main factors thought to influence teenagers to begin smoking. First, they tried to increase students' ability to cope with direct pressures to begin smoking. Second, they tried to reduce students' susceptibility to indirect influences such as advertising campaigns. Third, they tried to improve students' ability to deal with anxiety in

general based on the assumption that smoking is often used to relieve anxiety.

The intervention program, conducted by a specialist, lasted ten weeks and contained two main components. An informational component discussed smoking myths and realities and how to respond to false or misleading advertising. The skills component used modeling and behavioral rehearsal to deal with self-image, social skills, communication, and assertiveness. The results suggested that such a program can be very effective in reducing the number of new smokers. At the same time, to be effective the program needs to begin at or perhaps even before grade 8. The older the students, the less effective the program was in preventing them from beginning to smoke.

Perhaps the best known model is the one developed by Richard Evans. Evans's group (Evans, Smith, & Raines, 1984) developed informational films for junior high students that incorporated three important elements. First, the film narrators are age-mates. Second, the films deal with realistic psychosocial pressures that occur in everyday life. In so doing, the films aim to help adolescents resist such pressure. Third, the films point out that the student can make decisions to avoid situations and groups that might lead to undue pressure to smoke. In general, students who viewed these films were less likely to take up smoking than those who did not see the films.

Another research group compared various short- and long-term strategies to prevent cigarette smoking (Murray, Luepker, Johnson, & Mittelmark, 1984; Murray, Davis-Hearn, Goldman, Pirie, & Luepker, 1988). The results suggest that a short-term program conducted by peer models is the most effective means of preventing nonsmokers from beginning to smoke. Such a program may not be as effective, though, when the adolescent has already begun to experiment. This outcome is not unexpected based on the selection notion that once the adolescent has begun to experiment, he or she will select friends with compatible values and interests (Agnew & White, 1992).

Summary

In this chapter, we have considered one high-risk behavior, drug addiction, that unfortunately affords many gateways to a lifelong habit. The health risks are substantial even at low doses for many drugs of abuse. The decline in drug abuse, especially among smokers, is encouraging, but there is much yet to do to understand and treat drug abusers—and preferably prevent people from being caught in the cycle of addiction in the first place.

1. Definitions of addiction and dependency are still not universally accepted because both research results and direct observations of behavior do not match clinical criteria.

2. Drug abuse may be defined as a maladaptive pattern of substance use that continues for more than one month or recurs periodically over a longer period of time.

3. Drug dependence occurs when there is evidence of physiological dependence that goes on for more than one month. The three most common signs of dependence are intense craving, tolerance, and withdrawal symptoms.

4. Craving is an intense desire for the drug. Drug tolerance occurs when the user has to take a larger dose to achieve the same effect as before. If the person quits using a drug that has been used for a long time, she or he may experience a host of unpleasant physical and emotional effects, which are withdrawal symptoms.

5. Three models have been used to account for drug abuse, the medical, psychological, and social models. The medical model proposes that drug abuse should be regarded as a disease because of altered physical functioning. The psychological model invokes motivational, learning, and personality notions to explain drug abuse. The social model looks at environmental stressors, family, and peer affiliation process to explain drug abuse.

6. The dopamine depletion theory suggests that many drugs act to deplete dopamine in the nervous system. Studies of twins suggest that at least some of the variance in addiction is explained by genetic factors.

7. A rewarding brain center has been proposed as the physical site controlling drug abuse. This center may interact with dopamine to account for the powerful rewarding effects of many drugs.

8. The opponent process theory proposes that using drugs leads first to a strong emotional reaction, affective pleasure, and then to a strong after-reaction, affective withdrawal. The first reaction adapts quickly, leading to tolerance, whereas the second grows stronger with continued use.

9. Smoking now contributes to more than 400,000 deaths each year from cardiorespiratory illnesses, cancer, and other smoking-related disorders.

10. Nicotine is a stimulant that affects both the cardiovascular and central nervous system and loads the system with toxic by-products, such as carbon monoxide.

11. Cotinine is the favored marker for nicotine consumption, since it is the most sensitive and specific measure discovered to date.

12. Nicotine produces all the classic signs of dependence, including craving and withdrawal symptoms.

13. Social learning theory suggests that a constellation of conditioning and reinforcing processes, including peer modeling and vicarious reinforcement, may explain both initiation and maintenance of smoking behaviors.

14. Personality research indicates that smoking may be initiated and maintained because of its ability to reduce anxiety.

15. Passive smoking—inhaling sidestream smoke produced by other smokers—shows a clear dose-response relationship to increased risk of illness and lung cancer.

16. About 50% of all smokers have quit, but no more than 14% are able to quit in any one year, usually because there are substantial barriers to quitting.

17. One barrier is the concern for weight gain, but as many people lose weight as gain it after quitting smoking. To quit and not gain weight, the quitter must monitor the amount of sugar in the calories consumed and maintain an exercise program.

18. No single therapy program has emerged as the clear choice to help people quit. Most programs show an early success rate between 60% and 90% that rapidly declines below the 30% to 40% level.

19. Workplace intervention programs produce roughly the same rate of quitting that small-group or individual therapy produces.

20. Prevention may be the most viable long-term solution, getting into the schools prior to the 8th grade with information presented by peers about the short-term negative effects of smoking and the positive results of not smoking.

Key Words

affective pleasure
affective tolerance
affective withdrawal
concordance index
cotinine
craving
differential association
disease model
drug withdrawal
general strain theory
heritability index
macronutrient analysis
mainstream smoke
medical model
opponent process
  theory
opponent process
  (b process)

primary process
  (a process)
psychological model
sidestream smoke
smoking cessation
  stages:
  precontemplation
  contemplation
  preparation
  action
  maintenance
social control theory
social model
substance abuse
substance dependence
substance withdrawal
tolerance

Study Questions

1. What are the major strengths and weaknesses of the three main models of drug abuse: the medical, psychological, and social?

2. How is the information on brain reward centers and dopamine depletion consistent with a psychological explanation such as offered by Tiffany in his automatized action schema theory of drug abuse?

3. What are the major mortality and morbidity risks that accompany smoking?

4. What evidence is available to suggest that smoking is, in fact, physically addictive?

5. How are personality variables believed to be related to the risk for smoking?

6. What evidence suggests that passive smoking is dangerous?

7. If you wanted to quit smoking, but were afraid of weight gain, what two things should you do to avoid gaining weight?

8. What are the general findings from studies of smoking cessation?

Class Projects

1. Arrange a field trip to a nearby drug treatment facility if one is accessible.

2. Invite local experts, especially those actively involved in drug rehabilitation counseling, to speak to the class.

3. If possible, arrange for a psychiatrist, a psychologist, and a social worker to present the pros and cons of the different models of drug abuse.

Suggested Readings

Carmelli, D., Swan, G. E., Robinette, D., & Fabsitz, R. (1992). Genetic influence on smoking: A study of male twins. *The New England Journal of Medicine, 327,* 829–833.

Geist, C. R., & Herrman, S. M. (1990). A comparison of the psychological characteristics of smokers, ex-smokers, and nonsmokers. *Journal of Clinical Psychology, 46,* 102–105.

Klesges, R. C., & Shumaker, S. A. (1992). Proceedings of the National Working Conference on Smoking and Body Weight [Suppl.]. *Health Psychology, 11.*

Henningfield, J. E., & Woodson, P. P. (1989). Dose-related actions of nicotine on behavior and physiology: Review and implications for replacement therapy for nicotine dependence. *Journal of Substance Abuse, 1,* 301–317.

NIDA Research Monograph 84. (1988). *Learning Factors in Substance Abuse* (pp. 44–61). U. S. Department of Health and Human Services.

Prochaska, J. O., & DiClemente, C. C. (1983). Stages and processes of self-change of smoking: Toward an integrative model of change. *Journal of Consulting and Clinical Psychology, 51,* 390–395.

Tiffany, S. T. (1990). A cognitive model of drug urges and drug-use behavior: Role of automatic and nonautomatic processes. *Psychological Review, 97,* 147–168.

Wise, Roy A., & Bozarth, M. A. (1987). A psychomotor stimulant theory of addiction. *Psychological Review, 94,* 469–492.

WEBSITES   *Smoking and Other Addictions*

ADDRESS	DESCRIPTION
http://www.autonomy.com/smoke.htm	☆The Master Anti-Smoking Page—forums, links, tips, and software to help quit smoking
http://www.lungusa.org	American Lung Association
http://www.quitnet.org	☆Quitnet—a site devoted to helping smokers quit
http://www.ccsa.ca	Canadian Centre on Substance Abuse
http://www.cancer.org	SMOKEOUT—from the American Cancer Society
http://charlotte.med.nyu.edu/woodr/div28.html	APA Division 28—Psychopharmacology and Substance Abuse

Substance Abuse II: Use and Misuse of Alcohol

Few writers have captured the mind's imagination or stirred the heart's passions like the Welsh poet Dylan Thomas. In spite of fame, Thomas lived most of his life in poverty, often desperate to keep bill collectors from the door. He once said that he had "achieved poverty with distinction, but never poverty with dignity" (FitzGibbon, 1987, p. 240). Yet Thomas never lost hope that someday his poetry would earn the respect it deserved, and that he would earn then a comfortable, if not wealthy, life for his family.

Thomas's frustration with the injustice of life often colored his work. In these lines from "There's plenty in the world," there is a somber, even darkly prophetic tone:

> *But we, shut in the houses of the brain,*
> *Brood on each hothouse plant*
> *Spewing its sapless leaves around,*
> *And watch the hand of time unceasingly*
> *Ticking the world away*

Thomas brooded over, talked incessantly about, the frailty of his existence. He often reckoned that his life's candle would burn out long before he reached 40.

Thomas's most disabling physical liability was his weak lungs, which hemorrhaged and often kept him bedridden as a child. He had a tendency to bronchitis and asthma, but he added insult to injury by chain-smoking. Apparently, he picked up his smoking habit at a tender age since, by his own account, he had been chain-smoking for five years when he was still only 18 or 19. As a grown man, Thomas's "wheezings and hawkings and roarings [were] on a truly

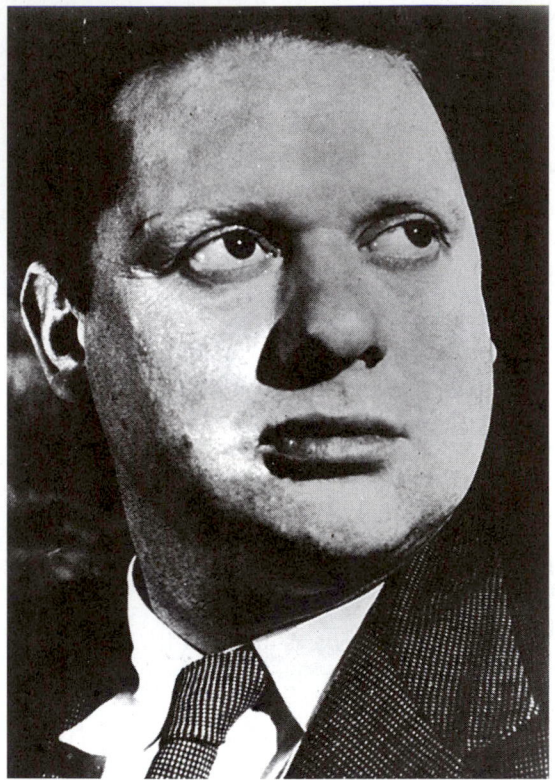

FIGURE 9.1   Dylan Thomas.

Wagnerian scale that frequently went on till he vomited" (FitzGibbon, 1987, p. 23).

The World's Drunkest Man: Thomas's Boast of Demon Alcohol

Thomas came from a family with a history of alcoholism, a fact they apparently tried to conceal. He once called his father a human beer barrel, and his father confessed a terrible addiction to alcohol. When his father died, Thomas penned in memorial the oft-quoted poem containing the line "Rage, rage against the dying of the light."

In Thomas's world, alcoholism was unknown; drinking was simply a lifestyle. In his cavalier fashion, Thomas defined an alcoholic as someone you don't like who can still drink as much as you.

Thomas's drinking bouts became as legendary as his notorious affairs. His social life revolved around the pub, often beginning before noon. He moved from pub to pub, drinking copious quantities of ale. Along the way, he collected a coterie of friends, maybe artists looking for a jolt from artistic lethargy, maybe thrill seekers hoping to impress friends with the story of an afternoon spent downing ale with the legendary Dylan Thomas. Evenings often ended in a blur; only the morning light would unveil a night spent with a woman whose intimacy meant everything at the time but whose name he could not then recall.

In a letter to a friend, Thomas bragged that he "managed to become drunk at least four nights a week" (FitzGibbon, 1987, p. 92). Small wonder, then, that he sometimes complained about being on the verge of delirium tremens. He feared that he had cirrhosis of the liver and tuberculosis. In 1946, just seven years before death, Thomas collapsed with alcoholic gastritis and nervous hypertension. There are signs he recognized that "demon alcohol" (Thomas's words) had been too long his close friend. Still, he would boast that he was the drunkest man in the world.

The end for Thomas came shortly after he returned to New York in October 1953. He was there for another series of speaking engagements and a theatrical production that excited him greatly. Already on the verge of another physical collapse, he received injections of the new drug, ACTH. His doctor warned that combining ACTH and alcohol could be dangerous, but it was not the type of warning Thomas ever heeded. Each night, he took sleeping pills to combat another bout of insomnia. During the day, his friends gave him pep pills to boost his energy for the frenzied cycle of rehearsals and meetings.

Thomas went out in the middle of the night on November 4th, to find a drink. When he returned 90 minutes later, he made a remark that may have been his last recorded for posterity: "I've had eighteen straight whiskies. I think that's the record" (FitzGibbon, 1987, p. 46). This was probably another of his exaggerations for effect. Friends concluded (after retracing his steps) that he had drunk only four or five. Still, another ACTH injection came in the morning, followed by the d.t.'s, and yet another afternoon injection—some believe of morphine. He lapsed into a coma, never to regain consciousness. The hand of time had ticked away Dylan Thomas's world, leaving the paradoxical legacies of alcoholic excess alongside his lyrical and memorable poetry.

Alcoholism: Definitions, Dependence, and Abuse

Although alcoholism did not exist as a diagnostic category in Thomas's time, the behaviors commonly associated with it were well recognized. Since then, clinicians typically have used the term in reference to loss of control over alcohol consumption with frequent episodes of prolonged heavy drinking ending in intoxication. **Episodic heavy drinking** occurs when a person takes five or more drinks in one session (MMWR, 1992, September 18). In this section, we will discuss the terminology used to describe alcohol abuse. We will consider some disputes about terminology and look at current diagnostic criteria.[1]

The label *alcoholism* has encountered several problems in recent years. For one thing, it has become burdened with negative value implications. Further, use of the label has not always been consistent with new scientific research. Finally, the label has lacked precision for clinical diagnosis. Tarter and his colleagues (1987) noted that the common multiple clinical criteria could produce 79,210 distinct groups of alcoholics. In addition, the criteria did not correlate strongly with objective measures of the amount of alcohol consumed, the consequences of con-

sumption, or self-reported drinking behavior.[2] These difficulties led to renewed efforts to reformulate the definition of alcoholism in more precise terms.

Recently, the National Council on Alcoholism and Drug Dependence joined forces with the American Society of Addiction Medicine to draft an up-to-date definition of **alcoholism** (Morse & Flavin, 1992):

> Alcoholism is a primary, chronic disease with genetic, psychosocial, and environmental factors influencing its development and manifestations. The disease is often progressive and fatal. It is characterized by impaired control over drinking, preoccupation with the drug alcohol, use of alcohol despite adverse consequences, and distortions in thinking, most notably denial. Each of these symptoms may be continuous or periodic. (p. 1013)

This definition includes several elements that require comment. First, the definition relies on the disease concept. In simplistic terms, the disease notion is that observable symptoms result from an underlying physical pathology.[3] Alcoholism probably does not fit the disease model in this simple sense. The authors address this issue when they stipulate that alcoholism is a primary, chronic disease: Alcoholism is not a symptom of an underlying disease state but the disease itself.

Second, the definition identifies probable etiological factors. These include biomedical and psychosocial factors. The definition then is highly compatible with the biopsychosocial model. Although the definition is an attempt to improve on older definitions, Morse and Flavin

---

[1] Several terms relevant to drug use, such as tolerance and dependence, were defined in Chapter 8.

[2] We should note that self-reported alcohol consumption has many validity problems. Fitzgerald and Mulford (1987) suggest a possible solution to this problem: Measure purchases instead of consumption. They provide evidence that purchases more closely match actual consumption. People may see consumption as more negative and thus reduce their estimates when reporting consumption.

[3] See Chapter 2 for a more detailed discussion of the disease concept.

(1992) cautioned that it is not a diagnostic standard by itself.

Finally, the definition notes that symptoms of alcoholism may occur continually or periodically. At one extreme are chronic alcoholics who drink heavily each day and do so for years. The binge drinker illustrates the periodic case. The binger may be abstinent for days, weeks, or even months but then go on a drinking binge that lasts days, weeks, or longer.

Diagnostic Criteria: Dependence, Abuse, and Withdrawal

The current most widely accepted diagnostic system, DSM-IV, does not talk about alcoholism. It talks instead about alcohol dependence,[4] alcohol abuse, alcohol intoxication, and alcohol withdrawal (American Psychiatric Association, 1994).

The signs of **alcohol dependence** are the same as for any type of substance dependence:

1. Increased tolerance
2. Withdrawal symptoms
3. Loss of control over amount and duration of consumption
4. Recurrent unsuccessful efforts to regain control or quit
5. Substantial time spent seeking alcohol
6. Interference with social, work, and family obligations
7. Continued use in spite of adverse consequences

If alcohol dependence develops at all, it usually does so within the first five years of regular use. Alcohol tolerance, though, can occur in a matter of hours or days for some. Tolerance and dependence do not occur consistently together (Miller, Dackis, & Gold, 1987). In any case, it takes substantially longer to become addicted to alcohol compared to either cocaine or nicotine.

---

[4] Note, though, that the criteria for alcohol dependence are roughly comparable to those conventionally used for alcoholism.

Compared to cocaine, the slower path to alcohol dependence may be because alcohol has some unpleasant aspects including a bitter taste, unpleasant hangover effects, and feelings of lethargy or drowsiness the next day.

It is revealing to compare prevalence statistics among these three drugs. Nearly 90% of the population have had some experience with alcohol, 55% with tobacco, and 12% with cocaine. Still, only 8% of the population suffer from alcohol dependence and 5% from alcohol abuse. In comparison, nearly 20% of the population suffers nicotine dependence, but only about 0.2% of the population suffers from cocaine abuse (American Psychiatric Association, 1994). Both alcohol and nicotine are socially accepted drugs, but the difference in rates of abuse suggests that nicotine may be much more addictive than alcohol.

Alcohol abuse is chronic maladaptive drinking that does not meet the criteria for dependence. Two major dependence symptoms do not occur in abuse: tolerance and withdrawal. Abuse is distinguished then by four signs. First, social, work, and family obligations suffer. Second, the person uses alcohol in dangerous situations such as driving. Third, there are recurrent legal problems because of alcohol use. Finally, the person continues to use alcohol in spite of recurrent adverse social and psychological outcomes.

Alcohol intoxication is a temporary state following recent alcohol intake. Overt signs appear such as slurred speech, impaired coordination and reaction time, unsteady gait, and impaired attention and memory. The most important criterion, though, is the appearance of maladaptive behavior such as increased aggressiveness or improper sexual conduct. Steele and Josephs (1990) suggested that such behavior occurs because of an **alcohol-induced myopia.** They believe that intoxication lowers the drinker's ability to process information outside a narrow range (myopia). This effect also helps to lower inhibition of impulsive responses. Innocent comments or glances then become signals for hostile aggression or unwelcome advances. A recent meta-analysis adds some support for this view (Ito, Miller, & Pollock, 1996).

Finally, **alcohol withdrawal** occurs when the person stops using alcohol after a long period of heavy drinking. Typical withdrawal symptoms include sweating, elevated pulse rate, hand tremors, nausea, sleeplessness, agitation, anxiety, and perceptual distortions. Clinical diagnosis requires that two or more of these symptoms be present.

Legal Criteria of Intoxication: Blood Alcohol Concentration, Behavior, and Cognitions

Clinical criteria do not necessarily serve well in the legal arena. For legal purposes, most states use blood alcohol concentration (BAC) as a quantitative index of intoxication. BAC can be reliably tested in the field with a breathalyzer, like the one in Figure 9.2.

Blood alcohol concentration is the ratio of alcohol to a standard volume of blood. The more alcohol in the blood, the higher the concentration. The amount of alcohol is measured in milligrams, a weight measure. The reference amount of blood is a volume measure, 100 milliliters. A simple analogy illustrates how this measure works. Imagine that you have an 8-ounce cup a little less than half full of coffee. That volume is about 100 milliliters (technically about 3.3 fluid ounces). Then add a standard sugar cube which weighs about four grams. The more cubes, the higher the ratio of sugar to coffee and the sweeter the coffee. Then imagine breaking the four-gram sugar cube down into 4 parts, one gram each. Then, break one of the 4 parts down into 1000 parts. Each part is a milligram. If you put 50 parts in the small cup of coffee, it would be the same ratio as a BAC of 0.05%.

Thus, if a police officer says you have a BAC of 0.05%, it means you have 50 milligrams of alcohol in a 100 milliliter blood sample. At this level, people typically feel light-headed and relaxed, and their inhibitions may be lowered. With 0.10% BAC (100 milligrams alcohol per 100 milliliters blood), sensory functions are noticeably impaired, speech slurred, reaction time markedly slowed, and coordination is very poor. At 0.20%, alcohol seriously impairs or even incapacitates most people. Coma and death may occur above 0.40% to 0.50%.

Still, individual's differ widely in the absolute BAC that results in altered mental and behavioral functions. Some people may experience adverse effects with just one or two drinks (low BAC). Others may not show adverse effects until they drink four or five cocktails (a higher BAC).

Further, several variables influence how much and how rapidly the body absorbs alcohol. These variables include sex, weight, rate of drinking, metabolic rate, amount and recency of food consumption. An adult female of 120 pounds might exceed the 0.10% level after drinking four or more drinks (1.2 ounces of 80 proof liquor or 12 ounces of beer) in a two-hour period. An adult male of 180 pounds might not exceed the 0.10% level until after five to six drinks in two hours.

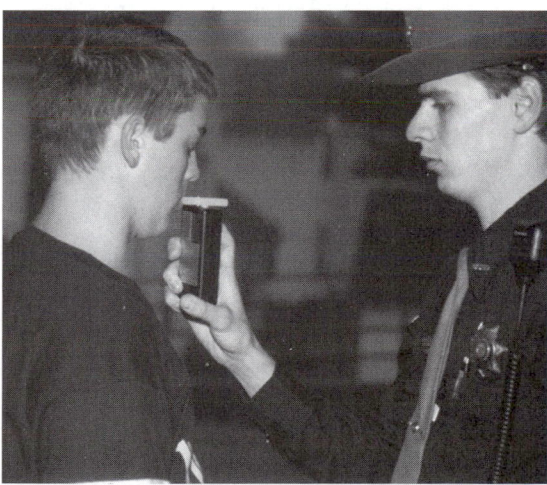

FIGURE 9.2   This portable breathalyzer is similar to the machines used in various settings, including field sobriety checkpoints, to obtain blood alcohol concentration readings.

TABLE 9.1   *Effects of different concentrations of alcohol in the bloodstream.*

BLOOD ALCOHOL CONCENTRATION	NEURO-BEHAVIORAL EFFECTS OF ALCOHOL
.05	Beginning effect on higher CNS functions; feeling of well-being; impaired judgment; lowered inhibitions
.10	Effects in CNS spread to lower centers; impaired psychomotor functions including reaction time and coordination; legal threshold of intoxication in many states
.15	Major increases in reaction time
.20	Marked depression in sensory and motor capability
.30	Stuporous but conscious; lacks general awareness of world around
.40	Almost complete cessation of CNS cognitive functions; coma
.50	Serious danger of death (although death may occur in rare cases at even lower levels)

Legal definitions of intoxication set some arbitrary threshold using BAC. Most states use a BAC around 0.10%. Now, there is pressure, based on health goals established under former Surgeon General Koop, to set an even lower limit, around 0.08%. The intent is to reduce it even further, to 0.04%, by the year 2000. This level is still higher than certain European countries where a BAC of 0.02% defines intoxication.

Effects of Alcohol: Physiology, Neurology, and Immunology

Many people continue to believe that alcohol is a stimulant, probably because they feel more sociable and carefree when drinking. Alcohol also may have positive reinforcing effects because it induces euphoria and lowers anxiety (Lewis, 1990). Yet alcohol is really a central nervous system depressant. The path from ingestion to CNS depression can be outlined as follows.

When alcohol enters the stomach, some of it passes directly into the bloodstream bypassing the normal digestion process. In so doing, alcohol changes permeability of the gastrointestinal tract. Unfortunately, this increases the amount of potentially infectious materials that can pass through (Watzl & Watson, 1992). The rate at which alcohol passes into the bloodstream depends on sex, age, metabolism, stomach contents, and type of alcohol. Beer, for example, contains some food content and must be partly digested. Therefore, it passes more slowly into the bloodstream.

After passing into the bloodstream, alcohol begins to work in the brain much like an anesthetic. It first depresses higher cognitive functions, such as judgment and reasoning, and shortly after, it begins to alter sensory-motor processes. Chronic alcoholism may lead to a condition referred to as amnestic disorder that includes long-term memory impairment (American Psychiatric Association, 1994).

Alcohol's Neurochemistry: Opioid Sites and Oxidation

Recent research has begun to uncover the neurological sites and processes involved in alcohol dependence. Blum and Trachtenberg (1988) suggested that alcohol acts on the opioid peptides to interfere with their synthesis and alter their brain concentrations. Alcohol—more accurately, alcohol's metabolic by-products—act as surrogates at opioid receptor sites in the brain. This process is shown in Figure 9.3. Possibly, then, the psychological feeling of well-being that occurs when drinking results from the substitution of alcohol at opioid sites,

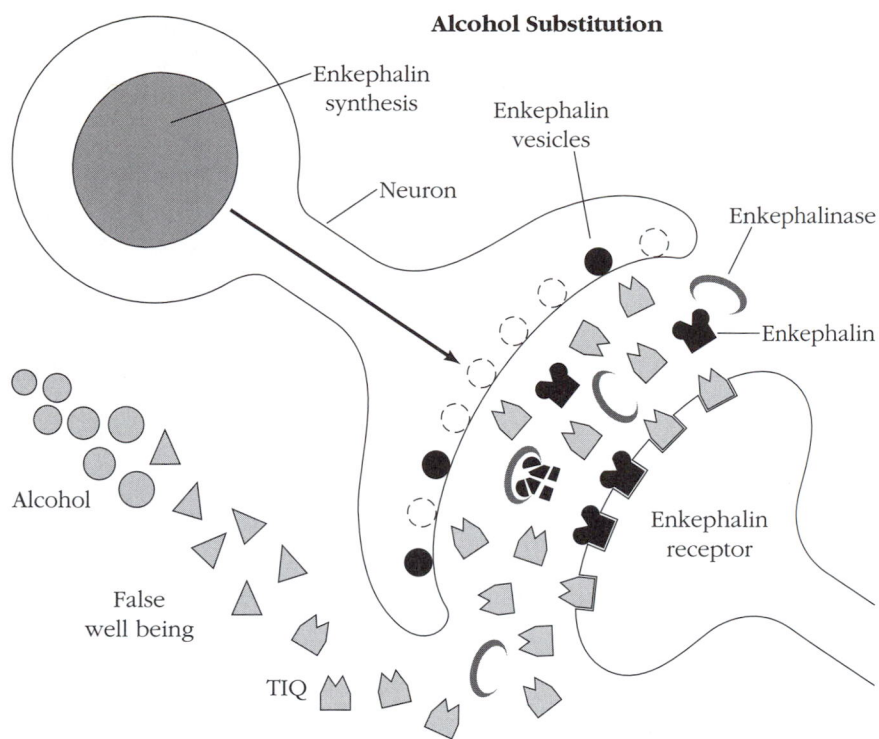

Alcohol Substitution

FIGURE 9.3   *This schematic diagram indicates how alcohol is converted to acetaldehyde (wedges) in the liver, then to tetrahydroisoquinolines (TIQs, dual pointed triangles). TIQs act as surrogates at the postsynaptic receptors, generating a false feeling of well-being (from Blum & Trachtenberg, 1988).*

but the exact mechanisms are not entirely clear. Other research reveals that alcohol may influence several neurotransmitters including GABA, serotonin and its precursor tryptophan, dopamine, noradrenaline, acetylcholine, and vasopressin, among others (Pihl, Young, Ervin, & Plotnick, 1987; Topel, 1985).

The effect of alcohol continues until it is fully oxidized. The oxidation process occurs mainly in the liver. Everything that goes into the blood from the digestive tract, pancreas, and spleen first goes through the liver before returning to the heart (Spence, 1989). On average, the system clears about 20 mg of alcohol per deciliter of blood each hour (Gershman & Steeper, 1991). A single drink may clear the system in 4 hours, but multiple drinks that produce intoxication may

not clear for 24 hours or more. Thus, alcohol puts a great strain on the liver.

One major effect of alcohol is that it changes food metabolism. In an alcoholic, ethanol may supply as much as 50% of dietary energy (Suter, Schutz, & Jequier, 1992), sometimes because of missed or partly eaten meals. The net effect is that alcohol changes the balance of nutrient intake, impairs absorption in the gastrointestinal tract, and then impairs utilization, storage, and excretion of nutrients. Over time, the alcoholic is vulnerable to malnutrition, vitamin deficiencies, and immunosuppression. The most common vitamin deficiencies occur with Vitamin A, C, and several B-group vitamins, including thiamine (B_1), folic acid, and niacin (Watzl & Watson, 1992).

Alcohol's Metabolism: Beer Bellies and Immunosuppression

There are two other important results from prolonged excessive alcohol consumption: alcohol alters fat storage and immune system function. A research group working in Luzanne, Switzerland may have discovered the basis for the legendary beer belly. Alcohol increases energy expenditure, but it also changes the way the body stores fat, especially when the alcohol comes from beer. More specifically, ethanol reduces lipid oxidation by 36% when added to the diet and 31% when substituted for food calories. Note that this change occurs only for lipids; alcohol does not change protein or carbohydrate oxidation (Suter et al., 1992).

The second effect, still under investigation, reveals that long-term alcohol consumption may contribute to immune system suppression. Infectious and contagious diseases are the most common cause of death in alcoholics (Watzl & Watson, 1992). Alcohol depresses production of leukocytes in the bone marrow. Animal studies show atrophy of the thymus and spleen, a result unconfirmed in humans. This atrophy may have a direct effect on T-cells, though results are inconsistent. One effect does seem clear: Alcohol interferes with the delivery of neutrophiles to sites of bacterial infections, resulting in increased frequency and severity of infections in drinkers. Watzl and Watson made a very important point, though: In well nourished alcoholics there is little or no evidence of immune suppression, but in malnourished alcoholics there is substantial evidence of immune system impairment. Nutrition appears to play the deciding role in whether immune suppression and vulnerability to infectious disease occurs or not.

Epidemiology of Alcoholism: Prevalence, Gender, and Culture

Approximately 70,000 to 100,000 Americans die each year from alcohol use. This statistic means that every year, about twice as many Americans die from alcohol as died in Vietnam in 16 years of war. Losses in wages and productivity are between $100 billion and $120 billion per year (Charness, Simon, & Greenberg, 1989; Reich, 1988; Rice, Kelman, & Miller, 1991). This amount includes costs for care plus losses due to morbidity and mortality. Hospitals treat in excess of 1.2 million people each year for alcoholism, 75% of whom are males and 69% of whom are white (Gunby, 1987).

In this section we will discuss several demographic traits related to alcohol consumption, including age, gender, and race. We will note the most typical and troublesome health risks, and we will consider emerging scientific explanations of the etiology of alcoholism. This discussion will take us again into the arena of genetics and neurotransmitters. Finally, we will consider several personal, familial, and social factors.

Prevalence Statistics: Gender, Age, and Race

According to information compiled by the American Psychiatric Association, about 35% of the population abstains from alcohol, and 55% drink fewer than three drinks a week. The most startling fact is that the remaining 10% of the population consumes fully 50% of all alcohol sold (American Psychiatric Association, 1987). Overall, the prevalence of clinically defined alcoholism is about 10% for men and 2% for women, with the highest rate occurring among people aged 18 to 44 (Myers et al., 1984). The rate declines rapidly after age 45. Alcoholism appears to be predominantly a male disorder.

Among high school students, about half the males and a third of the females reported using alcohol daily during the previous 30 days (Bachman et al., 1991). The rates were highest for white (48.1%), Mexican American (45.3%) and Native American (48.1%) males, and lowest for Asian American (19.4%) males and black (9.3%) and Asian American (10.7%) females. Figure 9.4 shows an encouraging drop in daily use of alcohol among adolescents over a 15-year period.

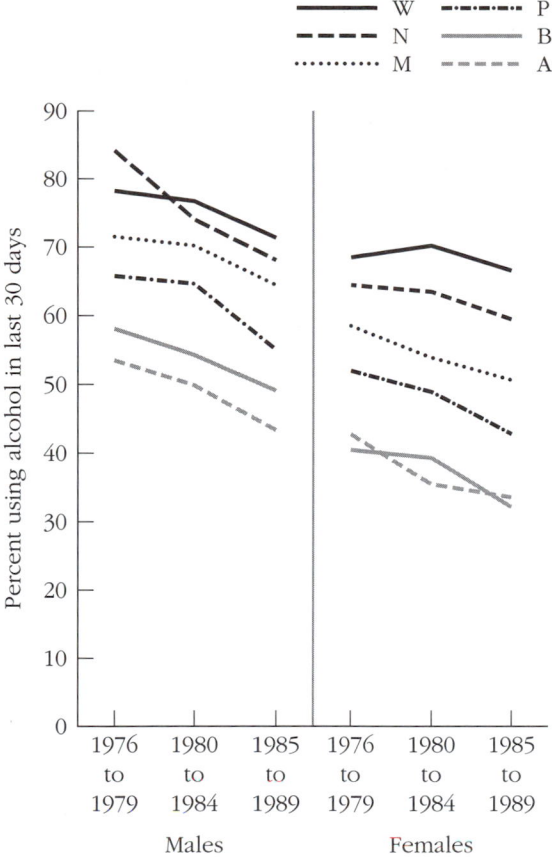

FIGURE 9.4   Decline in daily use of alcohol between 1976 and 1989; data are based on the Monitoring the Future study (adapted from Bachman et al., 1991).

Women and Alcohol: Prevalence, Risks, and Health

Even though women consume less alcohol than men and are less likely to abuse alcohol compared to men, women still may experience more alcohol-related health risks than men. There is evidence that women have a higher BAC after drinking the same amount of liquor as men even after controlling for body size.

Further, liver disease develops faster in women than it does in men, which may be linked to sex differences in gastric metabolism of alcohol (Frezza et al., 1990). Women gen-

erally have a lower gastric oxidation of alcohol compared to men, so more alcohol is left available in the body of a woman drinker, which may alter both biological and psychological functions. Further, both alcoholic men and women have lower gastric oxidation of alcohol than their nonalcoholic peers. Alcoholic women have almost no first-pass oxidation of alcohol, which places them at the top of the ladder for availability of alcohol in the system. The net result is to increase the vulnerability of women to the negative effects of alcohol consumption.

Black women are more likely to abstain from drinking (51%) compared to white women (39%), but are also more likely to engage in heavy drinking—38% for black women versus 11% of white women (Amaro, Beckman, & Mays, 1987). This difference still exists when controlling for socioeconomic status. Amaro's group could find no apparent differences in health beliefs, attitudes toward the sick role, going to the doctor, or worry about health to explain this difference. One personality variable was significantly different: black women had a higher sense of self-worth compared to white women. Black women seeking treatment did have one major problem: They had more limited financial resources for treatment, including third party payor arrangements, making it more difficult for them to obtain treatment.

Sociocultural Correlates: Ethnic Groups, Socioeconomic Status, and Occupation

Cross-cultural differences in alcohol use are highly visible. To illustrate, Jewish and Chinese people usually limit alcohol to special events. Mormons and Muslims have strong sanctions against the use of alcohol. Europeans have evolved a culture that supports the visible use of alcohol in daily routines, such as taking alcohol with meals. One outcome is that Europeans typically consume alcohol at a higher per capita rate than Americans. In spite of this, the rate of alcoholism is often notably lower in European cultures.

Ethnic groups also differ in systemic response to alcohol. One oft-cited difference is the flushing response in Asian people (Newlin, 1989). This response is usually unpleasant, even aversive, and may account for the lower total levels of drinking and alcoholism observed among this group. Conroy (1988) pointed to recent research suggesting that approximately 50% of Asian people lack an enzyme necessary to metabolize acetaldehyde, the first metabolic product of ethanol. Acetaldehyde metabolism affects the flushing response. The flushing response and the metabolic deficit occur in alcoholics with a positive family history of alcoholism independent of race. This suggests that the alleged cultural difference may be instead a differential distribution of a genetic trait linked through acetaldehyde metabolism to the flushing response.

Socioeconomic status (SES) also may contribute to problems with alcohol. Groups lower on the socioeconomic ladder are more likely to turn to bad alcohol when unable to obtain legal drinks. The active ingredient in legal alcohol is ethyl alcohol. Some products contain other alcohol distillates, such as the methyl (wood) alcohol found in rubbing alcohol. Methyl alcohol clears the bloodstream much more slowly than ethyl alcohol and is very dangerous. It can damage the optic nerve, produce blindness, and lead to death.

Further, there is an increased likelihood that lower SES groups will use alcohol as a food substitute. When this happens, they are at increased risk for malnutrition and more health problems due to increased vulnerability to infections (Watzl & Watson, 1992). Even in treatment, low SES continues to work to the detriment of the alcoholic. Low SES alcoholics are less likely to have social support networks, and they are more likely to be treated in public facilities or simply jailed and allowed to dry out on their own. Upon release, they are also less likely to have access to continued support that may be crucial to maintain abstinence.

Alcoholism and Health Risks: Cirrhosis, Accidents, and Fetal Alcohol Syndrome

Many health risks go with excessive alcohol use besides risk for malnutrition. One significant risk is cirrhosis of the liver. In 1989, chronic liver disease, including cirrhosis, caused 26,720 deaths, the ninth leading cause of death in the United States (MMWR, 1993, January 8). Of cirrhosis deaths, 46% were related to alcohol: 53% occurred among white males, 9% among black males, 29% among white females, and 5% among black females. The tragedy is that fully 90% of deaths attributed to cirrhosis are preventable through changes in lifestyle. If this cloud has a silver lining, it is that the death rate from chronic liver disease is on a downward trend.

The Alcohol, Drug Abuse, and Mental Health Administration (ADAMHA, 1989) reported that nearly 24,000 deaths and 534,000 injuries occurred in 1988 due to alcohol-related traffic accidents. Alcohol plays a role in about 48% of fatal accidents and 30% of traffic injuries. The good news is that alcohol-related traffic fatalities dropped to about 19,777 deaths by 1991 (MMWR, 1992, March 20), and the decline continued in all age groups through 1994, though at a slower rate than prior to 1990 (MMWR, 1995, December 1). (See Figure 9.5.)

One major risk among women is damage to the fetus. Women who drink during pregnancy are more likely to suffer miscarriage. Should the fetus survive to birth, it is more likely to have a low birth weight. If the mother takes more than three drinks daily during pregnancy, the risk triples that the child will have subnormal intelligence, for two reasons. First, alcohol ingested by the mother reduces oxygen supply to the fetus's brain (Streissguth, Barr, & Martin, 1983). Second, animal (rat) models of alcoholism show that ingestion of alcohol during pregnancy changes the growth and migration of neurons in the developing brain. This observation has some credibility for humans as well, since human infants with fetal alcohol syndrome (FAS) have

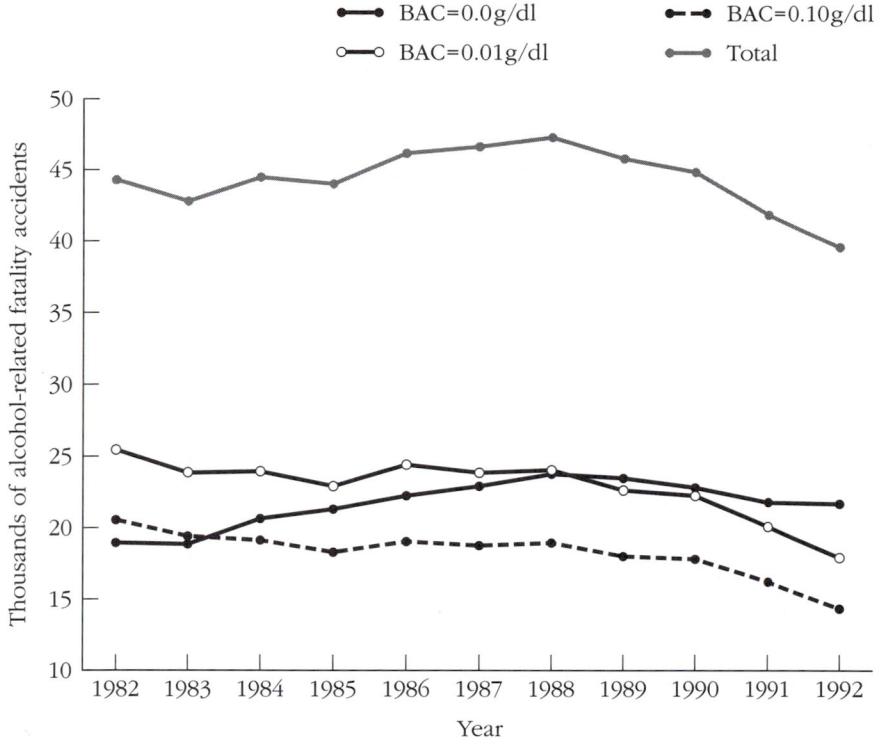

FIGURE 9.5   *Trend in alcohol-related fatality accidents from 1977 to 1989 (from MMWR, 1995).*

shorter and fewer neural dendrite branches (Miller, 1986).

The worst possible scenario is that the mother's drinking may produce a baby with **fetal alcohol syndrome.** FAS includes lower IQ, lower alertness, hyperactivity, and problems with both fine and gross motor performance (Barr, Streissguth, Darby, & Sampson, 1990). Victims of FAS carry the effects throughout their lives (Streissguth et al., 1991). A study by the Centers for Disease Control for the period from 1979 to 1992 set the prevalence of FAS at 2 per 10,000 births (Centers for Disease Control, 1993). Prevalence increased from 1 in 10,000 births in 1979 to 3.7 in 10,000 births in 1992.

One high-risk period for FAS occurs during the embryonic stage, when the mother may not even realize that she is pregnant (Sulik, Johnston, & Webb, 1981). Animal models sug-

gest another "temporal window of vulnerability" occurs *in utero* during the third trimester (West, 1993). The third trimester has a brain growth spurt period when neuronal populations complete their growth and differentiation. The brain appears to be highly vulnerable to alcohol during this time.

Although we have emphasized risks associated with alcohol consumption, there is evidence that moderate amounts of alcohol actually may promote cardiovascular health (Gaziano et al., 1993). The effect has been observed both in males and in females (Stampfer, Colditz, Willett, Speizer, & Hennekens, 1988). Moderate alcohol consumption is defined as drinking between 3 and 14 drinks per week, but less than 3 drinks per day. The beneficial effect appears to occur because alcohol intake increases levels of high-density lipoproteins (HDLs). Recall that HDLs are the good fats that act to remove large amounts of fatty deposits from the bloodstream.

The Etiology of Alcoholism: Genetics, Personality, and Family

As we observed in the last chapter, there are many different theories of addiction. The story is much the same with alcohol addiction. In this section, we will explore theory and supporting research that bears on the etiology of alcoholism.

The Genetic Model: Concordance, Tolerance, and Dopamine

Science has used various research designs and subject populations to confirm the genetic basis of alcoholism. Most animal models have used rodents and a self-administered preference test procedure. Even the lowly fly, *Drosophila melanogaster,* shows a partial heritability for ethanol tolerance, however (Geer, McKechnie, Heinstra, & Pyka, 1991). George (1987, 1988, 1990) and his colleagues showed that genetic factors are important in determining whether ethanol acts as a reinforcer in rats and mice (Ritz, George, de Fiebre, & Meisch, 1986). Further, George provided evidence that common biological factors influence drug-seeking for ethanol, cocaine, and opiates. Crowley and Andrews (1987) also found that monkeys showed alcoholic-like drinking with either flavored or unflavored alcohol.

Sufficient evidence now supports the genetic model, based on the fact that alcoholism runs in families. Identical twins have almost twice the concordance rate for alcoholism as fraternal twins. This concordance exists whether the twins grew up in the biological parents' home or in foster homes.

The classic concordance study of alcoholism was carried out in Denmark by Donald Goodwin's research group (1974; 1988). In this project, Goodwin found that either parent can transmit alcoholism to their sons but not to their daughters. Further evidence to support the genetic argument and diminish the environmental argument comes from two sources. First, adopted sons of alcoholic birth parents were at higher risk for alcoholism than other adopted children. Second, there were no significant differences between adopted sons of alcoholic birth parents and those who were raised by their alcoholic birth parents.

Cloninger's group used a cross-fostering analysis (Cloninger et al., 1981). Using data from adopted children, this analysis looked at the association between biological background (low to high risk of alcoholism) crossed with adoptive home environment (low to high risk of alcoholism). Compared to nonabusers, mild abusers had four times the amount of alcohol abuse when both genetic and environmental predispositions were present. In the group of moderate users, the biological fathers had low occupational status, criminal activity and convictions that began in adolescence, and recurrent alcohol use. The moderate user group had a ninefold greater risk for alcoholism compared to nonabusers. Further, environmental factors (adoptive home environment) did not add to the explained variance. In the severe abuse category, both inheritance and environment added small amounts to risk, but the results were not significant. Heritability indices ranged from 38% for mild abuse to 25% for severe abuse.

From this analysis, the Cloninger group proposed two types of alcoholism. Type I alcoholism is a milieu-limited late-onset type, in which both the biological father and mother contribute. There is evidence of mild alcohol abuse in both parents and some criminal activity. In addition, the postnatal environment influences both the frequency and severity of alcoholism. Type II alcoholism is a male-limited early-onset type. The biological father shows a history of severe alcohol abuse and criminality with extensive but failed treatments. The mother is normal, and the postnatal environment does not influence the risk. This type of alcoholism is highly heritable. Cloninger and his colleagues argued that the phenotypic expression of alcoholism may reflect both genetic heterogeneity and complex gene-environment interactions that result in clinical heterogeneity.

More recently, a group led by Roy Pickens studied 81 monozygotic (MZ) and 88 dizygotic (DZ) twins from the Epidemiological Catchment Area (Pickens et al., 1991). Pickens's group used serological analyses to confirm zygosity and the DIS to determine type and degree of drug abuse. The risk of becoming addicted to alcohol was 76% among MZ males.[5] Pickens's group estimated heritability for alcoholism to be .357 in males and .262 in females. These values are consistent with other analyses. The results are compatible with findings that sons of either alcoholic fathers or alcoholic mothers are at high risk for alcoholism. Additional analysis from this research team suggests that the genetic influences may be substantial only in early-onset male alcoholism (McGue, Pickens, Svikis, 1992). This finding is in general agreement with Cloninger's analysis.

Although most people now accept the genetic argument, there are still criticisms. Searles (1988; 1991) noted that formidable methodological problems beset many of these studies. One serious flaw continues to be the lack of clear diagnostic criteria. Even using the best standard tests and interview protocols, there is room for error in diagnosis of alcoholism. This ambiguity often leads to differences in comparability of results because groups defined as alcoholic may actually differ in important ways. Searles also noted that some studies had high rates of psychopathology in the foster parents. This could have a contaminating effect on interpretation.

Further, the finding that a disorder is genetic-familial says nothing about the specific mode of inheritance (Dinwiddie & Cloninger, 1991). As Cloninger's group noted, "susceptibility to alco-holism is familial, but its distribution cannot be explained by either genetic or environmental factors alone" (Cloninger, Bohman, & Sigvardsson, 1981, p. 861). In addition to probable differences in neurophysiology and ethanol sensitivity, alcoholics probably inherit differences in temperament, stress reactivity, impulse control, and learning styles.

Some investigators have begun to move on to probe the mode of inheritance. Schuckit (1985) argued that the phenotype is a high tolerance for alcohol that blocks signals to stop drinking. Le (1990) reviewed evidence showing that ethanol tolerance depends on complex interactions between genetic, pharmacological, and behavioral factors. Behavioral factors apparently include both experience and forms of Pavlovian conditioning, as we discussed in Chapter 8 (especially with regard to Siegel's work). There is also evidence that the brain's serotonin system[6] must be intact for organisms to become tolerant to the unpleasant effects of alcohol.

Blum and his associates provoked much excitement when they reported that they had found a strong association between the dopamine D_2 receptor (A1 allele) and alcoholism (Blum, Noble, Sheridan, & Finley, 1991). Their data showed that the A1 allele was present in 69% of alcoholics but in only 20% of nonalcoholics. Cloninger (1991) pointed out, though, that Blum's study analyzed only the brains of deceased subjects, and these were severe alcoholics who had experienced repeated treatment failures. Blum's conclusion since has been challenged by several groups who failed to replicate Blum's results (Gelernter et al., 1991; Comings et al., 1991).

Cloninger (1991) summarized results from six studies and found the implicated A1 allele was present in 45% of alcoholics and only 26% of controls. The prevalence of the A1 allele increases to about 60% in alcoholics with severe medical conditions. It appears now that the A1

---

[5] Stated in other terms, when one twin showed alcohol abuse or dependence, 76% of the time the MZ twin also showed alcohol abuse or dependence.

[6] The serotonin system is the medial raphe nucleus in the brainstem to the hippocampus, and the brain's noradrenergic system.

TABLE 9.2   *Association of the A1 allele of DRD2 with alcoholism in six case control studies of white subjects (from Cloninger, 1991).*

| | PREVALENCE OF THE A1 ALLELE | | | | |
| | ALCOHOLICS | | CONTROLS | | |
SOURCE	NUMBER	%	NUMBER	%	ODDS RATIO
Blum et al., 1990	22	64	24	17	8.8*
Bolos et al., 1990	40	38	62	33	1.2
Parsian et al., 1991	32	41	25	12	5.0*
Comings et al., 1991	104	42	108	22	2.6*
Gelernter et al., 1991	44	43	68	35	1.4
Blum et al., 1991	96	50	43	21	3.8*
All sources	338	45	330	26	2.4*

*Alcoholism significantly associated with A1 allele ($p < .05$).

allele modifies the expression of alcoholism, but that it is neither necessary or sufficient as a causal agent in the development of alcoholism.

Brain Behavior and Alcoholism: Deficits in Processing

Researchers have also considered the possibility that the genotype for alcoholism may be expressed in altered mental function. One group, headed by Henri Begleiter (Begleiter, Porjesz, Bihari, & Kissin, 1984; see Polich, Pollock, & Bloom, 1994 for a meta-analysis), found a brain wave anomaly that may help explain alcoholism. Begleiter's group argued that sons of alcoholic fathers have a primary deficit in information processing. They based their method and conclusions on two lines of evidence.

First, the investigators used the well-established clinical technique called evoked brain potential (EP). The EP method presents controlled stimuli while brain waves are recorded with common neurological instruments (for example, the EEG). In addition, the investigator assesses cognitive functions with neuropsychological instruments (for example, subtests from the WAIS or HRNB). Second, Begleiter linked his work to previous research showing that alcoholics have several cognitive abnor-

malities detected with the EP method and that concordance for EP waveforms occurs in monozygotic twins. Identical twins, in other words, show as much similarity in EP waveforms between themselves as a lone individual does from one testing to the next.

Begleiter targeted the **P3 waveform,** which reflects the amount of subjective information provided by an event (Johnston, 1979). The amplitude of P3 increases markedly when new information reduces uncertainty. Intoxication results in lower amplitudes of P3. Sons of alcoholic men show a changed P3 function compared to control boys without exposure to alcohol. This result suggests that the changed P3 function precedes and contributes to alcoholism. Begleiter's group suggested that the changed P3 function results in "a reduced capacity to assess significance or allocate the necessary neural resources for encoding a specific event." (1984, p. 1495)

Psychological Etiology: Personality, Anxiety, and Expectancy

Theorists have long sought to link personality and familial processes to alcoholism. Early research approached the issue from a solely descriptive point of view; in other words, it did little more than describe processes that distinguished alcoholics from nonalcoholics. It soon became apparent that this approach did not distinguish factors that initiate alcoholism from those that maintain alcoholism. As one example, anxiety, depression, and insomnia can occur after a single dose of ethanol (Miller, Dackis, & Gold, 1987). Some theorists argue, though, that anxiety and depression dispose one to alcoholism. The burden of proof is to show that these traits existed prior to exposure and contributed to the pattern of abuse. Researchers must show, in other words, that the traits are the cause of alcoholism, not the result of alcohol consumption.

According to Alterman and Tarter (1983), the predisposing factors (diathesis) include a genetically transmitted psychological vulnerability expressed as conduct disorders in childhood, plus hyperactivity and attentional problems. This pattern was replicated in work by Glenn and Parsons (1989). Precipitating factors (stress) include a disordered family with disturbed family interactions, association with certain types of peers, ethnic background (probably because of association with low income, discrimination, and so forth), and deprived environment. Drinking increases or decreases depending on the amount of current perceived stress. The fact that stress and ethanol consumption interact also has received support from animal models (Pohorecky, 1990).

A common portrait of the alcoholic suggests a person who has chronic distress, is externally controlled (Apao & Damon, 1982), avoids confronting problems (Rohsenow et al., 1989), and has weak or ineffective psychosocial skills (Nerviano & Gross, 1983). Difficulty in psychosocial skills usually revolves around feelings of personal inadequacy, higher levels of fear than normal, and problems with concentration. The alcoholic reveals these traits through conflict with authority figures, more frequent and intense expressions of hostility, and aggressiveness. This combination of factors often serves to reduce effectiveness on the job and disturbs social and intimate relationships.

In more recent work, Rohsenow's group focused on a variable called cue reactivity (Monti et al., 1993; Rohsenow et al., 1994). **Cue reactivity** is the tendency for the alcoholic to respond to alcohol use cues. Alcoholics appear to respond more strongly to the sights and smells of alcohol as measured by salivation and urge to drink. The stronger this tendency is, the more it is predictive of problems in controlling drinking.

One cognitive variable, the expectancy effect, appears to play a prominent role in alcoholism. Simply stated, the influence of alcohol depends in part on what the drinker expects. For example, children of alcoholics tend to expect more positive outcomes from alcohol use (Sher, Walitzer, Wood, & Brent, 1991). This effect is stronger in males than in females, and it is also significantly linked to negative affect. Cox and Klinger (1988) believe that positive expectancy is the motivational key leading to the decision to drink or abstain. Brown and Munson (1987) showed that when people have a positive expectancy, they tend to drink alcohol more frequently and in larger amounts.

The expectancy effect appears to interact with personality variables. In the Brown and Munson (1987) study, extroverted students expected more social and physical pleasure from alcohol. They also expected that alcohol would provide more relaxation and lower tension. Introverted students expected more power and aggression. Finally, students with more trait anxiety expected a broad range of positive changes including better sexual performance, social assertion, and increased power and aggression. These contrasts are shown in Figure 9.6.

A major concern in alcohol research is that expectancy effects may heighten risk taking when driving. McMillen, Smith, and Wells-Parker (1989) showed that high sensation seekers took more risks in a driving simulator when they believed they had just drunk alcohol. On the other hand, low sensation-seekers became more cautious in driving when they believed they had just drunk alcohol. Additional evidence

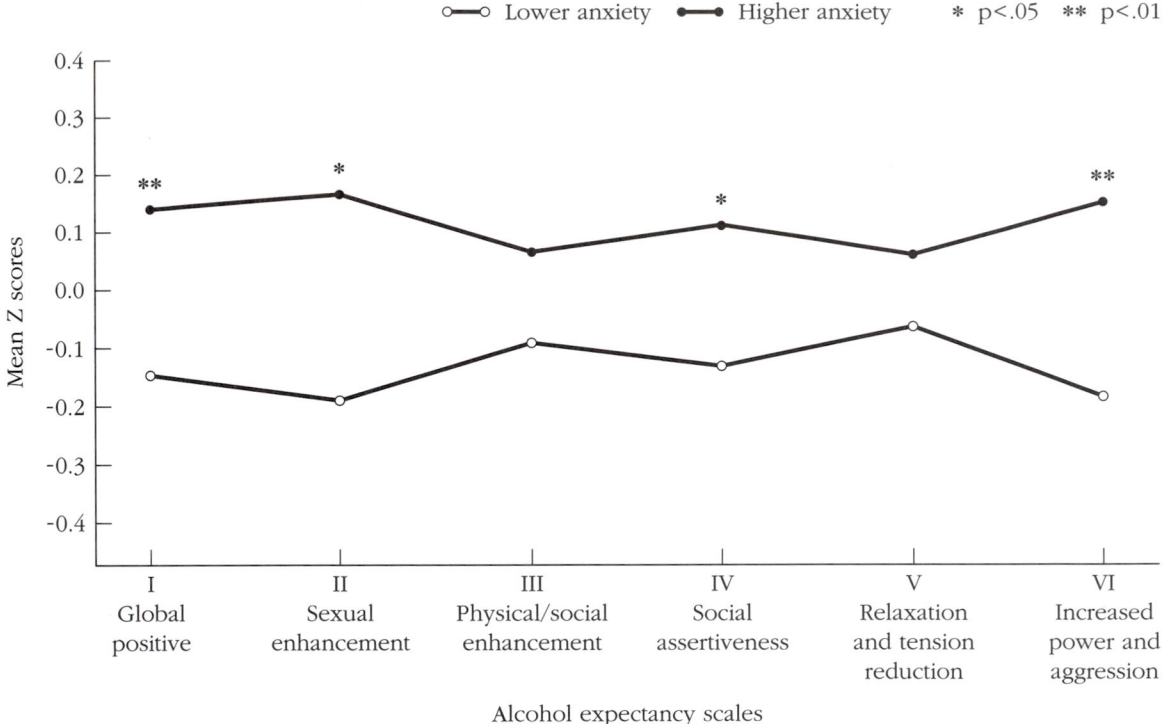

FIGURE 9.6   Contrasts of alcohol expectancy between low and high trait anxiety. High trait anxiety persons expect more positive benefits from alcohol (from Brown & Munson, 1987).

reveals that both drinking motives and location predict accident risk for males, but not females (Pang, Wells-Parker, & McMillen, 1989); that is, males who drink expecting to lower inhibitions and to meet females are at high risk for auto accidents. Finally, males appear to use the car more as a type of mobile bar, engaging in both more deviant behavior and heavier drinking while in their cars.

Social-Familial Etiology: History, Pathology, and Setting

The issue of family correlates of alcoholism continues to be of intense interest despite the surge of interest in genetic substrates. About one in eight children lives in a home where parenting is compromised because of drug abuse

(Kumpfer & DeMarsh, 1985). Although the evidence is sometimes inconsistent (Orford & Velleman, 1991; Pandina & Johnson, 1989), alcoholism presumably correlates with several family traits, and certain traits of the alcoholic may be linked in turn to the family history. For example, problem drinking occurs more often in those with low occupational status whose parents also were heavy drinkers (Parker & Harford, 1987).

Susan Glenn and Oscar Parsons (1989) carried out an extensive study to answer some questions in this area. They found that alcoholics generally had a higher density of familial alcoholism and a greater history of family psychopathology. More depressive symptoms, anxiety, and lower IQ scores occurred in those with a positive family history of alcoholism (FH+).

Marital problems were more evident among alcoholics, and job stability was a problem among those with a FH+. Glenn and Parsons concluded that a child reared in a home with a FH+ is likely to show various deficits whether that child becomes alcoholic or not.

To summarize, alcoholism has several roots. Genetic factors contribute substantially, but still explain only a small percentage of the variance in alcoholism. Environmental factors include family history of alcoholism, exposure through peers and role models, and stressors. These variables appear to contribute strongly to alcoholism. Finally, personality variables, such as anxiety and problem avoidance, also appear to contribute to alcoholism.

Clinical Treatment: Pharmacological, Behavioral, and Cognitive

Through the ages, society has used almost every imaginable form of treatment to combat alcoholism. The list of current interventions includes biomedical techniques, insight therapies, aversive therapies, cognitive-behavioral therapies, group therapy, and milieu therapy. Biomedical therapy usually attempts to control the discomfort and pain of withdrawal symptoms. Insight therapies try to deal with interpersonal conflicts, anxiety, and low self-esteem among other personality processes. Aversive therapies attempt to condition a negative association to alcohol so that it will produce appropriate avoidance instead of inappropriate approach. Cognitive-behavioral therapies may try to alter self-defeating thoughts, change beliefs and expectancies about alcohol, or instill self-control through a variety of procedures.

Along with the many therapies, there are many treatment issues that give rise to frequent debates. One issue is the success of treatment as measured by relapse. Another issue concerns whether training in moderation (controlled drinking) will yield more success or whether

complete abstinence is necessary for all recovering alcoholics.

Abstinence Versus Controlled Drinking: Point and Counterpoint

Perhaps no treatment issue has been more hotly debated than the temperance treatment approach, also called the controlled drinking model. Credit for this view is most often given to Mark Sobell and Linda Sobell (1978, 1987), but clinical efforts to produce controlled drinking appeared nearly two decades before the Sobells' work (Rosenberg, 1993). Space does not permit a replay of the extensive discussions on the Sobells' model or on accusations that they falsified data. It is sufficient to say that independent reviews verified the integrity of their data, and the model is considered a viable, though qualified, treatment option. It is qualified because both treatment goals and type of therapy should be selected in recognition of the client's unique situation and with the client's active involvement. The controlled drinking model should no more become the treatment of choice than should therapies based on a total abstinence model. The history of clinical interventions has shown that treatments are more or less successful to the extent that they match the unique traits, problems, and milieu of the client.

The controlled drinking approach suggests that total abstinence is both an unrealistic and unnecessary goal for many recovering alcoholics. It is unrealistic because the availability of alcohol and pressures to drink are pervasive in modern culture. Abstinence is unnecessary because it is based on two faulty notions. The first faulty notion is that once a person is an alcoholic, the person is always an alcoholic. The second faulty notion is that to take even a single drink will instantly and automatically return the person to uncontrolled drinking based on an unavoidable effect on the physical system.

Substantial evidence refutes both these ideas, however. Many people—perhaps 90% of the people who consume alcohol—do so in a controlled, nonproblematic way. Additionally, many alcoholics do recover to resume a normal life with controlled drinking (Rosenberg, 1993). Even in abstinence treatment programs, between 10% and 30% become controlled drinkers after treatment. It is noteworthy that the range for abstinence success in such programs is precisely the same, between 10 and 30%. Biomedical data based on individual differences in alcohol metabolism also refute the view that all people are equally vulnerable to the physiological effects of alcohol. Finally, to assume that one drink is sufficient to reinstate alcoholism is to deny the complexity of factors (biopsychosocial) that contribute to alcoholism in the first place.

Harold Rosenberg (1993) summarized several issues bearing on the controlled drinking controversy including some methodological problems. Through about 1980, the data suggested that controlled drinking was a viable treatment outcome for those whose drinking problem was of lower severity. On the other hand, those with an alcoholic self-image and more serious drinking problems generally needed a therapy that focused on abstinence.

Another factor that influences whether controlled drinking may be successful or not is persuasion. Very simply, treatment success may be related to the alcoholic's belief that abstinence is necessary versus the belief that temperance is attainable. To the extent that the mode of therapy and the activities of the therapist successfully convince the client one way or the other, the treatment may or may not be successful. Rosenberg noted that lower severity, belief in controlled drinking, stable employment, younger age, psychosocial stability, and female gender all predict controlled drinking as a successful therapeutic outcome.

Treatment Factors: Commitment, Depression, and Self-Efficacy

It is not uncommon for alcoholics to drop out before the fourth treatment session (Noel, Mc-Crady, Stout, & Fisher-Nelson, 1987). This has led clinicians to a search for the factors that predict not only persistence, but also successful completion of therapy. Several factors predict successful treatment. One is the personal motivation to change. It is almost a truism by now that therapy is less likely to be successful when the person is committed involuntarily. The flip side is that treatment is more likely to be successful as the person's motivation to change strengthens. In addition, people who finish treatment more often are only mildly affected by alcohol and are still involved in their social and vocational environment. Dropouts are more likely to be heavily involved in alcohol and affected by alcohol, anxious, and ambivalent about treatment, and they report many somatic and psychosomatic symptoms. Treatment refusers are more likely to be younger with a shorter history of drinking and involuntary referrals.

Depression is usually viewed as a negative characteristic, one that may even lead to treatment dropout. One research group, however, provided evidence that the presence of depressive symptoms may be beneficial to the therapeutic situation (MacMurray, Nessman, Haviland, & Anderson, 1987). According to this group, the higher the score on the Beck Depression Inventory, the longer the person persists in treatment. Conversely, the absence of affective distress predicted early withdrawal from treatment. It is possible, then, that depression is not directly related to treatment success, but that it plays a moderator role in association with other unknown variables.

Another factor that may be related to treatment success is self-efficacy (Bandura, 1977). As applied to alcohol treatment, self-efficacy presumably is related to such elements as persistence in therapy and the ability to withstand pressures from high-risk situations following treatment.

Support for this idea comes from a project showing that people higher in self-efficacy at intake persisted longer before relapse (Rychtarik, Prue, Rapp, & King, 1992). When high self-efficacy and strong aftercare were combined, survival analysis showed that almost 50% of the group met the criterion for successful treatment at 12 months' follow-up. This criterion allowed for two days of drinking during the 12 months following treatment—in other words, strict but not total abstinence. The study revealed a possible role for self-efficacy in relapse prevention, but the follow-up did not extend to 18 months so as to include the entire time frame (6–18 months) during which most relapse occurs. Further, most successful programs have found it necessary to incorporate maintenance therapy during this critical relapse period. Thus,

self-efficacy may help predict success in treatment, but it is probably not sufficient to produce success itself.

Treatment Methods: Antabuse, Cognitions, and Alcoholics Anonymous

Treatment programs often confront the problem of alcohol withdrawal—especially programs specifically designed to treat severe or emergency cases. An addict who goes through withdrawal cold turkey (by total abstinence) will

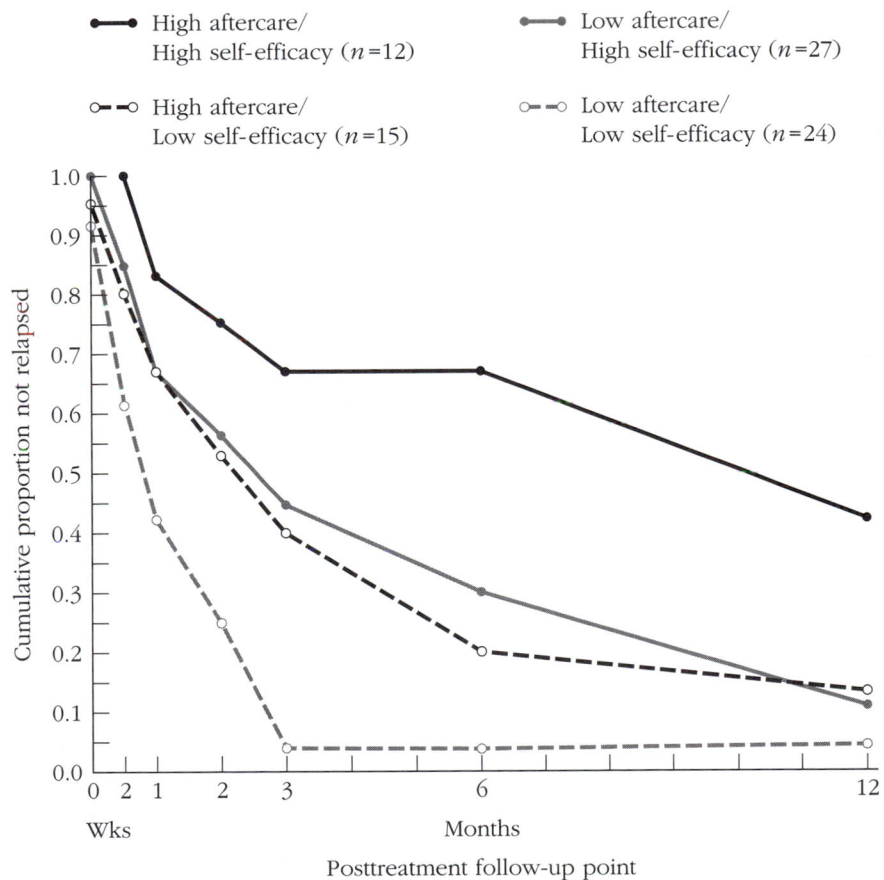

FIGURE 9.7 Cumulative relapse curves for subjects classified according to self-efficacy and aftercare duration (from Rychtarik et al., 1992).

likely experience a difficult and painful withdrawal. The degree of discomfort, though, depends on the severity of the addiction. Another method is medically aided gradual withdrawal, called **detoxification,** which uses a substitute drug to enable the body to clear itself of alcohol while reducing and controlling withdrawal discomfort and pain. Although several complications can occur in detox, it is now a routine practice with adequate safety.

Perhaps due to the long history behind detox programs, clinicians have begun to consider whether detox requires admission and treatment as an inpatient, or whether it can be carried out safely and effectively with outpatients. The concern is in part prompted by rapidly escalating treatment costs. A large-scale study directed by Hayashida (Hayashida et al., 1989) addressed these issues. The investigators assigned patients randomly to an inpatient group or an outpatient group. Then, they used oxazepam[7] in decreasing doses to aid detox. Although the inpatient group had slightly more severe alcohol problems, there were few differences at six months' follow-up. More inpatients (95%) completed treatment compared to outpatients (72%). Yet there were no differences in medical complications or in the number of patients who needed further alcohol detox or treatment. One factor was highly significant: The cost for inpatients over nine days of treatment ranged from $3,319 to $3,665, whereas the cost for outpatients over six days ranged from $175 to $388. The results suggest that detox may be carried out effectively with outpatients and at considerably reduced costs.

Antabuse: Biomedical Basis and Aversive Conditioning

Pharmacotherapy continues to arouse great interest as new medications come on line (see Schuckit, 1996 for a review). Still, the old

standby treatment is antabuse, otherwise known as disulfiram. Disulfiram (tetraethylthiuram disulfide) was a chemical used in the rubber industry. In 1947, someone noted that workers who absorbed it had increased sensitivity to alcohol (Royce, 1989). In 1950, after controlled medical trials in Denmark, the drug was brought to the United States. More clinical trials established safe dosage levels so that it could be used with few side effects. Most antabuse programs advise clients to take antabuse just once in the morning.

Antabuse is not psychoactive, so there can be no criticism, as with methadone, that the patient is simply trading one addiction for another. The mechanism of antabuse is simple: It blocks the enzyme process that breaks down acetaldehyde, the first metabolic by-product of alcohol. If the person does not consume alcohol, there is no problem. If the person consumes any alcohol, however, acetaldehyde builds up quickly, and a very unpleasant physiological change occurs. Among other symptoms, the person will experience a flushed face, rapid pulse, sweating, difficult breathing, and blurred vision. Most notably, there is a feeling of intense nausea and vomiting.

On the surface, antabuse seems to be a biomedical treatment, but the underlying process works more like aversive counter-conditioning.[8] Antabuse serves as an aversive UCS that becomes connected with the sight, smell, or taste of alcohol. These cues then function as conditioned cues to elicit an aversion response and thus prompt avoidance.

Several considerations are important to the decision to use antabuse. First, antabuse is an adjunct to therapy, not a complete treatment. Addicts must be counseled that other therapeutic activities need to be completed before long-term abstinence can be obtained and before they quit antabuse. Royce (1989) noted, though, that some recovering alcoholics believe that if diabetics can use insulin all their lives,

---

[7] Oxazepam is an antianxiety drug from the benzodiazepine group. See Chapter 5 for more details on this group of drugs.

[8] See Chapter 5 for details on aversive counter-conditioning.

alcoholics should be able to use antabuse the same way. Second, antabuse clears the system in about five days. This leads to potential problems in compliance, even deceit. It is widely known that addicts not fully committed to recovery may use antabuse to maintain sobriety for short periods. Then, they time going off antabuse so they can tolerate a weekend bender. Third, certain foods and medicines containing alcohol must be avoided. Fourth, some people do not absorb antabuse. As a result, they will not experience the unpleasant response that normally occurs, and their drinking is not likely to change. Finally, some people complain of other effects that may or may not be psychological. For example, some complain of impotence, but this effect may be because antabuse causes bad breath at first. The sex partner may react negatively, which could increase performance anxiety in the antabuse user.

Aversive therapy: promise and problems

Aversive therapies have enjoyed long-standing popularity for the treatment of alcoholism.[9] Modern aversive techniques used emetics such as apomorphine hydrochloride or emetine hydrochloride to produce nausea and vomiting. With proper timing, the nausea should coincide with ingestion of alcohol. In this way, the appropriate link between the CS (sight of alcohol) and the UCS (nausea) could be established. There was some initial expectation that this method could produce a quick and effective treatment, but the hope was short-lived. The procedure produced recovery rates in the 70% to 80% range, but abstinence rates were rarely any better at follow-up than several other methods. This approach had several drawbacks as well, not the least of which was the problem of controlling, collecting, and disposing of the vomit. Further, treatment often had to take place in a medical setting with a medical team available to give the injection and monitor possible complications,[10] all of which drove up treatment costs. Also, there are methodological problems with emetics. They have a slow onset, making it more difficult to optimize the CS-UCS association. Dosage also has to be adjusted to several of the patient's physical traits and conditions.

It is tempting to think that the use of shock would get around the problems that go with the use of emetics. Unfortunately, shock therapy does not work well for something like alcohol, a fact that studies in taste aversion support (Garcia & Koelling, 1966).

Alcoholics Anonymous: hope, drunkalogs, and the 12 steps

Based on sheer numbers of successfully treated alcoholics, no program rivals Alcoholics Anonymous (AA). Accurate statistics are hard to come by because of AA rules (participation is anonymous), but more than two million people may have completed the road to recovery through AA's famous 12 steps. Estimates of success rates are about 75% to 89%, but this figure allows for one relapse in the first year. AA meetings can be found now in 114 countries around the world (Royce, 1989). An alcoholic does not have to become a member to join or speak to participate. The program is first a fellowship of men and women sharing a common problem with the hope of full recovery. Second, it is a partnership between the alcoholic and a same-sex support partner. AA has overtones of a spiritual quest, but it is careful to avoid any appearance of sectarian affiliation and specifically prohibits endorsement of any religion.

There are four types of AA meetings: speaker, discussion, step, and study-group meetings (Royce, 1989). At a **speaker meeting,** members tell the group their stories about involvement with alcohol. They may share a "drunkalog," a recital of their worst personal abuses of alcohol. In a **discussion meeting,** members may talk about a variety of topics such as personal

---

[9] Refer to Chapter 5 to review details on conditioning models.

[10] Emetine, for example, could produce cardiovascular problems.

conflicts, resentments, success stories, and faith. In a **step meeting,** the group discusses in depth the 12 steps. Finally, in a **study-group meeting,** the members may take some of AA's materials, such as a few chapters from a book, and discuss their significance. Several psychosocial processes may be influenced through these meetings including alteration of cognitions, beliefs, and values; emotional catharsis and bonding; social networking and support; reframing of self-concept and development of self-respect; and increases in feelings of self-efficacy. Still, little systematic research is ever carried out on AA itself to discover the specific processes and components behind its success.

Although AA has shown both widespread acceptance and some measure of success, numerous criticisms of AA have been forwarded. AA is a social support system more than a therapy per se. It uses quasi-religious notions for motivation, and it does not have a systematic theory. The participants are anonymous, so no demographic, social-familial, medical, or intervention data are available. Finally, AA's criteria of treatment success do not coincide with those customarily used in medical and psychological treatment programs. All these factors make it difficult to test empirically the primary features that contribute to success.

Risk reduction: secondary prevention

In addition to multimodal treatment programs, several people have begun to look at ways to reduce risk in those who are currently drinking but not yet defined as problem drinkers. This is the realm of secondary prevention, since some signs of disorder are already present. The hope is that with early treatment, the risk for damage may be minimized or eliminated. Consider as an example an adolescent or young adult who may be on the verge of alcoholism. A psychoeducational program that successfully changes cognitive schemas about drinking and alters the person's behavior to a controlled drinking pattern could effectively prevent most of the damage that would accompany alcohol abuse.

Marlatt and his research group have been at the forefront of work on programs that seek to reduce risk.

In one such study, volunteers were randomly assigned to three different risk reduction programs (Baer et al., 1992). One program used a cognitive-behavioral self-management group instruction format developed by Marlatt's group in earlier studies. The class ran for six weeks. Another group used much the same material, but in a six-unit self-help manual. The third group received a single session that combined individualized feedback and professional advice.

At the conclusion of the program, participants rated the classroom instruction most helpful in changing drinking behavior, while they rated the self-help manual lowest. The programs were equally effective for changing lifestyle. Measures of drinking and estimates of blood alcohol showed a significant decline over the course of the program. The greatest decline occurred in the classroom instruction program. Baer's group discovered that subjects who were 19 years old at the beginning of the study relapsed to an even higher level of drinking at two years' follow-up. Those who were 20 years old at the beginning had a one-year relapse, but then dropped back to near post-treatment levels. The groups over 21 years and under 19 years maintained their gains even at two years' follow-up.

At the social policy level, former surgeon general Koop released information in 1989 containing ten recommendations to impact drunk driving (see Table 9.3). Efforts are also under way to develop more effective means to keep intoxicated drivers off the road. Such efforts include breathalyzers in bars, skin patch tests, and car lockouts to tell drinkers when they have had enough. Car lockouts require the driver to breathe into a breathalyzer-type device; the car will not start if the device detects a BAC above the legal limit. Another widely used method is the designated driver program, or arranging other transportation for those leaving a bar or party with high BAC. Assertive inter-

TABLE 9.3 *Recommendations from the Workshop on Drunk Driving, released May 1989 by then Surgeon General C. Everett Koop (ADAMHA NEWS, August 1989).*

1. Reduce the legal blood alcohol concentration from 0.10 to 0.08 immediately and to 0.04 by the year 2000.
2. Increase the federal excise tax on alcoholic beverages based on their alcoholic contents.
3. Increase funding by states for impaired-driving prevention programs.
4. Reduce the availability of alcoholic beverages.
5. Enact state legislation to allow "on the spot" suspension of driver's license of person found to be driving with a blood alcohol concentration above the legal limit.
6. Balance the level of alcoholic beverage advertising with an equal number of pro-health and pro-safety messages.
7. Restrict certain types of advertising and marketing practices, especially those addressing underage youth. Also extend warning labels.
8. Conduct public information efforts based on social marketing and communication strategies and on sound learning principles.
9. Conduct drinking and driving education within work sites, health care agencies, schools, and the community.
10. Increase the enforcement of drinking and driving laws, and expand the use of sobriety checkpoints.

ventions, such as the car lockout, work well in public settings where there is concern for drunk driving. In private settings, however, more passive interventions are called for (Hernandez & Rabow, 1987). Another approach is to develop a typology of DWI drivers. The intent of this approach is to help match alcoholics to treatment (Wieczorek & Miller, 1992).

After therapy: mortality, cohesion, and coping Finney and Moos (1992) carried out a ten-year study designed to determine the functioning and mortality of alcoholics following treatment. Patients received treatment in one of

five multimodal inpatient programs combining a medical component (antabuse), psychoeducational components (lectures, films, and therapy), and vocational and recreational elements. At two years following treatment, patients functioned better when they were in a cohesive and supportive family marked by low conflict and active recreational patterns. At ten years, mortality risk depended on several measures obtained at the two-year follow-up.

In brief, patients had higher risk of mortality when they had few confidants, depended on avoidant coping strategies, were unemployed, had lower incomes, were suffering from more medical symptoms, and took more medications. Conversely, positive life context and coping skills at two years predicted better functioning at ten years. People who lived in less stressful life situations with cohesive and well-organized families and who used active coping skills functioned better at ten years than those who did not show these characteristics.

Prevention Methods: Schools, Employee Assistance Programs, and Clinics

Efforts to prevent development of problem drinking include school-based prevention programs, employee assistance programs (EAPs), and special services comprehensive health care clinics.[11]

School-based interventions target a subgroup of students entering high-risk years for beginning alcohol consumption (Institute of Medicine, 1992). The focus is often on prevention (Jensen, 1992). These programs follow a logic similar to the smoking prevention programs described in Chapter 8. They typically integrate different skills believed necessary to keep adolescents from becoming trapped in an addictive

---

[11] EAPs may function to reduce risk (secondary prevention) as well as to help employees who have serious problems with alcohol (tertiary prevention).

pattern. These include problem-solving skills, decision-making skills, and cognitive techniques that help adolescents to resist the persuasive powers of peers and mass media campaigns. Further program units focus on coping skills, self-esteem, assertiveness, and interpersonal communication. More extended programs may include components for early identification of children at risk and lifestyle assessments to help students identify potential problem areas. Peer-conducted prevention programs seem to be very helpful, since peer clusters often play a role in adolescents' becoming involved in drug use (Oetting & Beauvais, 1987).

Another prevention approach provides comprehensive health care to adolescents in hopes that high-risk youths will be served and high-risk behaviors, including substance abuse, changed for the better (Earls, Robins, Stiffman, & Powell,

1989). Seven clinics in large cities from Boston to Los Angeles participated in a study designed to provide special services to high-risk adolescents. These clinics were compared to three clinics without specialized services. The funded special services clinics did not show any evidence of significantly changing behavioral and lifestyle problems. Further, instead of reducing heavy alcohol use and substance abuse, the proportion of clients with problems went up in the funded specialized services programs compared to the other clinics. The authors suggested that the goals of treatment for problem youths may need to be refocused on stabilizing community risk conditions instead of concentrating solely on behavior change.

Work site programs may be structured to serve individual needs or risk reduction at the group level. One randomized trial compared

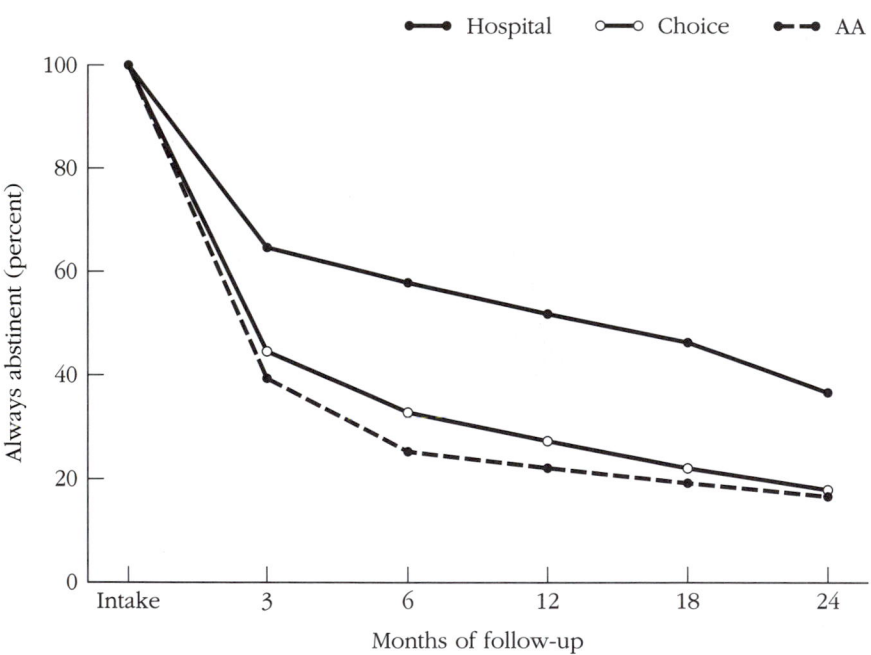

FIGURE 9.8   *Comparisons of three methods of treatment for workers referred from an on-site EAP: This shows months of continuous abstinence over the two-year follow-up (from Walsh et al., 1992).*

three groups of employees whose initial contact for alcohol problems came in established work site EAPs. One group received a standard medical inpatient treatment using a three-week intensive detoxification program. A second group went to local AA meetings, and a third group chose their own treatment (Walsh et al., 1991). Workers from all three groups were on job probation for a year after treatment. During this period, they were required to attend AA meetings, maintain sobriety on the job, and check in weekly with the EAP staff. Based on a continued abstinence criterion, the results suggested that those treated as inpatients fared best, the AA-treated group fared worst, and those who chose their own programs fell in the middle. Hospital treatment cost more than the other treatments, but continuous abstinence and sobriety measures and length of time to hospitalization for further treatment all favored the hospital treatment group at first. At two year's follow-up, though, there were no significant differences in 12 job outcome measures.

Summary

In this chapter, we have discussed the epidemiology and etiology of alcohol abuse. We have considered various theories that try to explain the origins of this habit, but have found again that single cause models are inadequate. In spite of growing confidence in the genetic model, psychosocial factors still play very important roles. The following are the major points made in this chapter.

1. Alcoholism is defined as a loss of control over drinking with frequent episodes of extended heavy drinking ending in intoxication.

2. Alcohol dependence includes prominent alcohol-seeking behavior, increased tolerance, repeated withdrawal symptoms, and continued use in spite of negative consequences.

3. BAC, or blood alcohol concentration, is used in the legal arena to get around subjective elements in clinical definitions. This establishes a level, usually 0.10%, at which the person is legally intoxicated.

4. Alcohol is a CNS depressant, not a stimulant as some people think. The feeling of well-being is related to the fact that alcohol acts as a surrogate in the brain's opioid receptors.

5. Alcohol changes food metabolism and contributes to malnutrition when it replaces food in the diet. Malnutrition may lead to immunosuppression and increased health risks in the alcoholic.

6. Current estimates suggest that as many as 100,000 people die each year from alcohol-related causes.

7. Alcoholism occurs predominantly in people aged 18 to 44 and is about five times more prevalent in men than in women.

8. Women are at increased risk for health problems from alcoholism because they have almost no first-pass oxidation of alcohol.

9. Cultural differences influence the rate of alcoholism and general patterns of drinking.

10. A major health risk from alcoholism is cirrhosis of the liver.

11. Alcohol probably has its most devastating effects on the road where 20,000 alcohol-related deaths and 534,000 alcohol-related injuries occur each year.

12. Fetal alcohol syndrome lowers IQ and alertness, and it contributes to hyperactivity and to problems with fine and gross motor control.

13. The genetic model of alcoholism is based on the observation that alcoholism runs in families, that identical twins have twice the concordance rate for alcoholism as fraternal twins, and that this difference persists whether the children are raised by their biological parents or by adoptive parents.

14. According to Cloninger's research, the genetic contribution is strongest in Type II alcoholism, or male-limited early-onset type.

15. Blum's work implicated the dopamine D_2 receptor (A1 allele). Later work suggests that this receptor modifies the expression of alcoholism but that it is not necessary or sufficient to produce alcoholism.

16. Psychosocial explanations of alcoholism point to a genetically transmitted vulnerability including conduct disorders in childhood, disturbed family interactions, family psychopathology, and chronic distress with weak psychosocial (including coping) skills.

17. Treatment programs may focus on achieving complete abstinence or on controlled drinking. The abstinence approach has been favored historically, especially by groups such as AA. Controlled drinking may be successful, and more realistic, with less severe cases. Either approach should be selected in recognition of the patient's unique history and situation.

18. Several psychological factors influence treatment success. People with more personal motivation, self-efficacy, and assertiveness are more likely to be treated successfully.

19. Detoxification programs use medical interventions, such as administration of oxazepam, to enable the body to clear itself of alcohol while reducing the pain and discomfort that often accompanies withdrawal.

20. Antabuse treatment associates an unpleasant stimulus, nausea, with consumption of alcohol. This presumably will lead to a conditioned aversion to alcohol. Although there are problems with the use of antabuse, it is still regarded as a viable treatment technique when combined with other therapeutic methods.

21. Alcoholics Anonymous, using its famous 12-step program, may be the most successful treatment program ever in terms of sheer numbers. AA generally works toward complete abstinence.

22. Secondary prevention programs try to reduce the risks for people who are drinking but may not be regarded yet as problem drinkers. The most successful approaches to date appear to be cognitive-behavioral programs that attempt to change attitudes and behaviors that support drinking.

23. Primary prevention programs usually work in the schools or with identified high-risk populations to try to keep problem drinking from developing in the first place.

Key Words

alcoholism	detoxification
alcohol abuse	discussion meetings
alcohol dependence	(AA)
alcohol-induced	episodic heavy drinking
myopia	fetal alcohol syndrome
alcohol intoxication	P3 waveform
alcohol withdrawal	speaker meetings (AA)
blood alcohol	step meetings (AA)
concentration	study-group meetings
cue reactivity	(AA)

Study Questions

1. What are the distinctions, if any, between alcoholism, alcohol dependence, and alcohol abuse? Why does one have to be careful in citing prevalence statistics based on the definition of alcoholism?

2. What is BAC, and how is it related to perceptual-motor and psychological impairment?

3. What are the basic steps involved in absorption of alcohol from the time it hits the stomach until it is fully absorbed? What organs are involved, and what damage may occur as the body tries to absorb alcohol? Does gender change the equation at any point? If so, how?

4. What are the potential changes that may occur in an infant born to a mother who has consumed too much alcohol during her pregnancy? In the worst case scenario, fetal alcohol syndrome, what are the symptoms?

5. What data is available to support the contention that alcohol abuse is, in part, influenced by genetics?

6. What psychosocial variables are related to alcohol abuse?

7. What are the most common methods for treating alcohol or cocaine abuse?

8. Is abstinence an absolutely necessary goal for treatment to be successful?

Class Projects

1. Locate material from your library that will allow you to construct a graph that relates the amount of alcohol drunk to BAC. Do this for the typical weight range of males and also for the typical weight range of females. Consider how these figures are related to patterns of alcohol consumption that you or your friends engage in.

2. Invite professionals from your community, including possibly local or state police personnel, to discuss problems that stem from alcoholism.

3. Locate support-treatment groups in your region and invite them to talk to your class about how they intervene in alcohol dependence or drug abuse in general.

4. If you can locate professionals in your community who support the controlled drinking model and the abstinence model, consider holding a debate on the pros and cons of each approach.

Suggested Readings

Blum, K., & Trachtenberg, M. C. (1988). Alcoholism: Scientific basis of a neuropsychogenetic disease. *The International Journal of the Addictions, 23,* 781–796.

Dinwiddie, S. H., & Cloninger, C. R. (1991). Family and adoption studies in alcoholism and drug addiction. *Psychiatric Annals, 21,* 206–214.

Institute of Medicine. (1992). Prevention and treatment of alcohol-related problems: Research opportunities. *Journal of Studies on Alcohol, 53,* 5–16.

Morse, R. M., & Flavin, D. K. (1992). The definition of alcoholism. *JAMA—Journal of the American Medical Association, 268,* 1012–1014.

Rosenberg, H. (1993). Prediction of controlled drinking by alcoholics and problem drinkers. *Psychological Bulletin, 113,* 129–139.

Sobell, M. B., & Sobell, L. C. (1987). *Moderation as a goal or outcome of treatment for alcohol problems.* New York: Haworth.

Watzl, B., & Watson, R. R. (1992). Role of alcohol abuse in nutritional immunosuppression. *The Journal of Nutrition, 122,* 733–737.

WEBSITES *Alcohol Addiction*

ADDRESS	DESCRIPTION
http://www.well.com/user/woa	☆ Web of Addictions—numerous links and excellent content for alcohol and other addictions
http://www.nwrc.org/	☆ National Women's Resource Center—substance and drug abuse
http://www.cts.com/~habtsmrt/	☆ Habit Smart—resources for destructive habits and addictions of all types
http://solar.rtd.utk.edu/~Al-Anon/eng.index.html	Al-Anon/Alateen—support for families and teenagers with alcoholic family members
http://alcoholics-anonymous.org	Alcoholics Anonymous
http://niaaa.nih.gov	National Institute on Alcohol Abuse
http://www.health.org.ncaditop.html	National Clearinghouse for Alcohol & Drug Information

Eating Behavior: Healthy and Unhealthy Habits

On the surface, nothing sets Al apart from most older men. At 88 years old, he lives in a retirement community near the Rocky Mountains. His only complaint is desperate loneliness since his wife died.

Throughout life, Al never drank or smoked excessively, and his physical health seems excellent for his age. He does suffer from recurrent bouts of depression. Still, this is not unusual for someone his age, especially someone deprived of a lifelong companion. There are signs of mounting problems though. It has become apparent to the community staff that Al is having more trouble remembering things. Recently, a medical examination revealed that Al is in the early stages of Alzheimer's disease.

Yet none of this, not even Alzheimer's, had anything to do with the medical community's interest in Al. What brought Al to medical research's attention was his unusual eating routine: he eats about 25 hardboiled eggs daily plus other foods. One large egg has about 31 grams of fat and about 213 mg of cholesterol.[1] This means that Al consumes about 775 grams of fat each day. While the prudent daily level of dietary cholesterol is thought to be no more than 300 mg, Al takes in more than 5000 mg of cholesterol a day. This is not healthy by any stretch of the imagination: Yet the startling fact is that Al has normal to low levels of blood cholesterol (Kern, 1991). Medical investigators believe that Al may be able to help them understand how

---

[1] All this fat and cholesterol are contained in the egg yolk; the egg white contains no fat or cholesterol.

some people can resist accumulation of fatty deposits whereas others struggle with problems of excess weight, high blood pressure, and high risk for coronary disease.

Al's lifestyle and medical status serve to illustrate important issues in diet and nutrition. First, it is clear that individuals differ in food tolerance. These basic individual differences probably are related to genetic factors that influence a host of variables in the body's food handling, storage, and utilization systems. As the nutritional and physiological sciences proceed, evolving theories also will reflect this complex matrix of factors. Then, it may be possible to link individual differences more precisely to both positive and negative health outcomes.

Second, guidelines established for a healthy diet do not predict individual success or failure. National guidelines use normative data that apply to the majority of people but do not cover various exceptions.

Finally, dietary guidelines often change to reflect new research. In the future, research may point out more precise markers from family and personal health history that foreshadow personal health problems. Then, public education programs may provide dietary information tailored to individual differences. This may relieve dietary pressure for some people like Al who are less vulnerable to dietary risks. For others, though, it may signal the need to control diets even more carefully.

This chapter summarizes what we know about the relations between diet and health. We will discuss techniques that may be useful to help people change lifestyle or manage troublesome eating habits. We will consider new guidelines for a healthy diet. In the process, we will discuss biomedical and psychosocial factors that influence the control of eating. Later, we will review the epidemiology and etiology of obesity. Then, we will look at clinical methods, both biomedical and psychosocial, that offer some promise of success, limited though they may be, in treatment of obesity. Finally, we will discuss briefly the disorders of anorexia nervosa and bulimia.

The Epidemiology of Eating: Healthy and Unhealthy Habits

A quick review of the history of diet and health reveals some startling contrasts. Not too long ago, most concerns centered on nutritional deficits and related illnesses. The great explorers roamed the seas early in this millennia subsisting on diets that did not provide nutritional balance needed for a healthy body. Often they were plagued by rickets, pellagra, and other diseases related to poor nutrition, especially the absence of vitamins and minerals. Some of these diseases were still evident in the early 1900s. Now, however, our concerns more often are related to dietary excesses—the consumption of too much food or of unhealthy foods.

Nutrition 2000: Goals for Nutritional Health

Nutrition research shows that adult humans need 46 nutrients to stay healthy. These nutrients cover six categories: water, carbohydrates, nine proteins, fat, 13 vitamins, and 21 minerals. The average woman needs about 1600 to 2400 calories to keep her weight constant. The average man needs about 2300 to 3100 calories for constant weight (Mayo Clinic, 1981). Table 10.1 shows the average range of energy needs for children and adults at different weights and heights.

A crucial fact often overlooked in dieting is that to obtain those 46 nutrients, most adults must average as a bare minimum about 1300 calories per day. Diets that restrict caloric intake below 1000 run the risk, indeed pose a very real danger, that the person will be nutritionally starved. Safe very low calorie diets (VLCDs), which provide about 200 to 800 calories per day, use high biologic quality protein supplemented with vitamins, minerals, and electrolytes to avoid danger (Blackburn, Lynch, & Wong, 1986).

The Surgeon General's office released a report in 1988 that resulted from an intensive

TABLE 10.1   *Recommended daily energy (calorie) intake for children and adults (adapted from Mayo Clinic, 1981).*

	AGE YEARS	WEIGHT LBS.	HEIGHT IN.	ENERGY NEEDS CALORIES
Youths	1–3	29	35	1,300 (900–1,800)
	4–6	44	44	1,700 (1,300–2,300)
	7–10	62	52	2,400 (1,650–3,300)
Males	11–14	99	62	2,700 (2,000–3,700)
	15–18	145	69	2,800 (2,100–3,900)
	19–22	154	70	2,900 (2,500–3,300)
	23–50	154	70	2,700 (2,300–3,100)
	51–75	154	70	2,400 (2,000–2,800)
	76+	154	70	2,050 (1,650–2,450)
Females	11–14	101	62	2,200 (1,500–3,000)
	15–18	120	64	2,100 (1,200–3,000)
	19–22	120	64	2,100 (1,700–2,500)
	23–50	120	64	2,300 (1,600–2,400)
	51–75	120	64	1,800 (1,400–2,200)
	76+	120	64	1,600 (1,200–2,000)
Pregnancy				+300
Nursing				+500

review of nutrition and health in the United States. These nutritional standards are still accepted today. The report contained five specific recommendations.

1. Fats and cholesterol: Reduce the consumption of fat to no more than 20% of daily calories and cholesterol to less than 300 mg daily.
2. Energy and weight control: Work to reach a desirable body weight. Then maintain that weight through regulation of caloric intake combined with regular exercise.
3. Complex carbohydrates and fiber: Increase intake of whole-grain foods, cereals, vegetables, and fruits so that about 50% of total calories are from complex carbohydrates.
4. Sodium: Reduce the intake of sodium by using foods low in sodium content and limit the amount of salt added to foods at the table.
5. Alcohol: Take alcohol only in moderation (two drinks per day maximum, no matter what type of alcohol) to reduce the risk of chronic disease (McGinnis & Nestle, 1989).

It is preferable to think of these goals as a package: Changing only one habit may have a small positive effect in its own right. Changing all the components should have a synergistic effect that is greater than the sum of the parts. Centuries ago, Hippocrates recognized the synergy between diet and exercise. He noted: "Eating alone will not keep a man well; he must also take exercise. For food and exercise, while possessing opposite qualities, yet work together to produce health" (Hippocrates, 1923, pp. 227–228).

We can see the interactive effects of diet by comparing diets across cultures. The Finns typically eat a diet that is high in saturated fat, but they also eat more cereals and high-fiber foods than other groups do. Finns take in about 32 grams of fiber each day, and they have low rates of colon cancer compared to other Western groups (Wynder et al., 1992). This example suggests that concentrating on one nutritional item alone will not have the impact desired. In contrast, adjusting total diet to balance nutrients can have a significant impact.

In summary, the essence of an ideal diet is

about 50% carbohydrate, 30% protein, and 20% fat. About 80% of carbohydrates should be complex. Saturated fats should make up no more than 10% of fat intake. Finally, the daily menu should contain about 25 grams of fiber (Gershoff, 1990; Wynder et al., 1992).

Diet and Health Risks: Heart Disease, Cancer, and Diabetes

Diet contributes to five of the top ten causes of death: heart disease, cancers, strokes, diabetes, and atherosclerosis (National Center for Health Statistics, 1988).[2] Also, Americans spend about $3 billion annually on packaged vitamins and nutrients, often taking megadoses on the assumption that more is better. They do so in spite of the weight of research showing that megadoses of vitamins often have adverse side effects (Gershoff, 1990) and that the body simply flushes these excess vitamins out in stools and urine.

Most Americans consume excess fats, with 40 to 45% of daily calories coming from fatty foods. This problem is magnified because the fatty foods they choose often have too many saturated fats. Compared to residents of the United Kingdom or France, Americans eat more red meat each week, consume more eggs, and based on the body mass index, are more obese (Retchin, Wells, Valleron, & Albrecht, 1992).[3] In Japan, the percentage of calories derived from fat has gone up from 10% in 1950, to 20% in 1980, to about 25% today (cited in Wynder, Weisburger, & Ng, 1992). Further, most people do not take in enough carbohydrates. They get fewer than 40% of their calories from this source, and even then too many of these calories are from sugars. One 12-ounce can of nondiet cola, for example, contains the equivalent of 10 teaspoons of sugar.

Based on recent estimates, nearly 34 million Americans, or about one-fourth the population, are overweight (McGinnis & Nestle, 1989). Many may be overweight because of poor diet, but the problem is also one of sheer overeating magnified by inactivity. Technologically advanced societies with abundant food supplies tend to be overconsumers in many areas including food. Nowhere is this overconsumption more evident than at the popular buffet meals where people continue to gorge themselves long after satiety cues have told the body, "Enough!" A marketing ploy to gain market advantage becomes the consumer's own worst enemy. In addition, many people are taught to eat till the last scrap of food is gone from their plate to avoid waste. The thought that consuming more than enough will end up as their own body waste—in other words, as fat on their waists—is somehow less important.

Weight Control and Exercise: TV, Couch Potatoes, and Inactivity

The lack of consistent activity contributes to eating-related weight and health problems. About 40% of the population are probably active at levels too low in intensity and frequency to control weight and improve cardiovascular fitness (Herbert & Teague, 1989). Further, television may be fostering more inactivity, and with it increases in the prevalence of obesity (Tucker, 1986). As Figure 10.2 shows, there is a direct relationship between the prevalence of obesity and the time spent watching television: the longer the time spent in front of the TV, the higher the prevalence of obesity (Dietz & Gortmaker, 1985).

In one study on television viewing habits, Larry Tucker and Glenn Friedman (1989) investigated health, obesity, and physical fitness among more than 6000 men. After controlling for several variables such as age, length of workday, and amount of exercise, they found that men who watched TV three or more hours a day were twice as likely to be obese as men

---

[2] Of the remaining five, excessive alcohol consumption contributes to three: unintentional injuries (auto accidents, for example), suicide, and chronic liver disease.

[3] The Quetelet index (kg/cm^2) is discussed later in this chapter.

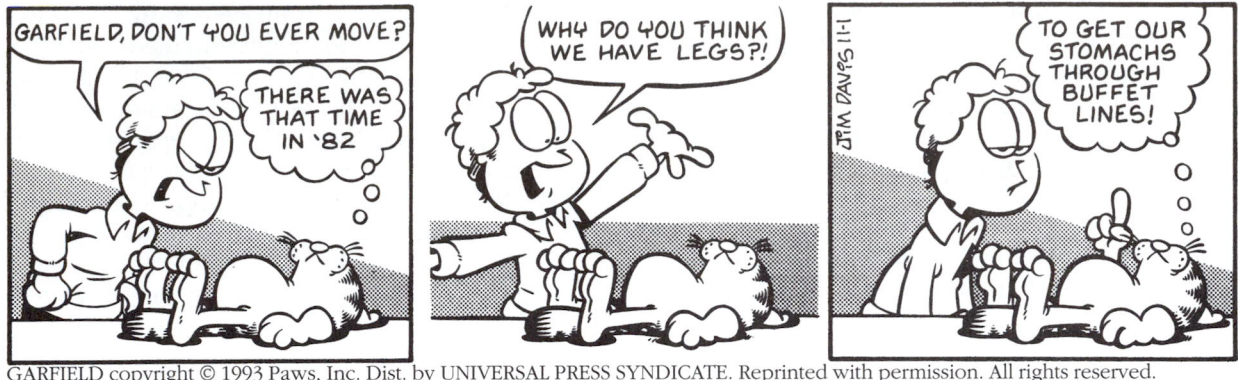

FIGURE 10.1   Garfield understands the attraction to buffet meals.

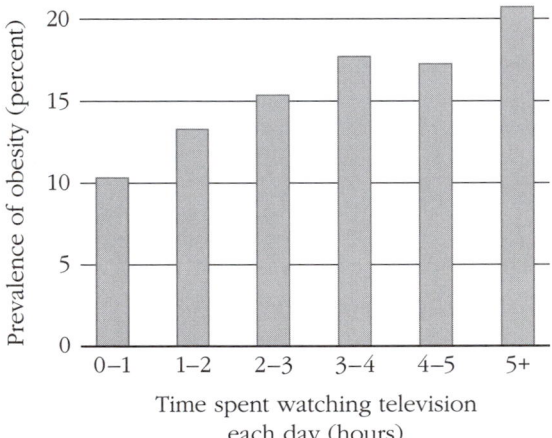

FIGURE 10.2   The prevalence (in percentages) of obesity in 12- to 17-year-old adolescents shows a near linear increase as time spent watching television increases (from Dietz & Gortmaker, 1985).

who watched less than an hour. It is, of course, possible that those who are obese watch TV longer because they cannot tolerate exercise.

In spite of these pessimistic notes, there are encouraging signs of change. Overall quality of diet in the United States has improved dramatically since 1965, and differences between racial and socioeconomic classes have disappeared (Popkin, Siega-Riz, & Haines, 1996). Further, compared to British and French samples, Americans have dramatically cut their consumption of eggs, red meat, and alcohol, and they are more often inclined to lose weight and engage in exercise to reduce risk (Retchin, et al., 1992). The food industry is also responding to the demand for healthier foods. Sales of health and fitness foods are growing rapidly and were expected to reach the $2 billion mark in the early 1990s.

Obesity: Signs, Origins, and Treatment

Beryl Markham was a pioneer woman aviator who spent much of her life flying supply routes in Africa.[4] Writing about her life in *West with the Night,* she told of a chat she had with an African friend from a nearby village, a young boy named Toombo. Toombo was heavy, but his attitude was one of quiet dignity and self-acceptance. Toombo said, "God makes fat birds and small birds, trees that are wide and trees that are thin. . . . He makes big kernels and little kernels. I am a big kernel. One does not argue with God" (Markham, 1983, p. 124).

---

[4] Beryl Markham was one of the few women to take up flying at a time that flight was still in its infancy, still very much of an adventure without navigational instruments, and still very dangerous. She was romantically linked, at least by innuendo, with Denys Finch Hatton, who was Isak Dinesen's lover in *Out of Africa,* a story that will have more relevance for us when we get to Chapter 13.

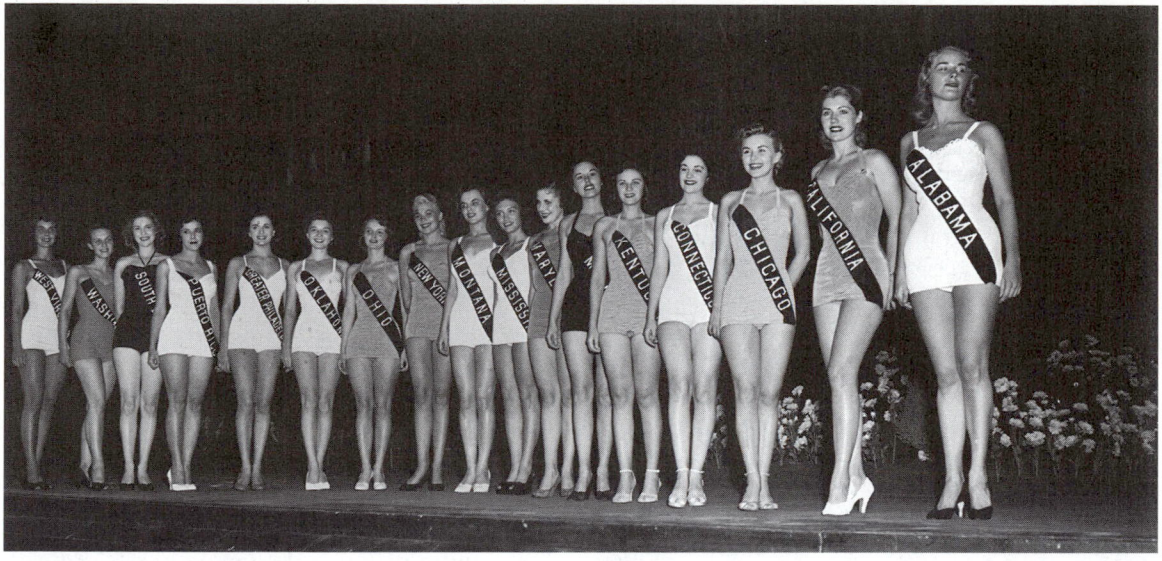

FIGURE 10.3   *Beauty pageant contestants in 1951 reveal fuller figures compared to modern contestants.*

Tolerance for obesity, in self or others, seems to be low in Western culture, however. Personal consequences of being overweight often include treatment similar to that reserved for the physically handicapped. Thinness is valued, and plumpness has become something of a physical stigma.

This was not always the case. Indeed, from the golden age of Greece all the way to the 17th century, plump men were seen as having attained position, power, and wealth—in a word, success (Polivy, Garner, & Garfinkel, 1986). In both Western and Eastern cultures, plump women were often seen as more healthy, attractive, even more erotic than their thinner peers.

The situation has changed dramatically. Polivy, Garner, and Garfinkel (1986) argue that increased health consciousness, fear of obesity, and changing social roles underly the current obsession with thinness. Compared to 17th century standards, men now appear to prefer women with smaller tummies and slightly larger hips (Singh, 1993). Singh noted that this trend is evident in recent Miss America winners and Playboy playmates. Further evidence reveals

that as recently as the 1950s and early 1960s, Miss America contestants and Playboy centerfolds were close to the average weight (only about 10% below average) for females their age. Today, the slender, almost anorexic women who compete in such contests are nearly 20% below the average for their age-mates (Sobal, 1990).

DeJong and Kleck (1986) argued that the term *obesity* is now loaded with stigmatizing connotations and suggested that the term *overweight* is preferable. George Bray (1986), however, cautions that being overweight is not the same thing as being obese. **Obesity** in Bray's scheme involves a surplus of adipose tissue, while being **overweight** involves excess weight based on some standard such as a weight chart or body mass index. Thus, a person can be overweight without being obese.

In summarizing the results of several studies on social stigma, DeJong and Kleck found three common victimizing stereotypes. The overweight person is seen as (1) lazy, (2) less intelligent and (3) less often chosen as a friend than people who are not overweight. Such stereotypes are often supported by the belief that overweight people are weak, lacking in

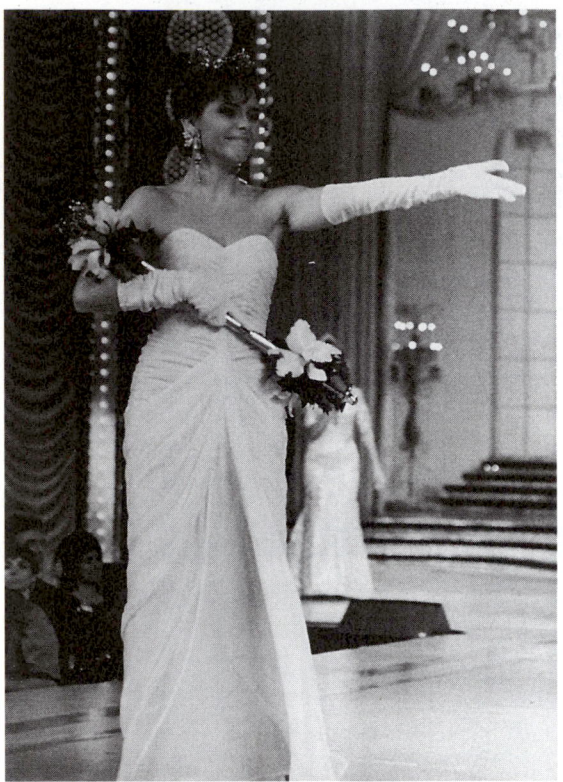

FIGURE 10.4   A recent, slender Miss America.

willpower, and self-indulgent. Whereas children with birth defects have an "excuse," overweight people are considered responsible for their condition. Finally, there is evidence that overweight people may be discriminated against in grading, college admissions, and employment.

Assessment of Obesity: Charts, Ratios, and Skin Folds

Several methods are used to determine whether a person is in a normal weight range or is overweight. These include standard weight charts, the body mass index (BMI), skin-fold tests, waist-to-hip ratios, and hydrostatic (underwater) weighing. Hydrostatic weighing, although the most accurate method by far, is also the most costly and thus far less practical. Here, we will discuss only the other four methods.

The most commonly used standard for many years was a chart developed in the insurance industry that related weight to height for men and women. In the 1959 Metropolitan Life Insurance version, types of body frame were distinguished to provide more precise estimates. This distinction was based on a not unreasonable assumption that someone with a large frame could carry more weight with fewer health risks than someone with a smaller frame. These charts changed in various ways over the years. One interesting change was that later charts provided for heavier weights compared to the 1959 Met Life chart. The charts were criticized on several grounds, including the unrepresentativeness of the sample and the charts' failure to use age, economic status, or body distribution of fat to determine risk (Callaway, Foreyt, Nuckolls, & VanItallie, 1992).

Definition of obesity by the chart method was based on a simple percentage criteria. If the person was up to 20% over the upper limit noted in the chart, the person was classified as overweight (Bray, 1986). If the person was more than 20% over the upper limit, the person was classified as obese. The National Research Council provided standards for height and weight that reflect more current thinking based on research into risks for chronic disease. This chart is shown in Table 10.2 using conventional pounds and inches.

In the 19th century, the Belgian mathematician Quetelet observed that a person with a normal build has a weight that is proportionate to the square of their height. This equation became known as the **body mass index,** or BMI for short, and is now the de facto standard for comparing degrees of obesity (Callaway et al., 1992). The index is expressed by the following formula:

$$\text{BMI} = \frac{\text{W(kg)}}{\text{H(m)}^2} : \frac{55(\text{kg})}{1.625 \ (\text{m})^2} = 21 : \frac{82(\text{kg})}{1.57 \ (\text{m})^2} = 33$$

The formula assumes metric values for both weight, in kilograms (kg), and height, in meters (m). To illustrate, a person whose weight is 55

TABLE 10.2   *Recommended weights for different heights and ages (from National Research Council, National Academy of Sciences [1989]).*

HEIGHT (FEET/INCHES)(WITHOUT SHOES)	WEIGHT (POUNDS) (WITHOUT CLOTHES)	
	19–34 YEARS	35 YEARS AND OLDER
5'0"	97–128	108–138
5'1"	101–132	111–143
5'2"	104–137	115–148
5'3"	107–141	119–152
5'4"	111–146	122–157
5'5"	114–150	126–162
5'6"	118–155	130–167
5'7"	121–160	134–172
5'8"	125–164	138–178
5'9"	129–169	142–183
5'10"	132–174	146–188
5'11"	136–179	151–194
6'0"	140–184	155–199
6'1"	144–189	159–205
6'2"	148–195	164–210
6'3"	152–200	168–216
6'4"	156–205	173–222
6'5"	160–211	177–228
6'6"	164–216	182–234

kg (120 lbs) and stands 1.625 m tall (64" or 5'4") has a BMI of 21. For either male or female, this is in an acceptable range. A person whose weight is 82 kg (180 lbs) and stands 1.57 m tall (62") has a BMI of 33. This is in the range of obesity.

The easiest way to compute BMI is with the nomogram (see Figure 10.5). This visual method connects a person's weight on one scale to height on the adjacent scale. The point at which the connecting line crosses the center BMI scale is the crude BMI value.

A range of 20 to 25 is optimal for health and longevity. The clinically important condition below this range is anorexia nervosa. BMI values between 25 and 30 generally reflect an over-weight condition. BMI values above 30 suggest obesity, and skinfold tests will almost always confirm this (Bray, 1986). Figure 10.6 shows BMI related to levels of obesity (Garrow, 1992).

A third set of measures, skin-fold tests, have emerged as a very popular way to assess obesity. They tend to provide a better clue to body composition than the weight chart or BMI. Body composition in this context means the ratio of fat to lean mass in the body. There are many different skin-fold tests, though not all have the same degree of precision and usefulness.

One method is to measure a skin fold on the back of the arm (triceps) and one skin fold beneath the shoulder blade (subscapular) using calipers. As Figure 10.7 shows, the calipers basically trap a double layer of fat for measure-ment. The more weight the person carries as fat, the larger this measure will be. Combining the two readings, the definition of obesity is be-tween 45 mm for men and 69 mm for women.

A more recent assessment technique is the **waist-to-hip ratio** (WHR). The WHR is very easy to obtain. First, measure the waist just

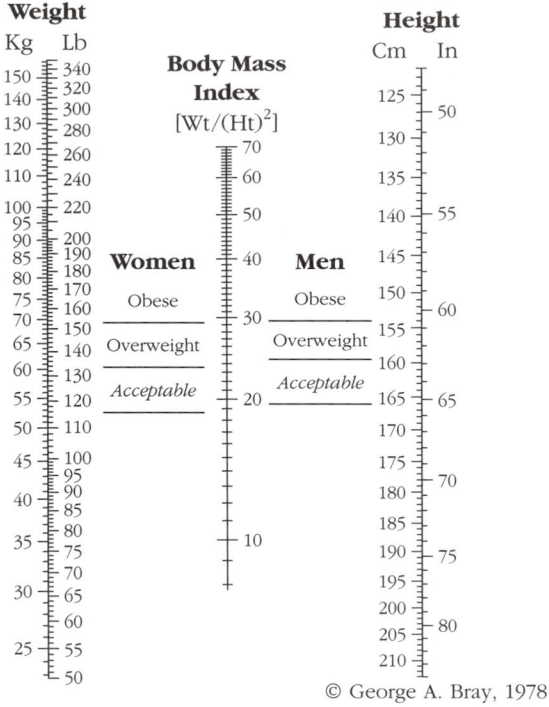

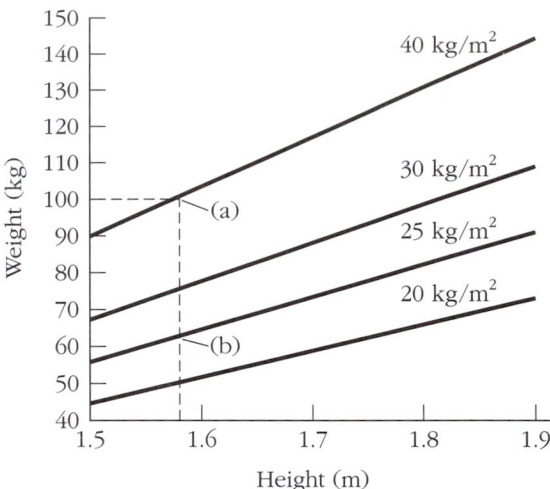

FIGURE 10.5   A nomogram to compute a crude BMI value. Any straight edge may be used to draw a line from weight on the left to height on the right; the BMI then may be read from the scale in the center.

FIGURE 10.6   The relation of BMI to levels of obesity. The desirable range is 20 to 25. Lines at 30 and 40 kg/m² show the boundaries between grades I, II, and III obesity. The broken line shows that a patient with weight of 100 kg and height of 1.58 m, is on the boundary between grade II and III (point a), and needs to lose 37 kg to return to a desirable weight (from Garrow, 1992).

above the navel while standing relaxed with normal stomach position. Then measure the hips at the largest point. Finally, divide the waist size by the hip size. For women, a WHR above 0.80 is considered high, and for men a WHR above 0.95 is considered high (Callaway et al., 1992).

This measure has become more important with the discovery that WHR more accurately predicts risk from obesity than any other measure. In general, the larger the waist relative to the hips, the higher the person's health risk because abdominal fat is far more atherogenic than any other type of fat (Bouchard, Bray, & Hubbard, 1990).

The large waist and small hip distribution pattern is called **male pattern obesity,** or abdominal obesity. Obviously, all males do not fit the male pattern obesity norm, but it is more common in men than in women (Laws, Terry, & Barrett-Connor, 1990). Male pattern obesity is associated with several health risks including heart disease, high blood pressure, diabetes (Morris & Rimm, 1991), and lower HDLs (Ostlund, Staten, Kohrt, Schultz, & Malley, 1990). Stated in other terms, as WHR goes down (and the abdomen becomes smaller relative to the hips), the good fats (HDLs) tend to go up. Note that male pattern obesity does occur in women, and when it does, it produces the same health risks as in men.

Females tend to carry more weight in the hips relative to the waist, a distribution that is called **female pattern obesity** (gynecoid obesity). This form of obesity does not carry the health risks that occur with male pattern obesity. In general, women have to be more seriously obese than men before they experience the same risks.

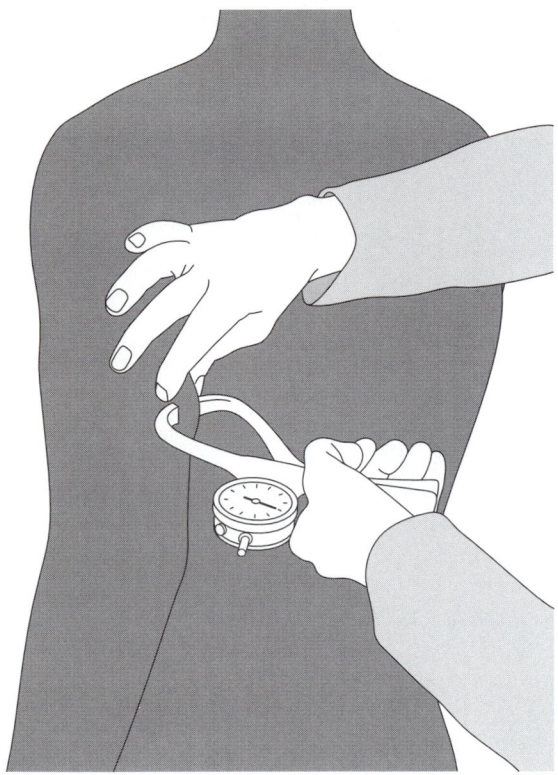

FIGURE 10.7   A common skin-fold test.

Distribution of Obesity: Epidemiology, Costs, and Risks

The estimated prevalence of obesity in the United States varies widely, but it is thought to be nearly 30% for men and nearly 35% for women (Colditz, 1992). Obesity also tends to be more prevalent among blacks and Mexican Americans than among whites. In absolute numbers, more than 35 million people may fit the clinical definition of obesity, and 12 to 13 million of these may fit the clinical definition of severe obesity. Concern is also increasing about obesity in childhood, because 14% of overweight infants become obese adults but just 6% of normal weight infants do (Epstein, 1986). In a 40-year study, Mossberg (1989) found that obese children had a mortality rate of 10.9% compared to 6.5% in a nonobese reference group. The primary health problem was cardiovascular dis-

ease, which occurred in 29.1% of the obese group compared to 14.7% of the nonobese group.

Being overweight involves both biomedical and psychosocial risks. Contemporary medical research reveals that mortality and morbidity increase with being overweight. This is true in adolescent males (but not adolescent females) as well as in adults (Must, Jacques, Dallal, Bajema, & Dietz, 1992). Figure 10.8 shows that excess mortality increases rapidly as BMI increases above 30. Based on data from the Framingham study,[5] there would be 25% less coronary disease if people maintained an optimal weight (Kannel & Gordon, 1976).

Beyond the commonly known cardiovascular risks, obesity is linked to kidney failure, gall-bladder disease, and several forms of cancer.[6] Obesity is also associated with lower pulmonary (breathing) function complications. Lowered pulmonary efficiency typically makes physical activity more difficult, which then becomes a major deterrent to beginning and staying with an exercise program. The short-term costs of exercise are high for an overweight person because all systems of the body are subjected to more stress while exercising.

Added to the physical health risks are several psychosocial costs. Graham Colditz (1992) estimated that the overall costs of treating side effects of obesity in 1986 came to nearly $40 billion, or 5.5% of all costs for illness in that year. Two chronic diseases, diabetes and cardiovascular disease, accounted for $33.5 billion of this total.

Steven Gortmaker's team carried out a longitudinal study of the social and economic outcomes of being overweight (Gortmaker, Must, Perrin, Sobol, & Dietz, 1993). The investigators began in 1981 with a sample of more than 10,000 men and women between the ages of 16 and 24.

---

[5] The Framingham Study is one of several long-term prospective studies of risks for coronary heart disease that continues to provide large-scale data for analysis by many investigators.

[6] See Chapter 14 for more information.

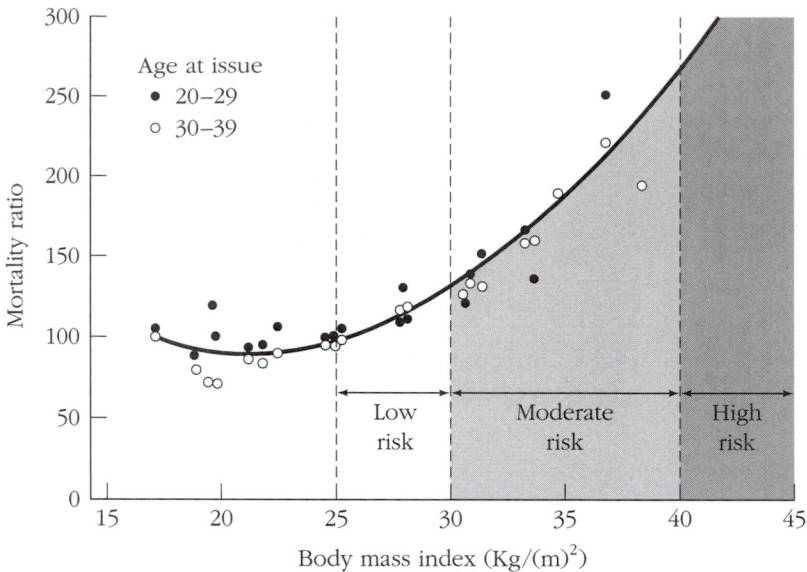

FIGURE 10.8   Relation of body mass index (BMI) to excess mortality in 20- to 39-year-old adults (from Bray, 1986).

From this group, 370 were overweight, and another 136 had chronic medical conditions such as asthma (73 cases). Women who were overweight had completed fewer years of school, and they were less likely to be married. Also, they had lower incomes and higher rates of poverty compared to their nonoverweight cohorts. These outcomes were independent of SES status or aptitude test scores. Men suffered fewer negative consequences, showing only a lower rate of marriage compared to more slender peers. Further, Gortmaker's group could find no evidence of these same negative consequences among a contrast group of chronically ill subjects.

Types of Obesity: Clinical Criteria and Causes

There was a time when obesity was just obesity, the common cold was just a cold, and cancer was cancer. Now the common cold refers to symptoms that may be caused by any one of scores of viruses, and the identified forms of cancer number about 250. Obesity, like those other disorders, can no longer be confined to a single category. The multiple forms of obesity may help dispel negative attitudes toward obesity. Just as important, the variety of types of obesity may serve to guide development of new treatment modalities as different etiologies are confirmed.

Mervyn Willard (1991) devised a classification scheme including seven discrete forms of obesity, each with distinct causes and treatments. The first type, **metabolic obesity,** presumably results from a low resting metabolic rate. In prospective studies, low metabolic rate appears to reliably predict future obesity. A low metabolic rate may be inferred when a person eats on a tightly controlled diet plan but still gains weight. In this case, treatment should adjust diet and exercise to the metabolic level of the client.

A second type of obesity, **environmental obesity,** is presumably caused by a number of lifestyle variables, such as a family that supports recreational eating, sedentary work, or leisure preferences that do not involve exercise. Because the etiology is environmental, and eating behavior is presumably controlled by food-related cues, a variety of behavior modification techniques seem appropriate.

Third, **endocrinopathic obesity** results from a disturbance (pathology) in the endocrine system. One of the more common endocrine pathologies that can cause obesity is hypothyroidism, in which the person has both a lower resting metabolic rate and reduced appetite.

The fourth type is **abnormal appetite regulation obesity.** This type of obesity has not been demonstrated apart from damage to the hypothalamic control system. Both this and endocrinopathic obesity should respond only to medical interventions to treat the underlying disease.

Fifth is **adipose cell proliferation obesity.** Here, adipocytes multiply to allow for continued storage of excess energy in the cells. A combination of psychosocial and medical interventions may be useful in these cases. Lifestyle changes may be necessary to help reduce health risks and maintain weight at a lower level. Further, lifestyle changes are important to avoid dangerous cycles of dieting and regaining weight. Surgical procedures include liposuction (female pattern) and gastroplasty (male pattern), but liposuction is primarily for cosmetic purposes. Typically, **gastroplasty**—surgical modification of stomach or intestines—is reserved for cases of morbid obesity that have not responded to other forms of treatment.

In the sixth type, **compulsive eating disorders,** presumably a psychological conflict or emotional disturbance leads to compulsive eating. Bulimia is the most notable example of this type of eating disorder. A second example is reactive eating, eating in response to high levels of stress or anxiety. In these cases, therapy may be combined with behavioral techniques to get weight under control and reduce the likelihood of recurrence of an eating disorder.

The seventh category is a **pharmacologically induced obesity.** In this case, the person gains weight because of a medication that brings about metabolic change. The appropriate treatment in this case is to switch to a medication that does not have the undesirable effect of weight gain.

Physiology of Obesity: Fat Cells and Triglycerides

The culprit in obesity is the fat cell, or the adipocyte. This cell unit transforms and stores excess energy as triglycerides. The triglycerides are housed in a lipid droplet in the cell, which then expands to accommodate new deposits (Björntorp, 1986). An enzyme known as **lipoprotein lipase** (LPL) sits on the cell surface and does the actual work to break down circulating fats (McMinn & Katahn, 1986). For this reason, LPL is called the gatekeeper of the adipocyte. As the process continues, cell metabolism actually speeds up and makes it easier to store even more excess energy.

Then, as a second step, new cells are recruited and added to store even more fat. These cells are probably pressed into service from the supply and support system. You might think of it as adding more safety deposit boxes to the bank vault. The net effect of these changes is that the system increases its capacity for storing fat. In morbid obesity, both the size and the number of fat cells increase markedly. Unfortunately, once cell proliferation begins, it cannot be reversed.

Further, it appears that the action of the gatekeeper LPL makes it difficult for the obese (especially those whose BMI ≥ 35) to lose weight. A study under the direction of Philip Kern at Cedars Sinai Medical Center suggests reasons (Kern, Ong, Saffari, & Carty, 1990). Kern's group used nine subjects whose average BMI of 43 indicated extreme obesity. After the subjects lost a substantial amount of weight but then stabilized, measures of LPL activity were obtained. This measure showed that weight loss resulted in an increase in LPL activity that was

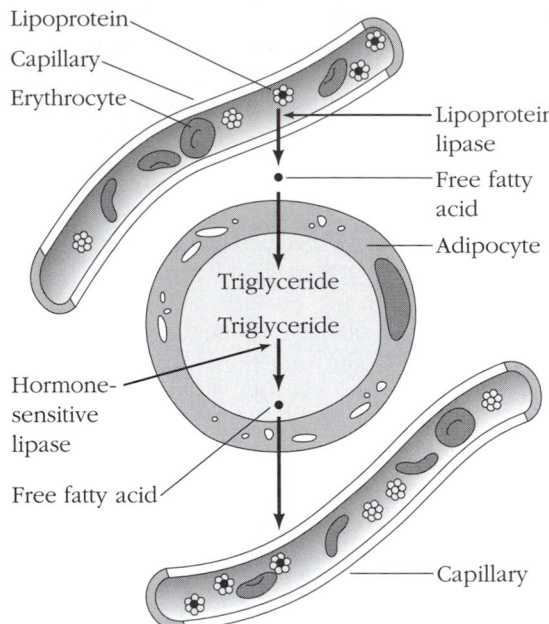

FIGURE 10.9   An adipocyte showing the metabolic process behind triglyceride storage in the cell (adapted from Willard, 1991).

varied according to the subject's BMI prior to weight loss. In other words, the higher the person's BMI was before the weight loss, the greater the increase in LPL activity following weight loss.

Kern's group suggested that overeating induces a perpetual state of LPL activation, which contrasts with the normal state of affairs in nonobese people. Under normal conditions, variation in LPL activity more or less follows caloric intake. LPL activity increases with more food intake and decreases with dietary restraint and weight loss. Dietary restraint reduces the tendency for more triglycerides to be stored in the adipocyte, which is, of course, the desirable outcome of efforts to lose weight. In the obese, though, LPL not only keeps on storing fat when calorie intake is reduced, but actually increases its activity to improve the process. Increased LPL activity also is suspected as the primary cause of strong urges to eat. For those wanting to lose weight, it seems a horrible injustice for nature to have concocted such a scheme.

Etiology of Obesity: Genetic, Behavioral, and Social Causes

The notion that obesity runs in families has a long history. As Ravussin and Swinburn (1992) point out, though, families share more than just genes. They share a common culture, diet, and some aspects of lifestyle. Thus genetic theory must be combined with knowledge of environmental influences (Grilo & Pogue-Geile, 1991). Here, we briefly consider the genetic, personality, and family theories of obesity.

Obesity as genetic predisposition   Evidence for a genetic contribution to obesity comes from several sources, including recent work that points to an obese gene and the classic twin and adoption studies. Using animal genetic models, investigators have found evidence for an **obese gene** that controls several physiological systems involved in obesity (Pelleymounter et al., 1995; Zhang et al., 1994). The altered systems include thermoregulation (resulting in lower body temperature), adrenal and thyroid function important to energy regulation, and numerous biochemical abnormalities. Mice with the so-called ob gene show morbid obesity, become diabetic, exhibit lower activity and reduced metabolism. Zhang's group also has succeeded in cloning the human variant of the ob gene. An interesting sidelight to the study by Pelleymounter and her group is that mice injected with ob protein showed reduced weight and increased activity, indicating that the condition may be in part reversible.

Grilo and Pogue-Geile (1991) provided summary figures based on review of many twin studies. In one twin concordance study, monozygotic twins showed a stronger concordance for being overweight than dizygotic twins did (Stunkard, Foch, & Hrubec, 1986). Further, when monozygotic twins were reared in separate homes (adoption studies), they showed more similarity to their biological parents' weights than to their adoptive parents' weights (Stunkard et al., 1986). But these studies may also provide the strongest evidence against an environmental hypothesis, since most correlations between adoptive parent and adoptee on any of several weight measures are close to zero.

Further evidence of a genetic contribution comes from studies of food absorption. At the beginning of this chapter, you read of an elderly gentleman, Al, who each day ate 25 eggs, containing about 5000 mg of dietary cholesterol. Fred Kern (1991), who conducted the study with Al, thought there might be differences in one or more of the energy regulation mechanisms that could explain why Al's cholesterol levels were nevertheless normal. Kern's logic was based on studies in animals that have identified several genetic determinants of energy regulation. Kern compared Al's absorbed cholesterol to five subjects on low and high cholesterol diets. While the normal subjects absorbed about 55% of the cholesterol on the low diet and more than 46% of the cholesterol on the high diet, Al absorbed only 18% of the cholesterol from his 25 eggs. He still absorbed more cholesterol per day than the normal subjects, but he disposed of about twice as much cholesterol in bile acids. These changes left little dietary cholesterol to raise blood cholesterol. These processes parallel those found to have genetic components in animal studies.

Bouchard and his group took a different approach to this issue. They overfed monozygotic twins for 84 days and monitored weight change (Bouchard, Tremblay, et al., 1990). They found that twins gained on average between 4.3 and 13.3 kg. Within twin pairs, though, the variability in weight gain was much less. In a review of weights from both identical and fraternal twins reared together and reared apart, Stunkard came to the conclusion that 70% of the variance in weight could be accounted for by the genetic factor, and the remaining 30% by environmental factors (Stunkard, Harris, Pederson, & McClearn, 1990).

One issue hotly debated over the past few years is whether weight gain follows reduced energy expenditure or, instead, lower energy output is a natural consequence of weight gain. This is the proverbial chicken and egg issue: Which comes first? Eric Ravussin's group studied a large sample of adult southwestern Native Americans (Ravussin et al., 1988). The researchers found that lower resting metabolic rate predicts weight gain. Further, they found that family membership predicts this low metabolic rate. Although Ravussin's study used data from an adult sample, similar conclusions have been drawn from observations of infants born to lean and overweight mothers (Roberts, Savage, Coward, Chew, & Lucas, 1988). Both Ravussin's and Roberts's studies suggest that low energy output is part of the metabolic process that leads to obesity, rather than a change that occurs once one has become obese.

Finally, early but incomplete data suggest that the predisposition to an eating disorder also has a genetic component. Anorexia nervosa and bulimia occur at a significantly higher incidence rate among first-degree female relatives of anorexic patients compared to the immediate families of control subjects (Gershon et al., 1983; Strober, Morrell, Burroughs, Salkin, & Jacobs, 1985). Further, monozygotic twins have a much higher concordance rate for anorexia than dizygotic twins (Crisp, Hall, & Holland, 1985).

Psychodynamic and personality theories   Psychoanalytic theory made many excursions into psychosomatic disorders, so it could not very well ignore obesity. Psychoanalytic theory proposed that obesity results from unresolved conflicts. Presumably the person turns to eating as an escape from a reality that is too harsh to bear. Unfortunately, this defense proves maladaptive and the person becomes trapped in a cycle of emotional frustration, self-doubt, and still more eating.

Clinical descriptions of the obese personality use such terms as neurotic, dependent, and in need of oral gratification. A typical personality profile paints the picture of a person with emotional frustration, a strong desire to be loved, passive dependence, and poor coping skills (McReynolds, 1982). One research team describes a subtype of obese clients who are obsessive-compulsive (Mount, Neziroglu, & Taylor, 1990). Others suggest that obesity is a self-handicapping strategy that gives an excuse for failure. Baumeister, Kahn, and Tice (1990) were unable to find evidence to either support or refute this notion. Another view is that eating is a response to depression or anxiety; this view also has little empirical support (Striegel-Moore & Rodin, 1986). Comparisons of obese and nonobese people show roughly the same distribution of traits in the two groups.

Robert Klesges and his associates used both cross-sectional and longitudinal analyses to look at relationships between psychosocial functioning and body fat in children (Klesges et al., 1992). The investigators assessed several esteem and cognitive variables plus family functioning. The only variable that consistently predicted higher levels of future body fat, however, was physical self-competence. In brief, as the child's reported level of physical self-competence went down, body fat went up on future assessments.

A number of investigators have looked at locus of control and obesity. **Locus of control** is the expectancy that personal actions will be effective to control or master the environment (Rotter, 1966, 1990). In Rotter's model, people vary on a continuum between two extremes called external and internal locus of control. Lefcourt (1976) defined an **external locus of control** as the perception that events are outside the realm of personal control. An **internal locus of control,** the perception that events are under personal control, may be associated with successful treatment of the obese. The prevailing notion was that the obese clients come into weight loss programs with an external locus of control. Mills (1992), however, reported that many obese subjects in his studies had an internal locus of control prior to entering a weight loss program. He argued that obese individuals may be internal with regard to most

of their life affairs even if they do feel that weight is beyond their control.

One widely discussed psychological theory of obesity was that proposed by Stanley Schachter and Judith Rodin (1974) based on notions of internal and external stimulus control. In this view, the person who manages to keep a normal weight starts and stops eating in response to internal stimuli that signal hunger or fullness. Obese people, though, presumably respond primarily to external cues. The clock, an advertisement on TV, the suggestion of a friend—"Let's go eat something"—all could trigger eating. Once started eating, the cues of sight, texture, and taste of the food keep these people eating long after internal signals have indicated that they have eaten enough.

When Rodin (1981) reviewed the stimulus control theory later, she asked the cryptic question of this hypothesis: "What went wrong?" Rodin noted that all overweight people are not externally responsive and that all normal weight people are not internally sensitive. Some over-

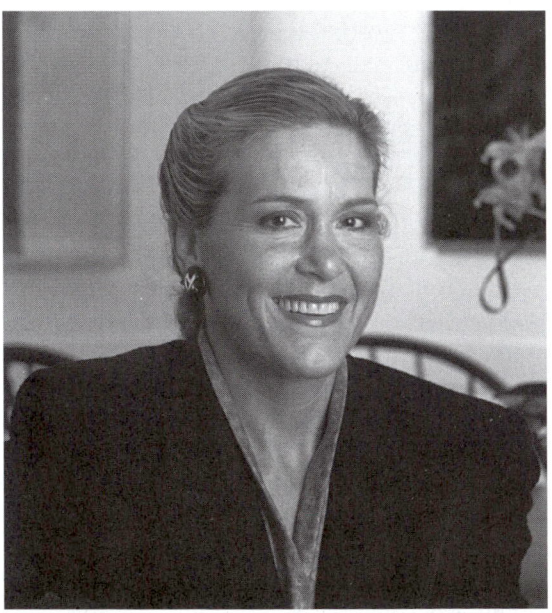

FIGURE 10.10   Judith Rodin, president of the University of Pennsylvania and respected research psychologist.

weight people are largely nonresponsive to external cues. Further, there were remarkably few differences between obese and normal weight people on a variety of eating behaviors. Both normal and obese people eat larger quantities when the food is tasty. Yet obese people tend to eat more food when it is not tasty (see review by Spitzer & Rodin, 1981). The internal-external theory became less and less tenable as investigators discovered more biological grounds for obesity.

Further, Striegel-Moore and Rodin (1985) reviewed a host of factors involved in the prevention of obesity. Their review suggests that feeding practices during infancy, childhood learning experiences including acquired food preferences and aversions, and problems with self-control skills are very important in developing and maintaining obesity.

During this same time frame, an alternative formulation called restraint theory began to emerge. Restraint theory suggested that many people, obese and nonobese, try to force their weight below a biological set point (Herman & Polivy, 1975). These people are referred to as restrained eaters because of their tendency to try to curtail food intake severely (diet) to control weight. The alternate group, unrestrained eaters, do not engage regularly in dietary restraint. A large body of data accumulated to support this distinction. Restrained eaters placed under stress or given a so-called preload, a milkshake, tend to eat much more. This tendency to eat more after having just eaten is called the counterregulatory effect. Cognitive processes, especially beliefs about caloric intake, are far more important in the counterregulatory effect than actual caloric intake. On the other hand, unrestrained eaters do not respond to stress by eating more. Further, they will eat far less after a preload than after no preload. This suggests that restrained eaters may lose control under certain conditions, whereas unrestrained eaters exercise good control.

Michael Lowe (1993) believes that restraint theory is far too simplistic to account for attempts to regulate weight. He suggested that dieting behavior has to be considered in the context of three general factors, including weight status, dieting history, and mediating processes. Weight status ranges from obese, to normal weight, to underweight. Dieting history includes previous cycles of dieting, current dieting, and weight suppression. Weight suppression is weight loss that is sustained over a long time. Mediating processes including psychological, biological, and sensory factors. Lowe argued that eating behavior displayed by restrained eaters (whether obese or nonobese) is a product of their frequent dieting and overeating, not cognitive restraint or current dieting practice. This approach may be applicable to eating behavior across the range of body types and weights, not just to the obese.

Weight Loss Strategies: Medical, Dietary, and Behavioral Methods

The benefits of achieving and maintaining normal weight are now well known. The exact benefit depends on how overweight the person is, how much weight they lose, how consistently they keep the weight off, and how they lose the weight. The more overweight, the greater the benefits assuming that the person uses a carefully managed program. Virtually all cardiac risk factors return to near normal as weight loss occurs (Bray, 1986), but gains may be seen with even 10% weight loss.

At any one time, 25% to 30% of adult Americans may be trying to lose weight through dietary restraint (Bouchard, 1991). A large-scale study in the workplace, using a point prevalence estimate, found that 13% of men and 25% of women were dieting (Jeffery, Adlis, & Forster, 1991).[7] Unfortunately, about 90% of dieters who lose 25 pounds regain most or all of the weight within two years (Pace, Bolton, & Reeves, 1991).

---

[7] Compare these findings to prevalence data showing that 30% of men and 35% of women are overweight.

When regaining weight becomes part of a long-term pattern of weight cycling, or yo-yo dieting, additional health risks arise. Analysis of data from the Framingham sample showed for both men and women that rates of total mortality, coronary mortality, and coronary disease morbidity increased as variability in body weight increased (Lissner et al., 1991). At one time, it was thought that weight cycling would lead to more depression or some other adverse long-term psychological outcomes, but this does not appear to be the case (Bartlett, Wadden, & Vogt, 1996; Foster, Wadden, Kendall, Stunkard, & Vogt, 1996). Still, weight cycling gives a poor prognosis for future meaningful weight loss.

Potential problems also exist in the weight loss industry, which has spawned hundreds of programs all over the nation. Some of these programs are well thought out and reasonably safe, but some are no more than marketing ploys to capitalize (in the most unsavory sense of that term) on what is now a multibillion dollar industry. Recent congressional hearings found that Americans now spend over $10 billion a year to try to lose weight (Wadden, Foster, Letizia, & Stunkard, 1992); others place the figure closer to $30 billion (Callaway et al., 1992). The industry is only minimally regulated in spite of the potential for significant harm, up to and including death, if weight loss is not managed properly.

The most prominent strategies to help achieve weight loss are medical-pharmacologic interventions that focus on reducing appetite; dietary restraint, to reduce energy intake; exercise, to increase energy output; and cognitive-behavioral strategies, to help people exercise a higher degree of self-control. It is now common wisdom that successful weight loss typically has to include at least a balanced intake-output strategy and some degree of environmental control. The day of simplistic explanations of obesity is past; the same goes for the one-shot intervention. Indeed, some data suggest that interventions for obesity must of necessity be long term (Kirschenbaum et al., 1992).

Pharmacotherapy of Weight Loss

Abuse of over-the-counter amphetamines for weight loss helped give pharmacotherapy strategies a bad name (Callaway et al., 1992). Nonetheless, some cases may justify use of appetite-reducing drugs. Fenfluramine HCL (Pondimin) was the last anorectic approved by the FDA. Fenfluramine is chemically similar to the amphetamines, but it works in a different way. It increases serotonin release and then inhibits reuptake. Since serotonin induces feelings of fullness, fenfluramine reduces the urge to eat. Another drug used to promote weight loss is fluoxetine (Prozac). Typically, patients receive fluoxetine only when depression and over-weight do not respond to other treatments.

Dieting for Weight Loss

It is hardly a revelation that dietary restraint is the most commonly used method for weight control and weight loss. Both self-directed and clinic-directed programs are used for these purposes. There are concerns that self-directed dietary restraint programs may lead to serious problems for the uninformed. The risks increase as the proposed diet plan becomes more severe either in reducing caloric intake or compromising nutritional balance. Add to this the possibility that people using dietary restraint may already have health problems, and the elements for a potential disaster are in place.

Thus it is all the more important to include nutritional education both in general health programs in the public school system as well as in formal weight loss programs. The American Dietetic Association takes the position that sufficient information must be provided to dieters to enable them to make their own informed choices (Pace, Bolton, & Reeves, 1991). In addition, long-term maintenance of weight loss depends on being able to manage several aspects of altered lifestyle, including planning a reasonable but controlled diet.

Nicholas and Dwyer (1986) pointed out three

more reasons why nutrition must be carefully considered before implementing a weight loss plan. First, after dieting has produced the desired weight loss, life goes on. One must plan as much for maintenance of reduced weight as for the actual loss. One way to do so is to plan for a transition diet that is still informed and wise in food choices after going off the weight loss diet and before resuming a more relaxed eating style. Since the typical diet lasts about six months and sometimes longer, there is usually ample time to build in a plan that aids transition.

Further, it is important to consider aspects of diet that influence motivation and compliance. The dietary composition can influence such variables as water retention, appetite, and satiety. If the person sees little significant weight loss because of water retention, motivation to continue will generally be lower. The same is true of hunger and appetite. If the foods do not provide for a comfortable level of fullness, the dieter will be constantly fighting urges to eat.

Finally, dietary needs change at different points in the life cycle. Thus, diets can have different effects at different times, influencing such critical processes as growth, sexual maturation, and fetal growth and development during pregnancy.

Fasting is the most extreme form of dieting, but it can be done in a variety of ways. Most often, fasting does not involve complete abstinence from food, and it is usually not done over an extended period of time. Fasting typically allows fluid intake and sometimes may be accompanied by bread or crackers. Some dangers in fasting need to be recognized, however. First, extreme fasting regimens can lead to potassium loss and muscle malfunction if strenuous activity takes place. Second, fasting can lead to dehydration and kidney malfunction. Finally, it can increase risk for infections and cardiovascular irregularities (Nicholas & Dwyer, 1986).

One problem in controlling a diet is that many people are very inept at calculating the size of the portions they are eating, and they are even worse at estimating both the caloric content and the nutritional content of what they are eating. Errors in estimates of weights of food are often on the order of 50% (Jensen, Wahrendorf, Rosenquisit, & Geser, 1984). There is some suspicion that this fact may be behind some dieting failures.

Steven Lichtman's group found evidence that obese subjects eat much more food than their self-reported diets showed (Lichtman et al., 1992). Subjects in one group reported taking in only 1028 kcal per day but their actual intake was 2081 kcal, a whopping 47% error in reporting. Further, they exercised a lot less than they said. In both cases, the energy imbalance—too much energy intake and not enough energy output—sustains weight. Rather than a deliberate attempt to deceive, these errors in reporting were probably related to inaccurate perceptions of the number of calories contained in food portions.

The conventional meal pattern of three meals per day—morning, noon, and evening—has evolved not out of biologic necessity, but to accommodate lifestyle and workdays. Yet studies of eating behavior suggest that the smaller the number of meals, the more likely larger quantities will be consumed. Further, people pressed by time in modern technological society tend to eat much faster than is desirable. All three of these factors—fewer meals, larger quantities, and faster eating—work against the body's natural energy balance mechanisms to increase the likelihood that more of the food will become fat.

These eating habits could be adjusted in a number of ways to help offset some of the negative consequences of this pattern. Because eating challenges the energy system, increases metabolism, and thus burns energy (some say wastes energy), a very simple intervention is to increase the number of meals, reduce the quantity of food, and slow down the rate of eating. It is, of course, easier said than done to make these changes. But solid evidence indicates that these changes can have beneficial effects, primarily in reducing risks related to cholesterol levels.

David Jenkins and his associates conducted a two-week study in which several men went on a nibbling meal plan while others stayed on the conventional three meal plan (Jenkins et al., 1989). The nibbling meal plan divided the three-meal quantity into 17 snacks. Thus, the nibbling group frequently ate small quantities. This is probably not a practical plan, but the authors forced the treatment to the extreme to get a clearer indication of what the effects might be. At the end of the two weeks, the nibbling group had reduced total cholesterol as well as LDLs. Further, they had lower C-peptide, serum insulin, and urinary cortisol compared to the three-meal group. These outcomes suggest that frequent intake of smaller quantities could help to reduce health risks related to being overweight.

Behavioral Methods: Reinforcement, Economics, and Habit

At the risk of beginning this section on an unduly cynical note, a comment made by Mark McMinn and Martin Katahn probably states the case for behavioral methods as concisely as it can be stated: "Behavioral treatments . . . provide a recent illustration of our lack of understanding, limited success, and our frustration" (1986, p. 89). In an earlier review of behavioral treatments for hyperlipidemia, the authors concluded that outcome research had failed to show behavioral strategies could be effective to maintain the necessary changes in diet and other behaviors to sustain clinically meaningful change over the long term (Carmody, Fey, Pierce, Connor, & Matarazzo, 1982).

Kelly Brownell and Thomas Wadden (1986) cited data showing that the average weight loss produced by behavioral methods was in the 10 pound range. The studies produced great variability, however, from only 2 pounds lost to nearly 19 pounds. Early programs most commonly used stimulus control and self-monitoring methods, though other techniques were tried off and on. Later modifications added cognitive restructuring, exercise, and social support. The

actual amount of weight lost went up but only because the length of the programs also increased. The per week average weight lost did not change. The most discouraging note was that weight loss could not be maintained by these methods.

Nonetheless, behavioral methods, either alone or combined with cognitive intervention strategies, have become the mainstay of weight loss programs. Typically, diet, exercise, social support, cognitive restructuring, and behavioral methods are combined. Behavioral techniques usually include stimulus control over eating behavior, self-monitoring, slower eating, and disruption of eating chains. The intent is to increase compliance with dietary restraints as well as to maintain consistent exercise. Cognitive restructuring includes goal setting, attitude changes, and coping techniques that will prevent relapse. Social support may focus on cooperation of spouse and other family members or people in the client's social network.

Judith Rodin and her colleagues combined cognitive behavioral methods with pharmacologic treatment (Rodin, Elias, Silberstein, & Wagner, 1988). The drug in this case was Tenuate, and the cognitive behavioral program lasted for 20 weeks. The experimental design called for a Tenuate plus CB therapy group, a placebo plus CB therapy group, and a CB therapy group. The cognitive component included instruction in eating behavior, the energy balance equation, exercise, self-cognitions and attitudes toward self, and relapse training, including coping skills and self-efficacy training.

Weight loss occurred for all groups during weeks 5 through 11; additional weight loss during weeks 11 through 16 occurred only in the Tenuate group. Although the Tenuate group lost the most weight, there were no significant differences between the three groups in the last weeks of the program. The research team took follow-up measures at six months and one year. The Tenuate group had regained a significant amount of weight in that time. Yet practically speaking, it only removed the slight difference that existed between the groups at the end of training. At the one-year follow-up, the CB therapy group showed better total sustained loss than the other two groups. These results suggest that cognitive-behavioral methods may be effective to sustain weight loss.

Anorexia Nervosa: Symptoms, Origins, and Treatment

At the pinnacle of her success, Karen Carpenter sang one song that seemed to me to be her trademark: "I'm on the top of the world." As she did with most of her hits, she sang it in a mellow, graceful style, filled with a sense of happiness. The style of her music and her public image seemed somehow to have their own harmony.

Karen was by most accounts squeaky clean, scrupulously avoiding the appearance of inpropriety, especially the twin sins of sexual promiscuity and drug use that were for many popular singers trademarks of their antiestablishment music.

But for about 12 years, Karen had kept a dark secret that most of her friends, many in her family, and certainly none of her fans knew. After reading a review that commented on her chubbiness, probably around 1970 or 1971, Karen became obsessed with her appearance and weight. At this time, her press pictures still showed the wholesome, beautiful, and vibrant Karen that everyone knew. A photograph taken just three years before her death in 1983, though, showed a gaunt, tired, and aged Karen.

Karen's closet illness was anorexia nervosa.

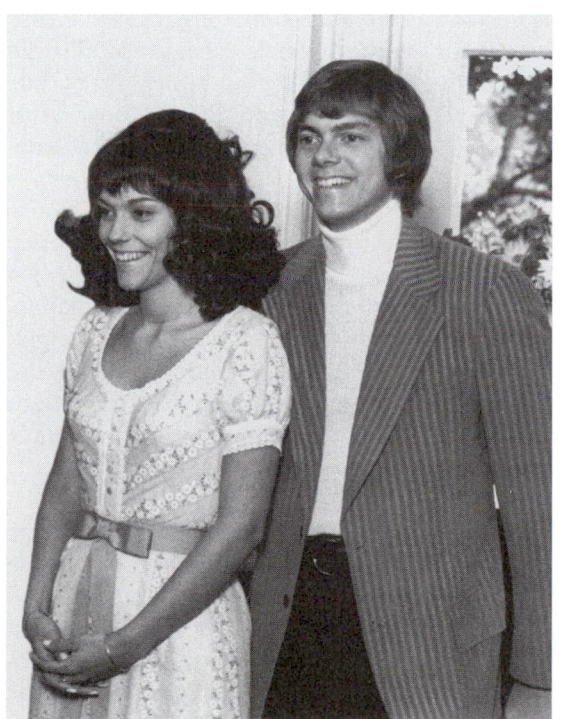 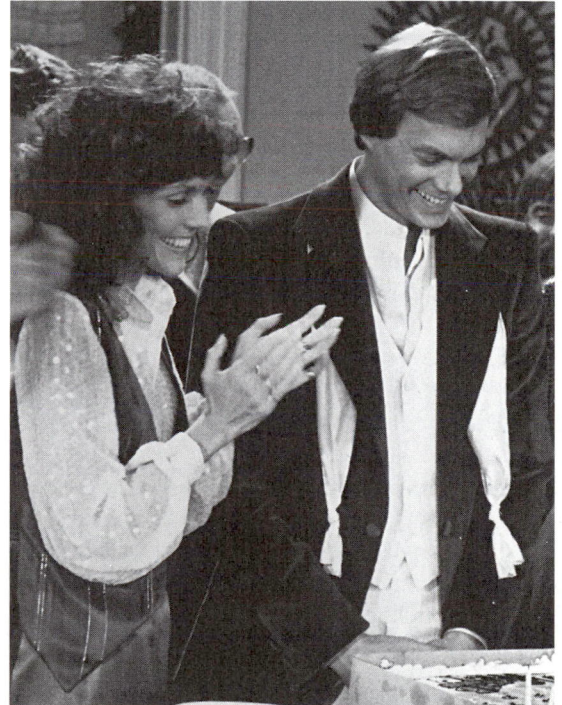

FIGURE 10.11 Karen Carpenter (left, early in her career; right, later in her career) kept her secret of anorexia nervosa hidden from public view, but her death called attention to the terrible ordeal that its victims may go through.

She abused her body, not as an addict would, but through an extreme starvation diet driven by her need to be thin. At one point, she weighed in at a skeletal 83 pounds (Diliberto, 1985). But no matter how much weight she lost, she still could not accept her appearance.

Therapy helped her restore some weight, and her therapist was convinced that she was cured. Before long, though, she returned to her old bad habits and tragically added to them as well. She began to use an over-the-counter drug called ipecac to help lose weight. In clinical terms, ipecac is an emetic, a substance that induces vomiting. Doctors sometimes recommend that parents keep ipecac in the medicine cabinet as an antidote should a child swallow poison. But, ipecac can cause irreversible heart damage if taken in large doses, and it can be lethal when taken regularly. Evidence obtained after her death revealed that Karen first increased her consumption of ipecac to several teaspoons following the evening meal, and later to a bottle or two at a time. This was apparently what led to heart failure and her death at age 32.

Anorexia Nervosa: Criteria, Subtypes, and Eating Patterns

Disordered eating patterns—including anorexia nervosa and bulimia—are not a modern phenomenon. Anorexia was reported as early as 1689 in one report (Jones & Nagel, 1992), and by 1874 binge eating and bulimia were also described (Johnson, 1987). The term *anorexia* refers to a loss of appetite, but it is somewhat of a misnomer since loss of appetite rarely occurs. It is, in reality, the refusal to eat due to fear of fatness. Many anorexics are obsessed with food, and they engage in a number of compulsive behaviors related to this obsession, such as hoarding food. The current diagnostic standard, DSM-IV (APA, 1994), uses four primary criteria to diagnose anorexia nervosa.

First, the person refuses to maintain a body weight over the minimum desirable weight for the person's age and height. DSM-IV defines the minimum desirable as 85% of the weight expected for age and height. Second, the person has an intense fear of gaining weight even when underweight. This fear is sometimes described in cognitive terms as obsessive. Third, the person has a disturbed body image and maintains a distorted perception of heaviness in spite of severe weight loss and even when confronted with external objective evidence. The fourth criterion, relevant only to women, is amenorrhea, the absence of three consecutive menstrual cycles. Efforts are underway to capture these criteria in a self-report format that will aid the diagnosis and study of eating disorders (Mintz, O'Halloran, Mulholland, & Schneider, 1997).

A few men do suffer from anorexia nervosa, but the disorder is still predominantly a disorder among young women. It occurs in about 1% of women aged 15 to 40. The average age of onset is 17 years. Probably no more than 1 male case occurs for every 20 female cases. Typically, the disorder occurred among the upper and middle classes. This distinguishing demographic factor has been disappearing over the past two decades.

Two subtypes of anorexia occur, distinguished primarily by the eating pattern they use to control weight. A person belonging to the first subtype, the **restricting type,** uses dieting, fasting, and vigorous exercise to lose weight. Someone belonging to the second subtype, the **binge/purge type,** has gone on eating binges and purges during the current episode and may binge and purge each week.

Typically, the anorexic greatly reduces total food intake and engages in strenuous exercise in order to lose the offending weight. These activities may be combined with self-induced vomiting, laxatives, and diuretics. When weight loss reaches severe levels, physical complications may become apparent as well. Most of the physical side effects result from extreme starvation and usually can be reversed with treatment.

Theories of Etiology: Family, Image, and Genetics

Observations of and attempts to explain anorexia are certainly not new. Psychoanalysts, such as Franz Alexander (1950), provided explanations of anorexia that seemed consistent with the classical theory of emotional conflict. In Alexander's view, the newborn child who stubbornly refused to suckle at its mother's breast was the prototype of anorexia nervosa. Further, psychoanalytic theory viewed the child as spiteful, one who wanted to manipulate and gain increased attention from the parents.

Current theories attempt to explain the origins of anorexia in terms of physiology, personality, or familial characteristics. Interestingly, lay people tend to think about anorexia nervosa in terms consistent with scientific theories even if they lack the details. Lay people tend to attribute anorexia nervosa to family disorder, social pressure, the problems associated with passage to adulthood, and conflicting roles and pressures on women (Furnham & Hume-Wright, 1992).

Biological theories propose that both genetic and biochemical mechanisms influence the emergence of anorexia nervosa. Both anorexia nervosa and bulimia occur at higher rates among first-degree female relatives of anorexic patients (Gershon et al., 1983; Strober, et al., 1985). Further, monozygotic twins have higher concordance for anorexia than dizygotic twins (Crisp et al., 1985).

A review of neurochemical abnormalities in eating disorders reveals that both anorexic and bulimic patients show disturbances in brain neurotransmitters (Fava, Copeland, Schweiger, & Herzog, 1989). Anorexic patients show lower norepinephrine activity and abnormalities in secretion of vasopressin. There are slight differences in the pattern of change in bulimic patients. Yet, these changes return to normal with refeeding and weight gain. This finding suggests that the brain neurochemistry changes in response either to the weight loss or to caloric deprivation or both. Another explanation is

possible, though. The neurochemical changes could alter mood, leading to changed eating patterns and anorexia nervosa. At this time, the data are not sufficiently unambiguous to allow a clearer interpretation.

Family systems theory, championed by Bruch (1973), suggests that the roots of anorexia nervosa lie in a disordered family environment. The family is sick functionally. The father and mother may show some form of psychopathology, but the anorexic member expresses the pathology for the entire family. Still, Bruch went beyond family dynamics. She recognized the need to monitor the anorexic's nutritional status and to observe her food intake attitudes and behaviors.[8]

Minuchin, Rosman, and Baker (1978) proposed that anorexic patients came from psychosomatic families. The traits of such families include (1) enmeshment, including intense family interactions; (2) overprotectiveness that hinders the child's progress to independence; (3) rigidity in family structure, rules, and resistance to change; and (4) lack of conflict resolution, including avoidance of conflicts. Although highly regarded as a theoretical model, Minuchin's theory has not stood up well in clinical tests (Hall, 1987).

In sum, a complete and clear picture of the etiology of anorexia does not exist in any of the theories taken individually. Anorexia nervosa appears to be a multiply determined disorder combining biological, psychological, and familial-social factors.

Treatments for Anorexia Nervosa: Medical, Cognitive, and Family

Treatment strategies attempt to restore normal weight through controlled refeeding and weight maintenance later. One perennial problem,

---

[8] Bulimic patients may not see the same degree of conflict that has been reported in families with anorexic members (Kent & Clopton, 1992).

though, is that anorexia nervosa patients usually do not seek treatment voluntarily and they do not want to be treated (Yates, 1989). They come to treatment because of family pressure and fear over severe weight loss, physical problems associated with weight loss, or psychological symptoms including suicidal thoughts. Therapies differ in the extent to which they focus on attitudes, behaviors, and family process as part of the treatment.

Since the work of Hilda Bruch, family therapy has been one of the primary therapies of choice. Family therapy provides support for all the family members and direction to help the parents manage eating problems in the patient. This approach has had inconsistent results, however. Hall (1987) reported that the family systems approach seemed to work only in intact families with younger patients when the entire family attended.

Inpatient medical treatment typically uses a controlled diet of 1200 to 1500 calories per day at the beginning. Rapid weight gain early in treatment is undesirable and can be life-threatening. Caloric intake is increased each week to about 3500 calories and then maintained until normal weight is achieved. Most therapy programs will include nutritional counseling to help the person achieve healthy daily eating habits. Several programs combine behavioral methods to encourage and monitor weight gain. Behavioral methods alone do not seem to be any more effective than other therapeutic interventions.

Pharmacotherapy has also had limited success. One antipsychotic agent, chlorpromazine, has been used on an inpatient basis because it tends to reduce anxiety and improve appetite (Yates, 1989).

Bulimia: Symptoms, Origins, and Treatment

If you sat beside Angela in comp class, you would have few clues to the problem hidden behind the facade she keeps up for all but one or two of her most intimate friends. On the surface, she seems to be a reasonably normal, energetic, inquisitive, and bright young woman. She is actively involved in school, has a part-time job, and does volunteer work for a regional crises intervention center. She is neat and well-dressed even when going casual, and her weight is about average for her height.

But if you could follow Angela through a week, you would see a pattern of behavior that reveals a disturbed self-image expressing itself in uncontrolled binges of eating followed by self-induced vomiting to get rid of the excess food eaten. Angela's binges occur as many as five or six times each week. She estimates that she takes in almost 4000 calories in most of her binges, but there are times when she consumes more than 10,000 calories in a single binge. Often, what she eats during these binges is anything but healthy. She may down a quart or more of rich ice cream laced with an entire pack of cookies and several cans of soda pop.

Angela has no apparent health problems yet, but she knows her behavior could lead to serious health consequences in the future. Most important, she is increasingly concerned about what the binges say about herself, her self-esteem, and her inability to control what is going on in this facet of her life. She has sought out information, discreetly, to try to get a handle on her situation, but as yet, she has not been willing to seek professional help or make any real effort to change. This pattern is typical of many young women who suffer from bulimia.

A Clinical Portrait: Binges, Purges, and Control

The modern era of clinical concern for bulimia can be traced to 1976. A large number of Cornell University female students sought counseling for a peculiar pattern of behavior that involved eating large amounts of food followed by forced vomiting, laxatives, diuretics, or continuous dieting to rid themselves of the unwanted consequences of their excess. The term *bulima-rexia* was first used at this time. Clinicians considered bulimia to be a rare disorder and they paid little or no attention to purging (Boskind-White & White, 1986). Later, when Russell (1979) described the syndrome, there was confusion over diagnostic criteria because of the use of overlapping samples of anorexics and bulimics.

In DSM-IV (1994), bulimia nervosa is recognized as a disorder with five distinguishing features:

1. There are recurrent episodes of binge eating when large quantities of food are consumed.
2. There is recurrent purging behavior using forced vomiting, laxatives, diuretics, dieting, or vigorous exercise to prevent weight gain.
3. The binge eating and purging occur on average twice a week for three months (severity criterion).
4. There is persistent and undue concern over body shape and weight.
5. The disorder does not occur exclusively during episodes of anorexia nervosa.

Several features distinguish bulimia from anorexia. The bulimic client is usually within normal weight range for body build and age, whereas the anorexic is typically below average weight. Some bulimics may even be at the upper end of the weight range. Many anorexics do not use the purging techniques that bulimics do. In anorexic patients, appetite is decreased because of unconscious emotional factors. In bulimia, appetite is exaggerated. Only rarely do organic factors play a role in bulimia. Finally, although amenorrhea is not listed as a primary diagnostic criteria, one study reported that it occurred in nearly half the sample investigated (Glassman, Rich, Darko, & Clarkin, 1991).

Current estimates of prevalence suggest about 1% to 3% of adolescent and young adult females fit the profile, although prevalence estimates vary greatly (Fairburn & Beglin, 1990; Johnson, 1987). The prevalence in males is about one-tenth that in females (American Psychiatric Association, 1994).

Etiology of Bulimia Nervosa: Opioids, Stress, and Cognitions

Ruth Striegel-Moore and her associates point out one problem in developing an etiological model of bulimia: the heterogeneity of the women who develop the disorder (Striegel-Moore, Silberstein, & Rodin, 1986). Explanations of etiology run the gamut from the biological, to the familial (Kent & Clopton, 1992), to the social.

A biological theory suggests that bulimia may be in part caused by abnormalities in endogenous opioids (Jonas & Gold, 1988).[9] The nature of the mechanism is still uncertain, but speculation centers on the notion that bulimia is a compulsive behavior with loss of control over eating behavior. The compulsive nature of bulimia shares some similarity to drug addictions. The theory suggests that purging bulimics have higher levels of beta-endorphins (a specific brain opioid), a point that has been supported by some research. The binge-purge cycle presumably leads to increased release of opioids, a consequent reduction in anxiety, and heightened feelings of well-being. Again, supporting evidence shows that the binge-purge cycle produces levels of beta-endorphins higher than those in normal subjects. Finally, the theory receives support from treatments that use naltrexone (Trexan), an opioid antagonist. More will be said of this work momentarily.

Psychological theories have focused on stress (Cattanach & Rodin, 1988) and on cognitive components of bulimia. The stress model suggests that bulimics perceive that they lack control, experience higher levels of anxiety, and have coping deficits that influence the origins and maintenance of bulimia.

Cognitive elements include overconcern with body weight, size, and shape; body image distortion; desire to be thinner; and perception of being out of control when eating. Body image

---

[9] Endogenous opioids are morphine-like substances that occur naturally (are endogenous) in the brain and serve to reduce the perception of pain. We will have more to say about these substances in Chapter 13.

is a psychological experience that focuses on one's attitudes and feelings toward one's body (McCrea, Summerfield, & Rosen, 1982). Heatherton and Baumeister (1991) suggested that binge eating in bulimics is supported by an attempt to escape from self-awareness. Cognitive distortions may be important in both the initiation and maintenance of bulimia.

Grissett and Norvell (1992) believe that several social variables play an important role in the emergence of bulimia. They used a sample of bulimic women from a university setting and carefully matched them to non–eating disorder control cases. Grissett and Norvell observed, first, that the bulimic women reported lower perceived social support from their network of family and friends. This finding is supported in the work of Wonderlich, Klein, and Council (1996), who found that bulimic females viewed parental relationships as disengaged and unfriendly, if not hostile. Second, in Grissett and Norvell's study, the bulimic women reported more negative interpersonal interactions and higher levels of conflict. Finally, the bulimic women reported lower social skills and social competence compared to the matched control cases.

Treatment of Bulimia: Naltrexone and Cognitive-Behavior Therapy

Many different therapeutic models have surfaced to help bulimia patients, ranging from individual psychotherapy to group cognitive therapies (Kettlewell, Mizes, & Wasylyshyn, 1992). We will describe the most representative efforts.

One biomedical theory already discussed proposes that endogenous opioids contribute to the etiology of bulimia. Based on this notion, Jonas and Gold (1988) conducted a study using naltrexone, an opioid antagonist, as a treatment for 16 bulimia clients. Naltrexone works to block the effect of opioids, which may then lead to more aversive qualities in the binge-purge cycle instead of feelings of well-being. About half the

subjects received a low dose (50–100 mg) of naltrexone, while the other half received a high dose (200–300 mg). At the end of six weeks, the high-dose group showed significant reductions in days of binge eating and purging. In contrast, the low-dose group showed little or no clinical improvement. Four of the subjects from the low-dose group elected to cross over—that is, to receive the high-dose treatment at the end of the regular study. When they did so, they also showed substantial reductions in days of binge eating and purging. The data presented in Figure 10.12 are adapted from Jonas and Gold. The sample is small, and thus the results must be interpreted cautiously. The crossover subjects (labeled "CO" in Figure 10.12), in particular, might have been more motivated to change, or to have had expectancy effects that further changed their behavior. Further, mere success of a therapy is not in and of itself proof of etiology.

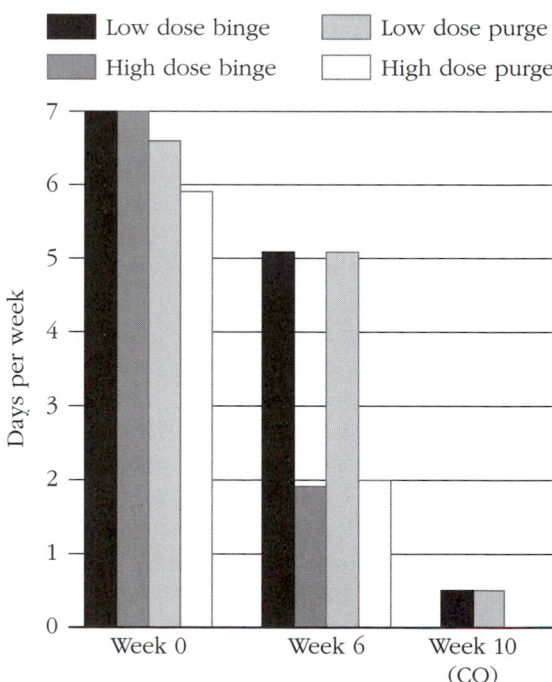

FIGURE 10.12   *The effects of naltrexone at two dose levels on days of binge eating and purging (n = 16) (data from Jonas and Gold, 1988).*

Cognitive-behavior therapy: binges, purges, and control One example of a behavioral technique is the exposure-response prevention (ERP) procedure developed by Leitenberg's group (Rosen & Leitenberg, 1982). This model is based on the notion that purging is maintained by the reduction of anxiety generated from fear of weight gain after bingeing. The technique then tries to prevent or delay purging after bingeing. Results of this approach have been mixed, however.

What predicts success in treatment? The answer may depend on whether you take success at the end of treatment as the criterion or whether you are concerned with success at a more distant follow-up point. Chris Fairburn and his colleagues addressed this issue in a closed follow-up design (Fairburn, Peveler, Jones, Hope, & Doll, 1993); that is, treated clients were not allowed to use alternative therapies during the follow-up period. They found that only two variables were associated with outcome: attitudes toward shape and weight, and self-esteem. In sum, the more residual disturbance in attitudes toward shape and weight and the lower the person's self-esteem, the poorer the long-term outcome.

Donna Thackwray led a research team comparing a behavioral treatment (BT) approach and a cognitive-behavioral treatment (CBT) method (Thackwray, Smith, Bodfish, & Meyers, 1993). Their design incorporated operationalized treatment manuals, formal manipulation checks, and multiple behavioral and psychological measurements.

The clinical design called for three groups. The first group received a nonspecific self-monitoring treatment (NSMT) with therapist contact and attention. The second group received a behavioral eating habit control program consisting of eight sessions. Early sessions gave the treatment rationale and educated the subjects on the link between dietary restriction and binge eating. Then, subject and therapist jointly developed a treatment plan. Later sessions focused on environmental structuring and stimulus control to identify circumstances leading to binge-purge events.

The cognitive-behavioral therapy group focused on dysfunctional cognitions and had substantial homework assignments. The components provided to the behavioral group were repeated with the addition of other CBT procedures. The latter included cognitive restructuring, challenging beliefs that perpetuate bulimic behavior, assertiveness, problem-solving skills, and relaxation training.

At the posttreatment assessment, all three groups, including the NSMT group, showed significant decreases in binge-purge episodes. The percentages of subjects free of binge-purge behavior were 69%, 100%, and 92%, for the NSMT, BT, and CBT groups, respectively. The success observed in the BT group is not a consistent finding, though, as Fairburn's project

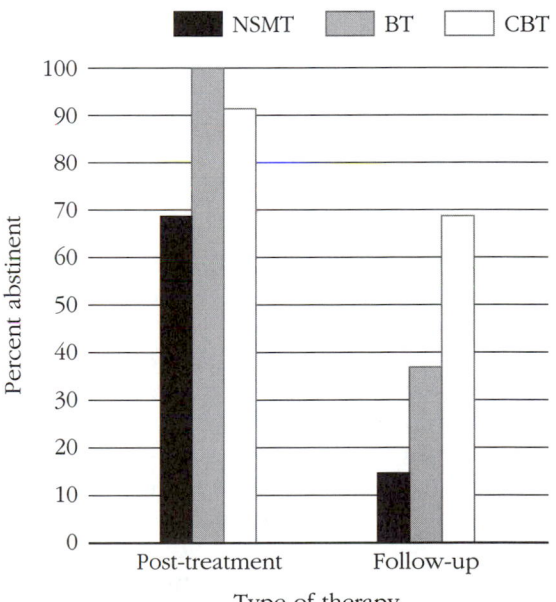

FIGURE 10.13   A comparison of two modes of treatment for bulimia showing the per cent of subjects free from binge-purge behavior at posttreatment and six months' follow-up (data from Thackwray et al., 1993).

showed very poor outcomes with BT (Fairburn et al., 1993). The improvement in the NSMT group is a reminder that merely having contact with a therapist and self-monitoring can sometimes produce impressive changes in behavior.

At follow-up, the superiority of the CBT treatment became apparent. At this time, the percentages of subjects free of binge-purge behavior were 15%, 38%, and 69%, for the NSMT, BT, and CBT groups, respectively. There were other notable differences among the groups. Although many of the BT subjects resumed binge-purge behavior, they did so at a rate averaging about 1 event per week, compared to a pre-treatment average of 5.5 episodes per week. Further, the NSMT subjects not only resumed binge-purge behavior, but they did so at rates that were higher than before. Thackwray's group suggests that the outcome provides support for the notion that dysfunctional cognitive processes must be addressed in therapy with bulimics and the CBT is more likely to lead to durable therapeutic changes than other interventions.

Summary

Developing healthy eating habits may be one of the most important lifestyle choices that can be made. Diet influences health in a multitude of ways; the continuing healthy functioning of the body depends on a continuing supply of nutrients. Conversely, abusing the body by eating too much food, by eating too much of the wrong type of food, or by extreme dieting practices will, sooner or later, lead to unhealthy results. Obesity, though it is due to several different causes, involves altered cell metabolism that presents complex nutritional difficulties. This chapter presented an overview of issues in healthy nutrition and some methods for dealing with obesity.

1. Diet is a contributing factor to 5 of the 10 leading causes of mortality in the United States.

2. Most Americans eat far more fat (about 45%) and consume fewer carbohydrates than is desirable. The target is 20% fat and 50% carbohydrates.

3. About 25% of Americans are overweight due to a combination of poor eating habits and inactivity.

4. In addition to reducing the overall amount of dietary fat, it is important to reduce saturated fats and to improve the ratio of good fat (HDL) to bad fat (LDL). This ratio can be shifted by both diet and exercise.

5. The common criteria for obesity is more than 20% over normal weight. Up to 20%, the person may be considered overweight but not obese.

6. Obesity appears to result in changes in the efficiency of fat storage that make it difficult to lose weight after the changes occur.

7. Obesity may be defined by standard charts, such as the National Research Council standard, by skin-fold tests, by waist-to-hip ratios, and through other means. One of the most commonly used measures is the Body Mass Index, which calculates the ratio of weight (kg) to height (m) squared.

8. Male pattern obesity, which involves a thick protruding waist relative to smaller hips, is a risk factor for heart disease, high blood pressure, and diabetes. Female pattern obesity, which involves larger hips relative to waist, is not linked to the risks that occur with male pattern obesity.

9. A genetic contribution to obesity may explain as much as 70% of the variance in obesity. It appears that low energy output is part of the metabolic process that leads to obesity.

10. In general, personality theories have not proved very helpful in explaining obesity. Even the once highly regarded view that obese people are controlled more by external cues has been abandoned.

11. Family dysfunction theory focuses on obesity as a metaphor for control. Such theories however, do not appear to help explain the origins of obesity.

12. The typical means of losing weight is through some form of dieting practice. Unless dietary restraint is combined with consistent exercise, there is danger of weight cycling— losing and then regaining weight. Weight cycling makes it even more difficult to lose weight in the future.

13. Pharmacotherapy for weight loss usually focuses on suppressing appetite. Usually, dietary constraint, exercise, and behavioral control principles are combined to provide one of the most effective means for weight loss.

14. Dietary restraint should reduce energy intake below energy expenditure without depriving the body of essential nutrients. It should supply all essential nutrients.

15. Behavioral methods generally have provided only modest weight losses. Yet these methods are still considered important in a complete weight loss intervention program.

16. Anorexia nervosa is a disorder characterized by significant weight loss, fear of gaining weight, and disturbed body image. It is primarily a disorder among younger women, but it occurs among men as well.

17. Bulimia is an eating disorder characterized by repeated binge eating and purging episodes. There is also excessive concern about weight, but the person may be in a normal to slightly overweight range.

18. Theories of anorexia nervosa and bulimia continue to focus on several possible causes, but no single satisfactory explanation exists for either disorder.

19. Treatment for anorexia nervosa typically uses a multimodal approach combining medical (pharmacological) therapy, cognitive-behavioral methods, and education to nutrition and dietary management.

20. Treatment of bulimia has focused on naltrexone as a pharmacological intervention, cognitive therapy to change self-defeating attitudes, and education. Inconsistent results make it difficult to say that any method or combination of methods has emerged as the most effective approach.

Key Words

abnormal appetite
 regulation obesity
adipose cell pro-
 liferation obesity
anorexia nervosa:
 binge/purge type
 restricting type
body mass index
 (BMI)
bulimia nervosa
compulsive eating
 disorders
endocrinopathic
 obesity
environmental
 obesity

female pattern obesity
gastroplasty
lipoprotein lipase (LPL)
locus of control:
 external
 internal
male pattern obesity
metabolic obesity
obesity
overweight
pharmacologically
 induced obesity
waist-to-hip ratio
 (WHR)

Study Questions

1. What are the five recommendations for nutritional balance and risk reduction related to diet?
2. How does exercise contribute to problems with diet?
3. What do cultural variations tell us about the effects of diet on health?
4. What cultural variations exist for tolerance or intolerance of obesity? How might these variations affect people for good or ill?
5. How is obesity defined? What are some common measures of obesity?
6. What are the major health risks from obesity?
7. What are the origins of obesity? Consider the different types of obesity and what this variety says about lumping all obese people in the same category.
8. Compare and contrast the different theories (genetic and psychosocial) of obesity.
9. What are the major methods of treating obesity? How do biomedical methods combine with psychosocial methods? How effective or ineffective are the different methods?

10. What is anorexia nervosa? What is bulimia? How are the two similar, if they are, and how do they differ?
11. What do current theories of anorexia nervosa tell us about the likely origins of the disorder? Likewise, what do current theories of bulimia tell us of origins?
12. What are the common methods of treating anorexia nervosa and bulimia? How effective or ineffective are these approaches for these two disorders?

Class Projects

1. Determine what educational and clinical services exist on campus for treatment of anorexia nervosa or bulimia. Invite people involved in these services to talk about current issues, successes and failures, and special needs on your campus.
2. Organize a roundtable discussion on biomedical versus psychosocial views of obesity. Include in the discussion information on new treatment programs from each perspective.

Suggested Readings

Brownell, K. D., & Foreyt, J. P. (Eds.). (1986). *Handbook of eating disorders: Physiology, psychology, and treatment of obesity, anorexia, and bulimia*. New York: Basic Books.

Garrow, J. S. (1992). Treatment of obesity. *The Lancet, 340,* 409–413.2.

Lowe, M. R. (1993). The effects of dieting on eating behavior: A three-factor model. *Psychological Bulletin, 114,* 100–121.

McGinnis, J. M. (1991). Health objectives for the nation. *American Psychologist, 46,* 520–524.

McGinnis, J. M., & Nestle, M. (1989). The Surgeon General's report on nutrition and health: Policy implications and implementation strategies. *American Journal of Clinical Nutrition, 49,* 23–28.

Polivy, J., Garner, D. M., & Garfinkel, P. E. (1986). Causes and consequences of the current preference for thin female physiques. In C. P. Herman, M. P. Zanna, & E. T. Higgins (Eds.), *Physical appearance, stigma, and social behavior: The Ontario Symposium* (Vol. 3, pp. 89–112). Hillsdale, NJ: Erlbaum.

Ravussin, E., & Swinburn, B. A. (1992). Pathophysiology of obesity. *The Lancet, 340,* 404–408.

Woods, S. C. (1991). The eating paradox: How we tolerate food. *Psychological Review, 98,* 488–505.

WEBSITES   Nutrition, Obesity, and Exercise

ADDRESS	DESCRIPTION
http://www.something-fishy.com/ed-f.htm	☆Website on Eating Disorders
http://nytsyn.com/live/Lead/	☆Your Health Daily—The New York Times site for fitness and health news
http://www.physsportsmed.com	☆The Physician and Sportsmedicine—A four-star site with information on exercise, nutrition, and rehabilitation
http://lifematters.com/	☆LifeMatters—four-star emphasizing holistic health
http://www.cnn.com/HEALTH/	☆CNN Food & Health News—a four-star site on current nutrition and health
http://www.psyc.unt.edu/apadiv47/	APA Division 47–Exercise and Sport Psychology

The AIDS Pandemic: A Behavioral Disease

Professional tennis has provided us with many models of fiery competitors whose manners, both on and off the court, were exemplary. The names of Rod Laver, Ken Rosewall, Virginia Wade, and Margaret Court come to mind. There is another, Arthur Ashe, who rightfully belongs with this group, and whose story of a lost battle with AIDS deserves to be told.

Arthur Ashe fought his way through racial discrimination to the top rank in tennis during the 1970s. He won three of the four grand slam events during his decade of excellence, and he became the first black man elected to the Tennis Hall of Fame. Ashe commented in his memoirs *Days of Grace* (Ashe & Rampersad, 1993) that for him, above all else, his humanity came first. Sportswriter Barry Lorge (1993, p. N32) noted that in spite of the millions Ashe made from tennis, he "learned that sportsmanship, dignity, and making a difference in human lives are priceless rewards."

Though terribly angered by the journalistic power play that forced him to make public his affliction, he struggled with AIDS with this same spirit of humanity and grace. His reflective intellect grappled with the heated debate in the press about the right to know versus the private lives of citizens. He concluded that the debate was one of the worthwhile things that grew out of his dilemma.

The opening line of his life story reveals much about the man: "If one's reputation is a possession, then of all my possessions, my reputation means most to me" (p. 3). What Ashe was fighting was the stereotypes, the questions, the unbridled speculations, and always the

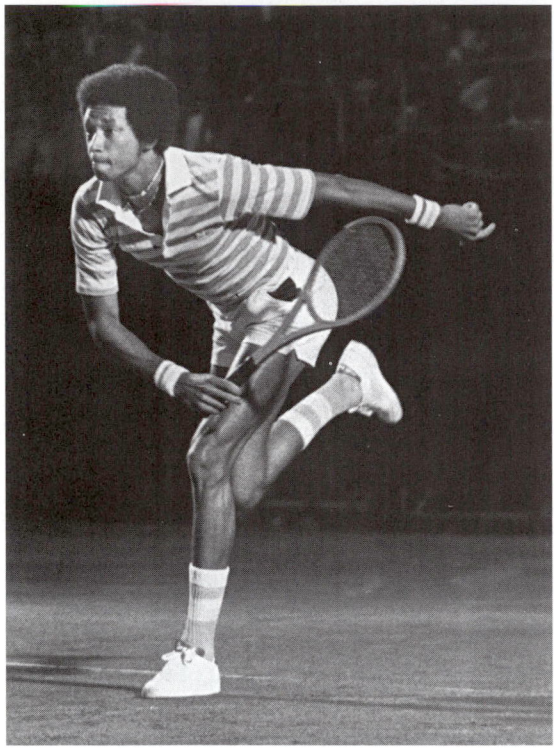

FIGURE 11.1   Arthur Ashe felt pressure from USA Today to reveal his exposure to AIDS.

stigma that seems to go with being identified as an AIDS carrier. For too long, the stereotypic AIDS victim was a white gay male or a minority male drug injector. The stigma, the blame heaped on AIDS victims seemed somehow justified because of behavior that did not measure up to society's most puritan norms. Arthur fit none of the stereotypes, but that did not matter to a press that was going through a journalistic feeding frenzy. In this context, Ashe watched "the quality of [his life change] irrevocably . . . Reason and rational thought are too often waived out of fear, caution, or just plain ignorance" (p. 17).

The story of how Ashe became infected is one of many horror stories in the AIDS pandemic. In 1979, Ashe's tennis career was first interrupted and then cut short by heart disease and quadruple-bypass heart surgery. For a short

while, he had hopes of returning to tennis. But that was not to be. From that time on, Ashe says he became a professional patient whose life revolved around hospitals, tests, treatments, more surgeries, and convalescence. Late in 1980, he announced that he could no longer compete in his beloved sport.

Some might think winning the Australian Open, the U.S. Open, and Wimbledon is all that one could ever ask for. Not so for Ashe, who now more than ever wanted to be taken seriously. Ashe was well-educated, widely read, and he loved art and poetry. Thus, he thought of himself as a gentle and reflective person. So he set out to get involved in activities that he hoped would make a difference. His involvement reflected his personal philosophy: "From what we get, we can make a living; what we give, however, makes a life" (p. 176).

He worked long hours writing a three-volume work on African Americans in sports, *A Hard Road to Glory* (Ashe, 1988). He served on boards including some that made him acutely aware of health care needs in the United States. Later, in the midst of his medical battle with AIDS, he also got caught in the politicized debate over the drug Kemron, which some held out as a miracle cure for AIDS. There were ghastly rumors afloat that a white conspiracy was keeping Kemron from public use. In his reflective style, Ashe said he would only take medicines that had been carefully tested and scientifically proven effective. A life crisis was not the time to let race issues sway judgment.

Just four years after his first surgery, he had yet another heart operation, this time a double-bypass. But this one was much more difficult and it left him weak and anemic. Offered the choice to wait or act instantly, he decided to act and had a transfusion of two units of blood. The immediate physical result was clearly positive and his recovery seemed assured. Yet the decision proved to be the beginning of his "descent into AIDS" (p. 87).

In late summer 1988, Ashe suffered a sudden paralysis of one arm. Immediate blood tests showed that he was HIV positive. Because the paralysis suggested a brain infection, his doctors immediately called for CAT scans and MRI tests. Doctors concluded that Ashe needed brain surgery. Subsequent tests revealed toxoplasmosis, one of the opportunistic infections that often results from AIDS.

It was only then, five years after that second surgery, that Ashe and his wife, Jeanne, discovered that the blood used in the transfusion was contaminated. Blame it on luck or fate. Blame it on the ignorance of health officials. Blame it on a slow response by the medical establishment, which did not begin testing blood until 1985. It really did not matter to either Ashe or to the nearly 13,000 other people who became AIDS carriers because of tainted blood.

Arthur Ashe died February 6, 1993, from another AIDS-related complication—PCP, *Pneumocystis carinii* pneumonia. Still, he continued to fight AIDS to the end with all the energy and willpower he could muster, supported by the unwavering love of his family and friends. Then in the finished record of his life, he left a legacy of what it means to confront a disease that is more than just a virus—a disease that is a social illness as well.

In this chapter, then, we will discuss the dread disease AIDS. We will look at the origins of AIDS keeping in mind that behind the identifiable virus there are identifiable behaviors that carry huge risks for contracting AIDS. Besides attacking the immune system, AIDS has serious neurological consequences.

As AIDS has spread, serious questions about the public health model and intervention strategies have been raised. We will look at both these issues later. Finally, as a logical outcome of these questions, we will consider issues in the prevention of AIDS. It is generally believed that the development of a cure is as yet so remote and the cost of care so huge (perhaps $65,000 annually per patient) that preventive measures must become the primary means of control. Still, there is renewed hope that breakthroughs in medical technology may bring effective treatments much sooner than many thought possible just a few years ago.

AIDS: Definition, Diagnosis, and Symptoms

Acquired immune deficiency syndrome, now simply called AIDS, is the name for a disease that does not itself kill but is nonetheless deadly. AIDS kills indirectly by threatening integrity of the immune system, the body's primary defense against bacterial, viral, and malignant diseases. Early in medicine's struggle to get control over AIDS, the Centers for Disease Control (CDC) referred to AIDS as a syndrome "characterized by opportunistic infections and malignant diseases in patients without a known cause for immunodeficiency" (cited in Seligmann et al., 1984, p. 1286). Intensive research in the early 1980s uncovered the cause, a virus dubbed the HTLV-III/LAV. Later, an international committee christened it the **human immunodeficiency virus** or HIV (Coffin et al., 1986).

Just as the HIV does not kill directly, it does not destroy the immune system, as one unfortunate early myth suggested. What it does is selectively attack the T_4 lymphocyte (CD4 T-cell), a white blood cell that is key to immune response (Burny, 1986). In simplified form, the virus works like this. The HIV is a **retrovirus,** an RNA virus with a viral enzyme that allows it to make a DNA copy of its own genetic material (Lee, 1989). It grabs on to host cells at vulnerable points and then takes over the cell by replicating its own code.

The T_4 lymphocyte cell has a large number of so-called CD4 receptors on the surface. These receptors are the Achilles heel of the T_4 cells. They are like handles the HIV can hold on to. Once attached to the cell, the HIV replicates itself and destroys the cells function. As the HIV continues to infiltrate, it produces several abnormalities in the immune system. Probably the most notable change is impaired cellular immunity through reduction of helper T cells.[1] The complete story of how the HIV brings about

---

[1] We discussed cellular immunity and T cells in Chapter 3.

destruction in the CD4 T-cells is not known but biomedical research is looking at several mechanisms (Greene, 1991).

In the body, the effects may be seen in opportunistic infections such as PCP, pulmonary tuberculosis, meningitis, and cancers such as Kaposi's sarcoma and cervical cancer. Further, the infected lymphocyte cells migrate to the brain, where the HIV has a specific affinity for CNS cells (Bridge, 1988). There, it can lead to CNS abnormalities that produce the AIDS dementia complex (to be described later).

Classifying AIDS: Symptoms, Severity, and Stages

AIDS presents several serious problems for diagnosis, tracking of progression, and treatment. It is a disease with a long latency, a large number of possible symptoms, and a period when the person is asymptomatic. Here, I will discuss the emerging scheme for classifying AIDS and what is known about the time course of AIDS.

In 1993, a revised classification system was adopted (MMWR, Dec. 18, 1992). In this scheme, shown in Table 11.1, the columns correspond to clinical categories related to patient symptoms, and they reflect increasing severity and number of symptoms. The rows correspond to lymphocyte counts per microliter of blood. These counts correlate with HIV-related immune dysfunction and disease progression. As the count drops, the disease becomes more serious.

In the most severe category, any of the symptoms of AIDS could appear, but the category represents appearance of the worst symptoms: Once a person reaches Category C, he or

she remains there. Category A is characterized as the asymptomatic or acute category. It involves one or more of the AIDS-related conditions, including asymptomatic HIV infection, a disorder of the lymphatic system called persistent generalized lymphadenopathy (PGL), and acute HIV infection. Category B is the symptomatic category. It consists of symptoms attributed to the HIV infection, including candidiasis (fungal infection), fever or diarrhea lasting more than one month, herpes zoster (viral infection), and peripheral neuropathy, among others.

Although the rate at which AIDS advances shows wide variability among people, the classification scheme is built on the notion of steady progression toward more severe symptoms. The progression and prototypical time course have been mapped by Pantaleo, Graziosi, and Fauci (1993; Fauci, Pantaleo, Stanley, & Weissman, 1996) as shown in Figure 11.2. Two markers are plotted, the gradual decline in CD4 T-cells and the presence of detectable virus in the blood. Immediately after the primary infection, CD4 T-cells drop by almost half and may be associated with acute HIV infections, the first signs that the AIDS virus is present. The fact that these first infections are acute (short in duration) may mislead people into believing the illness is just another common ailment. During this sinister window of opportunity, the victim can unwittingly pass the HIV to others.

The long latency between the time the person came in contact with the AIDS virus and the ability to detect the presence of the virus by blood test or by the appearance of symptoms is one major problem in combating AIDS. It makes the traditional case method approach used successfully in the public health arena for years largely unworkable with AIDS (National Commission on AIDS, 1993).

In the next stage, shown in Figure 11.2, the immune system does mobilize a credible though weak response, and CD4 T-cells rebound against the HIV infection. Still, the presence of the virus is almost undetectable during this clinical latency period. The CD4 T-cell count then begins an irreversible decline and sooner

TABLE 11.1   Revised classification system for AIDS (from MMWR December 18, 1992).

CD4+ T-CELL	(A)	(B)	(C)
≥500/mL	A1	B1	C1
200–499/mL	A2	B2	C2
<200/mL	A3	B3	C3

or later reaches a threshold level below which the body can no longer resist the appearance of symptoms. The median length of this latency period is 10 years. From this point on, physical symptoms and opportunistic infections may begin to appear. After this, it was once expected that the time course to death would take about two years. However, new drugs—the protease inhibitors—are dramatically changing this picture. A three-year prospective study by Peter Selwyn and his colleagues suggested that these signs do provide important clues in tracking the course of the disease (Selwyn et al., 1992).

AIDS and the Endocrine System: Adrenals, Pancreas, and Medications

Although the primary threat from HIV is to the immune system, AIDS has a pathologic effect in the endocrine system as well. It is now well known that an intimate two-way discussion occurs between the endocrine system and the immune system (Dion & Blalock, 1988). During immune response to challenge, for example in an infection and fever, the

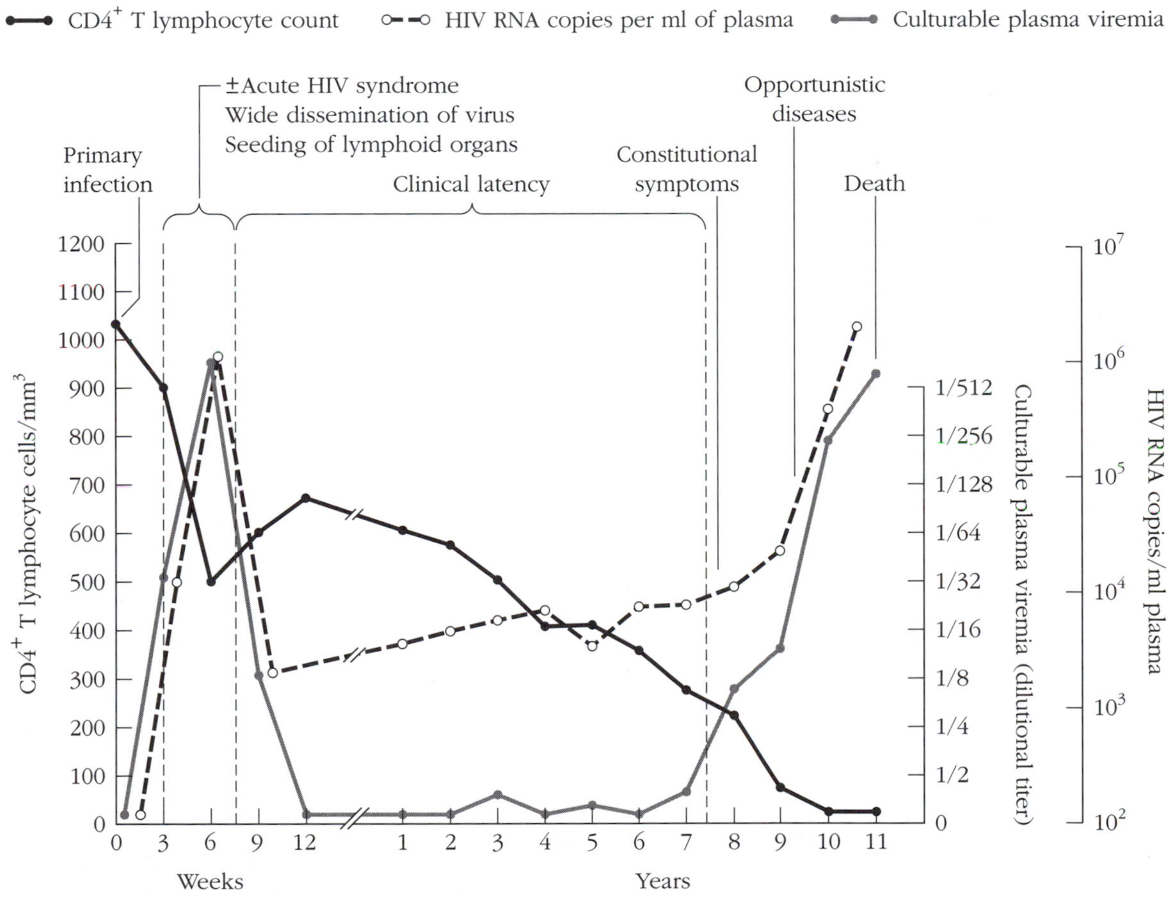

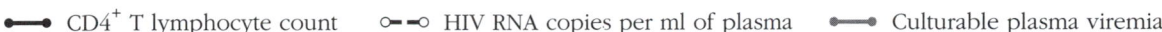

FIGURE 11.2   *Typical course of HIV infection showing the gradual decline in CD4 T-cells (dark circles) and the detectable presence of the virus in the blood (viremia) (from Fauci et al., 1996).*

hypothalamus-pituitary axes increases its activity, and glucocorticoid levels increase. These reactions appear to be triggered by feedback from the immune system.

AIDS can alter the endocrine system in various ways through infections, malignancies, or hemorrhages (Grinspoon & Bilezikian, 1992). It can also change hormonal secretions or interfere with their action due to the presence of antibodies or other active molecules that result from the infection. Finally, the various therapies the patient goes through may change activity in the endocrine system.

In their review of this area, Grinspoon and Bilezikian (1992) noted that the endocrine gland most often threatened by AIDS is the adrenal gland. Autopsies reveal that between 33% and 88% of patients show signs of adrenal viral infection. It is rare, though, for adrenal function to become so impaired that it adds to the patient's problems.

One area of interest is the link between cortisol and immunosuppression. This link has been widely studied because of early data suggesting that the physiologic system responds to chronic stress with hypersecretions of cortisol, which may in turn lead to immunosuppression. Presumably, AIDS as a biological insult and AIDS as an ultimate psychosocial stressor (the threat of death) could combine to further threaten immune competence. Evidence to date, however, suggests that AIDS does not markedly effect cortisol levels.

In summary, pathophysiological effects have been observed in the endocrine system during the course of the syndrome. Still, it is unclear what the overall role of such changes may be in the progression of AIDS.

AIDS and the CNS: Cognitions, Emotions, and Motor Control

The central nervous system is vulnerable to infections (HIV encephalitis), tumors, and vascular lesions. Bridge (1988) refers to AIDS as a neuropsychiatric disorder based on the type of neurologic and cognitive symptoms displayed. Subclinical signs of cognitive impairment may appear even in the asymptomatic stage (Category A) (Koralnik et al., 1990). The symptoms are believed to be secondary to brain infection caused by the virus. But the deficits observed in cognitive functions, motor control, and emotional balance have the potential to seriously impair daily functioning and erode the patient's quality of life.

In the cognitive domain, the person may show forgetfulness, slow processing and thinking, poor concentration, language impairment, and confusion. In the motor area, the person may show fatigue, loss of balance, and weakness or even paralysis in the extremities. Recall that it was this type of symptom that signaled to Arthur Ashe that something was terribly wrong. In the emotional area, AIDS patients often show signs of depression, paranoia, and hallucinations. In later stages, the **AIDS dementia complex** appears, typified by progressive global cognitive deterioration, personality change, and motor disturbance.

In a controlled study of neurological abnormalities, Koralnik and his colleagues found that 48% of the HIV-positive group showed one or more neurologic anomalies on standard clinical tests (Koralnik et al., 1990). In contrast, only 6% of the HIV-negative group showed neurological abnormalities.

Everall, Luthert, and Lantos (1991) wanted to pinpoint the actual pathophysiology that might explain the neurological abnormalities. First, they obtained samples of brain tissue from AIDS and non-AIDS decedents. Then, they compared the two groups on the density of neurons in frontal cortex tissue. They found evidence that loss of cognitive function probably results from actual loss of neurons. Keeping in mind that numerical counts of neurons are relative to a very small but equivalent sample of tissue, the HIV group had an average of 307 neurons, whereas the control group had 499 neurons, a highly significant difference ($p<.001$). This average represents a loss of 38% for the HIV group. Although the study brought us closer to the truth of what is going on in the CNS, Everall and his colleagues noted that the actual mechanism of CNS destruction was still not identified.

AIDS has powerful effects on several crucial body systems. It impairs immune function by attacking lymphocytes. HIV has some effect on the endocrine system, including some cases of adrenal insufficiency, but the effects are not as severe as once thought. There are also adverse side effects of medication, which add to biological insult and complicate treatment. Finally, the HIV migrates to the brain where it further attacks brain cells, producing a wide range of mood and cognitive effects.

The Epidemiology of AIDS: Plagues, Epidemics, and Pandemics

No health issue in the past half century has cried out for attention more than AIDS. Writing from a psychological perspective, Batchelor (1984) called AIDS "a modern day black plague." AIDS was unknown in the United States prior to 1977. It is thought to have entered the states via infected persons from Africa through Haiti (Bridge, 1988). Since then, it has traveled the world with little evidence that control might be possible until very recently.

In a special issue of *American Psychologist,* Stephen Morin (1988) wrote that AIDS was a three-stage epidemic that began with the insidious and silent onset of the disease. The second stage continued with intense case surveillance, and the third stage persists in sociocultural reactions to the epidemic. Today, the disease has become more than an epidemic: It is **pandemic**—a disease that has spread throughout the world. Thus has AIDS earned the dubious distinction of being the first disease to engulf the entire globe.

Tracking the distribution of AIDS by demographic traits and regions of the world is nearly a full-time job. Any report of current prevalence or incidence statistics is almost out of date as soon as it is printed. The best that can be done, then, is to provide time markers for any data presented.

In 1981, 189 cases were reported in the United States. Through mid-year 1984, 4431 cases were reported (Castro & Hardy, 1984). Just two years later, in early 1986, there were nearly 19,000 adult cases in the United States (Bakeman, Lumb, Jackson, & Smith, 1986), as well as numerous cases in Haiti and Africa (Kreiss et al., 1986). By late 1988, there were 65,000 cases, and worldwide reporting was coming on-line. Uganda, for example, reported 8000 cases that year (Goodgame, 1990).

When the CDC issued a report through September 30, 1991, there were 195,718 reported cases of AIDS in the United States and 126,159 AIDS deaths since the epidemic began in 1981. By October 1992, the count was at 233,907 cases and 158,243 deaths. By the end of 1996, there were more than 581,000 cases and 362,000 deaths (Centers for Disease Control, 1996). The projections to the end of this century are sobering: Possibly 30 million to 40 million people could be infected by then (Mann, 1991).

The nationwide prevalence rate is about 0.4% (cited in Gayle et al., 1990). Still, prevalence rates are highly variable, ranging from 0.02% in a sample of college women to as high as 57% among intravenous drug users. Data presented at the Seventh International Conference on AIDS suggested that prevalence rates are about the same in southeast Asia (Gilada, 1991).

At the present time, estimates of mortality indicate that between 40 and 50% of AIDS patients die from the disease. This figure is somewhat misleading since it is still assumed that AIDS is a fatal disease and that it is only a matter of time until the person will succumb to its effects.

During the first few years of the AIDS epidemic, the most vulnerable groups were male homosexuals, intravenous drug abusers, and African American and Hispanic men (Batchelor, 1988). These three groups constituted 90% of the cases, and they still represent the largest percentage of cases in the United States. Currently,

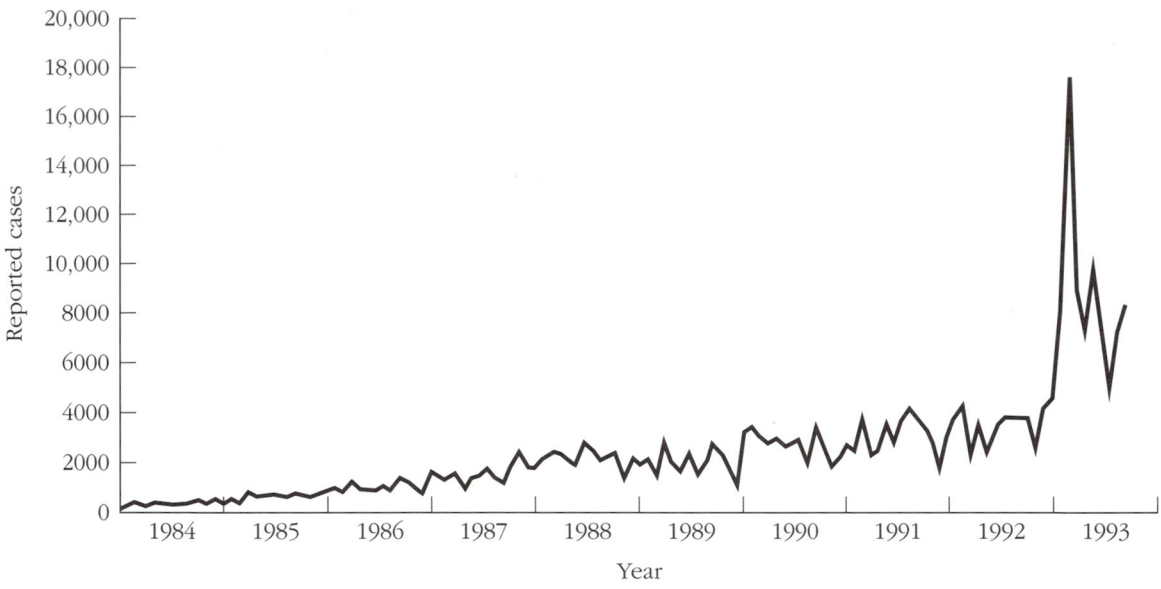

FIGURE 11.3   Growth in reported AIDS cases from the early 1980s to 1993 (data from Centers for Disease Control).

African-Americans make up 12% of the U.S. population, but they make up 29% of AIDS cases (St. Lawrence, 1993). In Thailand, less than a dozen HIV positive cases were reported in 1985. During 1986–1987, 1% of IV drug users were found to be positive. By 1988, 16% were HIV positive, and by 1989, 44% were HIV positive (Gilada, 1991). Fortunately, an intense public education program, including promoting condom use, has resulted in declines in the overall national rate of infections from a high of 12.5% in 1993 to 6.7% in 1995 (Nelson et al., 1996). Goodgame (1990) notes, however, that once HIV prevalence exceeds 10% in any community, the value of identifying risk groups greatly decreases.

By the middle of the 1980s, worldwide data began to accumulate showing that AIDS could be transmitted through heterosexual contact (Calabrese & Gopalakrishna, 1986). By 1989–1990, heterosexual behavior accounted for more new cases than homosexual or bisexual transmission (MMWR, Dec. 25, 1992). In Thailand, by 1989, 40% of the prostitutes were HIV positive.

In Bombay, the infection rate among prostitutes increased from 0.5% in 1986 to 30% in 1990 (Gilada, 1991). Now, 70% of new cases result from exposure in heterosexual activity (National Commission on AIDS, 1993), largely among sexually active adolescents and young adults with multiple sexual partners. Women now account for 11% of AIDS cases, and 53% are among minority women living in high-risk urban centers (Friedland & Klein, 1987; Kalichman, Kelly, Hunter, Murphy, & Tyler, 1993b). The death of many celebrities reinforces the notion that AIDS is no respecter of money, position, or nationality.

The fact that AIDS could spread in several ways required a major change in thinking. A very large segment of the population previously thought to have low vulnerability—namely women and adolescents—now had to be considered vulnerable. Perhaps 75,000 of the cases now reported are adolescents (cited in St. Lawrence, 1993). Recent statistics suggest that worldwide the fastest growing group of AIDS victims is female. Antonia Novello (1991), from

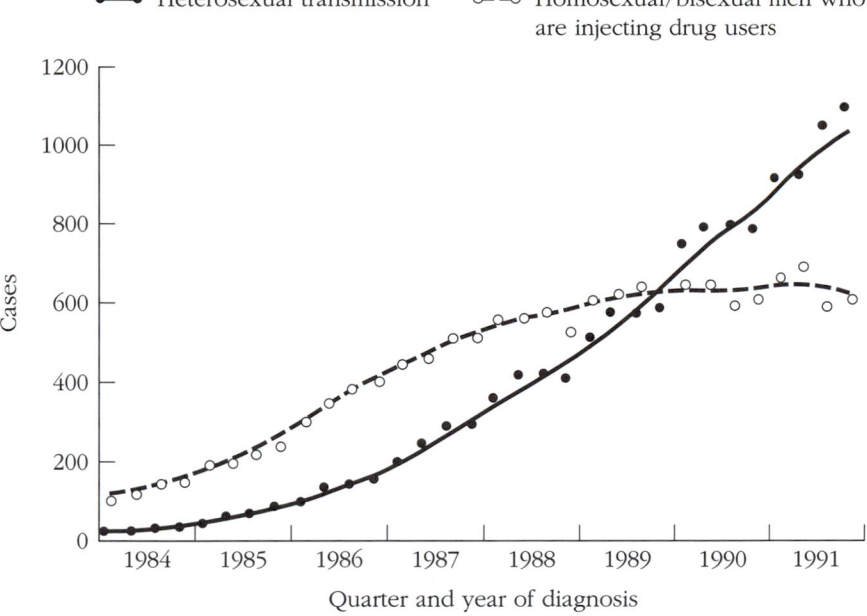

Heterosexual transmission ○--○ Homosexual/bisexual men who are injecting drug users

FIGURE 11.4   *Comparison of heterosexual with homosexual/bisexual mode of transmission of AIDS (from MMWR, December 25, 1992).*

the U.S. Surgeon General's office, noted that "there is no more age of innocence with women and AIDS" (p. 30).

The pattern of escalating cases and increased risk for women has prompted concern that risky behaviors among college students may provide AIDS with an all too easy inroad. College students are viewed as vulnerable to experimentation with sex and drugs, and they may hold attitudes about personal invulnerability that exposes them to even greater risk. The high rate of alcohol use is also believed to impair judgment and increase the likelihood of having unprotected sex.

To address this issue, Helene Gayle and her colleagues (Gayle et al., 1990) obtained blood samples from students at 19 universities nationwide. What they found was both surprising and encouraging. Among the nearly 17,000 specimens collected, Gayle's group found only 30 HIV-positive samples. The prevalence rate for men was 0.5%, and for women 0.02%. Recall that the U.S. prevalence rate is roughly 0.4%. The

authors suggested that although the AIDS virus is present on some college campuses, it occurs at a lower rate than that known to occur in high-risk groups. Further, the rate for women in this case was lower than predicted from worldwide trends.

In closing this section, a note on funding is in order. Federal funding for AIDS has grown as alarm has increased. In 1992, the U.S. government spent nearly $1.3 billion for research, $312 million for treatment, and $393 million for prevention. Even as the funding has increased, there are criticisms about timing, amount of support, and distribution of moneys. The government was generally slow to act in providing support for both clinical and research programs. Much of the increase in moneys was allocated in the biomedical arena with level funding in the social and behavioral science areas.

Critics of government policy point out that the medical model continues to drive most AIDS research and consume most of the federal dollar allocated for AIDS. Medical technology is still strongly driven by the lure of the magic bullet, the pill that will stop the disease in its tracks. Further, critics argue that the significant social and behavioral components of AIDS warrant more efforts to develop effective psychoeducational intervention and prevention programs. Still, government policy has slowed development of programs based on knowledge of the decisional-behavioral factors that lead people to ignore health risks and engage in behavior with potentially tragic consequences.

The Behavioral Origins of AIDS: Sex, Drugs, and Fluids

Since the AIDS virus was first identified, the great thrust in biomedical research has been to understand the mechanisms that allow HIV to wreak havoc in the body. This effort, of course, has been motivated by more than just a scientific need to understand the disease process. It has been an almost desperate quest for a cure, some clue that will solve the riddle of how to stop the onslaught, perhaps even reverse the process once begun. Note, though, that the incredibly

rapid early progress in understanding HIV was in large part due to basic biomedical research in retrovirology that had been going on for nearly a decade prior to the appearance of AIDS (Bridge, 1988).

Beyond the biomedical focus, AIDS has been characterized as a behavioral disease, because several behaviors contribute significantly to increased risk for AIDS. In this section, then, we will discuss the high-risk behaviors that can lead to exposure. As we do, keep in mind that the behaviors themselves do not cause AIDS. The HIV is the physical cause of AIDS. The behaviors are important because they provide the opportunities for contact with the virus.

The Behavioral Disease: Unprotected Sex, Multiple Partners, and Dirty Needles

The common avenues of AIDS transmission involve a few crucial high-risk behaviors. These avenues are most conspicuous in the lifestyles of high-risk groups: high-risk sexual behavior, sharing needles, and injecting drugs. A summary of risk variables is shown in Table 11.2 (Coates, Stall, Catania, & Kegeles, 1988).

TABLE 11.2   Variables associated with increased probability of HIV infection or AIDS-related high-risk behaviors (from Coates, Stall, Catania, & Kegeles, 1988).

VARIABLE	ASSOCIATION
Ethnicity	Blacks and Hispanics are at greater risk for AIDS and high-risk behavior.
Poverty	Poor are at greater risk for HIV infection.
Age	Older adolescents and younger adults are at greater risk for AIDS-related high-risk behaviors and for seroconversion.
Alcohol and drug use	Combining alcohol and drugs with sex increases risk for high-risk sex and HIV infection.
Knowledge of health guidelines	Knowledge may be related to change in the stages of the epidemic.
Health guidelines efficacy	The degree to which one believes information about methods for reducing risk is associated with reduction in high-risk behavior.
Costs	Perception of loss of pleasure and difficulty in changing are related to continued high risk behavior.
Perceived threat	Susceptibility to HIV infection predicts lower risk behavior.
Perceived efficacy	Belief that one has the skills necessary to reduce risk is associated with risk reduction.
Peer support	Belief that peers support low-risk sex predicts low-risk sexual behavior.

High-risk sexual activity is unprotected activity, whether homosexual or heterosexual, with several high-risk partners. The definition of a high-risk partner is one who is at risk for AIDS, has had a transfusion, is a hemophiliac, or is regularly involved in activities—such as prostitution and drug use—that increase risk of exposure to AIDS. The prevalence of multiple partners is about 7% overall and 9.5% in high-risk cities (Catania et al., 1992). These behaviors are influenced by social, cultural, and economic conditions (National Commission on AIDS, 1993). Although we describe several high-risk behaviors, remember that just one mistake is all it takes to expose a person to AIDS.

In a Florida study of pregnant women, Tedd Ellerbrock's research group (1992) tried to identify the major risk factors that predicted HIV status. In order of importance, the major risk factors among women were being black, having sexual intercourse with a high-risk partner, having had more than two sexual partners, and having used crack cocaine. The first factor, being a black woman, is consistent with observations that among women, minority status is a major risk factor. As we shall see later in this chapter, this may be due to several factors including misinformation about AIDS, attitudes toward AIDS, and stress associated with lower socioeconomic status and living conditions (slum living, crime, and so forth).

One of the most interesting outcomes of this study concerned condom use. HIV-positive women were more likely to have used condoms than uninfected women. Yet, only one of the women with AIDS reported using condoms more than 80% of the time. These findings highlight again the risks that occur when sexual activity occurs with multiple partners, especially high-risk partners, and when sex is more frequently unprotected than protected. The authors point out that the link between crack cocaine use and AIDS seemed due to the fact that drug use generally occurs in situations where unprotected sex with multiple high-risk partners occurs.

Recent studies suggest that adolescents may be very vulnerable both because increasing numbers of adolescents are sexually active and because age of first sexual experience is declining. Nationwide, there is evidence that many youths become sexually active during their high-school years, and some before they are 12 (St. Lawrence, 1993). Further, the percentage of sexually active youths is about 50% overall, while among minority groups about 80% are sexually active.

Susan Folkman and her colleagues investigated risky sexual behavior in the context of a stress coping model (Folkman, Chesney, Pollack, & Phillips, 1992). They noted prior evidence suggesting that some use sex as a tension relief strategy. This strategy may be associated with an increase in the number of partners.

Folkman's group conducted their study among gay and bisexual men in San Francisco, a city hit hard by AIDS with 10,000 recorded AIDS deaths by January 1993 ("San Francisco Notes," 1993). The investigators found no link between the amount of stress in a person's life and the tendency to engage in unprotected sex. Among those subjects who reported using sex as a coping technique to deal with stress, however, the researchers did find an increased tendency to engage in unprotected sex during periods of stress. Folkman's team interpreted this finding to mean that social aspects of coping are important to understanding when high-risk behaviors may take place. That outcome also suggested that intervention programs to prevent AIDS must account for unique coping strategies. By implication, intervention programs should provide training in alternative coping strategies that are likely to reinforce self-protective health behaviors.

Vehicles of Transmission: Blood, Birth, and Body Fluids

The high-risk behaviors just discussed share a common feature: exchange of body fluids. Three fluids are important: inoculated blood, sexual exchange of fluids, and perinatal transmission (Friedland & Klein, 1987). Blood inoculation can occur in a blood transfusion, by accidental puncture with a needle or sharp object, through an open wound, or through use of an unsterilized needle (common among IV drug users). Sexual exchange of fluids may be either homosexual or heterosexual from men to women or women to men. Finally, an infant born to an infected mother is at risk through exchange of fluids in the placenta and at birth through ingesting birth fluids. The infant is also at risk through ingestion of infected breast milk, though this mode of transmission appears to be rare. Friedland and Klein estimated that roughly 40% to 50% of infants born to infected mothers become HIV positive.

At the outset, many fears about AIDS were based on ignorance of how the HIV is passed on. Now substantial evidence exists that risk has been greatly reduced or is nonexistent in at least two areas. First, risk for contracting AIDS through blood transfusions has been greatly reduced because of improved blood screening (Lackritz et al., 1995). Based on a recent study of more than 4 million blood donations, investigators estimate that only 1 donation in every 360,000 was made during the so-called window period after the person had become infected but before the HIV was detectable. Further, they estimated that the risk of infection was no more than 1 in over 555,000 donations. This risk is substantially lower (by more than half) than previously thought.

Most family members of an AIDS victim have little or no risk of infection (Friedland et al., 1986). Friedland and Klein (1987) compiled data from several studies of people who were exposed to patients with AIDS or laboratory specimens from AIDS patients. In the first category were health care workers and family members. Among the 1,156 total subjects, only 2 tested positive for AIDS where no other risk factors were present. Among family members, the case can be stated simply: The only family members who have ever tested positive for AIDS are those who have been infected through blood, sexual activity, or birth. Further, epidemiological and clinical studies show that routine, nonsexual contact in offices, restaurants, or medical facilities does not transmit the virus. The virus is fragile and is easily killed by soaps and bleaches (Batchelor, 1988).

AIDS and Drug Abuse: Patterns, Mortality, and Morbidity

Intravenous drug use has always been one of the highest risk behaviors in the transmission of AIDS. Intravenous drug users (IVDUs) constitute the second largest infected group in the United States (Stephens, Feucht, & Roman, 1991). The riskiness of IV drug use holds true regardless of locale, as summary data from Asia shows (Gilada, 1991). When a drug user inserts a needle, it is not uncommon for the needle to aspirate (suck) blood back up the syringe. The next person to use the needle then injects the drug plus some tissue and blood residue from the previous user. In this way, the HIV can be passed to several users in very rapid fashion.

IVDUs appear to compound their risks in at least two ways. First, they abuse multiple drugs (alcohol, crack cocaine, marijuana, powder cocaine) at a higher rate than expected from drug use in general (Wambach et al., 1992). This drug abuse has both economic (higher costs) and physical effects (greater strain on the body). The pattern of use has the net effect of increasing risk for exposure through high-risk sexual behavior, such as a greater tendency to engage in sex with high-risk partners. Second, IVDUs more frequently engage in unprotected sex regardless of other drug use. This tendency appears to be a major contributing factor to infection in adolescent and young adult female IVDUs who end up trading sex for drugs or money to buy drugs.

Health care officials have been concerned that HIV-positive drug users might show higher mortality and morbidity rates compared to HIV-positive nondrug users. The data are somewhat mixed on this issue. Selwyn and his colleagues reported that HIV-positive drug users did not progress to AIDS any faster nor did they deteriorate more rapidly than others (Selwyn et al., 1992). They do, however, show a higher rate of more serious bacterial infections such as bacterial pneumonia, sepsis, and tuberculosis.

Finally, a behavioral ingredient receiving additional attention is alcohol use. Alcohol consumption typically increases the chances for indiscriminate sexual activity, including reducing the likelihood that condoms are used. Ralph Hingson and his coworkers surveyed more than 1,000 adolescents between the ages of 16 and 19 (Hingson, Strunin, Berlin, & Heeren, 1990). In this sample, 61% of the group were sexually active, but teenagers who were heavy drinkers or used marijuana were two to three times less likely to use condoms than those classed as light drinkers. Studies among IVDUs reveal that IVDUs who also use alcohol are more likely to share needles and to have multiple sex partners compared to IVDUs who do not drink (Saxon & Calsyn, 1992). These studies, correlational as they are, still do not provide explanations for the link between alcohol and sexual behavior (Cooper, 1992).

Correlational studies using samples of gay males have yielded mixed results (for a review, see Strunin & Hingson, 1993). Temple and Leigh (1992) reasoned that the mixed results found among gay males may be because the measures of drinking behavior and sexual activity were too general. They decided to look at more specific aspects of sexual activities in a sample of gay males. They asked subjects to report on two specific events: their most recent sexual encounter and their most recent sexual encounter involving a new partner. They found that encounters with new partners more frequently involved alcohol, but that alcohol was not significantly related to risky sexual behavior.

Psychosocial Aspects of AIDS: Attitudes, Stress, and Grief

Psychosocial processes play an important causal role in a person's decision to engage in high-risk behavior. Understanding these processes may have important implications for designing effective intervention programs. Further, AIDS may produce dramatic changes in the patient's psychosocial context. After being diagnosed with AIDS, the person typically experiences major changes in personal functioning and social relationships. These changes may include high levels of perceived stress, depression, overt signs of discrimination and rejection, and disturbed relations with family, friends, and coworkers. In this section, our focus will be on the role that health beliefs and attitudes play in high-risk behavior. We will first review some integrative theories that attempt to explain why people do or do not engage in behaviors that protect health.

Models of Health-Protective Attitudes: Beliefs, Protection, and Utility

As work has progressed on personal perceptions and attitudes that affect high-risk behaviors, many investigators have endeavored to provide more formally structured and tested theories. The health belief model (reviewed in Chapter 4) and the theory of reasoned action (reviewed in Chapter 8) have both been used in the context of AIDS.

Neil Weinstein (1993) noted similarities and differences between four theories used to predict health-protective behavior. These theories include the health belief model (HBM), the theory of reasoned action (TRA), protection motivation theory (PMT), and subjective expected utility theory (SEU). According to Weinstein, the theories all assume that when people perceive that a negative health outcome could occur, they will naturally want to avoid the outcome and will be motivated to engage in health-protective behavior.

Further, the theories all assume a person subjectively calculates the chances that the negative event will occur. For example, I might see a dark brown spot on my skin and immediately think of cancer. Then the thought might occur: "What are my chances of getting cancer?" Objectively, my chances might be 1 in 4, based on statistics that roughly one person in every family will be touched by cancer. But subjectively, I might reason that only one person in my family ever had cancer so my chances for getting it are virtually zero. If my family had a long history of cancer, however, I might be 100% convinced that the dark spot is cancer.

Next, all the theories assume that the motivation to act arises from a belief that taking action can reduce either the chances that the negative health outcome will occur or the severity of the damage should it occur. Finally, the theories assume that the benefits of taking action outweigh the costs. As we shall see in the next few pages, these assumptions are not very well supported when it comes to AIDS.

Blood Tests and AIDS: Screening, Fears, and Prevention

One of the early proposals to combat AIDS was to engage in massive blood screening. Japan, for example, reported one of the most massive screening programs ever undertaken when 110 million people were tested. From this massive effort, 400 AIDS patients were found and 1700 HIV-positive cases were detected (Gilada, 1991). In the United States, by the end of 1989, about 2.5 million tests had been carried out and 150,000 were positive (Roper, 1991).

The logic of blood test programs is fairly simple. From a medical point of view, screening makes it possible to offer people help that may improve immunologic status, manage symptoms better, prevent onset of opportunistic infections, and thus delay progression of AIDS (Levine & Bayer, 1989). From a behavioral point of view, it is assumed that if people know what their status is, they will want to change their behaviors to reduce the likelihood of infecting others. They will also tell their sexual or drug partners that they might be at risk. Their partners will then obviously want to be tested and tell their partners, and so on. It turns out, though, that this idealistic notion does not work in reality.

In numerous medical situations, patients seem to think that "no news is good news." For example, people who have chest pains but do not go to their doctors may be trying to avoid finding out about a potentially serious heart problem. It may be the same with AIDS: People fear hearing the bad news so much that they would rather not know the truth. Some may fear they could not cope knowing they were positive. People may also be in denial: They could not possibly be infected, so there is no point in being tested. These are among several reasons given for avoiding screening tests (Lyter, Valdiserri, Kingsley, Amoroso, & Rinaldo, 1987).

Landis, Earp, and Koch (1992) noted in one testing program that among those who tested positive for AIDS, 46% never returned for their results. And among those who did, less than 10% actually informed their partners of their condition. Gary Marks and his associates observed that disclosures by Hispanic males depended on severity of symptoms and closeness of confidant (Marks et al., 1992). Avoiding risk depends on knowing the HIV status of a partner, but if a partner chooses to act in a deceptive manner, even someone who wanted to act responsibly could still be exposed. In the final analysis, the various massive testing programs carried out have not produced the desired or expected effect in reducing high-risk behavior in many groups.

Attitudes about Sexuality: Pressures, Misinformation, and Risk-Taking

The attitudes and beliefs that underlie sexual conduct are extremely complex. Sexual behavior is an important part of a person's identity and involves powerful emotions that serve as drives to maintain sexual activity and increase risk. Most intervention programs include some assessment of attitudes and knowledge based on the assumption that both are related to the likelihood of taking protective steps. But several projects have been conducted just to find out what certain groups know or feel about AIDS without any intended intervention. The next few paragraphs focus on this type of study. Later, we will return to intervention studies.

Janet St. Lawrence (1993) asked some basic questions of African American adolescents in order to discover what they knew about AIDS and what attitudes most influenced their sexual behavior. She found that the adolescents often held a number of misconceptions about how AIDS is transmitted. For example, 32% of her sample thought that you could tell a person had AIDS because he or she would look sick. They thought they could protect themselves by avoiding risky behavior with people who looked ill, a misconception that could prove dangerous. AIDS may have a long latency period, during which time the carrier appears asymptomatic and looks as healthy as anyone else. The youths also thought that all sexually transmitted diseases are curable, and they generally thought that AIDS was a white gay male disease.

Ralph DiClemente and his colleagues compared public school youths with youths in juvenile detention (DiClemente, Lanier, Horan, & Lodico, 1991). All the youths were between 14 and 17 years of age. There was, as the saying goes, some good news and some bad news. First, both groups had high levels of knowledge about AIDS, correctly noting that IV drug use and unprotected sex were primary modes of transmission. There were major differences in perceived vulnerability and in the level of high-risk behaviors, however. Among the detained youths, more than 69% perceived they could be vulnerable, but only 45% of the school population thought of themselves as vulnerable. Health care officials tend to see lower rates of perceived vulnerability as undesirable. Yet these rates may reflect a more objective reality. Perhaps the youths in the public schools knew that they did not and would not engage in the behaviors linked to AIDS. A recent quantitative review of studies dealing with perceived vulnerability to HIV and precautionary sexual behavior suggests, though, that those who engage in high-risk behavior actually have higher estimates of their personal vulnerability (Gerrard, Gibbons, & Bushman, 1996). It appears, then, that the perception of vulnerability does not in itself play a crucial role leading people to adopt precautionary behaviors, but that a complex mix of factors interacts to lead to reduction in risk behaviors.

Further outcomes from the DiClemente study showed that all the detained youths were sexually experienced, whereas only 28% of the school youths reported sexual experiences. Among the detained youths, 52% reported their earliest sexual experience came around 12 years of age, compared to 26% of the school youths. This data highlights the need to target younger groups with crucial information on the modes of transmission and behavioral methods to reduce risk.

A final example comes from the work of Seth Kalichman and his associates (Kalichman, Hunter, & Kelly, 1992). Working at mass transit terminals in the greater Chicago area, Kalichman's group took a convenience sample of 272 minority and nonminority women. About 22% of the women reported what is considered high-risk behavior. There were substantive differences in attitudes towards AIDS as well as knowledge about AIDS. Minority women were less concerned about AIDS and perceived their risk to be lower compared to nonminority women. A possible explanation for this outcome is that minority women reported a much wider range of problems in living, including housing, employment, drugs and crime. They regarded these problems as more critical than the risk of getting AIDS.

In addition, minority women were more often misinformed about AIDS and the means of contracting AIDS. There were no differences, though, in rates of protected versus unprotected sex. The authors suggested that AIDS interventions to reach minority groups may have to be built into broader community programs addressing the serious socioeconomic problems confronted by many urban minority groups.

Attitudes Toward Condoms: Protection, Pleasure, and Control

The safest way to avoid AIDS is sexual abstinence or confining sexual contact to a single partner of known HIV status. Yet people who find this advice palatable probably already follow that standard for moral or religious reasons that have little to do with AIDS. In the meantime, reality suggests that a sizable segment of the population engages in multiple sexual liaisons from an early age in a social context where such behavior is almost normative. Under these circumstances, use of a condom is about the only way to provide protection.

Based on a nationwide probability sample, Catania and his associates observed a low overall rate of condom use. Among heterosexual subjects who had practiced anal intercourse, 71% never used a condom and only 19% always used protection (Catania et al., 1992). Among those with multiple partners, nearly 38% never used a condom, and only 17% always used them. Moreover, the condom is not a foolproof protection. Condoms have a known failure rate between 1% and 10% for preventing pregnancy, suggesting that condoms cannot be expected to do any better against HIV.

There are important gender differences in attitudes toward condom use. In St. Lawrence's (1993) study, girls were much more knowledgeable about AIDS than boys. Further, girls perceived themselves as having greater self-control than boys, and girls had more positive attitudes toward safeguard measures during sexual encounters, including use of the condom. This finding should not be at all surprising, since the woman typically suffers most from an unwanted and ill-timed pregnancy. Boys reported more sexual partners and more external control. But one prevailing stereotype seems to get in the way of condom use: that sexual pleasure is reduced when using the condom. Adolescents reported concern that using a condom destroys spontaneity and interrupts the flow of love-making.[2]

One problem that has been noted in regard to condoms is the tendency for use to be highest on the first sexual encounter and then to decline

with more encounters. Then, the condom seems to be perceived as useful primarily for contraception, not for AIDS protection (Træeen, Lewin, & Sundet, 1992). It has been observed that the more partners a person has, the less likely the person is to use a condom: The people who have multiple partners may be more impulsive risk-takers, anyway.

Perceptions of Risk and Behavior Change

We often assume that knowing the risks will alter behavior. Still, this assumption has been very often proved wrong. For example, we know that the highest risk for auto accidents is within five miles of home. We also know that wearing a seat belt significantly reduces the risk of serious injuries or fatalities. Yet many still refuse to wear seat belts on short errands even though they might wear seat belts on a long trip. Other factors, then, must influence personal estimation of risk and the way people decide to act.

Anna Kline and Jennifer Strickler (1993) were concerned with this issue when they undertook a study among women in drug treatment. They wanted to find out what factors most influenced the women's perceptions of risk and what changes in behavior might occur as a result. Kline and Strickler cited data from the New York and New Jersey metropolitan area that sharing contaminated drug equipment accounts for 62% of women's AIDS cases. The second most important factor is heterosexual activity, which accounts for 33% of the AIDS cases among women.

Kline and Strickler's sample included 242 women who were in treatment at methadone maintenance clinics or outpatient programs in the area. More than 76% of the women had injected drugs at some time in their lives. In spite of this high rate of intravenous use, more than 84% of the women thought they were unlikely to contract AIDS. Only 22% of the women used condoms more often than not, and 66% of the women never used them.

---

[2] Similar findings were reported from Madras, India (cited in Gilada, 1991).

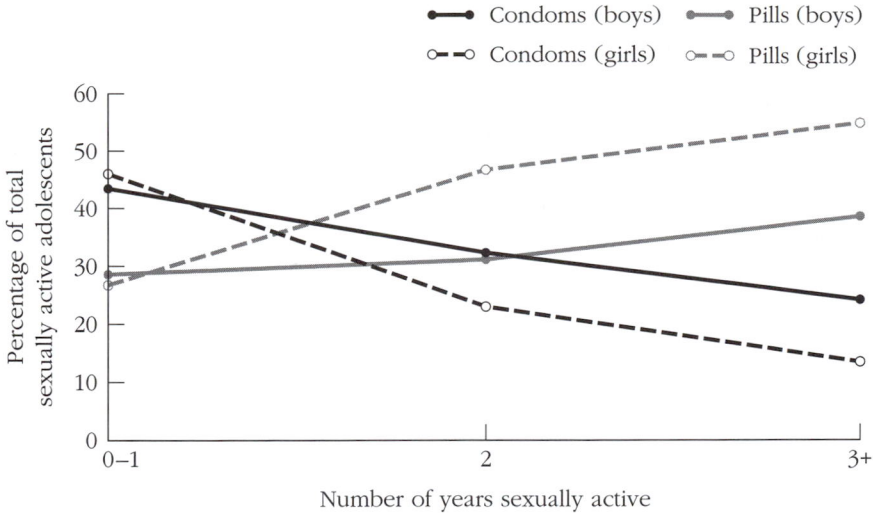

FIGURE 11.5   *Use of oral contraceptives and condoms for adolescent boys and girls. The trend over three years of sexual activity is for the use of the condom to decline while use of the pill increases. This trend suggests that the choices being made in regard to protection during sexual activity are perceived primarily as contraceptive, not protecting against AIDS (from Træeen, Lewin, & Sundet, 1991).*

Further, more than 47% of the women had no knowledge of their partner's HIV status. In fact, when Kline and Strickler tried to develop a model to show which factors could explain perception of risk among these women, the only useful factor was IV drug use. The women recognized that drug injecting was a high-risk behavior. But by statistical analysis, not one single sexual risk factor was important to their perception of risk. In explaining this outcome, Kline and Strickler noted that the women tended to focus on traits in their partners that generally have little relationship to actual risk. This error is consistent with information presented earlier that drug injectors will modify needle behavior to reduce risk, but modifying sexual behavior appears to be more difficult.

Gender Issues in AIDS Research: Status, Connection, and Abuse

The dramatic increase worldwide in the number of women infected with AIDS has drawn attention to gender issues in AIDS research and

treatment. Hortensia Amaro (1995) provided a thoughtful review of the flaws that existed in social policy for much of the first decade of the AIDS epidemic, when AIDS was viewed as largely a male disease. Most intervention and prevention research focused on male samples and provided little help for women. At the same time, the risk of a male-to-female transmission of the AIDS virus is nearly 12 times that of a female-to-male transmission. This disproportion obviously places the woman at substantially higher risk for infection in an intimate relationship. To make matters worse, the primary means of protection, the condom, often itself places women at risk because condom use depends on a male who might or might not be understanding and cooperative (as opposed to abusive) in negotiating the terms of the sexual activity.

Amaro went on to summarize several gender factors of great importance. First, social status and power continues to be unequally distributed between women and men. A woman's personal values and perceptions of power relative to her partner need to be considered. Second, social and intimate connection appear to be highly important as the core of a woman's identity and personhood. Thus the threat of disconnection may pose great difficulty for a woman when conflicts over intimacy and sexual protection become an issue. Third, the role of the male in a sexual partner's risk, the male's view of power, and male attitudes toward women must be more carefully considered as part of the web of risk factors for the woman. Finally, the woman's fear of abuse, whether emotional or physical, suggests that models of prevention and intervention must integrate general knowledge of violence, and specific history of violence, in intimate relationships. As Amaro noted in concluding her review, shifts in theory, research and practice to accommodate gender issues are important and necessary, but support for social change is also necessary to reduce the woman's risk.

AIDS and Moods: Anxiety, Grief, and Depression

In addition to the life-threatening nature of AIDS, early studies revealed that AIDS patients suffered from very high levels of stress. Some reported that they had contemplated suicide because of despair and endless depression brought on by their condition. These adverse effects were easily blamed on the life-threatening condition since AIDS was branded a lethal disease. But there was also uncertainty about the future and, at first, lack of a treatment procedure that offered hope of slowing the disease's progress.

Many people have suffered AIDS-related grief as their friends and loved ones died from the disease (Martin & Dean, 1993). Susan Folkman (1993) noted that three elements contribute to the meaning of death from AIDS among gay men. First, death occurs at a relatively young age; second, many grieve while coping with the fact that they are also HIV positive; and third, as time goes on, more people experience the loss of more than one friend.

Members of the gay community, for example, were reported to suffer from heightened anxiety, panic attacks, loss of self-esteem, fear of isolation from friends and loved ones, and loss of self-sufficiency (Morin, Charles, & Malyon, 1984). Many AIDS patients were victimized by the social stigma that often resulted in guilt and isolation (Dilley, Ochitill, Perl, & Volberding, 1985). Even gays diagnosed and found free of AIDS experienced high levels of stress. They were among the "worried well." There were dire forecasts that this "epidemic of stigma" could have serious negative health effects over the long term (Herek & Glunt, 1988). Some of the negative effects began to change, so that by about 1988 both stress and suicidal thoughts had abated somewhat (Kelly & Murphy, 1992). There is some evidence that the stigma associated with AIDS may be lessening as well (Levin & Chapman, 1993). Still, the stigma associated with AIDS apparently is greater than that experienced by individuals with comparable illnesses (Crawford, 1996).

As part of the San Francisco Men's Health Study, Robert Hays and his associates assessed depression in a large sample of gay males (Hays, Turner, & Coates, 1992). The mean depression score for this sample was 9.99 compared to a mean of 8.7 in the general population. The group was slightly more depressed than normal, but overall the depression was not clinically severe. Still, as the authors noted, 20% of their sample did score at a point that indicated clinical depression. The most important factors in buffering against stress and depression were the quality of social support received and the informational support provided.

In a more recent study, John Martin and Laura Dean (1993) tested an adaptation hypothesis. Using a seven-year longitudinal design, they focused on indicators of mental health such as grief following loss of a loved one, depression, stress, and suicidal thinking. Their sample consisted of both infected and noninfected gay males. At all times, males who were both infected and bereaved reported substantially more stress. Bereavement contributed to elevations in

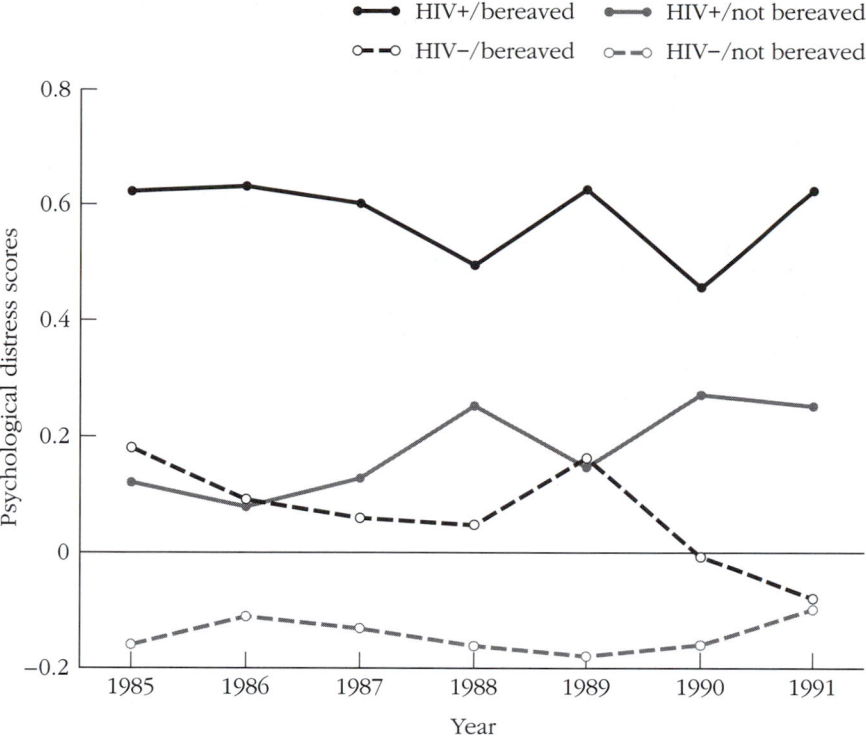

FIGURE 11.6   The combination of being HIV-positive and bereaved leads to high distress compared to control groups (from Martin & Dean, 1993).

depression, stress, and suicidal thoughts. Yet overall, the effects were not strong enough to suggest serious negative effects on mental health. Finally, the intensity and duration of bereavement effects decreased over time, supporting the idea of increasing adaptation to the negative effects associated with AIDS.

Stress, AIDS, and the Immune System

Questions have been raised about how the established connection between stress and the immune system may affect AIDS patients. Data to this point seem to suggest that stress does not substantively alter immune system competence beyond what occurs from the HIV. For example, Rabkin and his associates found no relationship between life stress and CD4 cells or other subsets of T cells in HIV-positive gay men (Rabkin et al., 1991).

Margaret Kemeny and her coworkers were concerned about gay men who responded to the loss of friends with depressed mood (Kemeny et al., 1994). The team reasoned that altered immune function might occur only in those who responded to loss with depressed mood. The investigators started with a large sample ($n = 1637$) from the Los Angeles Multi-Center AIDS Cohort Study (MACS). Then, they selected 45 men who agreed to participate and who had experienced loss of one or more close friends during the past year. The researchers excluded men who reported loss of a spouse or intimate partner because of the likely significance of the loss. Further, they selected a matched control group based on age and HIV serostatus; men in the control group, however, had not experienced loss. This control made it possible to compare bereaved to nonbereaved men where about half of each group tested positive for AIDS and half tested negative.

Measures included a POMS depression score and several tests of immune status. In addition, the investigators obtained data on several aspects of health behavior (nutrition, exercise, sleep, use of medications, and drug use). HIV-positive subjects differed significantly from HIV-negative subjects on several immune variables, as expected from their status. Bereaved men did not differ immunologically from non-bereaved men, however. Further, depressed men did not differ on immune function from nondepressed men.

Next, Kemeny's group carried out analyses with HIV serostatus combined with bereavement first and then HIV serostatus combined with depression. In design terms, these tests were for interaction effects. In both these analyses, the interactions did not predict immune function.

The surprise came when the team took the last step—combining HIV serostatus with both bereavement and depression. Remember that the research team predicted that immune function would change most in HIV seropositive men who responded to loss (bereavement) with depression. Yet, among HIV seropositive men, it was the *nonbereaved* subjects with higher depression who showed detrimental changes in immune function. Among bereaved HIV seropositive men, depression was not associated with any of the immune variables. This outcome was the opposite of what Kemeny's group had predicted. Finally, bereaved HIV seronegative depressed men did show detrimental changes in immune function. Kemeny and her coworkers pointed out that it is necessary, based on this and similar research, to distinguish between grief and depression. Grief alone does not appear to present problems, but when the person becomes depressed, physiological changes may occur that affect immune competence.

A number of health status behaviors (sleep, alcohol consumption, and exercise, for example) changed with depression. Kemeny's group did not find any evidence that these variables were related to immune status, however. Further, the analyses described in the previous paragraph did not change when these variables were used as controls.

These results point out the complexity of relationships that may occur in linking psychosocial variables to changes in immune function. The findings suggest that early notions of altered immune function following bereavement must not be generalized to different groups and situations without supporting data.

Intervention Strategies: Vaccines, Education, and Prevention

Even as hope continues that a wonder drug will emerge, the central mission of intervention programs is to change attitudes and behavior to defend against the spread of AIDS. There is some basis for optimism, but there is also reason for healthy skepticism. The success of many intervention programs is limited either in the amount of change produced or in the permanence of the change. In these concluding pages, then, we will review several noteworthy intervention and prevention programs.

Medical Treatment: Hopes and Promises

The medical community continues to search for treatments that will offer relief to infected patients or slow the progress of the disease. There is even hope that one day a vaccine will bestow protective immunity. The advent of a new class of drugs, the protease inhibitors, has brought renewed hope that the disease can be controlled.

The basis of this hope comes from work in molecular and cellular biology, scientific disciplines that have revealed much about the structure and regulation of HIV. For example, the life cycle of HIV has been studied, and scientists now know that it has a stage of vulnerability that may be its Achilles heel. This knowledge has not led as yet to any medication that can attack this weakness (Greene, 1991). Still, knowledge from this field has led to development of drugs to combat, at least to slow, the progress of AIDS. In addition, methods to better manage secondary infections help to reduce morbidity and to slow progress toward AIDS (Buckley & Schiff, 1991; Filice & Pomeroy, 1991).

One drug, **zidovudine** (AZT), has been the subject of several clinical trials to determine its effectiveness.[3] In general, zidovudine has prolonged survival and reduced both the frequency and severity of opportunistic infections in AIDS patients. It has also apparently slowed the progress of the disease in HIV-positive asymptomatic patients (Hamilton et al., 1992). Selwyn and his colleagues (1992) found that zidovudine given to HIV-positive IV drug users substantially slowed progress of AIDS. There are ongoing disputes in scientific circles about the limits of zidovudine's effectiveness, but it is probably the most effective therapy at this point.

In the first major study of zidovudine in asymptomatic HIV-infected patients, nearly 30% withdrew or were lost to follow-up (Fischl et al., 1990; Volberding et al., 1990). This rate of attrition is always disconcerting because it jeopardizes the generality of the findings. Still, the early results were encouraging. There were some unpleasant side effects such as bone marrow suppression, nausea, vomiting, and diarrhea. The AIDS Clinical Trials Group (Lenderking et al., 1994) concluded that any reduction in quality of life due to negative side effects approximately equals the increase in quality of life connected with the slower progression of HIV disease.

In a recent test of zidovudine, Neil Graham and his colleagues wanted to find out whether use of zidovudine for HIV-infected patients prior to the diagnosis of AIDS would prolong survival as well as delay the development of AIDS (Graham et al., 1992). The investigators found that zidovudine significantly reduced mortality in all follow-up periods through the two-year study period. The relative risks of death were 0.43 at 6 months, 0.54 at 12 months, 0.59 at 18 months, and 0.67 at 24 months.

One disturbing note comes from a Johns Hopkins study of the treatment of AIDS patients in the Baltimore metropolitan area (Moore, Stanton, Gopalan, & Chaisson, 1994). This study of 838 patients showed that blacks (48%) were much less likely to receive zidovudine (or one of two other similar drugs) compared to whites (63%). This difference remained even when other variables such as demographic factors (sex, age, income, education) and type of insurance were added to the analysis. In spite of the call for uniform access and treatment, then, the standard treatment guidelines for prescribing drug therapy do not seem to have been uniformly applied.

Advances in the molecular biology of HIV continue to spur hopes that a vaccine may be developed that will bestow protective immunity, much like the vaccines that eradicated some of the worst diseases of the past. The basis of this hope is that tests with monkeys at three research centers have produced protective immunity. Whether the same is possible in humans living in real-world conditions remains to be seen (Greene, 1991).

In the meantime, a new class of drugs has emerged, the protease inhibitors, which offers the best hope to date of controlling the disease (Deeks, Smith, Holodniy, & Kahn, 1997). The protease inhibitors (saquinavir mesylate, ritonavir, indinavir sulfate, and nelfinavir sesylate) act at a critical point in the early development of infectious (HIV) cells and prevent them from maturing. In general, the effect of the protease inhibitors has been to slow the progression of the HIV disorder, increase CD4+ lymphocytes, thus preventing the appearance of opportunistic diseases that present major problems for the AIDS patient.

---

[3] Zidovudine could be called an AIDS terminator: It works by terminating the chain of DNA replication when the retrovirus tries to replicate its own DNA.

Several cautionary notes are in order. First, the success of the protease inhibitors has only been demonstrated in short-term trials, so the overall long-term impact is not yet known. Second, these drugs impose more significant costs on patients and insurance providers. Current estimates indicate that the patient's drug costs will increase between $6000 to $8000 per year. Third, there are complex and troublesome side effects that include adverse interaction with other drugs commonly used to treat symptoms present with AIDS. Finally, there is concern that the drugs may be vulnerable to resistance effects: that is, after a period of time, the patient may not be protected by taking the drug. In spite of these concerns, the protease inhibitors have generated more optimism than virtually any treatment since AZT.

Nutrition in the Treatment of AIDS

One of the major symptom clusters that accompanies AIDS is the wasting syndrome, which is characterized by emaciation and extreme weight loss. The wasting process is not the same as starvation loss because fat tissue is not preferentially lost (Grinspoon & Bilezikian, 1992). AIDS patients may lose muscle protein as well as fat.

Fighting any illness requires a great deal of strength, but that strength is compromised if nutrition is not adequate during the illness. Unfortunately, AIDS victims fight many battles with fever, nausea, diarrhea, and digestive disturbances. Gastrointestinal infections can lead to damage of the stomach lining and impair absorption of vital nutrients. Medications and chemotherapy often complicate the picture, causing appetite suppression and alterations in taste and smell. The heavy emotional toll may reduce or eliminate any desire for food. The combined effect of these changes can bring irregular and reduced intake of food. Reduced energy intake appears to be a primary contributing factor to the wasting syndrome (Macallan et al., 1995). At the extreme, dietary deficiencies are believed to compromise integrity of the immune system and may serve to speed progress of the disease.

To address some of these problems, the American Dietetic Association (Collins & Garcia, 1989) drafted a position on the role of nutrition in the treatment of AIDS. The ADA stressed that nutritional support is important at all stages of the disease. In the asymptomatic stage (Category A), counseling the patient or family on nutritional needs strives to promote an adequate and balanced diet with two goals in mind: insofar as possible to prevent undue weight loss and to prevent vitamin and mineral deficiencies that can further compromise system integrity. Later stages of the disease may call for both enteral (intragastric) or parenteral (intravenous, for example) nutritional support.

In addition, nutrition counseling can serve to address some of the symptoms that patients find debilitating and immobilizing, such as severe diarrhea. Changing the balance of carbohydrates, fats, and fibers, for example, can positively change this symptom. As the disease progresses, the needs of the patient must be reexamined and adjustments made to provide a nutritional base to help fight the disease.

AIDS Counseling Programs: Patients, Partners, and Families

Since the beginning of the AIDS pandemic, many clinics have recognized the urgent need to provide counseling to AIDS patients and their families.[4] Counseling programs may differ somewhat depending on locale and unique needs of clientele. Nonetheless, some common features are shared by almost all counseling programs. In this section, I will outline one such counseling effort based on the work of Riva Miller and Robert Bor (1989).

---

[4] I use the term *family* to refer to both traditional and nontraditional units based on love and commitment. The term refers to the nuclear family of necessity but it may also refer to others.

Stages in AIDS counseling   Counseling may occur at any one of several stages. Some people may fear that they have come in contact with the HIV. They may want information about how to check out their status in the most discrete way without alarming others or compromising their work or family stability. Others may come after an AIDS test has come back positive. They seek help for the emotional trauma that goes with knowing they carry the seeds of a terminal disease. Still others may need help as the disease progresses. This help may include dealing with neurological impairments (AIDS dementia) and counseling caregivers on how to manage the patient at home. Finally, counselors may deal with some clients who are in the terminal stages of illness. They seek help in coming to grips with their impending death. They may want help to resolve relationship issues or help for family members who are grieving the impending loss. The latter issue extends beyond the death of the AIDS client, because loved ones often need continued help to adjust to their loss.

The goals of AIDS counseling   Beyond general counseling goals, several goals are specific to counseling AIDS patients. The relative importance of these goals depends on the client's AIDS status. One goal is to *provide information about AIDS and the HIV.* Many myths about AIDS cloud clear thinking and may affect mood, behavior, or both. For some, the suggestion that an HIV test might be wise could be enough to drive the person to despair and depression. Misinformation can influence both risk-taking behaviors and help-seeking behaviors. The counselor should clarify what information of the client's is accurate and build on that information while correcting misinformation.

Another goal is to *assess the impact of AIDS or HIV-positive status on the client's psychological well-being.* Often, this includes working with members of the client's family who may be shocked, angered, or dismayed by such news.

Third, the counselor should *arrange for some assessment of neurological and psychiatric impairment.* This may involve arranging for a colleague to carry out the assessment or for referral to an assessment center.

Fourth, the counselor needs to *be sensitive to several relationship problems* that can arise. These problems can and do occur between the client and lovers, friends, family members, and health care professionals. There may be issues of guilt in any one of several family members. Lovers may experience guilt if they feel responsible for the client's disease. Parents may feel guilty if they believe they have failed in their parental responsibilities. A parent with AIDS may be concerned about possible infections in a spouse or children. Often, problems in family continuity are involved, since most AIDS victims are young. In some cases, the counselor may arrange sessions that include one or more of these significant others.

An important aspect of counseling is to help the client think through important decisions and *make informed decisions about both risk-taking behaviors and help-seeking behaviors.* Finally, the counselor may need to *assess coping skills and provide training* to remedy deficits. Depending on the stage of the disease, the counselor can explore several issues with the client to help deal with AIDS-related stress. One area of great importance is the financial impact of AIDS. More insurance companies are providing early benefits (pre-death life insurance) to help the AIDS patient deal with financial emergencies. Emerging legal protections for AIDS patients prevent loss of access to schools, jobs, and other vital services. The counselor may remind the client of these benefits and help identify relevant regulations to obtain relief.

Psychoeducational Programs: Hopes and Promises

In the decade since AIDS made its presence known, many different strategies have been implemented. Many early intervention programs were developed to target specific high-risk groups in high-risk cities. Examples include interventions to reach infected gay males in San

Francisco or IV drug users in New York or Miami. Using both behavioral change strategies and educational strategies, such programs have typically tried to change attitudes and behaviors. Another focus has been on middle-school and high-school students' knowledge of AIDS, attitudes about preventive behaviors, and acceptance of condom use (Winter & Goldy, 1993). Programs at the college level have typically focused on increasing information and assessing attitudes toward preventive behaviors (Strauss, Corless, Luckey, van der Horst, & Dennis, 1992), but some have also attempted behavioral change as well. Mass media campaigns have also been developed worldwide to increase knowledge of AIDS and to try to increase awareness of vital health-protective behaviors that can reduce risk. The latter includes an AIDS hot line and clearing house that has filled more than 60 million requests for information in a three-year period (Roper, 1991). By 1987, 99% of American adults were aware of AIDS and most (more than 91%) knew the primary modes of transmission (Coates, 1990).

Margaret Chesney, in her address as president of the Health Psychology Division of APA, noted: "It is as though behavior change technology is being given a scientific treadmill test, and the limits of this technology are painfully apparent" (1993, p. 262). The most encouraging note from early data is that risk can be reduced (Des Jarlais & Friedman, 1988; Peterson & Marín, 1988; Stall, Coates, & Hoff, 1988). Still, as Chesney noted, the amount of change and rate of relapse is often less than desirable, especially among some of the highest-risk groups.

In spite of notable successes, there are still many frustrations. Many interventions are done on an informal basis rather than on the basis of a theory (Fisher & Fisher, 1992). Also, interventions frequently use a shotgun approach, mixing multiple components in the hope that some component will result in change. To make matters worse, evaluations of change seldom try to break down the components to find out which part of the package was most responsible for the change. For example, a clinic may provide its patients with individual counseling,

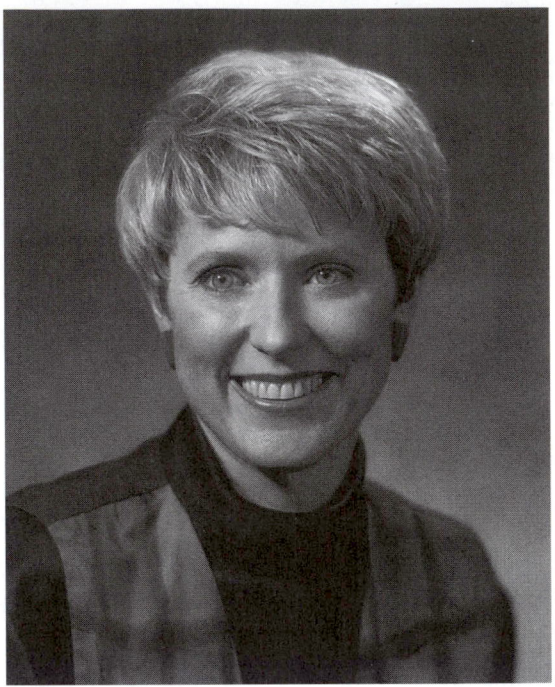

FIGURE 11.7   *Margaret Chesney, past president of the APA Division of Health Psychology and chair of the NIMH HIV Prevention Research Consortium, has contributed greatly to work on AIDS prevention research as well as women's health initiatives.*

group education programs, and stress management training, among other possible interventions. After a period of time, it may be possible to show that the patients have reduced the frequency of high-risk behaviors. The problem from a methodological viewpoint is what caused the change. Was it the counseling, the education, the stress management, or some combination of the treatments?[5]

The incredible pressures faced by many health care providers in the early stages of the epidemic may be partly responsible for this situation. Joseph Catania and his colleagues commented that the problem of balancing urgency and rigor was very real (Catania, Gibson, Chitwood, & Coates, 1990). Yet now that the

---

[5] We discussed this problem in more detail in Chapter 5.

panic has settled to some degree, there is renewed interest in evaluating intervention programs both in formal theoretical terms and in terms of the effectiveness of components (for example, Kalichman, Rompa, & Coley, 1996).

Barriers to adopting risk-reducing behaviors In their review of the problems confronted in getting people to change high-risk behaviors, the National Commission on AIDS noted some discrepancies between research outcomes and common sense notions about how to change behavior.

There is a notion that fear-inducing messages will get people's attention and that enough fear will motivate people to change. But a wide variety of research on persuasive communication shows that messages with too much fear content may lead people to tune out the message and continue to think of themselves as invulnerable. Australia used shock tactics in a mass media campaign to increase both concern about AIDS and knowledge of AIDS, but the campaign had little effect on either concern or knowledge (Rigby, Brown, Anagnostou, Ross, & Rosser, 1989). Other public health campaigns have shown that fear messages may increase awareness, but they do not necessarily change behavior (Chesney & Coates, 1990).

Further, getting behavior change to last is a significant problem. Relapse appears to be related to low self-efficacy, depression, drug abuse and alcohol use, and perceptions that

pleasure in unprotected sex is higher. Among women, low self-efficacy may also be associated with increased risk because the woman may feel that she has lower power in the relationship and cannot insist that her partner wear a condom (Worth, 1990).

A model of AIDS-preventive behavior
After reviewing much of the intervention literature, Jeffrey and William Fisher (1992) constructed and tested a model of AIDS-preventive behavior rooted in the theory of reasoned action. They suggest that the model has the potential to generalize across many different target populations. This model contains three factors: information, motivation, and behavioral skills. The information crucial to risk reduction concerns the modes of AIDS transmission and methods of preventing infection. Motivation directly affects whether a person will act on the basis of knowledge gained from informational media. Then, specific skills are required for the person to engage in risk-reducing behaviors. Examples of behavioral skills include bleaching works, putting on a condom, avoiding drinking or drugs prior to sex, and using assertive skills that may be required to adhere to health-protective behaviors. The authors noted that a person must be able to leave a situation in which safe sex cannot be negotiated.

In this model, information may act directly on preventive behavior, but only when the behavior is simple, such as avoiding sexual contact.

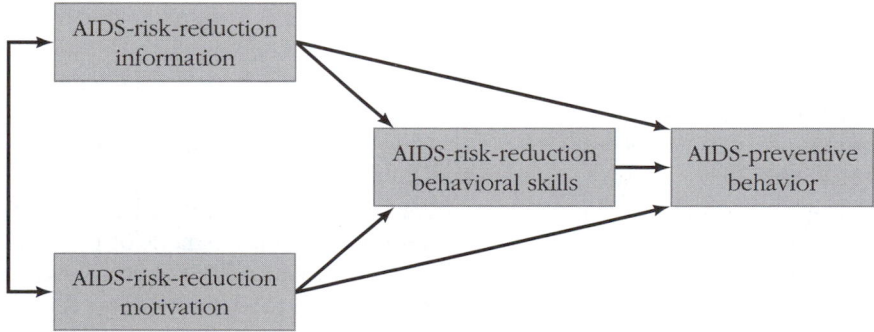

FIGURE 11.8   Three determinants of AIDS risk reduction proposed by Fisher and Fisher (1992).

Consistent with this, evaluations of programs among both drug injectors and gays show that information is necessary but not sufficient to change behavior (O'Keeffe, Nesselhof-Kendall, & Baum, 1990). As the behavior becomes more complex, such as buying and negotiating use of a condom on a regular basis, the behavior may need additional support from motivation change and skill acquisition before it will occur on a consistent basis. Fisher and Fisher provided data to show that the model is capable of explaining 35% of the variance in preventive behavior among gay males, but it explains only 10% of the variance in university students' preventive behavior. It is difficult to say whether the model will prove useful at this point, but it does provide a context of theory in which to test intervention programs.

Interventions to Reduce Risk from Sexual Behavior

Probably more effort has been expended on programs to reduce high-risk sexual behavior than for any other AIDS risk. Interventions that are broader in scope, including information, motivation, and behavioral skills training, tend to produce the best risk reduction (Fisher & Fisher, 1992). Substantive problems in methodology, however, including measurement errors and selection bias in subjects, make it difficult to interpret the studies (Catania et al., 1990).

Thomas Coates (1990), in reviewing strategies for changing sexual behavior, noted some remarkable successes. In one educational program in San Francisco, the rate of seroconversion and gonococcal proctitis (GCP) dropped over a four-year period after the program. In 1982, 13% of gay and bisexual males converted to HIV-positive status, but by 1986, the rate of conversion had dropped to 1%. At the first reporting period, there were more than 4000 cases of GCP, but by 1986 the number of cases had dropped to 390.

The San Francisco model is probably the most comprehensive program in existence and in-

volves much more detail than can be presented here. In brief, the model used a coordinated community-level program that involved seven different organizations to reach people at various levels of risk. The organizations involved the mass media, health care organizations, schools, work sites, drug abuse and family planning centers (including STD centers), community organizations (churches and clubs), and antibody testing centers.

Consistent with the notion that information, motivation, and skills are crucial components of risk reduction, programs were developed appropriate for use in the different centers. Educational information focused on modes of HIV transmission. Motivational components included models presented through the mass media, teen models in the schools, and co-workers at work sites, for example. Skill training was accomplished by mass media modeling of safe sex practices and safe needle behavior. At the different community sites, classes, videos, and models were used to teach risk-reduction skills.

In addition, the San Francisco model sought to publicize normative data that would create more awareness of the prevalence of high-risk behaviors and to create acceptance of HIV-infected persons in various walks of life. Finally, the San Francisco model used advocacy groups and social action groups to change policy at several levels. The intent of policy change was to change laws that would promote risk reduction but also reduce the stigma and discrimination that people with AIDS often experience.

As evidence of the success of the program, 60% of the sample in 1984 reported engaging in high-risk behavior, but by 1987 this figure had dropped to 30%. For one such behavior, 50% reported engaging in unprotected anal intercourse in 1984, but by 1987 only 12% reported this high-risk behavior. Assessment of the psychosocial processes that might explain changing high-risk behavior indicated that both perceived self-efficacy and peer support for low-risk behavior were important.

Interventions Among Drug Users

Intervention programs have encountered difficulty in persuading IV drug users to change high-risk behaviors. Paradoxically, IV drug users seem to be more aware of the risks that go with sharing needles than those that go with unprotected sex. They will adopt procedures to clean needles and cookers, but IV drug users continue to share needles, and they continue to engage in unprotected sexual activity.

In contrast, gay communities in several major cities have shown substantial changes in high-risk behavior. Ekstrand and Coates (1990) observed that unprotected anal intercourse dropped from about 35% to about 3% after an intervention program. This outcome must be viewed with guarded optimism, because evidence from other studies shows that changes may not persist very long (Kelly & Murphy, 1992).

Major differences between drug users and the gay community, however, may account for differences in interventions. Drug users probably do not share a sense of community with bonds of friendship, purpose, and reciprocal concern, as the gay community does. Further, use of illicit drugs places that behavior squarely in the law enforcement arena whereas the gay lifestyle, though still subjected to forms of discrimination, is not necessarily illegal. Finally, most drug users are distrustful of attempts at intervention mostly because of fear of detection, punishment, and possible incarceration.[6]

Stephens and his colleagues carried out an educational intervention with intravenous drug users in a one-on-one format (Stephens et al., 1991). They assessed numerous needle and drug behaviors both before and after the intervention. Among the needle behaviors they wanted to change were sharing needles or cookers, cleaning with bleach, and intravenous injections. Since the HIV is fragile, it can be killed very effectively, and needles and works can be decontaminated by washing them with bleach.

The educational program consisted of four components. The first was basic information on AIDS, the modes of transmission, and the typical course of progression. A film produced at the Taconic Correctional Facility by prisoners dying of AIDS—*AIDS: A Bad Way to Die*—presented most of this information. The second and third components focused on specific behaviors that needed to be changed, including both drug use and sexual behaviors. The fourth component was information on the HIV antibody test and encouragement to participate in an anonymous blood screening project.

Results from the study showed that six of the seven needle behaviors changed. A major decline occurred in the percentage of users sharing works, and a major increase occurred in the percentage who used bleach to clean their works. The intervention had a larger effect on needle behavior than on general drug use behavior although all of the drug use measures also declined. Compared to a nonequivalent control group, the treatment showed overall lower level of risk after the intervention. In addition, Stephens's research group took measures on three equal-sized subgroups (101 subjects each) at roughly three, four, and five months' follow-up. The evidence was not clear in regard to stability of the intervention: Although protective behaviors declined somewhat, the groups still were at lower risk than prior to the intervention. A five-month follow-up period is usually not adequate to judge the permanence of an intervention, however.

Virginia McCoy and her associates described a similar program to reach drug users, the Miami Community Outreach Project (McCoy, Dodds, & Nolan, 1990). Although data were not yet available to evaluate overall effectiveness, the program included some unique components not seen in the intervention just described. In the Miami project, an enhanced intervention provided intensive group counseling sessions designed to take clients through a sequence to obtain knowledge, develop skills, change

---

[6] I am indebted to the comment of a reviewer for highlighting the difference in community between these two groups.

attitudes and behavior, and develop a plan for such change.

Basic information was presented through the same film used in the intervention just described, *AIDS: A Bad Way to Die*. The second session provided practical information and demonstrations on safer sex practices, needle cleaning, and how the drug subculture lifestyle influenced risk behaviors, using two films, *Needletalk* and *Coat of Arms*. The third intensive counseling session was devoted to evaluating individual problem areas, then challenging clients to develop realistic goals and changes that could correct problem areas. Here, two films were used, one entitled *Black People Get AIDS Too* and a group exercise film called *Future Game Plan*. In addition, social reinforcers were brought into play in small group exercises. These exercises were designed not only to intensify the educational mission, but to bring peer group pressure into the social process. They also provided a way of introducing simulation of real-life circumstances for discussion and feedback. Further, positive role models delivered risk-reduction information. The project is designed to provide follow-up data at several points up to 18 months following intervention.

Mass media interventions

Mass media campaigns using public figures are considered useful, but only limited evidence of that usefulness exists. The disclosure by Magic Johnson that he was infected offered one group of investigators a rare chance to carry out a type of natural experiment (Kalichman, Russell, Hunter, & Sarwer, 1993). Prior to the announcement, television gave an average of three minutes per day to news and information about AIDS. The day of the announcement, TV devoted about two hours to AIDS information. From there on, coverage dropped until it was back at the three-minute average by two weeks after the announcement. There was evidence that between 20% and 33% of the people had misinformation about AIDS including modes of transmission. For example, about 33% incorrectly answered the item "Men cannot get AIDS from women."

Compared to white males, black males reported they were more strongly affected by Magic Johnson's announcement. Compared to a little more than 7000 phone calls in the preceding 90 days, the CDC received over 28,000 phone calls asking for information on AIDS the day after the announcement. Although difficult to assess its actual behavioral impact, the announcement may have had a significant impact on public awareness and knowledge about AIDS.

Kalichman and his colleagues believe that it is important to adapt media messages to the culture of the target group (Kalichman, Kelly, Hunter, Murphy, & Tyler, 1993). To this end, they tailored risk-reduction messages to African American women, who make up 53% of women with AIDS. One group of women viewed a public health message video prepared by former Surgeon General Koop, which used professional white broadcasters to deliver the information. The tape then was edited so that the information was presented in the same order, using the same graphics, and delivering the same verbal messages, but the information was delivered by African American women. Yet a third tape was developed that included three culturally relevant themes and examples obtained from focus groups. The three themes were cultural pride, community concern, and family responsibility.

Two weeks after viewing the video, women who had seen the cultural context video expressed both more concern and more fear than women who viewed the standard tape. They also engaged in more risk-reduction behaviors, such as getting tested for HIV antibodies. Few differences in either attitudes or knowledge appeared, however.

Public policy and partner notification

Another line of attack for prevention is partner notification. This effort assumes that if you know the person you are with has AIDS, you will be less likely to engage in unprotected sex or other high-risk behaviors involving that person. In the best of all worlds, people would be completely honest and forthright about their HIV status at all crucial times. But many social pressures as well as personal needs and conflicts influence the person's willingness to disclose information as potentially powerful as HIV status (Marks et al., 1992). Most states now have passed laws that require a person who has tested positive for AIDS to notify their partner(s).

One study examined such a program located in North Carolina and found less than positive results (Landis et al., 1992). This study used 74 subjects: 39 assigned to the provider notice group and 35 assigned to the patient notice group. In the first group, the counselors assumed responsibility to notify partners of the person's infection. In the other group, it was up to the patient to notify partners. Monitoring procedures showed that 50% (78 of 157) of the partners were contacted in the provider notice group, but only 7% (10 of 153) of the partners were notified in the patient notice group. Obviously, patient notification in this case was very ineffective. It would be preferable to have an even better record than the 50% that occurred in the provider notice group. But at the least, a large number of the partners could now make decisions about testing and health-protective behaviors that were not possible before. In this case, 23% of the partners notified and tested turned out to be HIV positive.

Summary

In this chapter, we have discussed the now pandemic disease AIDS. We began with the rapidly changing face of AIDS as the distribution across ethnic groups, gender, and sexual orientation have changed dramatically. The major points are summarized below.

1. AIDS is no longer just a disease for white gay males or minority intravenous drug users. It can afflict anyone who chooses to engage in any of several high-risk behaviors.

2. AIDS is caused by a retrovirus, the human immunodeficiency virus. It is able to attach itself to T_4 helper cells and then replicate its own DNA code in the host cell, destroying the integrity of the cell and weakening the immune system.

3. The HIV produces detrimental changes in the endocrine and central nervous system through infections, tumors, and indirectly through the side effects of medications.

4. The behaviors most often associated with risk of contracting AIDS are unprotected sex with multiple partners, injecting drugs, and sharing drug paraphernalia.

5. The fluids involved in transmission of the AIDS virus include blood, sexual fluids, and perinatal fluids.

6. Information and attitudes about AIDS contribute significantly to risks by shaping perceptions of vulnerability and lowering the likelihood of taking precautions against exposure. Minority groups often have less accurate information and feel less vulnerable than whites.

7. Resistance to condom use typically occurs because of the belief that condoms interfere with sensitivity and spontaneity. Use of condoms reduces risk substantially even though condoms are not foolproof.

8. Tests for AIDS are readily available but lack of concern or fear of knowing often keep people from finding out their serostatus. Even when they know serostatus, many do not tell their partners. Yet taking preventive steps depends heavily on knowing the serostatus of sexual partners.

9. AIDS produces many psychological effects including heightened anxiety, panic attacks, and depression. These changes may also make it more difficult for the person to maintain a healthy lifestyle.

10. Medical treatment relies on drugs, such as zidovudine, that try to stop the HIV from replicating. Other drugs are used to treat the side effects of AIDS, such as pneumonia and cancer.

11. Counseling objectives depend on where the person is in regard to AIDS. Pretesting objectives focus on information and emotional needs. Posttesting objectives, especially when the test is positive, may focus on emotional adjustment, growing mental and physical limitations, relationship needs, and practical (legal, financial) problems, among others.

12. Intervention programs include mass media informational programs, group programs to reduce high-risk drug or sexual behavior, and public policy interventions to change laws that impact the AIDS patient.

13. These programs have had some measure of success, but not enough to slow the onslaught of AIDS.

14. Misinformation, feelings of invulnerability, and perceptions about sexuality and personal freedoms continue to be major barriers to preventing AIDS.

Key Words

acquired immune deficiency syndrome
AIDS dementia complex
human immunodeficiency virus
pandemic
retrovirus
zidovudine (AZT)

Study Questions

1. How does the HIV weaken the immune system?

2. What changes have occurred in who is at risk for AIDS now as compared to the early 1980s?

3. What are the primary behaviors that lead to risk of exposure to the HIV?

4. What are the primary fluids involved in passing the AIDS virus from one person to another?

5. What attitudes are most likely to prevent changes in sexual activity to reduce risk of exposure?

6. What are some of the emotional outcomes of being diagnosed with AIDS?

7. Does AIDS-related stress weaken the immune system beyond that produced by the HIV? Explain your answer.

8. What is the major medical therapy for AIDS? How does it work? What are the pros and cons of its use?

9. How do nutrition and exercise impact AIDS progression and treatment?

10. Identify the core curriculum of the major programs to intervene in high-risk groups. How successful have these programs been in the short run? How successful in the long term?

11. What are some goals in counseling AIDS patients?

Class Projects

1. Some people argue that no research should be carried out until pressing social need demands it. Using the AIDS pandemic as an example, consider how a policy of this nature might have impacted the efforts to understand AIDS.

2. The relationship between alcohol and risk of exposure to AIDS is often overlooked. Set up a panel discussion on the role of alcohol in AIDS transmission.

3. If community resources permit, invite professionals to class to discuss the important needs of local AIDS patients. Include the legal issues of risks involved in being identified as an AIDS patient and protections available.

Suggested Readings

Ashe, A., & Rampersad, A. (1993). *Days of grace*. New York: Knopf.

Chesney, M. A. (1993). Health psychology in the 21st century: Acquired immunodeficiency syndrome as a harbinger of things to come. *Health Psychology, 12*, 259–268.

WEBSITES   AIDS

ADDRESS	DESCRIPTION
http://www.gen.emory.edu/MEDWEB/ alphakey/AIDS_and_HIV.html	☆ MEDWEB's alphabetized index (9 pages) to internet resources for AIDS-HIV
http://www.aaas.org/science/aidslink.htm	The American Association for the Advancement of Science—selected directory of AIDS sites
http://www.mic.ki.se/DISEASES/index.html	A top site for special section devoted to AIDS information
http://www.healthgate.com/choice/AMA/search. html	JAMA HIV/AIDS—AIDSLINE, AIDSTRIALS, and AIDSDRUGS
http://www.iapac.org/consumer/proinbk.html	Protease Inhibitors: An introduction to new AIDS medications
http://www.execpc.com/~corbeau/	Internet Depression Resources List—this could be placed in any one of the following chapters as well since depression is a common correlate of many illnesses
http://planetq.com/aidsvl/index.html	AIDS Virtual Library—comprehensive link site
http://gpawww.who.ch/ganews/ganews.htm	World Health Organization Newsletter

Coping with Chronic or Catastrophic Illness

As medical science has rushed to eliminate the epidemic killers of medieval days, new forms of disease have taken their place. Some of these—such as an increased rate of heart diseases—are often related to the affluent lifestyle that typifies technologically advanced societies. Physical effects may come on slowly but lead progressively to functional incapacity. Further, medical technology has reduced infant mortality and prolonged life for many people who might have perished in an earlier era at a much younger age. The gift of life, though, is often bought at the expense of living with a disorder that is partly or totally disabling.

The subject matter of the next three chapters, then, is chronic and disabling conditions. We begin with heart health, then consider pain, and finally discuss cancer and arthritis. Although various other chronic ailments could be discussed, these are at the core of current efforts to design psychosocial interventions. They also illustrate general methods that may be used with various chronic ailments.

In Chapter 12 on heart health, we will review the anatomy and physiology of the cardiovascular system. This review will help us understand how lifestyle choices can influence the physical system for better or for worse. We will look at heart ailments, including the myocardial infarct, better known as the common heart attack; coronary artery disease, or atherosclerosis; and high blood pressure, or hypertension. We will examine medical interventions for heart disease. These procedures often arouse anxiety and fear in patients, emotions that may influence the ease of operating and the course of recovery. Finally, we will examine several cognitive-behavioral techniques designed to help people prevent heart disease, adjust to difficult procedures before or after surgeries, or to rehabilitate themselves physically following a heart problem.

In Chapter 13 we will confront the perplexing problem of pain. Pain may be viewed from a physiological perspective: that is, as a sense receptor and neural response to physical trauma. Still, many people report pain in the absence of any known medical reason. Recent research suggests that subjective expectations and psychosocial context can influence a person's perception of pain. A variety of techniques have been developed to help pain patients develop more active coping skills and reduce negative thinking about pain. When these are implemented, subjective reports of pain tend to decrease.

Finally, in Chapter 14, we will discuss two major chronic disorders, cancer and arthritis. We will discuss current views of the etiology of cancer and describe the more common types of cancer. We will consider evidence on psychosocial processes involved in the course of cancer, all the while cautioning that cancer is a physical disease with known pathology that requires medical treatments. The common psychosocial interventions focus on helping the patient to adjust to the emotional strain of living with cancer, or to accept medical diagnostics and treatments with less anxiety. Arthritis has been a most perplexing disease for medical science. As yet, the cause of arthritis is not clear although there are promising new leads. Treatment generally is not curative but palliative—that is, offered to control discomfort and pain rather than to eliminate the disease.

CHAPTER *12*

Heart Health: Silent Killers and the Hurry Sickness

Imagine that you are on staff at a hospital in Los Angeles. It is just a few days before Christmas, but this night will be etched in your memory for years. An EMT squad has just called to report they are transporting a male heart attack victim. The symptoms are not good. The patient is coughing blood, a sure sign of congestive heart failure. The next ten minutes are a blur, getting the emergency room ready for the patient, expecting the worst but hoping for the best. Although it seems just a moment since the call, the siren's wail warns that the ambulance is rapidly approaching. Every effort is made to ensure there will be no delays when the patient arrives; even a few moments can make the difference between life and death.

The doors burst open for the onrushing stretcher. Instead of lying comatose, though, the patient sits up, calmly waves and grins at the staff, and says, "Gentlemen, I want you to know that you're looking at the darnedest healing machine that's ever been wheeled into this hospital."

The medical staff do not know exactly how to react. Is this person one of the last great optimists on the face of the earth? Is he somewhere a few mental miles off the deep end? The truth of the matter, as it turns out, is much closer to the former than the latter. This case is not fiction, but a very real life and death crisis and the story of a very unusual man, Norman Cousins. The record of those words straight from Cousins's mouth was made by his friend and physician Omar Fareed (Cousins, 1983, p. 264).

To know the man behind the words, we must go back years earlier. Shortly after World War II,

Cousins began his career with the *Saturday Review*. Under his leadership, the *Saturday Review* came to be regarded as a voice for reason and a champion for world peace. Aside from his hectic schedule, Cousins followed a reasonably healthy life style. He did not smoke or drink; he did not allow himself to get overweight; and he continued his lifelong interest in athletic activity. Thus, for much of his early life he had few health concerns. About 1954, though, at 39 years of age, he applied for life insurance and was turned down. The reason was a cardiogram that showed the presence of a silent coronary. Cousins began at this time to assert the patient's need to be self-informed about health and illness, and to be involved in health decisions as an equal partner with the physician.[1] In 1978, he joined the UCLA medical school to teach medical students about the humanity each doctor should possess. Still, he was never far from preaching Hippocrates' dictum that "the human body is the physician of its own illnesses" (Cousins, 1983, p. 160).

We come then to that night, December 22, 1980, when in that Los Angeles emergency room Cousins confronted another test of his view that a positive outlook is one of the greatest assets to healing. When asked a few days later to do a treadmill test, the results were shocking and discouraging. First, he had a strong emotional reaction to taking the test. Then, only a few minutes into the test, his heart rate went up, and his blood pressure dropped rapidly. This telltale sign usually indicates severe arterial blockage and typically leads to an angiogram. Still, Cousins would not consent because he also knew that an angiogram typically leads to coronary bypass surgery.

He insisted that they try a second time for a treadmill test. But this time, a very interesting

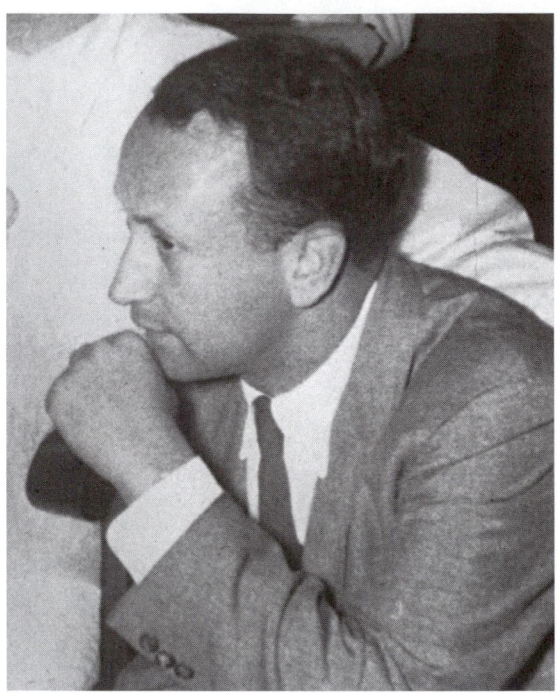

FIGURE 12.1   *Norman Cousins, former editor of the* Saturday Review, *was a champion of the notion that a positive mood is a powerful positive force for healing.*

event occurred on the way to the test room. He became dizzy just from the emotional panic that welled up as he thought about the test. His reaction parallels conditioned aversions that often occur in chemotherapy patients. Not until months later did he finally come to terms with the treadmill in a unique way. He thought if he could arrange the test to his own liking and run the controls that he would probably be less anxious. His doctor agreed, and the test went without a hitch.

In the meantime, outside the confines of the hospital, Cousins went on a strict diet of mostly salads, reducing his meat intake. He designed his exercise program in a carefully stepped fashion to increase time and pace gradually. By the end of January 1981, less than two months after the attack, he still could walk only a slow-paced half-mile without stopping and

---

[1] It should be noted that Cousins was as unique a patient as he was an individual. Many patients do not take the time to inform themselves at the level Cousins did. Cousins also confronted a serious collagen disease, an episode in his life that was detailed in Chapter 6.

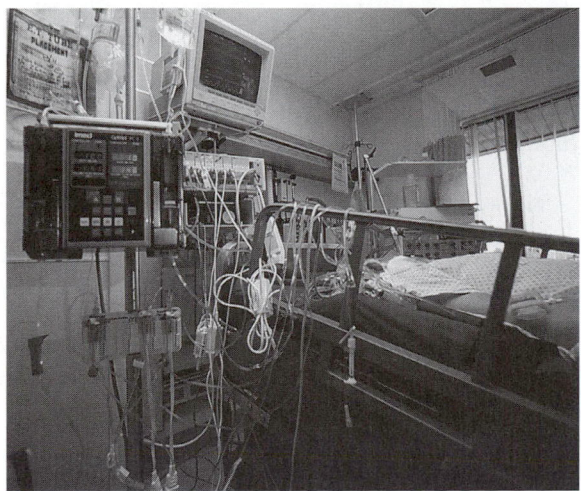

FIGURE 12.2   The ICU, or intensive care unit, can often be a depersonalizing and humiliating place. Medical staff are sensitized to the medical emergencies that can occur at any minute, and they may tend to overinterpret patient's behavior as fitting the model of a medical crisis.

without his pulse going above 94. By September, nine months after the attack, he could walk six miles each day, and his cholesterol and triglycerides were below the danger zone. Almost 2½ years later, having never gone through the angiogram or bypass surgery, he received a clean bill of health and his physician commented on the magnificent condition of his heart.

This story, told by Norman Cousins in *The Healing Heart* (1983), highlights many psychosocial factors that can influence the onset or course of heart disease. The purpose of this chapter is to consider risk factors for heart disease and psychosocial methods to prevent heart disease or restore heart health. We will look first at the normal heart as well as common pathophysiological processes. Then, we will consider some epidemiological data on the distribution of coronary disease.

The risk factors for coronary disease are many, including genetic traits, age, and gender. Among the more important risk factors are

choices about diet, exercise, and smoking. Some evidence suggests that dispositional traits such as anger and hostility can have a powerful influence on risk for coronary. Finally, we will consider several intervention programs designed to help coronary patients adhere to a strict regimen after an attack.

Biomedical Background: Physiology, Genetics, and Risks

In a normally healthy person, the heart does its work quietly and efficiently. We barely take notice of its operation unless some event occurs to stir it to stronger action. An attractive person may pass by causing the heart to flutter. A careless motorist whisks by dangerously close to our bike causing the heart to race, and perhaps anger to surge. At these times, we may be aware of the pounding in our chest or the tightness of the veins in our neck as the blood courses through. Then, for just a moment, we might ponder the small but mighty marvel that lies buried in our chest.

The heart is no bigger than a grapefruit, a mass of muscle that weighs between half and three-quarters of a pound. The heart beats day in and day out at a faithful pace, rarely missing a beat. The pulse rate of a newborn is around 120 to 140 beats per minute. In the mature adult, the resting heart beats between 60 and 90 beats per minute (bpm). Well-trained athletes may have heart rates as low as 40 to 45 bpm. Under stress, heart rate accelerates to much higher levels. During light exercise, for example, the rate may rise to around 100 bpm. In strenuous exercise, it may go up to around 200 bpm. Astronauts have pulse rates around 140 beats per minute during the most stressful periods of liftoff and reentry.

For some people, arousal in emotional situations may be one of the few times they really pay attention to their heart. But for others, the heart may constantly remind of its presence because it fails to function as it should. In this section, we will briefly review the physiology of the normal heart. Then, we will consider pathological processes that alter the cardiovascular system. This review will provide the background for understanding how risk factors can be modified by changes in lifestyle.

Heart Physiology: Pumps, Aerators, and Hoses

Superficially, the heart seems to be a simple pump that pulls blood in one side and pumps it out the other. But in reality the tissues that make up the heart, the vessels that make up the blood distribution system, and the neural system that supports its timing make a very complex system indeed.

In simplified terms, the heart can be viewed as a four-chamber organ divided into two upper receiving centers and two lower sending centers. The two sides perform a synchronized dance in which the right side mirrors at a lower pressure each step of the left side.

The heart's upper chambers are called atria and the lower chambers are ventricles. *Atrium* is an architectural term referring to a home's open entry way. A ventricle is a hollow cavity in any organ. On each side, the atrium and ventricle are connected by a single gateway that allows blood to move through, with a valve acting as gatekeeper. The tricuspid valve controls blood movement between the right atrium and ventricle. The mitral valve controls blood movement between the left atrium and ventricle.

In the **systolic phase,** the tricuspid and mitral valves close, the ventricles contract strongly, and both the pulmonary and the aortic valves open. The right ventricle ejects old oxygen-depleted blood through the pulmonary artery to the lungs. Here, carbon dioxide is removed, and fresh oxygen is infused into the blood. At the same time, the left ventricle ejects at high pressure about eight ounces of oxygen-enriched blood into the aorta. Normal systolic blood pressure is around 130 mm/Hg (the measurement refers to height of mercury in a standard tube), but this is in the left ventricle only, since the right ventricle works at a lower pressure. Further, when necessary, the heart can increase the amount of blood it pumps out each minute by a factor of 6 to 10 (Smith & Leon, 1992).

During the ejection phase, activity has been going on in the two artria. In the right atrium, used blood (oxygen-depleted blood) returns from the body. In the left atrium, oxygen-replenished blood returns from the lungs.

At the end of the ejection phase is the **diastolic phase.** During diastole, the ventricles begin to relax, pressure drops, and both the aortic and pulmonary valves close. The tricuspid and mitral valves open, and the ventricles refill with blood preparing for the next cycle. In the diastolic phase, blood pressure is around 70 mm/Hg.

Neural signals that control the heart's action originate in the brain stem region. These signals travel along the vagus nerve to the sinoatrial node located in the right atrium. Nerve impulses from the vagus cause atrial contraction. Then impulses travel to the lower region of the atrium where they stimulate ventricular contraction.

The sinoatrial node is the pacemaker of the heart. The stronger the vagus signal, the slower the heart rate. The parasympathetic system exerts dominant control over cardiac pacing in the early years, but strong fight or flight reactions and adrenaline release will weaken vagal signals and lead to more rapid heart rates. As the person ages, the parasympathetic control wanes, the sympathetic system exerts more control, the vagus signal weakens, and the heart rate increases.[2]

The technical name for heart muscle is myocardium. Before the heart can supply the rest of the body, it has to feed itself. The first arterial branches to split off from the aorta

---

[2] In this case, and with apologies to those who are older by this criteria than they think, *aging* means passing age 30 and beyond.

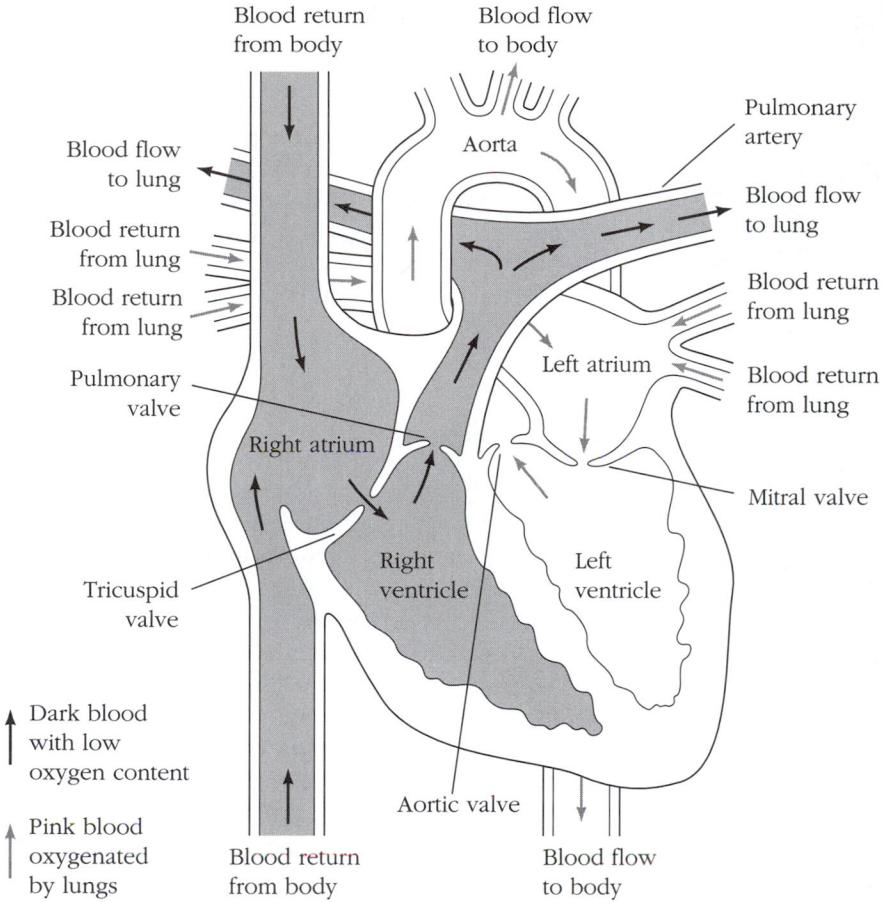

Blood return from body

Blood flow to body

Aorta

Pulmonary artery

Blood flow to lung

Blood flow to lung

Blood return from lung

Blood return from lung

Blood return from lung

Left atrium

Blood return from lung

Pulmonary valve

Right atrium

Mitral valve

Tricuspid valve

Right ventricle

Left ventricle

Dark blood with low oxygen content

Pink blood oxygenated by lungs

Aortic valve

Blood return from body

Blood flow to body

FIGURE 12.3   The anatomy of the heart shows the basic four-chamber structure as viewed from the front. On the right, the heart receives blood from the body in the right atrium. Blood then passes to the right ventricle. When the right ventricle contracts (pumps), blood is discharged through the pulmonary artery for aeration in the lungs. Reoxygenated blood returns through the pulmonary veins to the left atrium, and then to the left ventricle. When the left ventricle contracts, it forces blood out the aorta for distribution through the body (from Heller et al., 1996).

supply the heart. As Figure 12.4 shows, the right and left coronary arteries spread out, enveloping the heart in a rich network of supply lines. These arteries are also points of weakness where coronary artery disease wreaks havoc with the heart's own lifeline. These arteries are prone to the buildup of plaques that slowly narrow the opening, making it harder for the heart to get energy for its work. Here a heart surgeon may

put in substitute arteries to bypass blocked arteries.

The circulatory system consists of outgoing arteries, connecting capillaries, and returning veins. The blood vessels are composed of four tissue layers. The innermost layer is the smooth-muscle endothelium. The second layer is the intima, and the third is the media. The outermost layer is the adventitia.

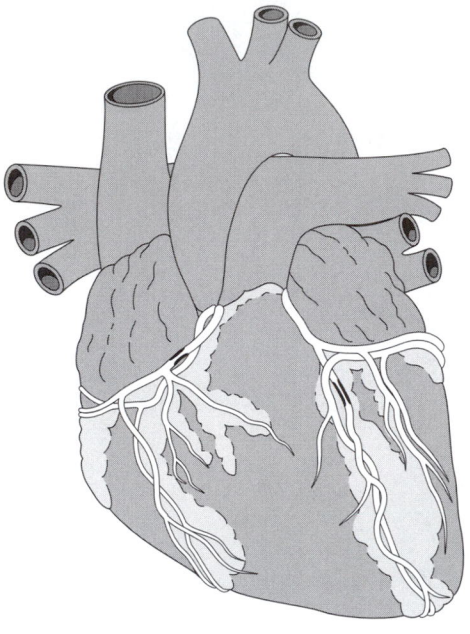

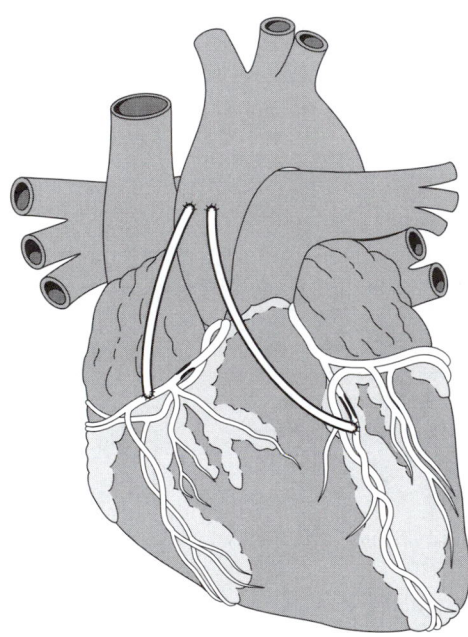

FIGURE 12.4   The build-up of plaques in the arteries leads to constriction that increases blood pressure and potentially blockage or moving clots that can cause death. The coronary bypass procedure, shown at bottom, is done to correct problems due to blockage of the coronary arteries.

Heart Pathophysiology: Cardiomyopathy, Arrhythmia, and Infarctions

The heart is vulnerable to several pathological conditions that affect both structure and function. Cardiomyopathies alter the size of the heart muscle or ventricle. Arrhythmias refer to changes in the pacing of the heart. Ischemia is an imbalance in the demand and supply of oxygen to the heart. A myocardial infarct, or heart attack, is the death of heart tissue because the heart cannot get enough blood to supply itself. The major culprit in coronary heart disease (CHD) is coronary artery disease (CAD), also known as coronary atherosclerosis. As we shall see later, however, atherosclerosis is only part of the story, since **thrombogenesis** (the formation of clots) is the most important contributing cause to heart attacks.

A **cardiomyopathy** is a disease that primarily involves the heart muscle (myocardium). There are two types of cardiomyopathy. In **dilated cardiomyopathy,** the left ventricle becomes enlarged and weakened. In **hypertrophic cardiomyopathy,** the left ventricle walls become much thicker than normal. Then, like a muscle-bound hulk, the ventricle does not perform its work as efficiently as it should. A related condition is **left ventricular hypertrophy,** a thickening of the left ventricle that is usually brought on by hypertension or some other cause (Frohlich et al., 1992). The condition becomes more severe with age, and it occurs more often in people with blood pressure readings above 160/95 mm/Hg. This condition has been the subject of intense press coverage because celebrity athletes, such as Hank Gathers, have died suddenly from the condition.

Another heart disorder is the cardiac arrhythmia. Typically, the heart beats at about 70 beats per minute. A heart rate below 60 bpm is referred to as **bradycardia,** although a slow rate is not a problem unless it becomes extreme. Well-trained athletes may have resting heart rates well below this range. For example, Miguel Indurain, five-time winner of the Tour de

France, is reported to have a resting heart rate of 42 bpm. **Tachycardia,** when the resting heart rate is above 100 bpm, is a problem. The atria or ventricles may contract very rapidly up to 300 beats per minute, a condition that is known as flutter. When the beats are not coordinated, it is called **fibrillation.** In some cases, the heart may need to be jolted to resume a normal rhythm. In this procedure, called **defibrillation,** small paddles (electrodes) placed on the victim's chest provide a path to deliver an electric shock. The intent is to restore a normal coordinated heart rhythm. Several psychological processes, such as emotional arousal, stress reactions, and conditioning, can lead to arrhythmias (Lynch, Paskewitz, Gimbel, & Thomas, 1977).

Angina pectoris means literally a pain in the chest, a term that fairly describes the location behind the sternum. Angina pain may spread out to involve other parts of the body such as the shoulder and arm. Angina occurs when the coronary arteries constrict and cut off the supply of oxygen to the heart.

Myocardial ischemia and infarctions: oxygen, blood, and attacks When the oxygen supply to the heart is not sufficient to meet demand, **myocardial ischemia** occurs. Ischemia occurs as a result of coronary artery disease. Ischemia can occur silently, in the absence of any pain, as Norman Cousins found out. Leisa Freeman and her colleagues studied the masking effects of stress that increase susceptibility to death from coronary (Freeman, Nixon, Sallabank, & Reaveley, 1987). She noted that more than 250,000 people die each year from heart attacks that have no preceding chest pain. Her study used 30 patients waiting for bypass surgery. Freeman's group observed that pain occurred along with restricted blood flow only one-third of the time. They also found evidence that stress hormones mediated this process. Specifically, when urinary stress hormones were at high levels, there was an increased likelihood of a silent ischemic attack. The reason may be that the stress hormones stimulate production of the brain's natural opioids which then mask pain. Additional data suggest that affective (anger control) and cognitive (external oriented thinking) variables are associated with silent myocardial ischemia during exercise (Torosian, Lumley, Pickard, & Ketterer, 1997).

One event that frightens most everyone is the heart attack, technically, the myocardial infarction (MI). A **myocardial infarction** occurs when the heart has been deprived of its blood supply for a prolonged time, usually about two hours.[3] Cells in the affected region are damaged or destroyed. From then on, that area of the heart gives signals different from the signals

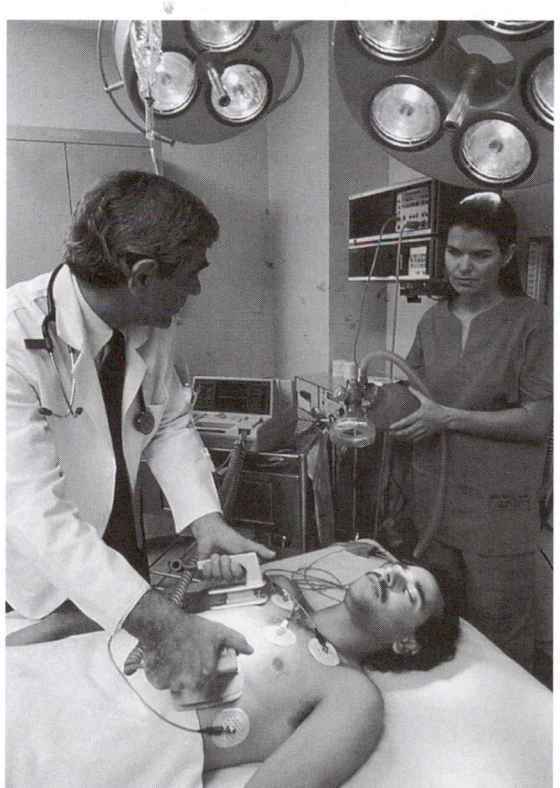

FIGURE 12.5 The defibrillation technique attempts to restore a normal heart rate.

---

[3] The term *infarct* comes from the Latin *infarce,* which means literally to stuff or to put out.

produced by healthy areas of the heart. The pain that results from infarction may resemble angina at first, but it soon becomes much more severe and it lasts for a longer time. It may last for more than 30 minutes and be accompanied by shortness of breath, weakness, nausea, and sweating (Smith & Leon, 1992).

Coronary artery disease: artery cracks, lipids, and plaques

Heart attacks do not just happen. They result from small insidious arterial changes taking place over many years. There is evidence that fatty streaks are present in the arteries of young adults. This suggests that atherosclerosis may begin early in life, perhaps as early as childhood (McNamara, Malot, Stemple, & Curring, 1971).

Two processes, atherosclerosis and thrombogenesis, are important in CAD. **Atherosclerosis** is an arterial disease in which yellowish lumps of fat become stuck in the inner lining of the artery, forming arterial plaques that reduce the size of the artery opening (Memmler & Wood, 1977). This blockage, or occlusion, restricts blood flow and leads to increased blood pressure. Even with substantial blocking, though, a person may show few if any symptoms. Smith and Leon (1992) note that arteries must be blocked by 70% or more before clinical symptoms typically appear. Further, the body grows new collateral vessels to compensate for any interference in blood distribution to the heart. In some people, this may occur at a level that is so adaptive, almost complete blockage may occur without harmful effects. More often, though, the process of resupply cannot occur at a level and pace adequate to prevent damage.

The formation of plaques is more complex than can be detailed here. In brief, **arterial plaques** are made up of lipids and other fibrous materials, presumably formed in response to damage to the arterial wall (Ross, 1986). The artery starts out as a very smooth tube composed of smooth muscle cells on the inner (endothelium) lining. Unfortunately, blood vessels suffer wear and tear just as any part of the body does. One way of visualizing this damage is to think of blood as a river flowing in narrow channels with bends. The flow is turbulent at bends or branches. Just as a river erodes a shore, blood flow erodes the endothelium. As blood pressure rises, the rate of damage increases. Damage may progress to the second layer, the intima, and even to the third layer, the media (Fuster, Badimon, Badimon, & Chesebro, 1992a). As damage occurs, the artery forms a type of scab to repair the erosion, somewhat like a badly scraped elbow forms a scab to close the wound. Unfortunately, these arterial plagues become loaded with lipids, or fats, and the stage is set for advanced atherosclerosis (Alpert, 1993).

In later stages, fibrous cells infiltrate the plaques and add to scar tissue on the artery wall. Calcium deposits harden the cell walls even more and narrow the corridor. The arteries lose their flexibility to expand and contract, hence the term *hardening of the arteries*. Blood must be squeezed through a much smaller space than normal, and the heart must work even harder. Just as a weight lifter develops larger muscles with increasing workouts, heart muscle also grows as it works harder. Unfortunately, the muscle grows faster than the supply network. The muscle that pumps blood to the rest of the body does not have enough of its own resource to stay healthy and the result is myocardial ischemia.

Still, the most crucial process is **thrombogenesis,** the formation of a blood clot. A plague can be viewed as a type of sack or capsule of lipid-rich materials. It can tear (plaque disruption) and reform, tear and reform, perhaps several times. This adds material to the plaque and leads to more complete blockage. A crude analogy is when you get a blister from hard work. It heals but forms a callous that becomes larger and harder with continued stress. The arterial plaque is like the callous that gets bigger and harder over time.

When the plaque bursts, it spills its contents into the bloodstream. The natural response is to repair the damage by means of a thrombus, a large blood clot. This clot can further close or completely block off the artery. When this happens, the heart's blood supply from the affected artery may be shut off completely.

Then, an acute coronary crisis is likely, in some cases, resulting in sudden death. After a plaque has formed, the three most important processes leading to a coronary crisis are plaque disruption, thrombosis, and vasoconstriction (Fuster et al., 1992a, 1992b). Thrombosis is, in actuality, the most frequent cause of heart attacks, and it can also lead to a cerebral vascular accident or stroke.

Physiology of blood pressure The foregoing description of heart physiology may make it appear that blood pressure results from the mechanical pressure applied by the heart when it contracts and relaxes. This notion is far too simplistic. In fact, blood pressure is determined by several interacting factors, including cardiac, neural, hormonal, and behavioral processes.

Two factors, blood volume and peripheral vascular resistance, have direct effects on blood pressure. Blood volume refers to the amount of blood the heart puts out. When blood volume increases, so does pressure in the circulatory system. When volume drops, in a condition called **hypovolemia,** the circulatory system compensates by increasing pressure. Vascular resistance relates to changes in the flexibility of blood vessels. At times, the blood vessels may be more dilated (stretched) allowing blood to pass through with lower pressure. At other times, blood vessels are constricted. When this occurs, the heart must work harder against the resistance and the effect is to increase blood pressure.

The wall of the heart contains **baroreceptors,** cells that monitor blood pressure. Further, the kidneys contain **blood-flow receptors.** If the baroreceptors sense a drop in blood pressure, they trigger release of ADH (antidiuretic hormone, also called vasopressin) from the posterior pituitary.[4] Simultaneously, blood-flow receptors in the kidneys sense the change in blood pressure. Together, the ADH and increased blood-flow receptor activity trigger re-

lease of an enzyme, **renin.** Renin in turn stimulates production of a peptide called angiotensin II. The release of angiotensin is the signal for peripheral blood vessels to constrict (Guyton, 1977). Angiotensin also signals release of **aldosterone,** a hormone that causes the kidneys to reabsorb sodium that would otherwise be lost in urine.

Activity in the hypothalamic-pituitary-adrenal axis and in the sympathetic system also can have profound effects on blood pressure. Increased levels of adrenaline lead to several changes in heart action including more forceful heart contractions and vascular constriction. With prolonged arousal (such as in stress reactions), overactivity in the CNS may lead to a **hyperadrenergic state** (continued high output of adrenaline) with resulting changes in cardiac volume and peripheral vascular constriction. Further, sympathetic activity acts directly on the kidneys to increase renin activity and sodium reabsorption by the kidneys. Elevation of blood pressure follows. These changes appear to play a formative role in the beginning of essential hypertension (Caris, 1985; van Hooft et al., 1991).

Diet also affects sensitive balances between sodium, calcium, and potassium, which are vital to regulating blood pressure. Using an animal model, Daniel Hatton and his coworkers showed that rats on a low-calcium diet had higher basal blood pressure levels and more extreme responses to epinephrine than did rats on a high-calcium diet (Hatton, Scrogin, Levine, Feller, & McCarron, 1993).

Epidemiology of Coronary Disease: Gender, Ethnic, and Social Differences

There is no mistake about the number one killer today: heart disease. In the normal population, approximately 1 out of every 162 Americans, or about 1.5 million total, will suffer a heart attack. Fortunately, this rate has been dropping for 30 years (Sytkowski, Kannel, & D'Agostino, 1990).

---

[4] We discussed vasopressin in our discussion of stress in Chapter 7.

Nearly 734,000 people died during 1989 from heart disease (National Center for Health Statistics, 1992). That is about 2010 people each day. Also in 1989, 145,551 Americans died from strokes. Nearly 7 million people are afflicted with coronary artery disease. Hypertension afflicts nearly 40 million people, and another 30 million are borderline hypertensive. Hypertension is a major contributing factor in heart disease. Although mortality is often the focus of statistical surveys, heart disease leads to both physical morbidity (including physical disability) and mental disability (chronic depression and anxiety, for example). When economic losses are considered, the yearly cost of coronary artery disease is nearly $95 billion (Leaf, 1991).

Ethnic and Cultural Differences: Risks, Delays, and Treatment

These numbers hide both gender and ethnic differences. Males are at higher risk for death from coronary compared to females, and blacks are at overall higher risk than whites. The death rate from CHD for black males is 273 per 100,000, compared to 206 for white males. The death rate for black females is 173 per 100,000, while it is 107 for white females.

Still, there are some discrepant findings. One regional study, the Charleston Heart Study, found that black males had slightly lower risk than white males (Keil et al., 1993). This is one of several inconsistent findings, and it indicates the need for caution when interpreting data of this nature. Investigators nonetheless accept as valid the findings from large-scale studies that continue to report ethnic differences. More important, whatever one's ethnic group, other risk factors are the same.

Differences in treatment and survival may be based on ethnic group membership. A Chicago study found that members of the black community were more likely to have a coronary attack out of sight of witnesses. Therefore, they were more likely to experience longer delays in getting help (Becker et al., 1993). Delays in obtaining initial treatment are crucial; they can mean the difference between life and death. About 30% who suffer their first coronary die within the first few hours, and about 50% of those who suffer a recurrent attack also die in the first few hours.

Once the call for help was made, though, the study found no difference in response time of EMT crews based on race of the victim. Still, blacks were less likely to receive bystander-assisted CPR and were more likely to have a less favorable heart rhythm when finally admitted to the hospital. These factors may have contributed to the fact that blacks were half as likely to survive a cardiac arrest compared to whites. This link between race and survival persisted even after other risk factors were controlled.

Gender Differences: Prognosis, Treatment, and Clinical Trials

Although women are at lower risk than men, coronary heart disease is still the most frequent cause of death among women. Myocardial ischemia causes 250,000 deaths annually among women, and it is the leading cause of death among women over 50 (Alpert, 1993). Heart disease usually strikes women about ten years later than men, but when it does strike it is typically more devastating (Legato & Colman, 1991). Further, CHD in women carries a worse prognosis than for men whether treated with medicines or surgery (Wenger, Speroff, & Packard, 1993). This difference may be due in part to the fact that heart disease typically is discovered later in women than in men, and less aggressive treatment is used for women.

Prior to menopause, women appear to have some protection against coronary artery disease due to estrogen production, but this protection rapidly disappears following menopause. Women who smoke heavily typically go through menopause five to ten years earlier than women who do not smoke. This effect may increase risk for women who smoke. Medical research has

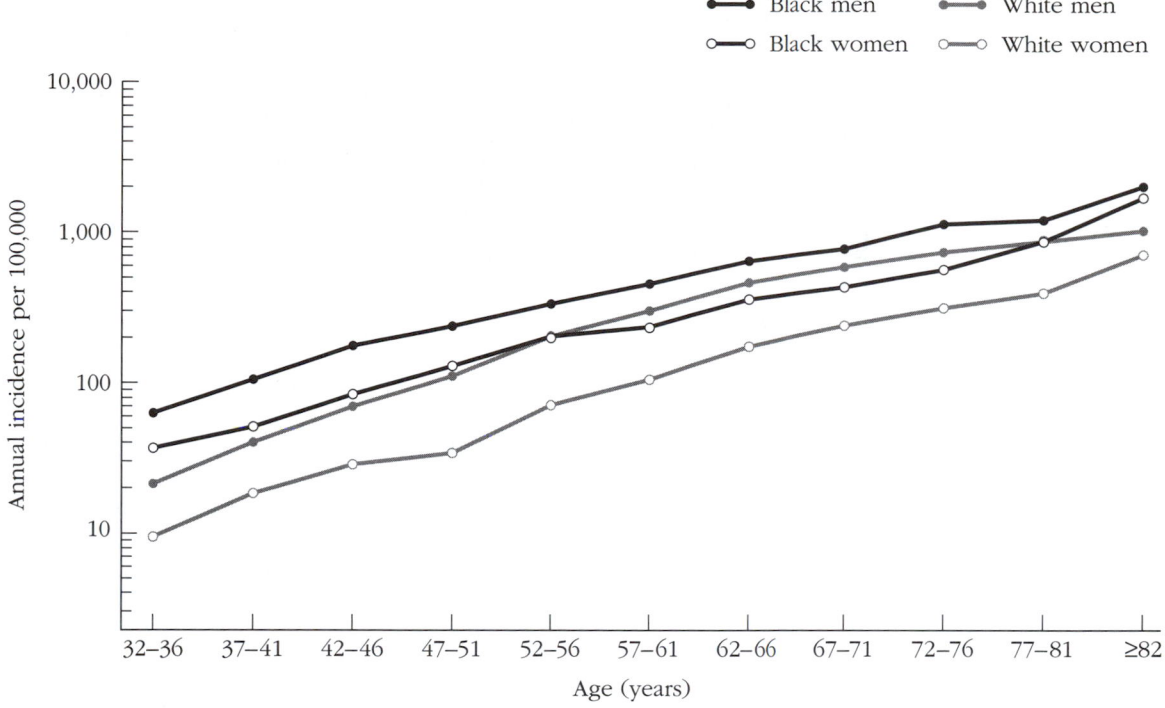

FIGURE 12.6   *Incidence of cardiac arrest according to race, sex, and age (data from the Chicago CPR Project (Becker et al., 1993).*

trials in process with estrogen replacement therapy (ERT) to discover whether some of the adverse effects of menopause can be reduced and the coronary protection extended. Analysis from one such trial, the Nurses' Health Study, shows that women using estrogen alone (or combined with progestin) had a better overall risk profile compared to women who never used hormones (Grodstein et al., 1996). However, using estrogen did not confer a benefit when stroke was used as the criteria. In fact, women using estrogen had a relative risk of 1.27 compared to women not using estrogen. Further, there is an ongoing debate about an undesirable side effect from ERT, that is, an increased risk for uterine cancer.

Women are also underrepresented in clinical trials, leading some to question whether treatments developed largely on males will be equally effective for women (Wenger et al., 1993). Less than 20% of the research funds provided by NIH go to women's health issues (Legato & Colman, 1991).

Women show poorer adherence to rehabilitation programs. This may occur because women more frequently have coexisting illnesses and face many pressures from work and family duties. Further, some women use low-yield cigarettes believing that they are safer than high-yield cigarettes. Yet the risk of myocardial infarction is the same among those who smoke low-yield as in those who smoke high-yield cigarettes.

Although much of this information may lead to pessimism, there is much good news. Over the past 30 to 40 years, heart disease has been declining gradually. This is due largely to significant changes in lifestyle that include diet,

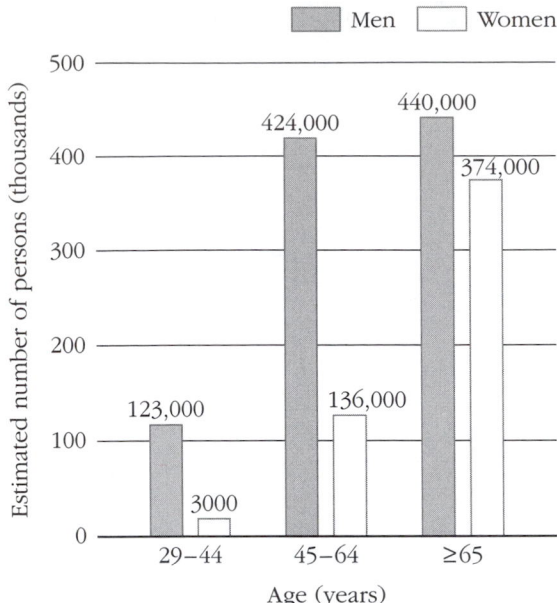

FIGURE 12.7   *Incidence of myocardial infarction in women and men in the United States (data from the Framingham Heart Study, in Rich-Edwards, Manson, Hennekens, & Buring, 1995).*

increased exercise, and gradual declines in the number of people smoking. In Western Europe, the decline in ischemic heart disease is between 10 and 14%, while it is about 25% in the United States (Retchin, Wells, Valleron, & Albrecht, 1992).

Unmodifiable Risk Factors: Genetics, Age, and Gender

Medical science has identified many risk factors for coronary disease. Information about risk factors makes it possible to identify those who are at high risk. With this information, it may be possible to design preventive programs that target groups most at risk. Preventive programs can pay big dividends by increasing individual survival, reducing economic loss to families and businesses, and cutting the social costs of disease incurred by both private and government insurance providers.

Physical risk factors include age, gender, family history of heart disease, hypertension, smoking, high cholesterol levels, diabetes mellitus, obesity, and inactivity (Rosenman et al., 1970). Logan Wright and his colleagues looked at these physical risk factors in a small group of male CHD patients (Wright, Carbonari, & Voyles, 1992). Their intent was to determine whether the factors show some grouping coherence as suggested by factor analysis. They found that family history, the genetic variable, stood by itself as a single factor. Exercise, weight control, diet, and blood pressure were major components in the second factor. Smoking and cholesterol were part of the second factor but at a nonsignificant level.

Another way to group risk factors is by clinical implications. Thus, risks have been classified as unmodifiable, major modifiable, and minor modifiable factors. The implicit bad news in this grouping is that certain factors cannot be modified. Three unmodifiable risk factors are genetics, age, and gender. Of these three, the genetic factor is often regarded as the most important. The process of aging cannot be reversed and it will inevitably produce some negative changes in the cardiovascular system.[5] Still, risks associated with aging can be slowed down or minimized through wise lifestyle choices (Berenson, 1993). Risks associated with gender also cannot be changed. Still, gender-linked risks usually work through mediating variables, such as lipid deposits and blood pressure mechanisms, which may be minimized or controlled through lifestyle changes and medical interventions.

On the positive side, three major risk factors—high blood pressure, elevated cholesterol, and smoking—can be significantly reduced by lifestyle changes. Simple adjustments to diet and exercise have positive effects on both cholesterol and blood pressure. As noted in

---

[5] See Chapter 16 on aging for more detail on both the biological changes that occur with aging and the lifestyle choices that can slow down the process.

Chapter 8, quitting smoking is not necessarily simple, but the positive heart health effects are just as undeniable as they are important.

Finally, certain factors—stress, Type A behavior, obesity, and physical inactivity—are considered minor risk factors. They can be modified, and well they should be, but they will not have as strong an impact on coronary risk as the major modifiable factors.

Genetic Risks: Tachycardia, Lipids, and Stress

Genetic factors contribute to overall risk for coronary heart disease (Marenberg, Risch, Berkman, Floderus, & de Faire, 1994), and for physical traits that influence coronary risk. For example, an autosomal dominant defect on chromosome 11 was found in one family for ventricular tachycardia (Mason, 1993). Hypertrophic cardiomyopathy may be related to a defect found on chromosome 14, but the exact mechanism is not as yet clearly identified (Cody, 1993). Hypertension shows a genetic predisposition probably related to such mechanisms as sodium sensitivity and hyperlipidemia among others (Frohlich, 1993).

The most common genetic influences are with lipid disorders that appear to be determined by single genes. Molecular biology has shown that the most common form of familial hypercholesterolemia is linked to a specific defect in the receptor for low-density lipoprotein. The suspect gene is on chromosome 11. **Familial hypercholesterolemia** is a group of diseases identified by an extremely high plasma cholesterol and a high risk for atherosclerosis and coronary heart disease. The rare monozygous form acts as a lipid storage disease, but afflicted persons usually die in their 20s (Berenson, 1993). The more common heterozygous form involves reduced or defective liver receptors that make it impossible for the liver to clear LDLs from the blood. Serum cholesterol levels may reach in excess of 400 mg/dl and LDL levels may be in excess of 190 mg/dl. The normal safe levels are 200 mg/dl and 130 mg/dl respectively (Leaf, 1991).

Debra Heller and her colleagues used data from the Swedish Adoption/Twin Study of Aging (SATSA) in an effort to separate the genetic influence on hypercholesterolemia from the environmental influence (Heller, de Faire, Pedersen, Dahlén, & McClearn, 1993). They used several lipid measurements including total cholesterol, high-density lipoproteins (HDL), triglycerides, and two apolipoproteins. Based on 302 pairs of twins, the investigators came to several conclusions that help to clarify this complex issue. First, they estimated that heritability for high serum cholesterol levels was 0.72 in younger twins. Second, monozygotic twins reared apart had much lower concordance for lipids than those reared together. This finding is important since it reveals that environment still plays an important role. Heller's group estimated that environment accounted for 15 to 36% of the total variance in lipid levels. Third, although all the cholesterol measures showed evidence of heritability, the most pronounced effect was on apolipoprotein B and triglycerides. Fourth, for most lipid measures, there were no gender differences in heritability. Genetics did play a more prominent role on apolipoprotein B in women than it did in men. Last, the heritability factor declined in importance with age. The implication is that, compared to genetics, environmental influences will play a more important role with advancing age in the expression of coronary disease.

Further evidence on the role of genetics in coronary disease comes from work on stress reactions (Rose, 1988). This work suggests that differences in the physiologic lability or hyperreactivity to stressors is influenced by genetic factors. Some people have more extreme autonomic arousal, stronger cardiovascular reactions, and elevated blood pressure in response to stressors than others (Krantz & Manuck, 1984). When a person faces chronic stress, it is possible that heightened arousal aggravates cardiovascular processes hastening the onset of CAD and CHD.

Gender and Coronary Risks: Hypertension, Contraceptives, and Stress

Since gender differences were highlighted earlier, only a few added comments are necessary here. Men have a higher risk for CHD, but women are more at risk for diabetes and hypertension (Alpert, 1993). Sudden death from heart attack is less common in women than in men. One physiologic change that occurs in almost all women who use oral contraceptives is an increase of 2 to 14 mm/Hg in systolic pressure and 1 to 8 mm/Hg diastolic pressure compared to women who do not use oral contraceptives. In spite of this increase, blood pressure levels remain within the normal range for most women. Only about 5% of users reach levels that qualify as hypertension (Caris, 1985). During pregnancy, women also may experience risks from hypertension including compromised personal health and risks to the fetus (Cunningham & Lindheimer, 1992).

Another factor of interest is the gender difference in response to stressors. Catherine Stoney and her colleagues reviewed several studies that point to a sex difference in physiological reactivity to stress (Stoney, Davis, & Matthews, 1987). Men show a substantially larger blood pressure increase in response to laboratory stressors compared to women. Women tend to be more reactive to natural stressors, however. The conclusion is that hyperreactivity to stress can alter the mechanisms that lead to coronary heart disease.

Modifiable Risk Factors: Hypertension, Cholesterol, and Smoking

Over the past few years, a great deal of attention has been paid to the major modifiable CAD risk factors. These are called the big three: hypertension, hypercholesterolemia, and cigarette smoking. Remember, though, that other modifiable factors, such as obesity and inactivity, may be less important relative to the big three, but they are not unimportant.

Hypertension: The Silent Killer

Hypertension is an elevation in blood pressure above accepted levels, no matter what produced it. Hypertension is the usual diagnosis when systolic blood pressure exceeds 160 and diastolic exceeds 120. Still, even slight increases in blood pressure above 140/90 predict increased risk of premature death (Taylor & Fortmann, 1983). Serious danger exists when systolic pressure reaches 200.

Hypertension is more common in blacks, and it has been identified as a serious condition in young black males. Among women of childbearing age, there are no significant differences between younger white and black women. As age increases, though, almost twice the proportion of black women suffer from hypertension compared to white women (Geronimus, Andersen, & Bound, 1991). The prevalence of hypertension is lower among Hispanic groups according to a large-scale study of Hispanic health and nutrition (Pappas, Gergen, & Carroll, 1990).

Hypertension is a contributing factor to kidney failure and stroke, and it is a major cause of congestive heart failure. About 75% of adults who become victims of congestive heart failure have had a history of high blood pressure (Caris, 1985). Hypertensive patients perform more poorly than normotensives on cognitive tests of memory, attention, and abstract reasoning (for a review, see Waldstein, Manuck, Ryan, & Muldoon, 1991). The differences do not seem to impair functional skills for daily living, though, and there is no evidence of a progressive decline.

A major problem is early diagnosis and treatment. Hypertension, the so-called silent killer, does not give loud warning signals and thus is easy to ignore. Nearly half of all hypertensives do not know they have the disease. Even then, among those who do know, only half will make the effort to get treatment.

Primary (essential) hypertension is hypertension of unknown origins. It may be due to higher peripheral resistance or increased cardiac output (Taylor & Fortmann, 1983). More than 95% of hypertension patients fall in this category (Frohlich, 1993). In **secondary hypertension,** which makes up only about 5% of the cases, a cause can be reliably identified. These causes are many and varied, including exogenous factors such as excess sodium or alcohol intake; use of drugs like cocaine, oral contraceptives, or nonsteroidal anti-inflammatory drugs; endocrine disorders such as hyper- or hypothyroidism; renal disorders; or CNS lesions (Caris, 1985).

The hallmark of hypertension is increased peripheral resistance. Normally, a renin-angiotensin-aldosterone mechanism helps regulate sodium and potassium balance and fluid balance to maintain proper blood pressure. This mechanism is altered in hypertensives. As hypertension progresses, however, structural properties of the cardiovascular system also change. These alterations include changes to left ventricular mass and vascular wall thickness.

One issue of interest to behavioral researchers is how genetic-constitutional factors influence hypertension during stress situations. To help answer this question, Jorgensen and Houston (1989) compared a group of people with a family history of hypertension to a group with no family history of hypertension. The investigators found higher resting systolic and diastolic blood pressure in those with a positive family history. The researchers also observed higher systolic blood pressure (SBP) and diastolic blood pressure (DBP) under conditions of laboratory stress. The link to life-event stress, though, was different for men and women. Men showed higher resting SBP with more negative stress events. Women showed higher resting SBP with fewer negative events.

Cholesterol and Cardiovascular Risk: Good and Bad Fats

Cholesterol is a lipid that appears as a white waxy fat. The liver produces all the cholesterol the body needs. Thus, a diet that is rich in fats adds a load to the system. Risk for CHD

increases as cholesterol levels increase above about 180 mg/dl. The recommended safe level is 200 mg/dl (NCEP, 1993). Moderate risk occurs at 200–240 mg/dl, and high risk occurs above 240 mg/dl. Absolute levels do not tell the complete story though. A higher ratio of good fats (high-density lipoproteins or HDLs) to bad fats (low-density lipoproteins or LDLs) confers some protection against coronary disease. HDLs help keep the cardiovascular system clear of fats that otherwise would leave deposits and build plaques in the bloodstream. Thus, people with higher HDLs have less risk of heart attacks (Pekkanen et al., 1990). Further, inactive people do not clear fats from the bloodstream as efficiently as active people. They carry more of their fat as LDLs (Gutlin & Kessler, 1983).

Michael Klag and his associates used data from the Johns Hopkins Precursors Study, started in 1947, to assess the relationship between serum cholesterol and later cardiovascular disease (Klag et al., 1993). This study provided strong evidence that high cholesterol contributes to risk for coronary disease. During a 30-year follow-up, Klag's team found 125 cardiovascular disease events, 97 of which were due to CHD. Then, the researchers conducted a proportional hazards analysis that included several variables such as age, exercise, smoking behavior, diabetes, and hypertension. A difference of 36 mg/dl in serum cholesterol at about 22 years of age nearly doubled risk for cardiovascular disease (morbidity) at a later age (RR = 1.72). Risk for death (mortality) from cardiovascular disease was slightly more than double (RR = 2.02) with the same early difference in cholesterol. The risks were similar whether the coronary event occurred before or after age 50. One flaw in the study was that serum cholesterol levels were not assessed throughout the follow-up period.

Smoking and Cardiovascular Risk: Toxins, Arteries, and Oxygen

The relationship between smoking and risk for coronary is simple and direct: Incidence of heart attacks and sudden cardiac death is directly related to the number of cigarettes smoked on a regular basis. The underlying mechanism is increased rate of cholesterol deposits in arteries. A strong dose-response relationship exists: The more cigarettes smoked, the more severe the atherosclerosis.

Smoking has several other negative effects in the cardiovascular system. First, smoking elevates heart rate and blood pressure (MacDougall, Dembroski, Slaats, Herd, & Eliot, 1983). Smoking also interferes with the oxygen-carrying capacity of blood, so that the same volume of blood is not as rich in oxygen as it would otherwise be. Further, smoking can produce instability in the bioelectrical control (pacing) of the heart. Finally, smoking increases the tendency to platelet aggregation and clot formation. Clots increase the potential for thrombosis and a fatal coronary (Smith & Leon, 1992).

There is some evidence that stopping smoking will reduce the risk for coronary substantially within about 5 years and that the risk will be near normal within about 15 years. Rosenberg, Palmer, and Shapiro (1990) provided evidence that the risk of a heart attack declines rapidly after women quit smoking, and the risk is largely gone after about two years. These data are consistent with findings among males who quit smoking. Data from the British Region Heart Study suggest that the decline in risk may not be so rapid or complete, however (Cook, Shaper, Pocock, & Kussick, 1986). Even after 20 years of smoking cessation, there was some increased risk of a heart attack, but it is much less than what it would be with continued smoking.

Synergistic Effects in Cardiovascular Risk

Any one of these three factors exerts a very powerful negative influence on the cardiovascular system even in the absence of the other two factors. Combined, though, the effect is not simply additive: It is synergistic. In other words, combining two or more of these factors amplifies risk above what would be expected from a simple addition of the factors (Perkins, 1989).

Psychosocial Factors: Behavior, Personality, and Exercise

The physical risk factors described above are considered most important in predicting coronary disease. Yet, even when all the physical risk factors are combined, they account for only about 50% of coronary events (Jenkins, 1988). Therefore, investigators are looking at other variables that might help predict coronary risk. Variables under consideration include stress, the Type A behavior pattern, and exercise.

Stress and Coronary Risk: Chronic Arousal, Blood Pressure, and Heart Rate

Several aspects of the stress response influence risk for atherosclerosis. First, stress activates the HPA complex and arouses the fight or flight response under sympathetic control. Further, the system increases circulating catecholamines, or stress hormones that also act to prepare the system for emergency. This arousal elevates heart rate and blood pressure, increases blood volume to peripheral muscles, and raises respiration rate. Prolonged stress hastens damage to the arterial walls. Although stress research often relies on laboratory stresses (complex mental tasks, for example), naturally occurring stressors, such as marital discord with hostile interactions, appear to be sufficient to increase blood pressure in women, but not in men (Ewart, Taylor, Kraemer, & Agras, 1991).

When atherosclerosis is already present, the system is less resilient to stress. Alan Yeung and his coworkers asked a group of patients to carry out a mental arithmetic task during cardiac catheterization (Yeung et al., 1991).[6] Yeung's group observed a clear difference in vasomotor response to the mental stressor. In smooth vessels, the typical stress response is to either

---

[6] Note that catheterization, described in more detail a little later, is a highly stressful procedure in its own right.

dilate or remain unchanged. This was the response pattern in patients without atherosclerosis. In patients with atherosclerosis, however, the occluded coronary arteries showed constriction under stress. Further, the constriction was more severe as atherosclerosis was more pronounced.

Another stress reaction may have an adverse effect on coronary function. During periods of stress, the sympathetic system stimulates the release of free fatty acids. In emergency conditions, these fatty acids would be burned as part of the increased metabolic requirements for meeting the crisis. However, most modern stressors require little in physical activity, so the free fatty acids become surplus blood materials. These acids appear to have an adverse effect on cardiac function, and they may increase production of atherogenic LDL cholesterol (Bloom & Herd, 1983).

Type A Behavior: Competitiveness, Hurry, and Hostility

The notion that personality is somehow related to a disease entity seems to have been a recurrent theme in psychoanalytic and psychological theory. Over the last 25 years, probably no aspect of coronary risk has received more attention among behavioral scientists than the Type A behavior pattern (TABP).

The **Type A behavior pattern** was first described by two doctors, Meyer Friedman and Ray Rosenman (1974). In their scheme, Type A people are time-driven, impatient, insecure of status, highly competitive and aggressive, generally hostile, and incapable of relaxing. The time driven component led Rosenman and Friedman (1974) to call it "the hurry sickness." In contrast, Type B people tend to cope with their environment in a more relaxed style.

In addition to looking at components of Type A behavior, several investigators have focused on physiological differences that might explain Type As' higher risk for coronary. Besides the major cluster of traits described by Rosenman and Friedman, a secondary cluster of depression combined with high levels of anxiety has been observed (van Doornen, 1980). Nancy Frasure-Smith and her colleagues found that depression and anxiety independently predict coronary events and severity of cardiac disease (Frasure-Smith, Lespérance, & Talajic, 1995). It is reasonable to assume that where there is anxiety there is autonomic arousal. Several research groups found just this connection (Goldband, 1980; Harbin, 1989; Irvine, Lyle, & Allon, 1982). Type A people typically show heightened sympathetic reactivity, elevated heart rate, and higher blood pressure. (See Jorgensen, Johnson, Kolodziej, and Schreer, 1996, for a meta-analysis of blood pressure and personality traits.)

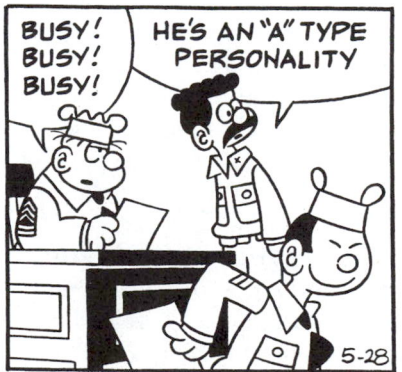
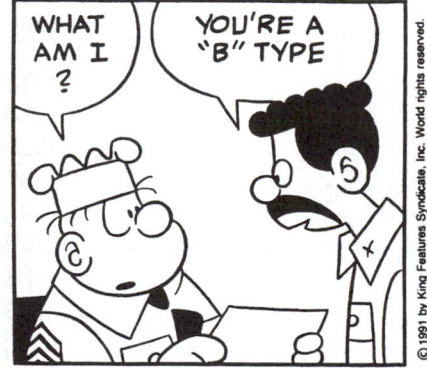
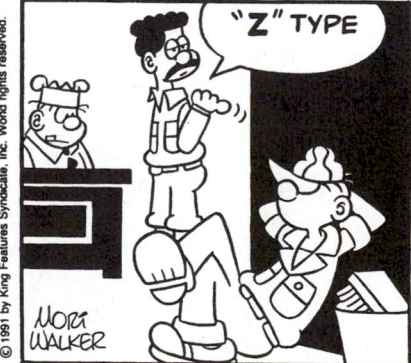

Reprinted with permission of King Features Syndicate.

FIGURE 12.8   Beetle Bailey as the antithesis of the Type A personality. Reprinted with special permission of King Features Syndicate.

A recent meta-analysis confirmed these outcomes (Lyness, 1993). Lyness concluded that the greatest cardiovascular reactivity in Type As occurred in situations that contained feedback evaluations, whether positive or negative; social aversive situations loaded with criticism or verbal harassment; and in playing video games. This work has prompted the suggestion that Type A people have an increased risk for several stress-related illnesses, not just coronary.

Type A people report more stress symptoms than do Type B people. They also smoke more and exercise less (Howard, Cunningham, & Rechnitzer, 1976). Further, Lovallo and Pishkin (1980) observed more blood clotting, higher cholesterol levels, and increased triglyceride levels under stress in Type A people. These factors are known physical risk indicators. Based on this type of evidence, some investigators suggested that coronary victims do not experience any more stressful events than healthy subjects, but they may translate emotional upsets into bodily symptoms more frequently through autonomic hyperreactivity.

Type A and coronary risk From the beginning, Friedman and Rosenman suspected that Type A behavior is related to increased risk for coronary disease. This was based on the classic longitudinal research project, the Western Collaborative Group Study (WCGS), involving 3500 subjects (Rosenman et al., 1964). This and other research initially suggested that the Type A behavior pattern could predict coronary disease better than all of the other physical risk factors combined. Compared to Type B males, middle-aged Type A males were 6.5 times as likely to have a heart attack (Suinn, 1975). Rosenman and Friedman (1961) reported a three-fold to seven-fold higher rate of diastolic hypertension in Type A women (34.8%) compared to Type B women (4.5%).

Over the past 15 years, views on the Type A behavior pattern changed dramatically. The most important reason for this is fairly simple: The alleged relationship between Type A and coronary began to evaporate after about 1977.

The findings for the WCGS could not be replicated in the Multiple Risk Factor Intervention Trial (MRFIT) (Kuller, Neaton, Caggiula, & Falvo-Gerard, 1980). Further, unexpected findings showed that although Type As might have a higher risk for coronary, they also had lower mortality after a first coronary event than Type B patients (Dimsdale, 1988). Ragland and Brand's (1988) data provided some of the most shocking negative data showing that Type Bs had twice the mortality rate of Type As after a first coronary. Finally, it is apparent that some people not classified as Type A still suffer CHD (Contrada, 1989).

Following a meta-analysis of this literature, Todd Miller and his coworkers provided some reasons for these negative results and for continued viability of the link between Type A behavior and CHD (Miller, Turner, Tindale, Posavac, & Dugoni, 1991). First, the authors suggested that many of the null results were subject to a disease-based bias, which occurs when the study selects only diseased subjects. Second, they observed that null results were found often when self-report measures (such as the Jenkins Activity Survey) were used as opposed to the structured interview method. Third, they observed that null results were obtained for all studies that used myocardial infarction as the disease criterion. Fourth, they noted that more Type As (70%) were found in diseased populations than in healthy populations (46%). This outcome is consistent with the conclusion reached by two other investigators (Booth-Kewley & Friedman, 1987). Finally, Miller's group observed that when the results of many studies are combined, Type A people are twice as likely to suffer from CHD as their Type B peers.

The toxic core of Type A behavior
These unexpected reversals posed a challenge to both the theory of the Type A behavior pattern and the methods used to assess it. The common measures of TABP are the Structured Interview (SI) and the Jenkins Activity Survey (JAS) (Jenkins, Zyzanski, & Rosenman, 1965), a

paper-and-pencil self-report test. Research on these scales showed that they tap a complex set of traits combining several behavioral and emotional components (Wright, 1988; Matthews, Glass, Rosenman, & Bortner, 1977). Still, there is a debate over the value of the JAS as a measure of TABP (Boyd & Begley, 1987). In addition, Scherwitz and his colleagues showed substantial variations in scoring speech traits with the SI that make it difficult to compare Type As from one study to Type As from another (Scherwitz, Graham, Grandits, & Billings, 1987).

The theoretical issues at stake had to do with the principle components of Type A. During the 1980s, researchers collected a mass of data

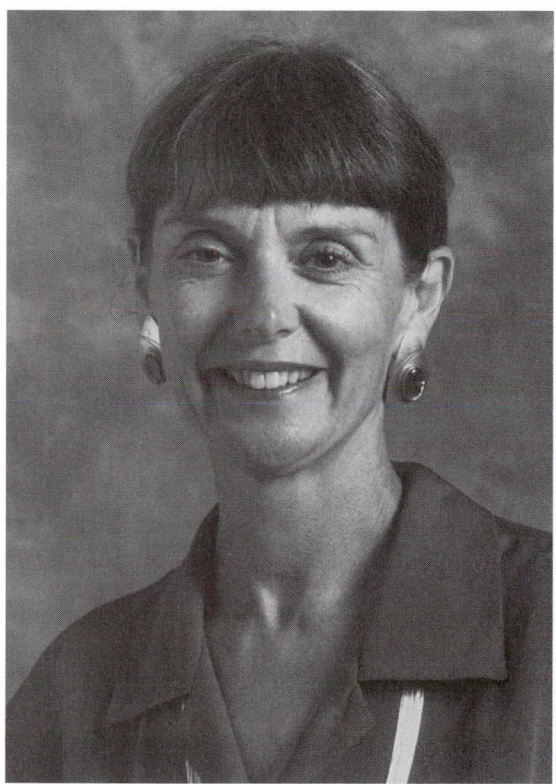

FIGURE 12.9   Karen Matthews, past president of the APA Division of Health Psychology as well as past president of the American Psychosomatic Society, has focused much of her work on behavioral risk factors in cardiovascular disease.

suggesting that the toxic core of Type A was hostility and anger (Blumenthal, Barefoot, Burg, & Williams, 1987; Dembroski & Costa, 1987). Hostility is defined as "a stable predisposition to respond to a broad range of frustrating circumstances with varying degrees of anger, irritation, distrust, contempt [and] resentment" (Dembroski, MacDougall, Williams, Haney, & Blumenthal, 1985, p. 230). The Western Electric Study showed that high-hostility men had five times the incidence of CHD (Shekelle, Gale, Ostfeld, & Paul, 1983). Matthews and her colleagues provided evidence that male adults and male children had higher hostility scores than female peers (Matthews et al., 1992). The authors suggested that this difference might account for males' higher risk for CHD. A recent meta-analysis of 83 studies pointed to negative affect as the most important ingredient, although depression also emerged as a strong component (Booth-Kewley & Friedman, 1987).

One program conducted by Logan Wright (1988) followed this anger-hostility lead with great tenacity. Wright and his colleagues identified three factors that accounted for more of the variance shared between TABP and coronary risk than either global measures or single components. The first of these factors was the traditional time urgency trait. Wright named the other two factors chronic activation and multiphasia.

Chronic activation is a tendency to be wired, to run at a high level of arousal, on a long-term basis. This translates to muscular tension and hormonal flooding, both key components of sympathetic arousal. A key point, though, is that the hormones associated with anger may be metabolized (shed) without damage when a large muscle response is possible. If anger is bottled up (no large muscle response), though, the hormones are believed to promote arterial damage and increase coronary risk.

The third factor, **multiphasia,** is the tendency to have multiple activities occurring at the same time, a type of double-timing to crowd more and more into less and less time. Examples include a business manager who takes work along on vacation, or the student who works on a term paper while attending a recital.

Although these clusters provided a better prediction of CHD than global Type A measures, they did not confirm the anger-hostility factor found in other studies. Wright's group thought that anger might have to be broken down into finer components. They used a variety of measures to tap anger directed inward and anger directed outward. Anger directed inward proved to be the strongest element predicting risk for CHD.

Recent work by Karin Helmers and her colleagues continues to point to repressed hostility as an important predictor of coronary risk (Helmers et al., 1995), and an extensive meta-analysis suggests that hostility is an independent risk factor for coronary disease (Miller, Smith, Turner, Guijarro, & Hallet, 1996). Helmers's group classified subjects as high or low in repressed hostility (measured by the Cook-Medley Hostility Inventory) and high or low in defensiveness (measured by the Marlowe-Crowne scale). Defensiveness was defined as the tendency to deny undesirable traits in oneself. In a series of three studies, coronary patients were monitored during a treadmill exercise, during a mental stressor test, and in natural ambulatory activity over 48 hours. In all three conditions, patients with high levels of defensive hostility showed more ischemic events than any of the other groups.

Remember, though, that coronary disease is multicausal. Wright's (1988) program, for example, identified five separate paths to coronary artery disease: inherited risk based on family history, risks that accrue from personal lifestyle choices such as overeating and lack of exercise, anger directed inward, anger directed outward that is combined with a sense of time urgency and chronic activation, and finally, the traditional Type A pattern identified by Rosenman and Friedman. Where anger and Type A behavior are concerned, the probable mechanism of biologic insult is through the chronic heightened physiological arousal that promotes atherogenic and thrombogenic alterations in the cardiovascular system.

Exercise and Coronary Risk

Exercise has positive effects on the cardiovascular system that reduce risk for coronary artery disease and myocardial ischemia. Exercise tends to reduce heart rate; it improves the efficiency of the heart; and it reduces blood pressure. It improves efficiency in the respiratory system so that oxygenation of blood and supply of oxygen to muscles is better. Because exercise also usually reduces weight, there is a beneficial effect on cholesterol, triglycerides, and the ratio of HDLs to LDLs.

Using data from the MRFIT study, Leon and his associates looked at the relationship between exercise and coronary risk in a high-risk group of men (Leon, Connett, Jacobs, & Rauramaa, 1987). When the men voluntarily exercised between 30 minutes and about an hour each day, they had $\frac{1}{3}$ fewer fatal coronary attacks than those who exercised less than 30 minutes per day. Additional increases in exercise activity did not further reduce mortality risk but did reduce the risk for nonfatal coronary events. When Leon's group controlled for other risk factors, the link between exercise and risk for coronary was still evident.

Biomedical Interventions: Bypass, Angioplasty, and Aspirin

It is an understatement to say that medical technology has taken the treatment of heart disease to new heights. It does not seem that long ago (1967) when Christiaan Barnard carried out the first heart transplant to the amazement of the entire world (Raithel, 1987). Coronary bypass surgery is almost passé, and angioplasty provides less intrusive means of altering occluded arteries. The range of medicines and surgeries is now truly astounding, but technical details are beyond the scope of this book. Still, an overview of what is involved in some of the more common treatment approaches is essential to psychologists who become involved in helping patients to accept invasive diagnostic and surgical procedures or to adhere to a long-term treatment program.

Coronary Interventions: Pharmacology, Bypass, and Angioplasty

Medications such as nitroglycerin tablets, beta-adrenergic blocking drugs, and calcium-channel blocking agents are used for a variety of purposes. Among the more common uses for medications is to manage angina pain and to reduce blood pressure and cholesterol.

One of the most widely discussed medicines is the common nonprescription drug aspirin. It is possible that aspirin reduces the atherogenic processes and thus may reduce the incidence of CAD and CHD (Fuster et al., 1992b).

The Physicians' Health Study was designed to test aspirin as a primary prevention to reduce mortality from cardiovascular disease (Steering Committee of PHSRG, 1988). This study was a randomized, double-blind placebo control trial comparing 325 mg of aspirin (Bufferin) to placebo. The treatment was cut short because "a statistically extreme beneficial effect on nonfatal and fatal myocardial infarction had been found" (p. 262). The study used a sample of 22,071 physicians, about half of whom received aspirin and half received a placebo. Relative risk of a fatal myocardial infarction was 0.25 for those using aspirin, and 0.56 for a nonfatal myocardial infarction. There was one down side, however: The relative risk for stroke in the same study was 3.0 for those using aspirin (although the number of cases involved was very small).

A large number of clinical trials have been and continue to be conducted on therapeutic interventions for heart attacks. A recent summary of these trials used a unique meta-analytic approach (Lau et al., 1992). Instead of conducting a one-time-only meta-analysis, the research team set up their procedures in such a way that when any additional data came in from a new trial, the results could be added to the existing analysis. In this way, the investigators hoped to be able to spot trends in the clinical trials more rapidly than by waiting for another entire meta-analysis. Their results showed significant reductions in mortality associated with several of the thrombolytic agents, anticoagulants, and beta-blockers. But their results also suggested that some treatments (such as lidocaine and calcium-channel blockers) either had no beneficial effects or could be harmful to the patient.

Beyond the pharmacological preventions and interventions, three invasive procedures are commonly used. These include cardiac catheterization, percutaneous transluminal coronary angioplasty (PTCA), and coronary artery bypass grafting (CABG).

Cardiac catheterization is a diagnostic X-ray procedure that is widely used to confirm the presence of coronary artery disease. A catheter (tubular device) is inserted into the right and left main coronary arteries (Smith & Leon, 1992). Insertion occurs either at the femoral artery in the thigh or the brachial artery on the inside of the elbow. Patients may report a burning sensation of pain as the catheter moves up the artery into the heart region. Then, the heart specialist injects a radiopaque dye through the catheter into the artery. The dye permits the X-ray pictures to show the anatomy of each artery. If there are arterial plaques, the picture of the artery will show the location and the amount of blockage. There are risks involved with this highly invasive procedure, and cardiologists may differ in their interpretation of degree of occlusion. Nonetheless, it is regarded as the gold standard for revealing clinically significant coronary artery disease.

Given the widespread use of catheterization and the anxiety that it often induces, it should not be surprising that psychologists have become involved in trying to help patients cope with the procedure. In one such program, Robin Ludwick-Rosenthal and Richard Neufeld (1993) studied a group of 72 first-time cardiac catheterization patients. They assessed the patient's desire for information, their desire for control, and their tendency to cope with stress by either avoiding or seeking out threat-relevant information. Outcome measures included state anxiety, subjective stress, and behavioral and physiological measures during the procedure. Finally, the authors manipulated the amount of information that subjects received. In the high information condition, subjects received a rationale for the procedure, a step-by-step process description, details about the operating environment and equipment, and information about sensory aspects of the procedure. The low-information subjects received a standard cursory medical explanation of the procedure. When the subject's level of information matched their desire for information, there was less behavioral anxiety during catheterization. There was more problem-focused coping and less emotion-focused coping under these conditions also. One interesting outcome was that desire for control did not affect the outcome. This suggests that patients may be better prepared for invasive surgical procedures if the information provided matches their desire for information.

Percutaneous transluminal coronary angioplasty (PTCA), or angioplasty for short, is a procedure that is like putting a balloon in a collapsed straw, blowing the balloon up, and then removing the balloon. In the arterial system, it has the effect of enlarging the opening at the site of arterial blockage without the trauma caused by coronary bypass surgery.

Coronary artery bypass grafting (CABG) is a surgical procedure that involves removing a section of vein from the leg and grafting it as a bypass from the aorta to the original coronary artery past the point of the blockage (this procedure was shown in Figure 12.4). CABG requires that the patient be maintained on a heart-lung machine during the procedure. The surgery usually leads to pre-operative anxiety and substantial post-operative distress. In spite of some concern that alternative treatment approaches may be overlooked, it remains one of the top choices for intervention with severe arterial occlusions (Bates, 1990).

As we noted earlier, there are race differences in incidence of coronary disease and cardiac arrest. There is also a difference in the use of invasive cardiovascular procedures, at least in Veterans Administration hospitals (Whittle, Conigliaro, Good, & Lofgren, 1993). Jeff Whittle and his colleagues looked at treatment of 882,508 veterans admitted for cardiovascular disease or chest pain during a four-year period from 1987 to 1991. Whittle and his colleagues found that more whites (18%) underwent catheterization compared to blacks (11.8%). Angioplasty (PTCA) was performed on 1.8% of white patients and 0.8% of black patients. Finally, bypass surgery was carried out on 5% of white patients and 1.6% of black patients. These disparities did not disappear when the analyses were carried out with controls for coexisting morbidity, demographic characteristics, or differences in the treating hospital. These results suggest that even granted equal access to medical care, there are differences in the equity of treatment that may be race related.

Interventions in Hypertension: Steps, Lifestyle, and Biofeedback

Since hypertension is a major modifiable risk factor for CHD, it makes an ideal target for preventive efforts. The National High Blood Pressure Education Program recommended four changes in lifestyle to help prevent or manage hypertension. These are weight control, reduced salt intake, increased exercise, and moderate alcohol consumption. Although other techniques (such as dietary supplements, biofeedback and stress management) may help control hypertension (Shapiro & Goldstein, 1982), these procedures have not received enough empirical support to warrant recommendation.

The first objective in treating hypertension is to reduce diastolic blood pressure (DBP) to a safe level, below 90 mm/Hg, and then to maintain it at this level.[7] This objective may not be feasible in some patients with severe hypertension, but even reducing blood pressure into the 90 to 100 mm/Hg range will still provide some benefit (Caris, 1985). Medical treatment usually follows a four-stage, stepped-care anti-hypertensive medication program combined with lifestyle changes.

Step 0 monitors the four lifestyle changes mentioned above for about six months. Step I uses one of four anti-hypertensive drugs: a diuretic, a beta-blocker, a calcium antagonist, or an angiotensin converting enzyme (ACE) inhibitor. At Step II, either a different class of drugs is added, or the dose of the Step I drug is increased, or another drug is substituted. Step III takes Step II to another level, either adding a third drug to the complete treatment regimen or substituting a second drug. Step IV may require additional evaluation, or other drugs may be added.

Some still argue, though, that it is better to control blood pressure through behavioral means if at all possible. Pharmacological treatments may have negative side effects, including some that may lower blood pressure but raise cholesterol and blood sugar levels. Anti-hypertensive medicines are also costly. This sentiment is a worthy one, but it tends to be practical only with milder cases of hypertension. Despite the usefulness of several behavioral methods including stress management, few would ever consider treating essential hypertension in isolation from pharmacological interventions.

The most effective first step (Step 0) to combat hypertension is to keep a normal body weight. This method alone will either prevent hypertension from developing, delay its onset, or reduce the severity of existing hypertension.

Reducing salt intake is another method to reduce blood pressure. The recommendation is to cut salt intake to no more than four to six grams. This recommendation is made because it is difficult to sort out who will and who will not benefit from salt restriction, and because reducing salt intake does not have harmful side effects (Smith & Leon, 1992). Still, reducing sodium intake does not always work. It appears that people vary on a dimension from salt-resistant to salt-sensitive. Only a small percentage of those who are salt-resistant develop hypertension. Conversely, only about 40% of patients with essential hypertension respond favorably to reduced sodium intake (Caris, 1985).

Additional steps that help manage blood pressure include such things as reducing alcohol intake, quitting smoking, and increasing physical activity. The recommended alcohol intake is no more than one ounce per day. Although exercise is generally recommended to help manage hypertension, the benefits of exercise usually work through weight reduction (Frohlich, 1993).

Numerous studies have compared behavioral and pharmacologic methods of treating hypertension. McCaffrey and Blanchard (1985) reviewed studies that compared pharmacotherapy to stress management in treatment of essential hypertension. They concluded that pharmacotherapy is clearly superior to stress management in the treatment of hypertension.

One high-tech solution, biofeedback, seemed to offer some promise for a nonpharmacologic intervention.[8] Early work suggested that biofeedback and relaxation procedures were probably both equally effective in reducing blood pressure and that both maintain lowered blood pressure up to a year after treatment (Peters, Benson, & Peters, 1977; Walsh, Dale, & Anderson, 1977). Meditation, a type of relaxation technique, reduced subjective distress for laboratory stress tests, but it raised systolic blood pressure compared to a relaxation-control group

---

[7] There is a controversy about whether DBP should be lowered more than this because some studies suggest that lowering DBP too much increases risk (Fletcher & Bulpitt, 1992).

---

[8] See Chapter 5 to review details of clinical biofeedback procedures.

(Sawada & Steptoe, 1988). Another group found that biofeedback could help subjects reduce blood pressure more than relaxation, but both procedures still provided some benefit (Engel, Glasgow, & Gaarder, 1983).

Probably the most extensive work on the potential usefulness of biofeedback for treating hypertensives has been carried out by Blanchard's research group (Blanchard et al., 1986, 1989). For their studies, they used hypertensive patients already on medications. They obtained a highly significant result showing that thermal biofeedback was successful in 65% of the cases as compared to 35% of those on relaxation training. One problem has confronted these efforts. Blood pressure could be reliably reduced by statistical criteria, but the changes were often of little clinical importance. In general, the reductions were on the order of 5 to 15 mm/Hg. If the patient was borderline hypertensive, these changes might bring the person back down closer to the normal range. But such changes in a severe hypertensive do not reduce risk sufficiently to be medically consequential.

Community Prevention Programs: Medicines, Surgeries, and Lifestyle

Numerous community-based programs have been developed to prevent development of CAD and CHD. Such programs target large segments of the population in contrast to more specialized programs that target high-risk individuals or families. Community-based programs may be run through the mass media, at the school level, through local HMOs, hospitals, and clinics, or through health clubs. Research on these interventions shows encouraging results.

The Lipid Research Clinics Coronary Primary Prevention Trial (LRC) found that reduction of total cholesterol through reduction of LDLs led to an overall decrease in CHD. Each 1% reduction in serum cholesterol led to a 2% reduction in mortality, and the overall reduction in CHD was 17% (Lipid Research Clinics Program, 1984).

The Helsinki Heart Study (Frick et al., 1987) was a five-year randomized, double-blind study that tested the effectiveness of gemfibrozil (a fibric acid) in raising the good lipids, HDLs, while also lowering the bad lipids. This trial resulted in an overall 34% reduction in risk for coronary heart disease.

Perhaps the best known program is the North Karelia Project, a mass media education program conducted in a rural county, North Karelia, in Finland. Dietary changes were recommended, cooking practices discussed, and the importance of quitting smoking was emphasized. Groups to facilitate smoking cessation were formed where possible. The program was effective in lowering blood cholesterol, blood pressure, and overall risk for CHD. These and other studies suggest that educational efforts to impact risk factors can have a significant impact on the incidence of coronary disease.

Cognitive-Behavioral Programs: Screening, Knowledge, and Action

Health psychologists may be involved in designing programs that seek to prevent coronary artery disease or that seek to offset damage done after a coronary event. Smith and Leon (1992) outlined several goals of behavioral interventions with coronary patients. The coronary patient may need help first to adjust emotionally to the coronary crises. Second, as we have seen, several stressful diagnostic tests require invasive procedures. Third, surgical procedures entail both pain and risks. Patients may need help understanding the importance of diagnostic and surgical procedures, and they may need help to understand the gravity of the risks described. Once the treatment program has been implemented, patients may need help in sticking to the program. Compliance may be crucial to the extent of recovery and the quality of life that can be enjoyed following a coronary event. Finally, appropriate adjustments in lifestyle may reduce the likelihood of a recurrent attack (Ornish et al., 1990). To accomplish these objectives, behavioral scientists have used a variety of preventive and cognitive-behavioral techniques.

Modifying risk in high-risk individuals typically depends on primary care physicians working with allied health professionals (Berenson, 1993). Although the rules remain much the same, the nature of the interventions change. Screening programs may be implemented for children and other family members who come from high-risk families. A nutritionist may become involved in more careful meal planning and monitoring for a time, ultimately restoring control to the individual or family. A specialist in exercise may help design a program of physical activity with built-in means to monitor progress. This means more than just improving physical fitness indicators. Coronary fitness and blood lipid indicators must also show signs of improvement. If necessary, an addiction counselor may become involved to help break a nicotine habit.

Behavioral interventions to reduce coronary risk may be effective in both young and old. Heather Walter and her colleagues conducted a five-year school-based intervention with a large sample of children in and around New York City (Walter, Hofman, Vaughan, & Wynder, 1988). They found that changes in dietary intake and health knowledge occurred during the study. The positive effects on blood cholesterol were small but significant in one school system, and favorable but not significant in the other school system.

The current interest in gender differences in cardiovascular disease also has prompted questions about gender differences in intervention strategies. Kris-Etherton and Krummel (1993) reviewed data on CHD risk factors in women. They noted that several of the risk factors (lipid levels, body weight, and hypertension) respond positively to dietary interventions. They estimated that 27% of all women and 50% of women aged 55 to 74 years are candidates for dietary intervention to reduce coronary risk. Still, investigators do not know for certain that dietary

interventions are more effective for women than for men.

As might be expected from research on Type A behavior pattern and coronary risk, interventions to change TABP have emerged. Price (1988) provided an overview of both recent efforts to modify TABP as well as insights into several problems that plague research on TABP interventions. Three long-term projects have been carried out to evaluate intervention strategies. The first is the Recurrent Coronary Prevention Project (RCPP) conducted under the leadership of Friedman. The second is the United States Army War College (USAWC) study. The RCPP carried out interventions over a 4½-year time frame, and the USAWC over nine months. The focus of change was time urgency and hostility, and the projects targeted the cognitive, behavioral, physiological, and environmental correlates of these two core features.

In the RCPP, Type A counseling led to significant reduction in hostility, time urgency, and impatience (Mendes-de-Leon, Powell, & Kaplan, 1991). Also, there was a 44% reduction in the rate of recurrence of myocardial infarction among those who went through this counseling compared to controls not receiving such counseling.

The third project, the Montreal Type A Intervention Project (MTAIP) compared three intervention strategies including a cognitive-behavior (stress management) approach, aerobic exercise, and weight lifting. Roskies's group reported reductions in behavioral reactivity of 13 to 23% below baseline values in the cognitive-behavior treatment group, but no changes in the other two groups (Roskies et al., 1986). No changes in physiological reactivity occurred in any of the groups.

Price (1988) noted four basic limitations of TABP clinical research conducted to that time. First, the studies often used very short interventions (some on the order of a few hours). It is highly unlikely that a behavior pattern so deeply ingrained as the TABP could be expected to change with such brief interventions. The RCPP went on for 4½ years, and the USAWC went on for nine months. Second, early studies often used only generic stress reduction strategies (relaxation training, exercise, and coping strategies, for example) without regard to the core of Type A risk. More recent studies have been more precise in targeting specific TABP components. Third, clinical studies often did not use appropriate measures of Type A behavior or did not use Type A measures at all to evaluate the success of therapy. In addition, there was so much variability in the types of measures used that it was often difficult to compare outcomes. Finally, many of the studies have not included follow-up data to determine the treatment's efficacy over the long term. The RCPP used a three-year follow-up period.

Summary

Eradication of killer diseases and changes in lifestyle have brought to light new killers, including the number one modern disease, coronary heart disease. Although a genetic component is involved, coronary risk is significantly influenced by self-controlled choices, including smoking, diet, and exercise. The major points discussed in this chapter are summarized below.

1. In the United States, more than one death occurs each minute from coronary heart disease. Males and blacks are more at risk than females and whites. Still, coronary disease is the number one killer of both men and women.

2. The heart is vulnerable to several pathological conditions, including arrhythmias (irregular pacing) and ischemia (lack of adequate oxygen supply).

3. The heart attack is technically called a myocardial infarction. It is caused by cutting off blood supply to the heart muscle.

4. A major cause of heart attacks is coronary artery disease, or atherosclerosis. Coronary artery disease occurs when the arteries become clogged with fatty deposits and plaques from damaged interior walls of the blood vessels.

5. The unmodifiable risk factors for coronary disease are genetics, age, and gender.

6. The three major modifiable risk factors are hypertension, hypercholesterolemia, and smoking. Other modifiable risk factors include diet, exercise, stress, and the Type A behavior pattern.

7. Hypertension is an elevation in systolic blood pressure above 160 and diastolic blood pressure above 120 (read as 160 over 120). Borderline hypertension is 140 over 90.

8. Hypercholesterolemia is elevated levels of cholesterol in the blood. To be safe, cholesterol should not exceed 200 mg/dl.

9. One important indicator of risk is the ratio of HDLs (good fats) to LDLs (bad fats).

10. Smoking damages the linings of the arteries and increases the rate of cholesterol deposits. Smoking elevates heart rate and blood pressure and leads to diminished oxygen carrying capacity.

11. Psychological factors thought to contribute to risk for heart disease include stress and components of the Type A behavior pattern.

12. Stress increases the production of the stress hormones, which increase heart rate and blood pressure.

13. The Type A behavior pattern has been linked to increased risk for coronary disease. The toxic core of Type A is now thought to be hostility.

14. Medical interventions for heart disease have increased in number and sophistication, including coronary bypass procedures and angioplasty. One very simple preventive medicine may be aspirin, which seems to reduce risk substantially.

15. Intervention in hypertension includes use of anti-hypertensive drugs, reducing weight, cutting down on salt intake, increased exercise, and moderate alcohol consumption.

16. Cognitive-behavioral interventions may be used to change lifestyle habits (diet, exercise and stress), to help patients prepare for invasive surgery, or to help clients adhere to medical regimens following a coronary attack or surgery.

Key Words

aldosterone
angina pectoris
angioplasty (PTCA)
arterial plaques
atherosclerosis
baroreceptors
blood-flow
   receptors
bradycardia
cardiac
   catheterization
cardiomyopathy
   dilated
   hypertrophic
chronic activation
coronary artery
   bypass grafting
   (CABG)
coronary artery
   disease (CAD)
defibrillation
diastolic phase
familial hyper-
   cholesterolemia

fibrillation
high-density lipo-
   proteins (HDLs)
hyperadrenergic state
hypertension
   primary (essential)
   secondary
hypovolemia
left ventricular hyper-
   trophy
low-density lipoproteins
   (LDLs)
multiphasia (Type A)
myocardial infarction
myocardial ischemia
percutaneous trans-
   luminal coronary
   angioplasty (PTCA)
renin
systolic phase
tachycardia
thrombogenesis
Type A Behavior
   Pattern

Study Questions

1. What are the major anatomical components of the cardiovascular system?
2. What ethnic and gender differences exist in risk for coronary disease? Are there biomedical or psychosocial explanations for the differences that do exist?
3. What are the unmodifiable risk factors? Why are they viewed as unmodifiable?
4. What are the modifiable risk factors? How do these factors influence coronary risk if they are ignored?
5. Describe the Type A behavior pattern. How has the notion of Type A behavior and coronary risk changed over the years? What value if any does the notion of personality have in explaining coronary risk?
6. What are the common biomedical methods of intervening in coronary risk?
7. What is the step/lifestyle notion of managing hypertension?
8. What are the major psychosocial methods of promoting heart health? How successful is the effort to change Type A behavior?

Class Projects

1. Consider inviting community health professionals, including one cardiovascular specialist, to discuss issues in managing hypertension or treating coronary patients. The discussion can focus on how psychosocial factors interact with physical components to influence success in treatment.
2. Have a discussion on the Type A behavior pattern, but also focus on defining the Type B person. What are the alleged strengths and weaknesses of each type? It may be of interest to look at cross-cultural variations in Type A.
3. Present recent information on cognitive-behavioral and community intervention projects aimed at improving heart health. Focus especially on information that suggests what components of the interventions have the most direct impact.

Suggested Readings

Ayanian, J. Z., & Epstein, A. M. (1991). Differences in the use of procedures between women and men hospitalized for coronary heart disease. *The New England Journal of Medicine, 325,* 221–225.

Blumenthal, J. A., Barefoot, J., Burg, M. M., & Williams, R. B. (1987). Psychological correlates of hostility among patients undergoing coronary angiography. *British Journal of Medical Psychology, 60,* 349–355.

Booth-Kewley, S., & Friedman, H. S. (1987). Psychological predictors of heart disease: A quantitative review. *Psychological Bulletin, 101,* 343–362.

Cousins, N. (1983). *The healing heart.* New York: Norton.

Dimsdale, J. E. (1988). A perspective on Type A behavior and coronary disease. *The New England Journal of Medicine, 318,* 110–112.

Horovitz, E. (1988). *Heart beat: A complete guide to understanding and preventing heart disease.* Encino, CA: Health Trend Publishing.

Kris-Etherton, P. M., & Krummel, D. (1993). Role of nutrition in the prevention and treatment of coronary heart disease in women. *Journal of the American Dietetic Association, 93,* 987–993.

Leaf, D. A. (1991). *Exercise and nutrition in preventive cardiology.* Dubuque, IA: Brown & Benchmark.

Legato, M. J., & Colman, C. (1991). *The female heart.* New York: Simon & Schuster.

Smith, T. W., & Leon, A. S. (1992). *Coronary heart disease: A behavioral perspective.* Champaign, IL: Research Press.

WEBSITES Heart Health

ADDRESS	DESCRIPTION
http://www.amhrt.org/	American Heart Association
http://www.wellweb.com/	☆ Wellness Web—designed by patients, caregivers, and health care professionals
http://www.heartinfo.com	☆ Heart Information Network—huge online set of resources and information
http://www.pitt.edu/HOME/GHNet/ GHWomen.html	☆ Women's Health page from the Global Health Network—special section devoted to heart disease
http://sln.fi.edu/biosci/heart.html	☆ The Heart: An Online Exploration—a four-star site with multimedia sounds and images

CHAPTER 13

The Problem of Pain: Headaches and Low Back Pain

"I had a farm at the foot of the Ngong hills." Those words from *Out of Africa* have been a haunting echo since I first saw the film. Still, those words only hint at the many remarkable accomplishments of Danish author Karen Blixen. In *Letters from Africa* she revealed that "a certain love of greatness, . . . could not be quelled, has kept a hold on me, has been 'my daimon.'" (Thurman, 1982, p. 254)[1] She struggled to run a 4500 acre coffee farm near Nairobi, Kenya, while her philandering husband pursued personally more exciting pastimes. Her words revealed a melancholy almost certainly traceable to her farm's failing and her departure before her passion for Africa's adventure could be exhausted. Yet another side to Karen Blixen's story was only partly told in *Out of Africa:* For nearly 50 years Blixen suffered terrible pain as a result of syphilis contracted from her own husband in Africa.

Many people know Karen Blixen not by this, her married name, but from her chosen pen name, Isak Dinesen. This man's name was symbolic in one sense of the freedom she sought for herself. It was also, by her calculation, a way to escape the sexist oppression that made it difficult for women to publish in the male-controlled industry of that time. She had begun already at a tender age to cultivate the art of oral and written storytelling, and she perfected it more during her time in Africa. She would not be denied the chance then to share her stories with

---

[1] This brief biography of Karen Blixen is based, among other sources, on Judith Thurman's masterful and literary biography *Isak Dinesen: The life of a storyteller.*

the world, though by all accounts the literati of Europe were not pleased with her deceptive maneuvers. After her return to Europe, her stories became world acclaimed; one, *Babette's Feast,* later became a compelling movie.

Karen left for Africa at the end of 1913 arriving early in 1914, where she concluded a prearranged marriage to the wealthy nobleman, Baron Bror von Blixen. For Karen, their marriage was more a union of childhood friends than the result of romantic love. Bror was supposedly the mold for Hemingway's original great white hunter in *The Short and Happy Life of Francis Macomber* (Thurman, 1982). He joined the military as an intelligence officer patrolling the border with German territory at the outbreak of WW I. At great risk and with tremendous effort, Karen led an ox-train to set up a supply camp for his unit. Apparently, it was during this time that he infected her with syphilis. Though friends can only guess, he probably contracted syphilis through his many indiscriminate liaisons with nearby Masai women where syphilis raged in near epidemic proportions.

According to her Danish physician, Karen probably first learned that she had syphilis later in 1914 (Thurman, 1982). The symptoms became most apparent near the end of the year: loss of appetite, inability to sleep, apathy, fever, headaches, and pains in the joints. During this time, her frustration with insomnia led her to take a nearly lethal dose of sleeping powder.

Though she survived this near calamity, she was sometimes her own worst enemy. Karen had long desired to be among the thinnest people in the world and thus she had little interest in food. Later, she tried to get by on oysters and champagne, a diet no nutritionist would ever recommend. To be afflicted with a disease that decreased her appetite even more could not possibly be a worse combination. To make matters worse, when she needed extra energy she got it by taking large doses of amphetamines.

Karen's particular form of syphilis was **tabes dorsalis,** or syphilis of the spine. This undoubtedly caused the cramps and vomiting that she

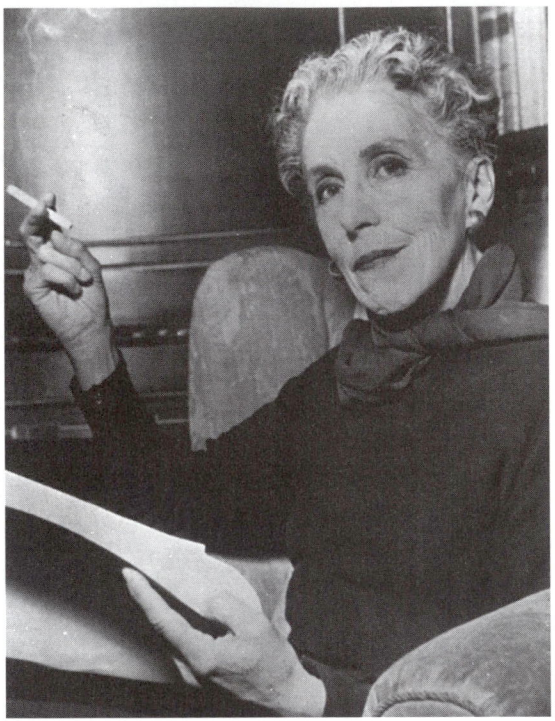

FIGURE 13.1   Isak Dinesen, *author of* Out of Africa.

often experienced. Later, along with anorexia, she was distressed by ulcers. As she aged, she showed more symptoms—an impaired sense of balance and unsteadiness of gait called **ataxia.** She was treated first with the only medication available, mercury tablets. Later, in 1925, she received Erlich's compound 606,[2] also known as salvarsan, and she had every reason to believe that she was cured.

When she returned to Europe in 1931, she had lost nearly 35 pounds. At that time, she believed her health problems were probably due to amoebic dysentery, an illness that was common among European settlers in Africa. To check this out, Karen and her brother Thomas proceeded to a clinic in Montreux. There, they found that her ruin was complete. Not only had

---

[2] The history of Erlich's work and compound 606 was presented in Chapter 2.

she lost her beloved farm, her adventure, her freedom, but syphilis had flared again now "beyond arrest or treatment, even by the most modern drugs" (Thurman, 1982, p. 256).

Later, in 1946 and again in 1955, surgeons cut some of the pain fibers, but even this radical invasive treatment did not bring her the relief from pain she desperately sought. There were times, as Thurman reports, that she was seized by such pain that she would slide out of her chair onto the floor howling and writhing in pain. Although she continued to write into her last years, more often than not, she did so from the floor or while in bed by dictating to her secretary. She tried to present a stoic front, but the pain had a powerful disabling effect on her, as revealed by a note Clara, her secretary, found. This simple brief phrase told all: "forfeited my claim to a real human life" (Thurman, 1982, p. 441).

During her last months, she was so weak she could barely stand without support, and she was so emaciated that she bruised at a touch. She wrote to a friend that she could not get her weight above 70 pounds. When she died on the evening of Friday, September 7, 1962, the cause of death was listed as emaciation. She herself had earlier mused that "by the time I had nothing left, I myself was the lightest thing of all, for fate to get rid of" (Thurman, 1982, p. 443).

The Problem of Pain: Perspectives, Definitions, and Issues

To theologians, philosophers, and ethicists, pain has always been more than a physical sensation. Even the Greek and Latin words for pain mean punishment. Pain is contrasted to pleasure as though they are polar opposites, like evil and good, dark and light. Pain and pleasure are considered basic emotional responses to events that comprise the burdens and the gifts of life. This suggests that pain is a complex phenom-

enon with the potential to affect people in many different ways.

Our purpose in this chapter is to explore the issue of pain, a sensory-affective experience that is viewed generally as a sign of physical disorder. It is also considered an important index of the quality of life: The more pain is present, presumably, the lower is the quality of life. I say "presumably" because some argue from high moral ground that pain may be associated with exceptional achievements and that it bestows a quality to life not granted those who know little of its purifying fire.

Further, in the course of this chapter we will consider how pain is defined and what its features are. We will review the physiology of pain and two mechanisms—neural and biochemical—that can serve to lower the scream of pain to a mere whisper. Numerous disorders' central feature is pain, but two pain disorders will occupy center stage here: headache pain and low back pain. Finally, we will discuss methods used to treat pain such as the stimulation method transcutaneous electrical nerve stimulation (TENS), cognitive-behavioral techniques, and meditative and hypnotic techniques.

Pain as a Biomedical Problem

Pain is understandably a serious biomedical problem. For clinicians treating a burn patient or an amputee, pain does not usually raise issues of moral value. The urgent objective is simply to provide immediate relief.

Further, medical science's forays into pain have as a primary goal to unravel the mystery of pain as mediated in neural and biochemical systems. The hope is to find a path that medicines can follow to reduce or eliminate pain. There is also the problem that pain is not a reliable sign of how severe a person's illness is. On the one hand, a cancer patient in the early stages may suffer little pain, but the health consequences of early versus late detection can be literally a matter of life or death. On the other hand, an impacted wisdom tooth can produce unbearable pain even though the health consequences are far less grim.

Still, in the absence of pain, people are not as likely to seek medical help, and common tests that could detect an emerging health problem may go undone. Finally, medical practice confronts the problem of how to manage different types of pain, such as arthritis, migraine, and chronic low back pain. Each presumably has a different pathophysiology that should justify different physical treatments. Yet, many cases of pain have no identifiable physical pathology and raise doubts about the best course for treatment.

Pain as a Psychosocial Problem

Pain may also be considered a psychosocial issue, one that transcends the mere physical switching of neural circuits and brain chemicals. In this view, pain wears many masks, altering its look to be gentle and uplifting at one time, hideous and distorting at another. The issues involved relate to tolerance and perceptual, cognitive, behavioral, and cultural processes. For Isak Dinesen, pain was the difference between merely holding on to a torturous existence and the capacity to live a real human life.

Many years ago, Beecher (1956) compared difference in pain perceptions between a group of 215 soldiers injured in the line of duty and civilians undergoing surgeries for comparable injuries. Only 25% of the soldiers wanted a narcotic for pain relief. But 80% of the civilians asked for a narcotic. Beecher concluded that the context in which the wounds occurred led to crucial differences in meaning for the two groups. For the soldiers, a wound received in service to one's country meant a ticket out of the battle zone and possibly a return to civilian life. For civilians undergoing surgeries following accidental maiming, though, the event was a real calamity and the pain significantly worse.

People differ in their tolerance for pain. Some of this difference is undoubtedly due to constitutional differences in people's physical threshold for pain, but some appears attributable to differences in learning and culture. People learn to use distracting thoughts or internal imagery to control pain. An ancient Chinese story, perhaps only a mythic event, tells of a military man who was treated by a venerable physician. It seems that during surgery, the general played chess and never displayed any signs of discomfort (Lyons & Petrucelli, 1978). According to Jane Howard (1984), Margaret Mead lived much of her life with chronic muscle pain, but her parents taught her to mentally dissociate herself from pain. Paradoxically, it never occurred to Mead that she might not have to suffer pain. Seeking medical help was a sign of weakness, like caving in to pain.

From a behavioral view, people show pain in a variety of ways. Pain behavior is defined as

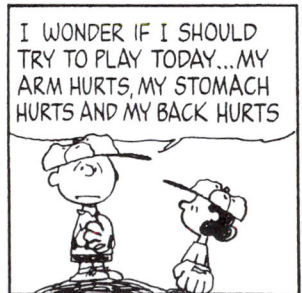
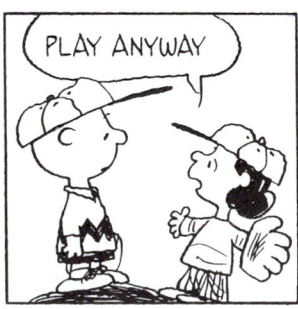
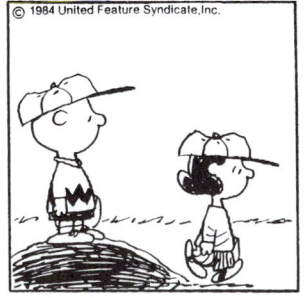
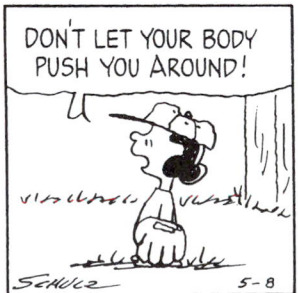

FIGURE 13.2   *Charlie Brown confronts the dilemma of pain and staying active. PEANUTS reprinted by permission of United Feature Syndicate, Inc.*

"the things people do when they suffer or are in pain" (Fordyce, 1988, p. 278). People may grimace, whine, moan, cry, or howl. They may change body stance to protect a painful injury. One research group found that pain behaviors could be grouped into four clusters: (1) distorted ambulation and posture, (2) negative affect, (3) facial/audible expressions of distress, and (4) avoidance of activity (Turk, Wack, & Kerns, 1985).

Conversing About Pain: Perceptions, Conditions, and Definitions

Even talking about pain can be a difficult task because so many different terms and definitions are involved. To make some sense of the bewildering array of pain terms, Melzack and Torgersen (1971) compiled a list of 102 pain words. The investigators then listed each word on a card, and subjects sorted these cards into piles based on their perceptions of similarity or belongingness of words to groups. From this, Melzack and Torgersen thought they could represent pain in three unique dimensions.

The first dimension they labelled the **sensory quality** of pain. Words expressing sensory dimensions included *flashing, shooting, burning,* and *itchy* pain. The second dimension, the **affective quality,** used words that describe emotional responses to pain, such as *annoying, sickening,* or *terrifying.* Melzack and Torgersen called the third dimension the **evaluative quality.** This refers to our tendency to attach some quantitative judgment of how mild or intense the pain is. Words such as *mild* or *excruciating* reflect this dimension. This process led Melzack (1975) to develop the McGill Pain Questionnaire. In a more recent survey, healthy subjects most often used the words *sharp, throbbing,* and *annoying* to describe pain while pain patients most often spoke of pain as *sharp, aching,* and *severe* (Salovey et al., 1992).

Although this three-dimensional view of pain is still commonly accepted, Fernandez and Turk (1992) suggested that only the sensory and affective dimensions can be reliably distinguished. The evaluative dimension probably is part of the affective dimension. The authors arrived at their conclusions through comparing results across a wide range of methodologies and scores of pain component studies.

Defining pain   The glut of pain definitions indicates both the confusion and the complexity that surround attempts to define pain. It has been defined in terms of physical tissue damage, psychological experience, and a combination of both (Fernandez & Turk, 1992). Definitions in terms of tissue damage rely on known physiology of the body's pain sensors (free nerve endings called **nociceptors**), and neural transmission of pain signals to the CNS, a process called **nociception** (Loeser, 1980).

Definitions that emphasize the subjective-affective component usually rely on patient reports that they feel hurt or damaged and experience sensations that are best described as aversive. Fordyce (1988) suggested that we must distinguish between pain as the sensory component and suffering as the affective component. In this view, **suffering** is an affective or emotional response triggered by a nociceptive-pain event or some other aversive stimulus. In contrast, Lazarus (1991a) argued that pain is a nonemotion. Our appraisal and subjective response to the pain sensation add the emotional component.

A behavioral component may be included based on the notion that emotions prompted by aversive events provide a strong motivational urge to escape or avoid the aversive events. These responses serve to protect the person from further harm with escape behavior, or from any harm at all with avoidance behavior. We can do little, then, to improve on the definition of pain first proposed by Merskey (1979) and adopted by Wall and Jones (1991, p. 28): "Pain is an unpleasant sensory and emotional experience associated with actual or potential tissue damage, or described in terms of such damage."

Types of pain   These dimensions of subjective experience are not adequate for diagnosis and treatment. Clinical work typically depends on making distinctions based on clusters of symptoms. The most common distinction is between acute pain and chronic pain. **Acute pain** is typically defined as a pain that lasts for a short time, usually less than three months (International Association for the Study of Pain Subcommittee on Taxonomy, 1986). Toothache pain, common headache pain, postoperative pain, and burn pain may be considered in this category. Even when the person has severe pain from surgery, it is still regarded as acute because the pain typically ends at a time that coincides with the wound's healing.

In **chronic pain,** the person experiences pain for more than three months, or pain lasts beyond the normal time for healing (International Association for the Study of Pain Subcommittee on Taxonomy, 1986). The pain may be mild or severe. It may be continuous or intermittent. It may be felt in muscles, joints, or tendons. It may be due to compression injuries, tears, or inflammation. It may be caused by a vascular disturbance as in migraine headache. Still, chronic pain may occur in the absence of tissue damage. The companions of chronic pain are prolonged distress, loss of sleep, irritability, and loss of physical ability to perform work or other activities. Depression may occur more frequently in chronic pain patients than among patients with other chronic medical conditions (see Banks & Kerns, 1996, for a review). A useful mnemonic is the three Ds: disruption, depression, and disability. The person's life is disrupted by the symptoms, mood is altered, and the person may be physically disabled.

Some chronic pain conditions, such as low back pain, may occur even when it is difficult to identify any tissue damage. The term for this type of pain, **chronic intractable benign pain,** emphasizes that the pain does not respond to treatment (it is intractable), but it is not progressive and does not threaten the person's life (it is benign). In contrast, cancer and arthritis pain are typically chronic and continuous. They present underlying pathologies that are progressive leading to a serious erosion in quality of life and threat to life itself. This type of pain is called **chronic progressive pain.**

The differences between acute and chronic pain can be clinically important. As we will see later, acute and chronic pain patients show different psychological profiles. Chronic pain may involve ongoing psychological conflict and distress because of an uncertain prognosis. Further, chronic pain has the potential for secondary gain: The pain behaviors may persist because they yield many rewards. Secondary gain presents many problems for diagnosis and treatment. Finally, pain interventions may work well with acute but not chronic pain.

Although these clinical descriptors have been in vogue for some time, Turk and Rudy (1988) thought it might be important to look at how chronic pain patients cluster in ways that could guide cognitive-behavioral interventions. To this end, they developed an empirical taxonomy or classification scheme for chronic pain patients.

Based on a study of 140 consecutive referrals to an outpatient pain clinic, the researchers found that patients fit three different profiles: They were dysfunctional, interpersonally distressed, or minimizing or adaptively coping. The *dysfunctional* group reported more severe pain than the other groups. They also indicated that pain interfered significantly with their ability to conduct their affairs in normal fashion. The *interpersonally distressed* group generally reported that they perceived family and friends as largely unsupportive. Thus, pain seemed to create distress in interpersonal relations among this group. Finally, compared to the other two groups, the *minimizers/adaptive copers* reported lower levels of pain and lower affective distress, and they perceived that pain did not interfere much in their lives. Further, they felt that they had higher daily activity levels and control over their lives. Whether this scheme will prove useful to design tailored treatment interventions remains to be seen.

Another pain type is **referred pain,** when there is a physical basis for the perception of

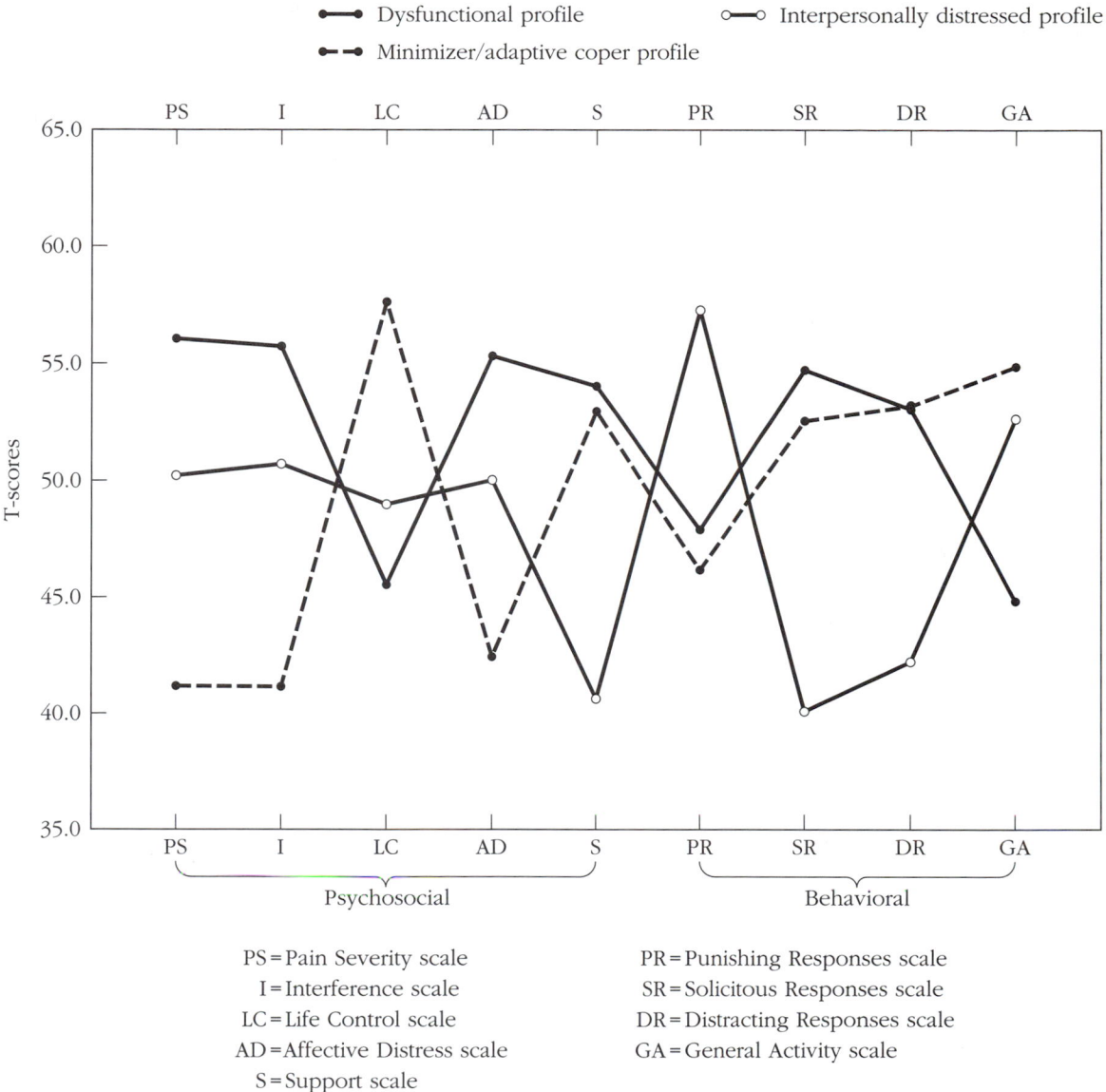

FIGURE 13.3 Differences on the Multidimensional Pain Inventory suggesting that three profiles may be identified among chronic pain patients (from Turk & Rudy, 1988).

pain, but the pain is felt in a different part of the body. My knowledge of this type of pain became much more personal not long ago when I had to have an impacted wisdom tooth removed surgically. For a short time after surgery, I had severe pain above the temporomandibular joint in the region of my left ear—even though the surgery had been on the lower jaw and forward from the joint. Referred pain usually occurs when sensory signals use the same pathways to the sensory cortex. Then, the person cannot tell precisely where the pain comes from.

Two other reported conditions are neuralgia and causalgia. In **neuralgia,** the person feels severe and unremitting pain. The pain is generally attributed to viral infections in peripheral nerves, to nerve degeneration associated with diabetes (among other illnesses), or to circulatory problems. Neuralgia is more common among older people, which may be related to degeneration in peripheral nerves associated with aging.

Causalgia is burning pain, unrelenting and of high intensity. This type of pain is usually caused by a high velocity object (such as a bullet) striking or penetrating the body. It is reported by about 25% of people as long as one year after their wounds have healed. In this case, physical damage produced the pain in the first place, but the perception persists long after the basis for the pain is gone.

The Epidemiology of Pain: Problems, Prevalence, and Costs

Pain seems to be everywhere and it is commonly associated with many medical disorders, from the everyday headache to the crippling heart attack. Yet, pain is singularly absent from some of the most devastating attacks, such as strokes, and it plays no role in the so-called silent sickness, hypertension. Thus, arriving at estimates of prevalence and costs of pain become complicated by the problem of setting limits on what conditions should be included.

The customary approach is to use direct care costs and indirect costs due to disability and premature mortality among those disorders for which pain is the dominant symptom or for behaviors in which pain relief is the primary intended outcome. Disorders commonly treated as pain disorders include headache pain, low back pain, orofacial pain, and arthritic pain, among others. Certain disorders, such as sickle-cell anemia and burns, may have significant pain symptoms but are not considered pain disorders per se (Platt et al., 1991). Pain behaviors include missing work because of disabling pain, purchasing pain-relief medicines, and seeking treatment specifically for pain relief.

Although estimates vary greatly, probably 33% of Americans have recurrent or persistent disabling pain that requires medical attention (Ball, 1984). Among the nearly 70 million pain sufferers, about 7 million suffer low back pain. Pain victims account for 8 million doctor visits each year, and about 80% of all doctor consultations are pain related. Pain sufferers spend more than $50 billion each year to control their pain (Salovey et al., 1992), including nearly $4 billion annually on pain relief medications purchased as over-the-counter drugs. The net economic effect is about 700 million lost work days per year, amounting to an annual economic loss of nearly $100 billion.

Note that the more people report stress and hassles, the more they also report the presence of pains. The Nuprin report revealed that people with moderate stress (38% of the sample) and with high stress (8% of the sample) also had higher prevalence of pain (Sternbach, 1986). As just one example, only 7% of the low stress group reported headache pain, but 17% of the moderate stress and 25% of the high stress groups reported headache pain.

The Physiology of Pain: Receptors, Neurons, and Analgesics

Imagine that you have been out riding your bicycle enjoying the sounds of waves and nature's sweet aromas as you ride along a lakefront road. You go down a hill around a sharp bend, perhaps a little too fast. Suddenly a car pulls out in front of you and you react swiftly to avoid a collision. Unfortunately, you overcorrect, the bike flips out, and you crash and burn over the rock-hard road surface.

When the dust has settled and you have pulled yourself back together, as it were, you realize that something is wrong. There is throbbing pain from your hip where you landed, and gnawing pain from your elbow which is also bleeding from a bad road scrape. You check more carefully to make sure that nothing is broken and then get back on your bike and return home. You notice for a while that the pain seems to be less than it was immediately after the crash. Later, as you settle in for a quiet evening, the pain returns, gets even worse, and begins to seem intolerable.

What is the physical process involved in transmitting pain signals to the brain from the bruise on your hip and the scrape on your elbow? Why did the pain subside for a while and then return? The overall process involves sensory receptors, neural fibers that both ascend and descend from the CNS, several brain centers, and the brain's natural analgesics. The details can only be briefly outlined, but they provide some clues to understanding how the physical and subjective components of pain come about.

Pain Receptors and Neural Messengers: A and C Fibers

To begin, the bruise on your hip and the road scrape on your elbow damaged tissue in underlying muscle and skin. In the process, the extreme pressure stimulated the body's pain sensors, called **free nerve endings** or nociceptors. Pain receptors are liberally scattered beneath the skin's surface, in muscles, and in viscera. Free nerve endings are so-called because they do not have specialized receptor mechanisms like other cutaneous receptors or like the eye and ear. The number of nerve endings stimulated and the strength of the stimulation both contribute to the intensity of pain sensations.

Free nerve endings can be viewed as tentacles that extend from neurons connecting into the ascending spinal pathway. Actually, there are two types of free nerve endings, and differences in structure and function seem to be related to differences in quality of the pain experience. The first type is a heavily myelinated large diameter neuron called the **A-delta fiber** (Kimble, 1988). A-delta fibers typically conduct impulses at about 15 meters per second, but they are capable of rates up to 30 meters per second. Immediate pain, or pricking pain, is mediated by these large fibers.

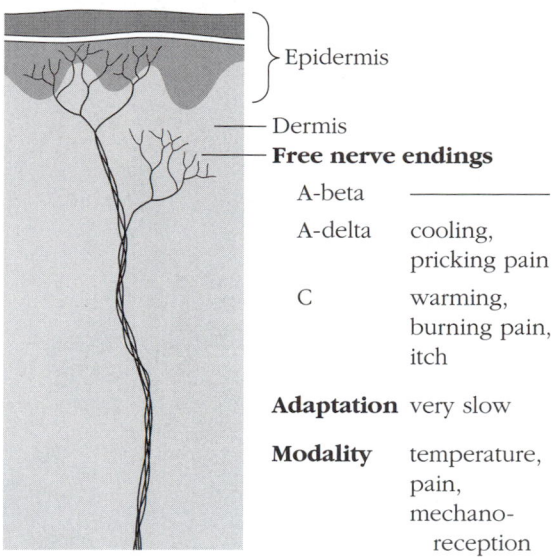

FIGURE 13.4   *Free nerve endings scattered liberally beneath the skin surface are the body's pain receptors.*

The second type is the **C-fiber,** also called the small fiber. As the name suggests, it is a small-diameter unmyelinated fiber. Small fibers conduct information at a slow rate, typically less than one meter per second. C fibers are responsible for the slow, burning pain that seems to last.

Both A-delta and C fibers are first-order neurons with their cell bodies in the dorsal root ganglia and with projections into the dorsal horn of the spinal column. These fibers synapse almost immediately with second-order neurons.

Regardless of their type, pain fibers adapt very slowly. Between the two fibers, though, we may have an explanation for the very quick pain reaction (A-delta fiber response) to something like a razor or paper cut that is followed shortly after by a persistent throbbing pain (C fiber response). This was probably behind your immediate perception of pain when you hit the road and persistent pain in the first few minutes following the crash.

From the dorsal horn, pain messages make their way up the primary pain highway in a tract called the **ascending anterolateral pathway.** This pathway really consists of three separate

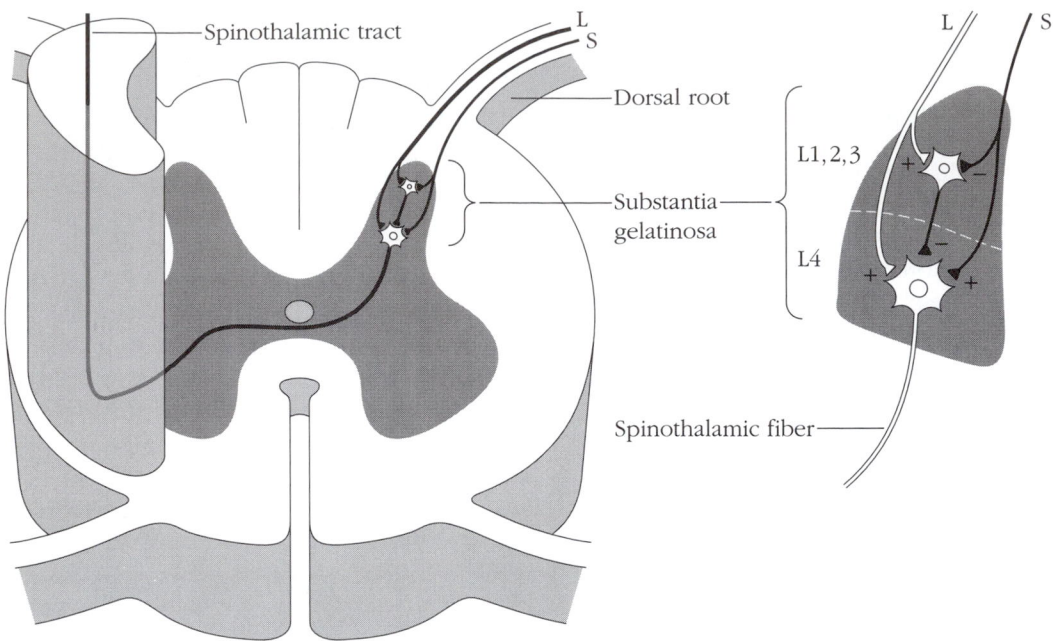

FIGURE 13.5   *Pain fibers synapse in the dorsal horn gray matter. As suggested by the gate control theory of pain, at this site descending pathways may shut pain gates. Also at this site, electrical stimulation such as TENS may block the perception of pain.*

second-order neuron tracts, each named for the point in the brain where it ends. Thus, the **spinothalamic tract** projects to the thalamus, and the **spinoreticular tract** projects to the reticular formation. The third tract, the **spinotectal tract,** projects into the tectum, or colliculi, in the midbrain. The primary purpose of the anterolateral pathway is to carry information about temperature and pain. Once in the brain, these second-order neurons synapse with third-order neurons that terminate in the sensory cortex. Thus, pain messages are processed in several different CNS areas, including the reticular formation, the thalamus, the sensory cortex, and the periaqueductal gray area (PAG).

Neural transmission of pain information also depends on two types of chemical neuroregulators, small-molecule neurotransmitters and large-molecule neurotransmitters (also called neuromodulators). Pain neurotransmitters may be either excitatory or inhibitory, but they work primarily at the synapses of individual neurons.

One neurotransmitter, substance P, is thought to be an excitatory peptide involved in transmission of pain signals to the CNS. If substance P is low or not available, then the pain signal may be reduced or blocked altogether. Substance P may be involved in cluster headaches as we shall see later (Sicuteri et al., 1990). Neuromodulators modify neuronal activity. They seem to act indirectly by modifying the action of neurotransmitters. This way of acting suggests that they may work over a large region of neurons instead of at particular synapses. The brain's natural opioids, endorphins, are examples of neuromodulators (Whipple, 1987).

Pain Centers in the Brain: The Thalamus and Limbic System

On the one hand, the brain has no clear-cut centers that unquestionably lead to pain when stimulated or that lead to pain cessation when cut out (Pinel, 1993). On the other hand,

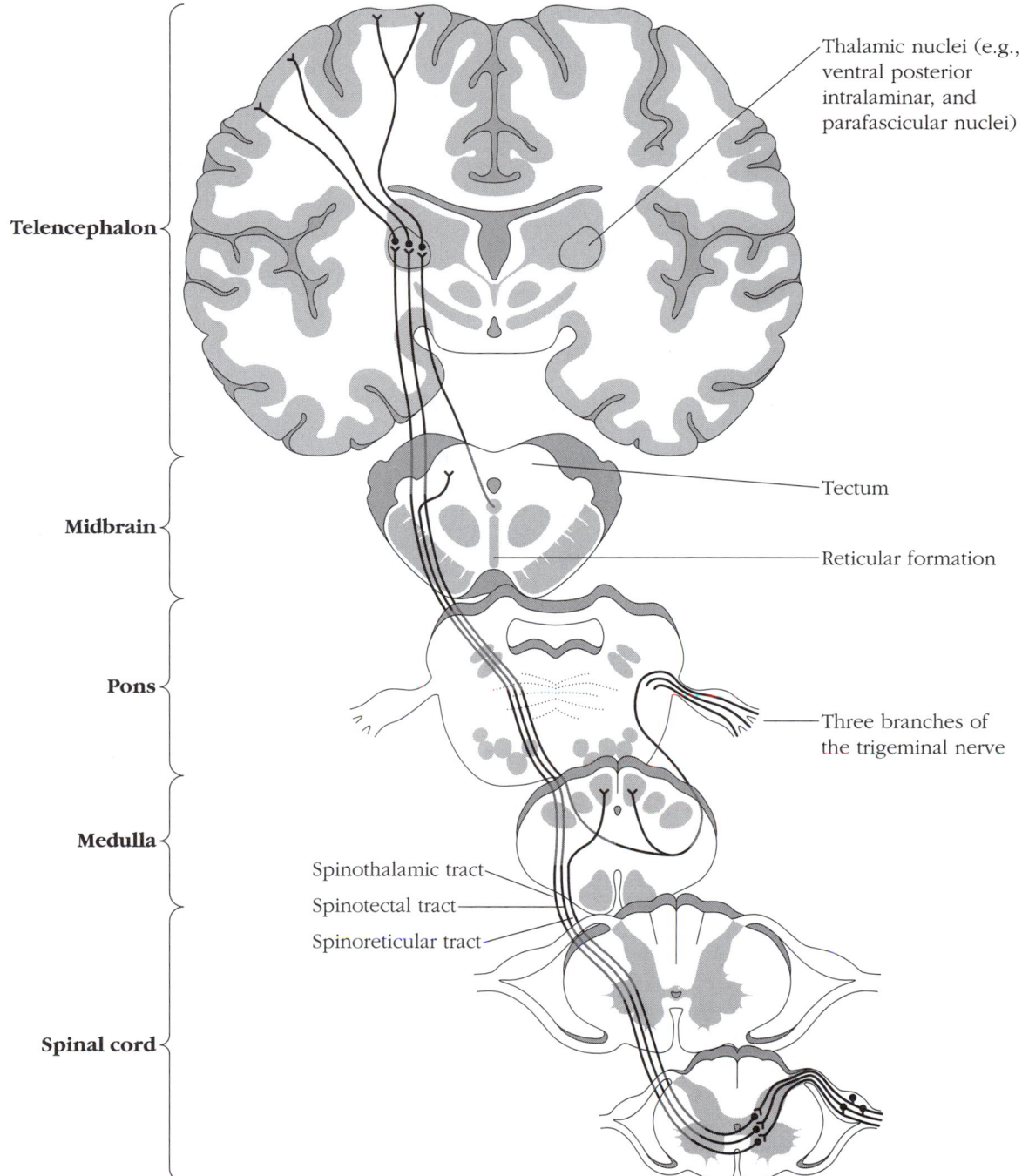

FIGURE 13.6   *The ascending pain pathways are composed of second-order neurons. They receive their information from the first-order sensory neurons in the dorsal horn. Second-order neurons then synapse with third-order neurons in the central nervous system and ultimately project to the sensory cortex where the perception and discrimination of pain occurs.*

Figure 13.6 makes it clear that some CNS centers are more important than others. The beginning of pain awareness and the quality of the pain experience seem to be jointly controlled mostly by the reticular formation and thalamic centers. The reticular formation is the brain's gating system. When you got back on your bicycle, the immediate demands of getting safely back home may have attenuated (reduced) pain signals.

The thalamus is the heart of the limbic system, which regulates many aspects of emotional sensitivity. This connection seems especially apropos since pain is usually connected with negative emotions: The connection may produce an amplification effect that increases sensitivity to pain. When you sat down later in the evening and had nothing to distract you, your emotional aversion to pain might have made the pain seem worse even if the level of pain signals was unchanged.

The somatosensory area located in back of the central fissure is the primary projection area for integrating information from the peripheral senses including pain. Each part of the body has its own area allocated in the sensory cortex, so that you know that the hip and elbow hurt, not the thigh and hand.

Descending Pain Pathways: The Periaqueductal Gray Area

Although we tend to think of pain largely as an arousing and irritating experience, the body has two built-in mechanisms to control or reduce the effect of pain. One is a descending neural pathway that seems capable of shutting the gates of pain. The second is the brain's built-in analgesic system.

It is an oversimplification, but we may think of the descending pathway as originating in the area called the **periaqueductal gray** (PAG). The importance of this area was first recognized in 1969 when Reynolds used intracerebral electrical stimulation to produce analgesic effects in rats. Reynolds actually was able to carry out surgery with no other anesthesia besides stimulation to the PAG area. This raised the question

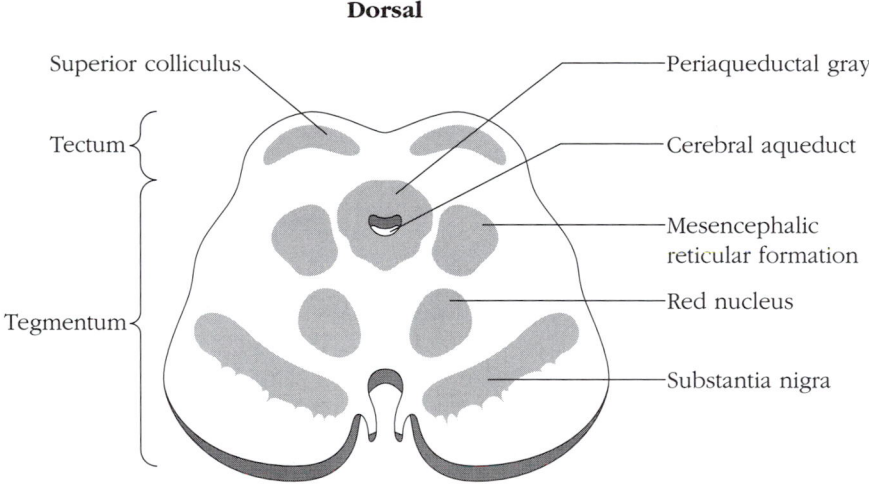

FIGURE 13.7   *The periaqueductal gray area located in the midbrain tegmentum region appears to be capable of reducing the perception of pain for some time after stimulation has stopped.*

of what was going on in the PAG area that could account for the reduction in pain. The answer turned out to be connected to the brain's natural opioids.

The PAG area is loaded with opiate receptors. When opiates bind at these receptor sites, they increase the activity of descending neurons in the medulla. These neurons then project to the dorsal horn precisely at the point where the A-delta and C fibers connect with the second-order ascending pain neurons. Activity in the descending neurons seems to close neural gates so that ascending pain signals cannot go through (Basbaum & Field, 1978). In more technical terms, excitatory signals from free nerve endings are countered by inhibitory signals from descending neurons. Under certain circumstances, the inhibitory signals may become strong enough to block most of the pain signal.

Pain Chemistry: The Brain's Natural Analgesics

Consider again the ill-fated bicycle ride. For most people, such a close call is a highly stressful event. There is not only the immediate and direct perception of pain, but also the meaning of the event—what might have been. Under stressful conditions the brain appears to increase the level of endorphins in the pain region. This term, **endorphin,** means literally the morphine within[3] and refers to a group of endogenous morphines that serve as pain killers. These natural opioids are not watered down, either. They are powerful enough to produce an analgesic effect roughly comparable to that of morphine (Stephens, 1980). Further, the process whereby a stressful event increases the level of endorphins has been observed in a variety of situations, and it is now called **stress-induced analgesia** (SIA). Combined with cognitive distractors, SIA may have helped

to reduce the level of pain you felt during the ride back home.

At one time, the brain's opioids were only poorly understood, but more information is becoming available all the time. It appears that neural cells in the brain and pituitary construct no less than three different types of opioids. Opioids are then concentrated in the lower and middle regions of the brain, such as in the thalamus and limbic system, and they are liberally distributed in the PAG area.

An Integrative Approach: The Gate Control Theory of Pain

An outline for the view of pain described in the last few pages, the *gate control theory,* was laid down in rudimentary form many years ago by Melzack and Wall (1965). Many technical details have been added that were unheard of at that time, but it is as though Melzack and Wall had a type of scientific crystal ball that allowed them to see the essential truth of the process. The theory has proved remarkably durable, and it has flexibly integrated more precise details as they became available (Melzack, 1993).

In brief, Melzack and Wall proposed that a spinal gate exists in the dorsal horn of the spinal column. This gate is opened or closed depending on relative activity in the A-delta (large-diameter) and C (small-diameter) fibers. Large fiber activity tends to close the gate (inhibit transmission), whereas small fiber activity tends to open the gate (facilitate transmission). A descending pathway can modify pain signals in the gating mechanism. Higher cortical centers are involved in an interpretive role that assigns meaning to both context and body condition. If the event is judged as painful because there is obvious tissue damage, then neural pain gates open and transmit pain signals to the brain.

This theory makes it clear that pain is not just a physiological process, with the person a passive sensor. Instead, it is a complex process in which psychological processes play a very important regulatory-mediating role. Gate

---

[3] The name *morphine* itself comes from the god of sleep and dreams, Morpheus (Kimble, 1988).

control theory integrated cognitive processes with the physiology of pain, but it still could not explain certain pain phenomena. Paraplegics with spinal cord transections still experience pain from the body area below the spinal cord damage, and amputees feel pain in missing limbs. This phenomenon, the phantom limb phenomenon, has been particularly troublesome for pain theory (Melzack, 1990; 1992).

Phantom Limbs: Pain in the Absence of Sensory Input

The **phantom limb phenomenon** refers to an amputee's impression that a leg or arm amputated years before still feels as though it is there. It may feel numb, or hot, or as though it has been cut with a knife. In short, a full range of sensory impressions is possible. Pain episodes may last only a few seconds or continue for several days. They may occur less than once a month or persist on a daily basis with constant pain (Bowser, 1991).

According to Jensen and Rasmussen (1989), there may be as many as 500,000 amputees in the United States. In a review of the phantom limb phenomenon, Margaret Bowser (1991) noted that between 84% to 98% of amputees perceive that the missing limb is still there. Between 69% and 85% of amputees experience painful sensations from the missing limb. Further, in nearly half of those who experience phantom limb pain, the intensity of the pain does not diminish over time. Finally, phantom limb pain does not respond to conventional pain treatments. Success rates may be as low as 1% and rarely exceed 30%.

The dilemma is obvious: A limb that physically is not there still hurts. How can this be? One explanation suggests that recurrent pain perceptions result from the amputee's poor emotional response to loss of the limb, an explanation that is not particularly helpful (see Bowser, 1991). Another explanation suggests that pain neurons still located in the stump fire signals that provide a neural basis for the pain perception. It is also possible that cortical events, memories stored for that limb, may trigger neural activity in the related sensory cortex that then invokes a subjective pain experience for the missing limb. These explanations, though, are at best still speculative.

Gate Control Theory Revisited: Neuroscience, Neuromatrix, and Self

To deal with this issue, Melzack (1993) extended gate control theory to include notions derived from neuroscience. Melzack argued from the data on paraplegics and amputees that pain cannot be the direct result of receptor activation. Instead, pain stimuli must act only as triggers for patterns of neural activity that underlie our perception of pain. According to Melzack, these patterns of neural activity occur in an extended neural network called the neuromatrix.

In normal circumstances, pain experiences arise from interaction between psychological processes in the neuromatrix and physiological processes in the nociceptors, the spinal gate in the dorsal horn, and ascending and descending neural pathways. In extreme conditions, such as those experienced by paraplegics and amputees, the neuromatrix perpetuates the experience of the body-self as a unity. The person may continue to feel those physically or neurally detached parts of the body because of activity in the neuromatrix. The existence of the neuromatrix is also somewhat speculative, yet Melzack began to provide evidence for its existence. He also pointed to data from neuroscience research to support his arguments. This model, if it passes more rigorous tests, may also provide a way to explain pain when no current physical pathology exists to explain the pain, as occurs in some chronic pain conditions. In this way, gate control theory continues to be elaborated as an integrative theory to account for the interaction of psychological (perceptual, emotive, and cognitive) processes and neurophysiological systems in the human experience of pain.

Etiology of Pain: The Biomedical View

If we focused only on the neural physiology of pain, the model just described could be considered a biomedical model of the etiology of pain. To be completely detailed, though, the biomedical model would also describe specific physical pathology. In some pain disorders, this turns out to be a fairly simple task. A bone break, for example, is a common structural pathology, and vascular constriction or a coronary attack are common functional pathologies that underlie a patient's perception of pain. In this view, expressed pain is merely a symptom of an underlying disease process that is the cause. To get rid of the symptom (pain), the cause (pathology) should be located, treated, and removed. At the same time, modern medicine may use methods that simply prevent the transmission of pain signals, as when doctors prescribe painkilling medications, provide corrective surgery, or prescribe neural stimulation. These techniques do not directly cure underlying pathology, but they are based on well-known principles of pain physiology.

The Psychology of Pain: Learning, Stress, and Depression

The psychosocial view of pain readily accepts the demonstrated physiology of pain but suggests that the medical model accounts for only one part of the pain experience. The medical model does not explain the phantom limb phenomenon, the lack of identifiable pathology in chronic pain disorders (perhaps 85% unidentified pathology in low back pain), and the relationship between psychosocial rewards and frequency of pain behaviors. Several psychoso-

cial processes may influence pain, including learning, modeling, individual differences, belief systems, stress, and depression.

A Learning Model of Pain: Reinforcers, Caregiving, and Policy

Perhaps the most clearly articulated psychosocial model comes from the work of Wilbert Fordyce (1976). In this model, pain behaviors are attempts to communicate to others the pain and suffering the person is currently feeling. Pain behaviors may increase because they lead to caregiving behaviors from family and friends. In the simplest possible terms, pain behavior becomes an operant that changes based on rewarding events in the environment. A high density of rewards for pain behaviors will make those behaviors increase in frequency. If this process goes on long enough, the pain behaviors may become functionally autonomous, persisting on their own long past the original pathology. If the density of rewards is only modest or low, then pain behaviors may stay at a stable level or decline, depending on other factors. In addition, pain behaviors appear to be functionally related so that attempts to intervene in one may influence other behaviors in the group (Kalsher, Cataldo, Deal, Traughber, & Jankel, 1985).

The learning model does not deny the sensory physiology that explains pain's pathway into and through the central nervous system. The model contends, though, that since pain is a very private experience, the report of pain may or may not be related to actual physical pathology. Since we cannot observe a person's pain from the outside, we are always at the mercy of the person reporting. In most cases, there is no good reason to believe that people willfully misrepresent their feeling of pain—that is, they truly believe pain is present even though an injury has long since healed. But their perceptions may be tainted by a number of expectancies about the likelihood of rewards.

The rewarding events that may support pain are many. For example, families are generally disposed to react to a member's pain with many caregiving behaviors, such as expressions of sympathy and other forms of tender loving care (Fordyce, 1976; Romano et al., 1992). Typically these care behaviors do not occur as often in the absence of pain. This cycle probably has been repeated for most adults many, many times from childhood and carries over into their own conduct as parents and spouses. Children learn about pain by watching their parents and significant others. Even before experiencing direct family reactions to their pain, children may have formed both cognitive and emotive impressions of what pain is about and what to expect when pain occurs. Finally, pain behavior may be strengthened by negative reinforcement when the person seeks to avoid activities that arouse a fear of pain.

A Cognitive Model: Appraisals, Beliefs, and Expectancies

The cognitive model suggests that beliefs and expectations can influence reactions to many stimuli, including psychosocial stressors and aversive or painful events. David Williams and Francis Keefe (1991) conducted an intriguing study of pain beliefs and their relationship to coping strategies. In this study, subjects responded to both a pain belief inventory and a coping strategies questionnaire. Using a statistical technique called cluster analysis, Williams and Keefe found that the subjects could be placed in three subgroups based on shared views about pain. The first group felt that pain was enduring but understandable. Another group believed that pain was long lasting and mysterious. This group was more likely to engage in what Ellis called catastrophizing behavior, and they were less likely to view their pain coping strategies as effective. The third group felt that pain was short-term and understandable. They did not engage in catas-

trophizing behavior like the second group, and they were also more likely to see their pain coping strategies as effective.

Karen Gil and her associates have obtained evidence that cognitive processes mediate the experience of pain (Gil, Williams, Keefe, & Beckham, 1990). Based on clinical data, Gil's team made a reasonable guess that during pain flare-ups, patients typically have some negative thoughts. These negative thoughts in turn may influence the person's perception of pain and distress. The investigators used three chronic pain groups, including people with sickle cell disease, rheumatoid arthritis, and chronic pain. The 185 adult subjects filled out an Inventory of Negative Thoughts in Response to Pain (INTRP), the Symptom Checklist (SCL-90-R), and a coping strategies questionnaire. A factor analysis discovered three components: negative self-statements, negative social cognitions, and self-blame. Gil's team found that subjects reported more severe pain and distress when they also had high scores on negative self-statements and negative social cognitions. This confirms the suspicion that negative thoughts may influence a person's pain perceptions. Further, subjects who lived with chronic daily pain had more frequent negative thoughts during pain flare-ups than those who lived with intermittent pain.

The Personality Factor: Anxiety, Self-Efficacy, and Depression

Repeated attempts have been made to connect a disease state with some personality variable. Similar questions have been raised with regard to pain with few consistent or useful findings. Acute pain patients may show personality profiles with increased agitation and anxiety as psychological reactions to the aversive quality of the pain experience.

Chronic pain patients usually present a different psychological profile. They have higher MMPI scores on hysteria, hypochondriasis, and depression (Jamison, Ferrer-Brechner, Brechner,

& McCreary, 1976). This difference in profile is thought to have some as yet undemonstrated importance for treatment, but it is not considered relevant to either etiology or persistence of pain behaviors. Unfortunately, many methodological problems exist in studies of this nature. These problems make it almost impossible to decide whether personality traits preceded and influenced the pain, or the pain preceded and contributed to the personality profile (Love & Peck, 1987).

Several studies point out that self-efficacy moderates the perception and tolerance for pain (Lackner, Carosella, & Feuerstein, 1996). One study from Bandura's lab illustrates this point (Bandura, O'Leary, Taylor, Gauthier, & Gossard, 1987). One group received instruction in cognitive coping skills designed to increase their self-efficacy for pain tolerance and reducing pain. A placebo group and a no-treatment control group were also used. Both the coping and the placebo group showed increased self-efficacy in tolerating pain, but only the coping group showed an increased self-efficacy for reducing pain once it started.

Pain disorders are seldom strongly related to personality traits. Burn victims, though, may represent one exception to the rule (Patterson, Everett, Bombardier, Questad, Lee, & Marvin, 1993). Studies focusing on premorbid psychological adjustment of burn victims reveal a consistent pattern of dysfunctional behavior. In general, people with premorbid psychopathology were more likely to sustain burn injuries, and these people were more likely to require longer and costlier recovery periods. The most common traits found were depression, character disorder, and alcohol and drug abuse. Burn injuries often resulted from suicide attempts.

We have discussed a number of psychosocial processes that bear on pain. To summarize, pain behaviors may be learned by observing others or through rewarding interactions in the family setting. Pain is influenced by the person's expectancies and beliefs. Finally, when subjects developed self-efficacy combined with pain coping skills, they were better able to manage and reduce pain compared to controls.

Two Pain Disorders: Headaches and Low Back Pain

If depression is the common cold of mental illness, headaches are the common colds of pain. Probably 90% of the U.S. population is afflicted with headache pain at one time or another during the course of a year, although the majority do not experience disabling pain. However, recent data indicate that 25 million people regularly experience migraine headaches that can disable them for short periods (Salovey et al., 1992).

Based on the Nuprin Pain Report, back pain may afflict from 55% to 60% of the adult population enough to interfere with functioning one or more days per year (Sternbach, 1986). Back pain may strike 2 to 7 million people at levels sufficient to impair functioning for longer periods of time, making health care costs very formidable (Deyo et al., 1990; Salovey et al., 1992).

The next few pages will describe the basic symptoms and etiology of these two conditions. A few specialized treatment approaches will be discussed, but general pain treatment strategies will be reserved for later.

Headache Pain: Migraine, Tension, and Cluster Headaches

In reality, there are about 14 types of headaches, 10 of which are biologically based. These different types of headaches have different origins, symptoms, and severity. They often have different recommended treatments. The four most common headaches include acute, tension, migraine, and cluster headaches.

The **acute headache** is the everyday headache that hits for a short time and is gone almost as suddenly as it appeared. The origin of acute headaches is not clear, but they may be related to stress, among other things. Acute headaches may respond to drugstore remedies such as aspirin, ibuprofen, and other specially formulated painkillers.

Tension headaches are generally attributed to muscle tension, which is why the alternative name *muscle-contraction headaches* is sometimes used. The core feature is a steady, dull pain that is evenly distributed over the two hemispheres. The onset is gradual, but the pain can last from a few hours to several weeks. Muscle contraction headaches occur in children in roughly the same form as in adults (Labbe, 1988). Tension headaches were thought to be classic stress headaches associated with emotional conflict. Permanently elevated levels of EMG frontalis muscle tension seem to distinguish both tension and migraine headache patients from normal controls (Flor & Turk, 1989). Further, vasoconstriction, the presumed core of migraine, has been found also in tension headaches.

Migraine headaches can bring on excruciating pain, thought to be caused by vascular disturbances, probably vasodilation and constriction in the temporal artery (Cohen et al., 1983). The headache is described as an episodic, throbbing, and unilateral attack (Welch, 1993). Although the attack most often begins with pain on one side, it can become bilateral. In addition to severe pain, migraine is marked by a cluster of related symptoms including nausea, vomiting, and irritability; visual disorders and an aura that often precede the attack; dizziness and sweating; duration of about two to eight hours; and a family history of migraine (Solomon, 1993). The aura probably occurs in no more than 10 to 15% of migraine patients. Finally, migraines are typically aggravated by physical activity.

Cluster headaches (CH) occur most frequently in males who describe their attacks as extremely painful with a subjective experience of sharp, stabbing pain, like an ice pick in the eye. Involvement of the eye is a central feature of the cluster headache (Sicuteri et al., 1990). Patients are typically restless during an attack, but they may also become violent and occasionally threaten suicide. The cluster headache, like a migraine, is a one-sided headache. It consists of two components, though, the pain itself and autonomic symptoms such as sweating, tearing, and nasal secretion (Sjaastad, Salvesen, Fredriksen, & Antonaci, 1989). The autonomic component is probably not linked to the origin of the headache, but it may be part of an anxiety reaction to the attack itself.

At one time, the cause was listed as unknown, but recently both biomedical and psychogenic theories have emerged. Psychosocial stressors and emotional conflict serve to initiate CH attacks, but CH is now more widely accepted as a headache with a firm organic basis (Sjaastad et al., 1989; Sicuteri et al., 1990). One notion is that there is impaired opioid blocking of pain signals (Sicuteri, 1986). Another theory suggests that the basic CH pathophysiology involves the trigeminal vascular system, with pain initiated in a cyclical fashion (Mathew, 1992). Sicuteri and his group provided evidence for this view: The trigeminal nerve stimulates secretion of substance P, thus facilitating pain signal transmission. In addition, the release of substance P in the eye creates a powerful contraction of the iris sphincter muscle, which feeds back as sensory information (via the trigeminal-ophthalmic nerve branch) to the CNS. This feedback may then amplify the perception of pain directly or by stimulating further release of substance P, or both.

Treatment of Headache Pain: The Biofeedback Debate

Treatment for headache pain covers a wide range of strategies including pharmacologic, surgical, cognitive-behavioral, biofeedback, relaxation, and hypnosis. In practice, most clinics use a combination of treatments rather than relying on only one strategy. We will discuss pharmacologic and cognitive-behavioral methods among general pain intervention strategies later. At this point, an extended debate on the merits of biofeedback for headache treatment requires some review.

The debate centered on the idea that each type of headache has its unique pathophysiology, that biofeedback could be used to correct the disturbed physiology, and that distinct biofeedback treatments could be matched to the different pathophysiologies. The conventional wisdom was that EMG biofeedback should be used for tension headaches, and skin temperature (thermal) biofeedback should be used for migraine headaches (Budzynski, Stoyva, & Adler, 1970).

The rationale for EMG biofeedback for tension headaches was simple: The headache occurs because of muscle tension. Reduce muscle tension, and the headache pain should pass. The rationale for skin temperature biofeedback is less obvious but still fairly simple. Skin temperature is a function of blood flow. The more blood flows in a region of the body, the higher the temperature will be. Vasoconstriction means less blood flows, and vasodilation means more blood flows. If migraines are the result of vasoconstriction, then thermal biofeedback could correct the problem by inducing vasodilation.

Many studies failed to provide support for these distinctions, however (Chapman, 1986). Further, different types of treatment may be equally effective in improving headache pain. For example, a meta-analysis looked at the outcome of 60 clinical trials using propranolol or relaxation/biofeedback. There was no consistent advantage for either method, and both showed identical success (43% reduction) in reducing headache pain (Holroyd & Penzien, 1990). Blanchard's group compared relaxation and biofeedback in treatment of three headache groups (Blanchard et al., 1982). Subjects treated with relaxation alone showed significant reductions in headaches regardless of type of headache. Biofeedback led to significant additional gains for all the groups. Yet, the fact that both relaxation and biofeedback produced improvement regardless of headache type is inconsistent with the idea that distinct pathophysiology requires distinct treatments.

Chronic Low Back Pain: Centers in the Brain

Chronic back pain has been attributed to disorders of the skeletal muscles, vertebrae, or invertebrae disks of the lower back. Neural disorders, such as nerve-root irritation, and degenerative conditions may also cause back pain. Improved diagnostic and evaluation procedures, such as MRI, are also providing clearer indications of subtle pathologies where previously no pathology could be found (Hoon, Feuerstein, & Papciak, 1985). Pain may be present even without clinically identifiable tissue damage, however. Richard Deyo (1991) cited statistics indicating that up to 85% of patients with low back pain cannot be given definitive diagnoses.

Psychosocial factors seem to play an important role in low back pain by magnifying existing pain or sustaining pain even after an injury has had ample time to heal. Psychological risk factors include monotonous job routines, boredom, and job dissatisfaction. There is some evidence that chronic back pain patients are hyperreactive to personally relevant emotional stressors and that EMG tension is prolonged following stressors compared to normal controls (Flor & Turk, 1989). Depression is about three to four times more prevalent in back pain patients compared to the general population (Sullivan, Reesor, Mikail, & Fisher, 1992). Low back pain patients may have less effective coping strategies, increasing their psychological distress. Keefe's research team found that one coping factor in particular, helplessness, could explain 50% of the variance in psychological distress and 46% of the variance in depression (Keefe, Crisson, Urban, & Williams, 1990).

Fordyce (1988) also noted that the number of reported back pain cases varies as social policy for disability claims changes. Disability, as Fordyce argues, differs from physiological pain (a physical state) and from suffering (a psychological state) because it is essentially a social policy judgment. In Sweden, back injury disability claims increased 3,800% in a 30-year period, supporting the view that psychosocial forces influence the rate of pain reports. A noted orthopedist responded to the explosion in disability claims by saying that "physicians should not treat back pain; nor should psychologists. Politicians should" (cited in Fordyce, 1988, p. 278).

In recent years, there has been a shift away from traction and bed rest as treatments for back pain, to active treatments including nonsteroidal anti-inflammatory drugs, muscle relaxant drugs, TENS,[4] and exercise. Back pain patients may benefit from either pharmacological or psychological or combined treatment for depression (Sullivan et al., 1992).

Treatment of Pain: Biomedical and Psychosocial Models

Treatment of pain has proved one of the more frustrating efforts for clinicians in either medicine or psychology. As you might surmise from the description of pain physiology and psychology, the reality of pain is indisputable for the person seeking help. At times, though, pain can be very elusive for the service provider to identify. Pain has led health care providers to develop a wide array of treatment methods. The next few pages will discuss the more common biomedical methods for pain relief, then expand on psychosocial strategies.

Biomedical Pain Treatments: Medication, Stimulation, and Surgery

Medical specialists have developed four methods of pain treatment. The most common strategy by far is to use some general painkiller medication, but specialized pain relief drugs have also been developed. A second method is TENS, the nonintrusive surface stimulation technique discussed on the next page. Third, in

certain cases, electrodes can be implanted in the brain's pain centers to block the perception of pain. This approach is by no means common. Fourth, surgical operations may cut pain fiber pathways in cases that have not responded to less intrusive measures.

The medicine cabinet: analgesics and narcotics   People usually look to the medicine shelf as the first choice of therapy when they get headaches. The number of medicines devoted to relief of aches and pain is truly astounding. Two groups of drugs are most commonly used for pain control: the narcotics and the analgesics.

Narcotics bind to opiate receptors in the CNS, triggering an inhibitory effect in the transmission of pain signals (Aronoff, Wagner, & Spangler, 1986). Codeine and morphine are common narcotics, the former being used in small amounts for some common drugstore cough syrups. They affect both the perception of pain and reaction to pain. They are useful for short-term pain control such as after a surgery, but medicine generally does not regard them as appropriate for chronic pain management because patients tend to develop tolerance for them, and they may become addictive. Certain cases, though—such as intractable pain in cancer—may justify use of a narcotic regardless of the addictive potential.

Analgesics are drugs that actively interfere with the neural transmission of pain signals or reduce the cortical response to pain (Whipple, 1987). The common analgesics—aspirin, acetaminophen, and ibuprofen—are superior to placebos in relieving migraine, but they are widely used for headache pain in general and other types of body aches. They work by reducing inflammation at the site of a wound, but they also inhibit the synthesis of neurochemicals that are needed to transmit pain signals into the CNS (Winters, 1985).

Nonsteroidal anti-inflammatory drugs (or NSAIDs) may be the first choice of treatment for mild to moderate migraine attacks. In Welch's (1993) review of drug therapy for migraine,

---

[4] See page 375 for more detail on the TENS procedure and its success in treating low back pain.

several clinical trials found that naproxen, an NSAID, proved effective in reducing severity of attacks, but results were inconsistent on other symptoms. Some trials showed reduced vomiting and duration of headaches, but other trials did not.

The stimulation approach: brain centers and control

In the time since the physiological principles of pain became clear, several methods demonstrated the practical utility of this knowledge. For example, TENS has been used successfully in the treatment of low back pain. It is a low-cost and effective treatment for this condition. TENS works in a very simple fashion that also illustrates the importance of the gate control theory described earlier. In a typical application, small electrodes are placed across the lower back muscles just about at or above the belt line and down the muscle slope toward the spinal column.[5] The electrodes are connected to a small portable stimulator (typically about the size of a small personal radio) that is worn on the belt (see Figure 13.8). When the stimulator is turned on, it delivers a pulse that feels somewhat like a repeated poke with a blunt pin. Some might describe the sensation differently, but this is the way it felt to me when I wore a TENS module for nearly 30 days following a biking accident which resulted in a faceted disk in the lower back and excruciating pain. A small dial, almost like a volume control on a personal radio, allows the patient to increase or decrease the intensity of the stimulation. Presumably, the stimulation closes the neural gate in the dorsal horn of the spinal column (as described earlier), so that the patient's perception of pain is significantly reduced if not blocked completely.

The efficacy of TENS is born out by research, and because of its low cost and ease of use, it is one of the more popular treatment choices. Still, recent research suggests that some placebo

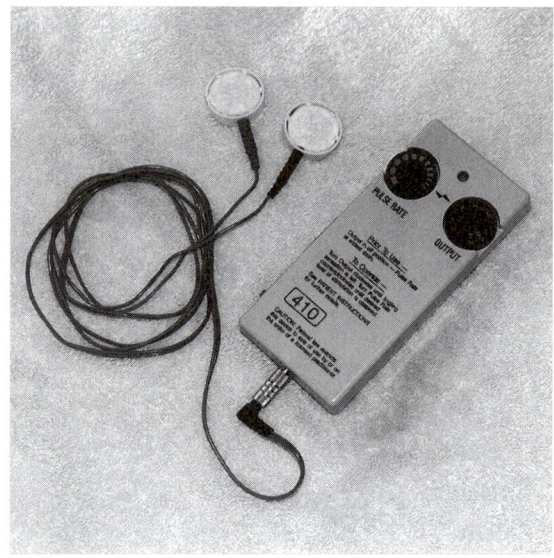

FIGURE 13.8 The TENS method for treating chronic low back pain.

effects (belief in the treatment) may be involved in the efficacy of TENS.

Deyo and his colleagues, for example, compared use of TENS to simple exercise (Deyo, Walsh, Martin, Schoenfeld, & Ramamurthy, 1990). Deyo's team followed four groups of patients through a brief one-month treatment period. One group received TENS while a second group received sham TENS. A third group practiced stretching exercises, and a fourth group practiced stretching exercises while receiving sham TENS. After one month, there were no statistically significant changes in pain reports in the TENS group compared to the sham TENS group. But the exercise groups, with or without sham TENS, showed significant drops in pain. Deyo's group noted, though, that the patients quickly abandoned their exercise program after treatment, at which point the pain returned. This underscores the importance of educating patients to understand the connection between health and activity and activating compliance strategies to achieve long-term success. Technologically sophisticated cultures seem to prefer convenient and effortless solutions (popping a pill or wearing a TENS pack) to effortful

---

[5] The electrodes can be moved for varying locations of pain, but this is one of the more common arrangements.

solutions. It is not surprising, then, that these patients quit exercising.

Another example of the stimulation technique to control pain is intracranial stimulation. One group of investigators confronted the problem of unmanageable pain in terminally ill patients. In this type of situation, medicinal preparations often lose effectiveness as the disease progresses and the severity of pain increases. To counteract the escalating pain, the dosage often has to be stepped up to a point that the patient is more or less comatose, not from the illness, but from the pain medication. At this point, of course, the patient's quality of life is virtually nil, and meaningful contacts with family and friends are lost.

In this study, though, the investigators implanted electrodes in several pain centers in the brain. These electrodes were brought out to small consoles at the patient's bedside. Then, the patient could turn any one of the electrodes on as their experience of pain dictated. With the exception of one patient, who died before the study was completed as part of the natural disease progression, all the patients reported that they could more effectively control the pain this way compared to medication. Most important, they felt that their quality of life significantly improved because they were able to reduce or completely eliminate the pain. But at the same time, they were able to carry on their important intimate family relations.

The surgical route   Surgery is used less often for pain treatment now than it has been in the past. When it is used, it is first and foremost because other means of pain control have failed. In addition, there must be good reason to believe from localization of the pain that a specific pathway is involved, increasing the likelihood that surgery will be successful. Still, there is no guarantee of success.

You may recall that Karen Blixen's pain from syphilis was so severe and unrelenting that surgeons tried on two separate occasions to relieve her pain by cutting pain fibers. From this perspective it is easier to see why their efforts failed. In general, surgical interventions may not succeed because of the complexity and resilience of the neural system itself. Pain signals appear to be transmitted by a complex network that is capable of rerouting signals. As a result, it may only be a matter of time until the signals have found a new pathway and the pain returns.

Psychosocial Interventions: Behavioral, Cognitive, and Meditative

Psychosocial interventions for pain have usually been based on the notion that pain behavior is subject to principles of rewarding or aversive control, or that the pain experience is subject to cognitive mediation through expectancies and beliefs. The distinction between what is behavioral and what is cognitive sometimes becomes blurred and may depend on the therapist's viewpoint. For example, Cautela's (1977) covert positive reinforcement was usually cast as a behavioral method even though it used mental imagery and thought stopping. Behavioral methods include contingency management, self-monitoring, self-reward, and social reward, among others.

Cognitive-behavioral methods   Cognitive interventions attempt to alter negative thoughts and self-statements that may aggravate pain conditions. Cognitive restructuring, modeling, imagery, and distraction techniques are often listed among the cognitive strategies. Some therapists prefer to teach coping strategies to help clients deal with pain. Inspecting the content of coping strategy sessions reveals a combination of standard cognitive and behavioral techniques. Techniques derived from stress coping programs, such as stress inoculation procedures, also may be added (Turk, Meichenbaum, & Genest, 1983). The coping approach is often targeted to clients with chronic and intractable pain such as in arthritis, but it has been used successfully with children suffering from recurrent abdominal pain as well (Sanders et al., 1989). This array of methods may be the subject of entire books, so I will focus here on just a few of the more revealing efforts at pain management through the cognitive-behavioral approach. We begin with a detailed comparison of a behavioral method with a cognitive-behavioral approach. Later, we will look at how the cognitive approach fares when compared to pharmacological interventions.

Judith Turner and Steve Clancy (1988) compared an operant behavioral treatment approach to a cognitive-behavioral approach for the treatment of chronic low back pain. A wait-list control group also provided a reference standard for the active interventions. Outcome measures included the McGill Pain Questionnaire, the Sickness Impact Profile, and observer and patient ratings of pain. Measures were obtained pretreatment, posttreatment, and at 6 months' and 12 months' follow-up. The trained observers, who were blind to group assignment, viewed videotapes of the clients going through a protocol of walking, standing, sitting, and reclining.

The operant method was based on a plan originally proposed by Fordyce (1976). Treatments were conducted in group format in two-hour sessions held weekly over eight weeks. Both patients and spouses were educated to the idea of pain behaviors and the role that social reinforcers play in maintaining such behavior. Spouses were taught to ignore pain behaviors and reward well behaviors. Also, patients and spouses kept daily diaries of pain behaviors and spouse responses. Additional components of the program focused on direct communication and on behavioral goals such as regular exercise.

The cognitive-behavioral component began with training in progressive muscle relaxation and imagery. Clients were also taught to identify negative emotions, stressful events, and maladaptive thoughts related to pain episodes. Finally, clients were taught how to generate adaptive thoughts and instructed to keep daily records of emotions and thoughts related to pain.

The results are useful for what they tell us, not only about the treatments, but about follow-up and change months after active intervention. Both the operant and the cognitive groups changed significantly across the period of active intervention, but the operant group showed the greatest change. In the follow-up period, however, the operant group leveled off while the cognitive group continued to improve. By 12 months' follow-up, the cognitive group had matched the operant group in degree of change and was still on an improvement trend. Finally, the cognitive group indicated higher satisfaction with treatment than did the operant group. We can only speculate from Turner and Clancy's data, but the continuing improvement in the cognitive group suggests that this method may carry long-term benefits beyond the confines of therapy.

We turn our attention now to a comparison of cognitive methods with pharmacological methods. Because of the extensive use of medications in pain treatment, it is useful to determine when alternative therapies may provide equivalent pain relief. One word of caution is in order, though. Certain severe pain disorders, such as burns, make medication absolutely necessary (Patterson, Everett, Burns, & Marvin, 1992). In these cases, psychological interventions should be considered only as adjuncts to medical therapy. When investigators compare medical and psychosocial interventions, several assumptions support the venture. Among these are that the pain has not responded to medical treatment, there is no detectable pathophysiology, the pain is chronic, or the pain appears to be psychogenic.

Herta Flor and Niels Birbaumer (1993) were concerned about the muddled picture of success in pain management that has been drawn from previous outcome studies. Like Carroll's dodo bird conclusion that all have won and all must have prizes, these investigators argued most studies have not adequately distinguished criteria for success. In particular, previous outcome studies have not disentangled the three levels of pain behavior that are relevant to chronic pain. These three behaviors are the verbal-subjective, motor-behavioral, and physiological-organic.

The researchers used one group of patients that suffered from chronic back pain (CBP) and another group that suffered from temporomandibular pain and dysfunction (TMP). Three different treatments were provided: EMG biofeedback (BFB), cognitive-behavior treatment (CBT), and medical treatment (MED). Flor and Birbaumer believed that patients with marked psychophysiological reactivity should respond best to BFB, whereas patients with pronounced negative self-statements should respond best to CBT. Finally, patients with marked medical findings should respond best to a medical treatment.

The BFB group received training in EMG biofeedback until they achieved a 90% reduction in muscle tension compared to baseline. Flor and Birbaumer introduced one important variation in this training: They used the specific pain site as the focus for tension reduction. According to their analysis, many of the studies reporting little or no success with BFB have used a nonpain site for tension reduction. The CBT group received training in progressive muscle relaxation, stress management, identifying pain-evoking events, problem solving, distraction, and positive self-statements. The MED group received the best available medications for their condition. This group also received a number of other interventions that could confound interpretation, however, such as physical therapy, spa, massage and chiropractic treatments.

The results indicated that all three groups showed improvement at posttreatment, but the BFB group improved most. At six months' and two years' follow-up, only the BFB group maintained the changes present at posttreatment. This marked superiority of BFB was inconsistent with other results, but Flor and Birbaumer suggested that their focus on the specific pain site may explain this finding. When results were analyzed by subgroups, Flor and Birbaumer found evidence that supported their notion on matching therapy to clients. In other words, the presence of marked psychophysiological reactivity predicted success with BFB, whereas the presence of negative self-statements predicted success with CBT. This result suggests, again, that successful pain treatment may require more precise matching to patient symptoms and physiological processes that underlie the pain.

Distraction and pain management   Distraction techniques have often been advocated as a cognitive means for coping with chronic pain. It is by no means clear that the technique is effective or under what conditions it might be effective. But recent studies have attempted to shed some light on this issue (Holmes & Stevenson, 1990).

Robert Baron and his associates wanted to find out whether sensory or emotional focus during root canal procedures would affect the patient's pain reports (Baron, Logan, & Hoppe, 1993). These investigators fit their work into the context of Leventhal's theory that if stressful stimuli are processed in terms of an emotional schema, the stimuli will be more aversive. In the context of pain, using an emotional focus should prove more aversive, whereas a sensory focus should prove less aversive. Subjects also filled out a dental control scale to indicate how much control they would like to have while in the dentist office, as well as how much control they felt they actually had. Patients in the emotional focus group were instructed to pay attention only to their feelings while the root canal was in process. Patients in the sensory focus group were instructed to pay attention only to physical sensations in the mouth.

The results, provided in Figure 13.9, show that the perception of pain varied depending on the differences in feeling about control. When subjects wanted a lot of control but felt they had little, an emotional focus pain coping strategy was ineffective. In fact, this strategy produced the highest reported pain levels. In this group, the sensory focus produced better results. In contrast, when subjects did not want control and felt they had little control, a sensory focus produced higher pain reports, whereas the emotional focus was effective in reducing the reported level of pain. These results indicate that strategies used for pain coping combine with personal traits and expectancies to determine how effective the strategy will be.

Kevin McCaul and his colleagues are skeptical of claims for the efficacy of distractors (McCaul, Monson, & Maki, 1992). These researchers carried out four studies under laboratory conditions using a cold-pressor task. The distractors were reaction time tasks that varied the degree of required attention. There were no changes in reported level of distress as the distractor task became more demanding. Mc-Caul's group considered several explanations for their results. The investigators suggested, though, that the lack of change in pain perception during systematic changes in the attention requirement is strong evidence against the distraction notion. In the end, they made the bold contention that distraction quite simply does not work as a pain control technique. Further, they

suggested that in those procedures where distraction seems to work, a component analysis would probably reveal the operation of another variable that is the true effective ingredient. One example is distraction procedures that also tend to evoke a pleasant emotional state. It may be the arousal of the emotional state, not the distraction per se, that leads to the reduced pain report.

Meditation, hypnosis, and humor   Meditation as a method of pain control may be considered either a variation of the relaxation method, a cognitive focusing technique that may distract from pain, or both. One group headed by Kabat-Zinn used a method called mindfulness meditation as a way of coping with chronic pain (Kabat-Zinn, Lipworth, & Burney, 1985). In one study, they trained 90 subjects over a ten-week period to use this technique. The investigators found that subjects reported lower levels of pain, fewer pain-related emotions, and used fewer pain killing drugs. Quite often, therapists see the reduction in painkiller use as an outcome that is every bit as desirable as the

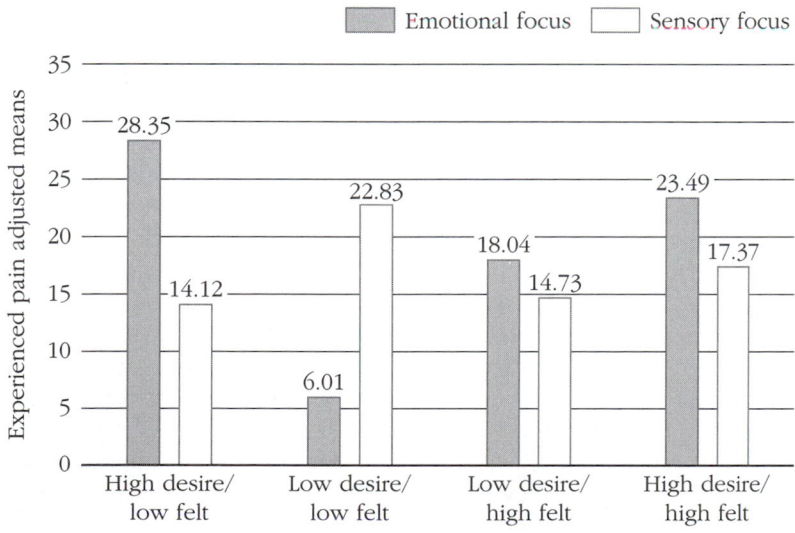

FIGURE 13.9   *Patients' report of pain during root canal surgery as a function of type of focusing strategy and desire for control (from Baron et al., 1993).*

reduction in pain itself. Kabat-Zinn's group used a small contrast group of 21 subjects who received traditional medical treatment for chronic pain. There were no reductions in the same pain-related measures among this group.

Traditionally, hypnosis has been viewed as an altered state of consciousness, a trance-like state in which perceptions are shifted dramatically from personal veridical reality to whatever pseudo-reality the inducer might create. A second view is that hypnosis is a channeled state of attention in which a person is susceptible to suggestion. Recently, hypnosis has been viewed from a cognitive-behavioral perspective (Chaves, 1993). In this view, the active elements of hypnosis include combinations of relaxation, distraction, suggestion, and cognitive restructuring.

David Patterson and his colleagues tested hypnosis under controlled conditions with 30 hospitalized burn patients (Patterson et al., 1992). Conservative estimates are that nearly 2.5 million people seek treatment for burns each year, that 100,000 require hospitalization, and that 12,000 burn victims die each year from their injuries (Deitch, 1990). Medical technology has made many gains in treatment of burn patients. Whereas prior to World War II, 50% mortality occurred with just 30% body surface burn area, now 50% mortality occurs only when 65% to 75% of the body surface has been burned.

In Patterson's study, the hypnosis treatment group consisted of ten subjects. An attention-information control group with ten subjects and a no-treatment control with ten subjects provided internal control. Subjects in the attention-information group were led to believe that they were going to be hypnotized without going through an actual induction. Several findings are of interest. First, the hypnosis subjects' self-report of pain showed a significant decline from pre- to posttreatment. In addition, they were significantly lower than the pain reports of the other two groups at posttreatment. In spite of the positive effect on self-report of pain, use of pain relief medications did not drop. Patterson's

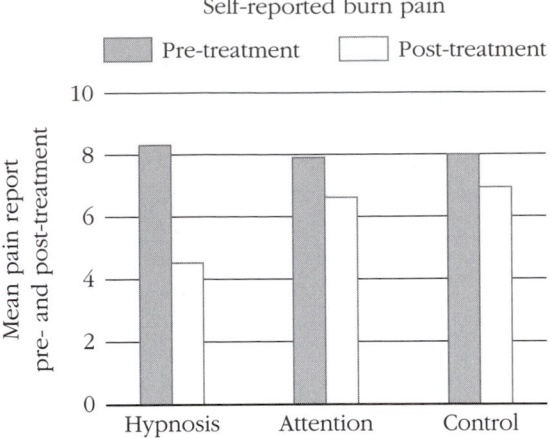

FIGURE 13.10   *Patient self-reports of pain using a visual analog scale following treatment with hypnosis compared to an attention-information placebo group, and a no-treatment control group (adapted from Patterson et al., 1992).*

group does not suggest that hypnosis should be used as a primary intervention, but as an adjunct that may facilitate treatment and recovery in burn patients.

A few therapists have also wondered how useful humor might be as a pain coping strategy. Certain physiological changes occur during laughter that may evoke protective body responses, such as activation of the body's natural opiates. Humor may work also at the cognitive level, serving as a simple distractor to take the person's mind off the pain. It may serve to change the sensitivity threshold for aversive stimuli. Finally, humor may facilitate cognitive reframing, or reinterpreting aversive events in a more positive way.

Elizabeth Adams and Francis McGuire (1986) reviewed a small body of literature on humor in pain management as a prelude to carrying out their own study. They noted cross-cultural and anecdotal evidence in support of the notion, but they were especially concerned about increased perceptions of pain reported among the elderly. Then they had one group of elderly subjects watch humorous movies over a six-week period and another group watch non-humorous movies. While both groups improved during the observation period, the humorous movie group showed significantly more improvement than the nonhumorous group. One problem encountered by Adams and McGuire may be related to novelty. That is, subjects showed increasing boredom and began to drop out of the study before the allotted time was up. This result suggests that rather than the humor per se, the novelty of the stimuli may have led to lower perceived pain. This conclusion is consistent with the idea that humorous videos serve as distractors that work only as long as the novelty of the stimuli can be maintained.

To summarize, we have reviewed behavioral, cognitive, meditative, and hypnotic interventions for pain. These methods claim some measure of success. Still, as we saw in Flor and Birbaumer's work, the client's physical and cognitive traits may determine how successful the intervention is. Behavioral methods may work best with clients who are highly reactive physiologically, whereas cognitive methods may work best with those who have ingrained thought patterns that undermine coping. Finally, we saw that many of the methods that go by different names may have common cognitive components that contribute to success. While research and theory will continue to deal with these issues, the range of psychosocial interventions provides clinicians with valuable tools to help clients confronting the problem of pain.

Summary

This chapter presented one of the more perplexing problems for health psychology and medicine: the problem of pain. Although we often think of pain only as something that results from physical hurt, pain is known to occur in cases where there is no physical injury, as well as long after an injury that first aroused pain has healed.

The major points made in this chapter are outlined here.

1. Pain may be described in various ways— for example, as burning pain, sickening pain, or mild pain. These different descriptions tend to reflect first the sensory quality, second the affective quality, and third the evaluative quality of pain.

2. Pain has been defined as an unpleasant sensory and emotional experience associated with actual or potential tissue damage, or described in terms of such damage.

3. Pain is categorized in terms of its duration as acute pain (short-term) or chronic pain (long lasting). Chronic pain presents many difficulties for a patient, including the triad of disability, disruption, and depression.

4. Pain is a core feature of many injuries and disease processes, and it is often associated with invasive medical procedures. At any one time, perhaps 33% of Americans have recurrent or disabling pain.

5. Typically, pain begins with stimulation of free-nerve endings called nociceptors. Large A-fibers signal immediate pain, whereas small C fibers signal slow, burning pain.

6. The ascending spinal tract for pain actually consists of three tracts that project to different brain areas: the thalamus, the reticular formation, and the midbrain.

7. Endogenous opioid substances in the brain work to reduce the level of pain, while a descending pathway (beginning in the PAG) is able to influence pain signals at the dorsal horn of the spinal column.

8. One integrative theory, the gate control theory, attempts to summarize both biomedical and psychosocial data on pain. It suggests that a pain gate exists in the spine's dorsal horn. Large fiber (A-delta) activity tends to close the gate, whereas small-fiber (C fiber) activity tends to open the gate. The brain's descending pathway also modifies pain signals at the gate.

9. The phantom limb phenomenon seems to require more than an input model of pain, since about 50% of amputees experience pain in a limb that is missing.

10. Biomedical theories of pain typically focus on structural pathology as in broken bones, or functional pathology as in a coronary attack.

11. Psychosocial theories of pain focus on processes such as learning and caregiving that contribute to pain behaviors. In this view, pain behaviors may increase because of the rewards received when in pain.

12. The cognitive view of pain suggests that beliefs and expectations influence the subjective experience of pain.

13. Recurrent negative thoughts are often correlated with reports of increased frequency of pain or increased severity of pain.

14. Several factors may influence pain, but two seem to be very important: coping skills and self-efficacy. People who adopt effective coping strategies and who have higher self-efficacy tend to report less pain or less severe pain.

15. The most common causes of pain are arthritis, headaches, and low back pain.

16. Besides the common acute headache that appears briefly and then disappears, three types of headaches are identified: tension, migraine, and cluster headaches.

17. Biomedical methods of treating headaches typically focus on medications, including aspirin, acetaminophen, and ibuprofen, or surgical interventions.

18. Psychological treatment methods for headache may use EMG or temperature biofeedback, relaxation, and cognitive methods.

19. One biomedical treatment for low back pain is TENS, which uses an electrical stimulation procedure to close the pain gate in the spinal column.

20. Psychological interventions for low back pain may depend on patient characteristics. Patients with high psychophysiological reactivity appear to respond to biofeedback better than to other methods, whereas patients with negative self-statements appear to respond better to cognitive interventions.

21. Distraction, hypnosis, and humor have been suggested as possible treatment methods.

Key Words

A-delta (large) fibers	free nerve endings
acute headache	migraine headache
acute pain	narcotics
affective quality	neuralgia
analgesics	nociception
ascending anterolateral	nociceptors
pathway	periaqueductal gray
spinoreticular tract	area (PAG)
spinotectal tract	phantom limb
spinothalamic tract	phenomenon
ataxia	referred pain
C (small) fibers	sensory quality
causalgia	stress-induced
chronic pain	analgesia (SIA)
intractable benign	suffering
progressive	tabes dorsalis
cluster headache	TENS
endorphin	tension headache
evaluative quality	

Study Questions

1. How do biomedical and psychosocial views of pain differ? Does the definition of pain provided integrate both views or does it favor one view more than the other?

2. Describe in detail the physical system involved in the sensation and perception of pain. What are the differences between the large and small pain fibers, and how do these differences relate to different pain experiences?

3. What processes work to reduce pain? Consider both opioids and descending pathways.

4. Describe the gate control theory of pain. Why may it be considered an integrative theory?

5. What is the phantom limb phenomenon? Why is it a problem for a physical theory of pain?

6. What personality and cognitive traits influence the pain experience? How does depression relate to pain?

7. What are the common types of headache pain? What are the symptoms of each?

8. How are headaches treated under the biomedical model? What are the common psychosocial treatments for headaches?

9. How is low back pain treated under the biomedical model? What are the common psychosocial treatments for low back pain?

Class Projects

1. If your community is large enough to support a pain treatment center (or a burn center), invite members of the professional staff to discuss current issues and problems in treatment of pain. Ask them to address issues of psychosocial factors in pain, especially in chronic pain.

2. Have interested class members research and present brief reports on the etiology, symptoms, and treatment of pains other than those discussed in the chapter. One example might be sickle cell anemia.

Suggested Readings

Gil, K. M., Williams, D. A., Keefe, F. J., & Beckham, J. C. (1990). The relationship of negative thoughts to pain and psychological distress. *Behavior Therapy, 21,* 349–362.

Harbeck, C., & Peterson, L. (1992). Elephants dancing in my head: A developmental approach to children's concepts of specific pains. *Child Development, 63,* 138–149.

Holmes, J. A., & Stevenson, C. A. Z. (1990). Differential effects of avoidant and attentional coping strategies on adaptation to chronic and recent-onset pain. *Health Psychology, 9,* 577–584.

Holroyd, K. A., & Penzien, D. B. (1990). Pharmacological versus non-pharmacological prophylaxis of recurrent migraine headache: A meta-analytic review of clinical trials. *Pain, 42,* 1–13.

Keefe, F. J., Crisson, J. E., Urban, B. J., & Williams, D. A. (1990). Analyzing chronic low back pain: The relative contribution of pain coping strategies. *Pain, 40,* 293–301.

Melzack, R. (1992, April). Phantom limbs. *Scientific American, 266,* 120–126.

Melzack, R., & Wall, P. (1965). Pain mechanisms: A new theory. *Science, 50,* 971–979.

Sullivan, M. J. L., Reesor, K., Mikail, S., & Fisher, R. (1992). The treatment of depression in chronic low back pain: Review and recommendations. *Pain, 50,* 5–13.

Wall, P. D., & Jones, M. (1991). *Defeating pain.* New York: Plenum Press.

Wall, P. D., & Melzack, R. (Eds.). (1989). *Textbook of pain* (pp. 508–521). New York: Churchill & Livingstone.

WEBSITES *Pain Conditions*

ADDRESS	DESCRIPTION
http://www.headaches.org/	☆National Headache Foundation
http://www.cmhc.com/guide/pro10.htm	Mental Health Net—includes resources on neurofeedback and biofeedback
http://www.wellweb.com/pain/pain.htm	☆Wellness Web—special section devoted to pain management
http://www.aapb.org/index.htm	Association for Applied Psychophysiology & Biofeedback
http://www.achenet.org/	☆American Council for Headache Education
http://www.healthreport.com/Referral/ Npain.htm	Pain and headache site from Tufts University
http://www.scup.no/journals/en/j-220.html	Cephalalgia—Official online journal of the International Headache Society
http://www.spinenet.com	San Francisco Spine Center—provides information about back pain and spinal injury

CHAPTER 14

Chronic Illness: Cancer and Arthritis

In its own version of the quest for the Holy Grail, biomedical science has been on an intense search to unlock the mystery of life. One part of the quest has been to discover how information is encoded at the heart of the cell allowing it to control replication and make a faithful copy of itself. By the end of WW II, scientists were devoting much attention to a complex compound, DNA, which is now known to contain the genetic map for each living creature. At that time, the riddle's solution remained beyond science's grasp. Then in 1953, working at Cambridge University, James Watson and Francis Crick made a stunning announcement: They had unlocked the code. They were the first to see the mystery revealed. Their work is regarded as one of the great stories of science, "because the explantory power of the discovery itself cannot be overestimated" (Judson, 1986, 58).

Watson and Crick told the world of their momentous discovery in a paper that was no more than 1000 words long (Watson & Crick, 1953). The secret resided in the three-dimensional double helix structure of DNA and the sequence of four nucleotide bases arranged like ladder rungs between the two spiral backbones. In honor of their superb work, Watson, Crick, and a third player, Maurice Wilkins from King's College, received the prestigious Nobel prize in 1962.

One woman, Rosalind Franklin, also played a crucial role in this quest. Later, she became the focus of an intense debate over women's struggle for equality in the sciences. Less well-known is the fact that she carried on her passion for science while fighting a losing battle against

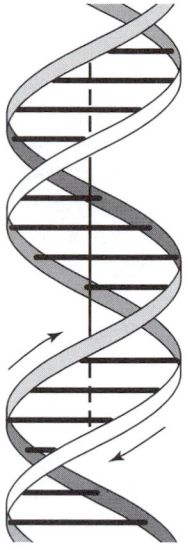

FIGURE 14.1 *The double helix represents Crick and Watson's view of how DNA provides the genetic code that is necessary to replicate a cell.*

one of life's great enemies, cancer, the uncontrolled replication of cells that consumes and ultimately destroys the body.

Rosalind Franklin: Passion, Logic, and Impatience

Rosalind Franklin was a scientist as passionate about her profession as she was passionate about life itself.[1] What Franklin did, she did with great energy and purpose. What she thought about, she thought about with focused intensity. Her intensity sometimes led people to see her as formidable and unapproachable. She seemed to see the path before her with such single-minded clarity that most other intrusions were just that: annoying trespasses that detracted from the task at hand. Someone said that genius does what it must, talent what it can. For Franklin, there was

[1] This short biography is based on several works but primarily on a book by Ann Sayre (1975).

never any question that her genius did what it had to; all else was secondary.

Rosalind Franklin was born July 25, 1920, the second child of Ellis and Muriel Franklin. Her parents were descended from an old British-Jewish family with many ties to politics and social life in and around London. They were a family dedicated to public work and activism for human suffrage. Apparently Franklin was supposed to follow this tradition, but the attraction to science was too strong to be denied.

Franklin received an excellent education at St. Paul's Girls' School. By the age of fifteen she already knew that science would be her life. In 1938, she entered Cambridge, a bastion of science education and research, to begin her studies and launch her research career.

Her path through Cambridge was not always smooth. WW II occupied many teachers, who were needed for war research. Less supervision, however, allowed her to work more independently, and this she did with fervor, devoting more than eight hours each day to lab work. The war forced its attention on her in another way for a very simple reason: safety and survival. During the countless bombing raids, she was obliged to hide in the air raid shelters, a situation she doubly detested, first because she was mildly claustrophobic and second because the raids constantly disrupted her work. Still, the war had raised vital energy questions that led to several publications based on her work in physical chemistry. This physical chemistry research was also the foundation of her professional progression to X-ray crystallography, a technique crucial to Watson and Crick's later insight into the structure of DNA.

After the war, still only 25, Rosalind moved to Paris and a government laboratory where she learned and developed her skill in X-ray crystallography. Her three years there were apparently among the happiest and contented of her life. During this time, she often could be found outside work hours frequenting the inexpensive bistros of Paris with her society of colleagues. These newly formed and lasting friendships provided her with support for her work as well as great intellectual stimulation. The papers she published during this time were among those that founded the science and technology of carbon fibers (Judson, 1986).

Her Paris crystallography experience led her back to King's College where she began working with DNA in 1951. This period was as productive for Franklin as it was turbulent. She improved the technique of photographing DNA so that it could be seen with much greater clarity than ever before, although mathematical models were still needed to decipher the overall structure. She also published 11 scientific papers from 1950 to 1956, producing meticulously detailed work that contributed important scientific information. Typical of the meticulous scientist, though, Franklin continued to suspend judgment on the structural nature of DNA, waiting for the data to reveal their secrets. She was still debating the merits of different solutions, never realizing that there was any race to be first, when Watson and Crick made their announcement.

Franklin worked for the most part under a cloud, the result of an unfortunate clash with her supervisor, Maurice Wilkins, that led to "instant hate" (Sayre, 1975). For her part, Franklin was impatient with, perhaps even insensitive to, the political protocols that often are intertwined with the scientific enterprise. For his part, Wilkins seems to have misinterpreted Franklin's intensity for brashness, and he found her mere presence intimidating. This situation left Franklin without the support that would have been so valuable to her work and Wilkins somewhat removed from understanding how far she traveled in so short a time. Later, without Franklin's knowledge or permission—still, perhaps without malice—Wilkins showed Watson the crucial photographs and provided an unpublished report that is known to have led Watson and Crick to their final elegant solution.

It is no small measure of Franklin's character and grace that when she saw the double helix model for the first time, she instantly recognized its essential accuracy and greatly admired Watson and Crick for the work they had done. In turn, Watson and Crick gave no more than a brief footnote in their paper admitting in an oblique way that their work had been stimulated by unpublished results and ideas provided by Wilkins and Franklin. This slight became a rallying cry for feminists convinced that Franklin had been mistreated. Franklin herself never seemed interested in feminism in the activist sense, however. She apparently could not conceive of women and men as anything but equal, and she never complained of mistreatment at King's College.

Whether Franklin would have discovered DNA's secret herself is little more than Monday morning quarterbacking. She was already moving on to Birkbeck College when Watson and Crick made their announcement. It did puzzle her, though, that Randall, the director at King's College, told her she must stop thinking about DNA. At Birckbeck, she began the last phase of her career with work on some potentially deadly viruses. She published 17 articles during the period between 1953 and 1958, even though she knew that her career and her life were slipping away.

Franklin had always been a stoic where illness and pain were concerned, and she preferred to ignore it as much as possible (Sayre, 1975). She knew already in the autumn of 1956 that her health was failing, and it must have been a great shock to learn that it was cancer. Still, her research was the most important thing, and she continued to work as long as her health allowed. Some have suggested that her long-term unprotected work with X-rays may have been a contributing factor to her cancer. Others have suggested that her willingness to work with deadly viruses in the last years of her career was in part because she already knew that the viruses could do her no more harm than what cancer was already doing.

Some who suffer chronic illnesses may accept their fate with resignation. They may yearn for an end, perhaps, with Keats, "Half in love with easeful death." Indeed, Franklin had every reason to give up after one operation when her surgeon told her "how mad and bad and sad it was" (Sayre, 1975, p. 185). Instead, Franklin was greatly angered, still clinging passionately to life and the hope that somehow she might survive. A close friend and physician, Mair Livingstone, said that she had "known people in greater physical distress, but never in greater anger about the unwanted, inconvenient, unjust and cruel sentence of dying young. She [Franklin] was indignant that there was not the technical skill available to avert death" (Sayre, 1975, pp. 186, 187).

No matter how hopeless her situation, Franklin rarely spoke of her illness and never asked for sympathy. Quite the contrary, she was almost apologetic for being a burden to family and friends during the few times she needed to stay with them while trying to fight the sickness. She spent her last days at Royal Marsden Hospital, unable to eat and too feeble to lift her head, yet she never lost sight of the humor present in the foibles of everyday existence. When she died on April 16, 1958, she was just 37 years old. It is no small irony that the work Franklin did at that time was part of the path that biomedical science had to traverse in order to understand the malicious nature of the disease that killed her.

Chronic Illnesses: Definitions, Types, and Distribution

A **chronic illness** is a disorder that persists for a long time and is either uncurable or results in pathological changes that limit a person's ability to function daily in a normal way. Among the various adult chronic illnesses are cancer, diabetes, arthritis, ALS, asthma, chronic obstructive pulmonary disease, multiple sclerosis, Parkinson's disease, muscular dystrophy, and sickle cell anemia, to name just a few. Some chronic diseases, such as arthritis, cannot be cured yet, but only treated to relieve symptoms. Other chronic diseases, such as diabetes, may be medically controlled. In any case, a chronic illness has the potential to force profound

changes in the person's lifestyle with resulting serious damage to quality of life.

This chapter considers the problem of coping with a chronic illness. We will look at the psychosocial processes believed to influence the course of and adjustment to chronic illness. Several factors may play a role, such as attitudes and beliefs about the illness, personal traits such as depression and optimism, coping strategies, compliance with prescribed regimens, and social support.

Since there are scores of chronic illnesses, we will consider only the two most common chronic conditions, cancer and arthritis. Both conditions involve the immune system, but the specific etiologies and pathophysiologies are very different, as we will see. Chronic illnesses are also discussed in several other chapters. Chapter 12 considered heart disease and hypertension. Chapter 15 will look at asthma, diabetes, and cystic fibrosis. These chronic illnesses have their onset in childhood or adolescence, and they have the power to affect health status across the life span. Finally, in Chapter 16, we will look at Alzheimer's disease, a disorder that impairs the memory of older people.

Epidemiology of Chronic Diseases

As control over epidemic diseases improved and the population aged, chronic diseases became much more important health concerns. In 1979, then secretary of Health, Education and Welfare Joseph Califano reported that the infectious diseases rampant at the turn of century—pneumonia, influenza, diphtheria, and tuberculosis, among others—accounted for 580 deaths per 100,000 people. By the late 1980s, these diseases accounted for only 30 deaths per 100,000. Simultaneously, there were dramatic increases in the prevalence and incidence of chronic diseases. Cancer, for example, accounted for nearly 133 deaths per 100,000 in 1989 (NCHS, 1992).

Taking all chronic conditions together, at any given moment 50% of the population suffers from a chronic illness requiring some form of

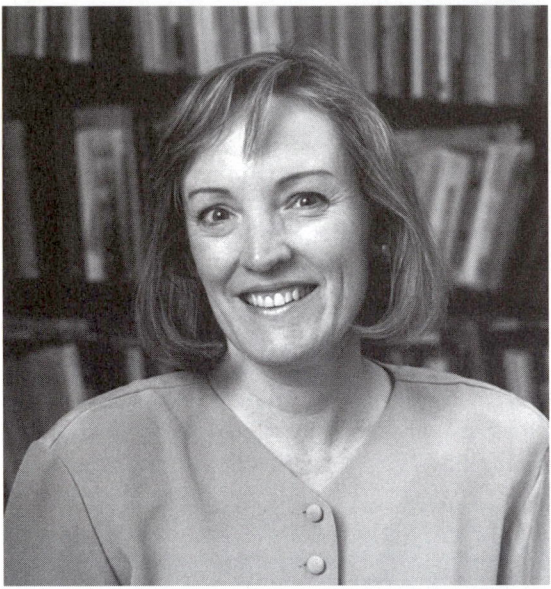

FIGURE 14.2   Shelley Taylor, a prominent health psychologist, has contributed to our knowledge of stress coping as well as chronic illness.

medical intervention (Taylor & Aspinwall, 1993). Among the most significant chronic illnesses, arthritis afflicts nearly 37 million people. Possibly 12 million Americans suffer from asthma. Chronic obstructive pulmonary disease (COPD), the fifth leading cause of death, afflicts at least 15 million Americans each year (Redline, 1991). The likelihood of death from COPD is 1.8 times higher in males than females, and 2.8 times higher in whites than in blacks (MMWR, 1989). It is estimated that 82% of COPD mortality is attributable to smoking, a modifiable behavioral risk factor. Diabetes, the seventh leading cause of death, is responsible for nearly 300,000 deaths per year.

Most estimates suggests that one in four Americans will be affected by some form of cancer at some time. Cancer accounts for more than one million new cases and nearly 500,000 deaths each year (National Center for Health Statistics, 1992). The average life expectancy of people who die from cancer is 15 years less than a person without cancer.

The distribution of new cancer cases is virtually identical for males and females, but the distribution of deaths is just slightly higher for males than for females. The encouraging news is that overall cancer mortality rates have been decreasing among Americans under the age of 55. Between 1983 and 1985, mortality declined by 6% for white males, 8.1% for black males, 6.1% for white females, and 15.2% for black females.

The four most deadly forms of cancer—lung, breast, colon, and prostate cancer—accounted for 55% of cancer mortality in 1990 (Henderson, Ross, & Pike, 1991). Lung cancer continues to be the number one cause of cancer deaths, leading to nearly 160,000 deaths annually. The number of deaths from lung cancer among males increased each year until the early and mid 1980s, when it began to level off. Unfortunately, lung cancer is still on the increase among older females.

Breast cancer has increased about 1% each year, and it led to nearly 151,000 new cases in 1990, with more than 44,000 deaths. Based on statistics compiled from 1983 to 1987, 12% of women will be diagnosed with breast cancer, and 3.5% will die from the disease (Harris, Lippman, Veronesi, & Willett, 1992a). Although white women are more likely to get breast cancer, African American women are 2.2 times more likely to die from it. This fact appears to be related to delayed diagnosis and treatment only after the cancer has already advanced (Eley et al., 1994).

Much of the data presented here have concerned case counts or mortality. Mortality data are more often reported than morbidity data, but morbidity data may actually be more informative (Wahrendorf, 1986). A strong argument has been made that quality of life measures should be included in research on chronic disease (Kaplan, 1989). Quality of life measures typically consider overall life satisfaction: capacity to enjoy work, love relations, and leisure time activities. Other possible contributors to quality of life measures include amount of time bedridden; loss of functional skills such as mobility, self-care, and ability to lift objects; and amount of time in pain or severity of pain.

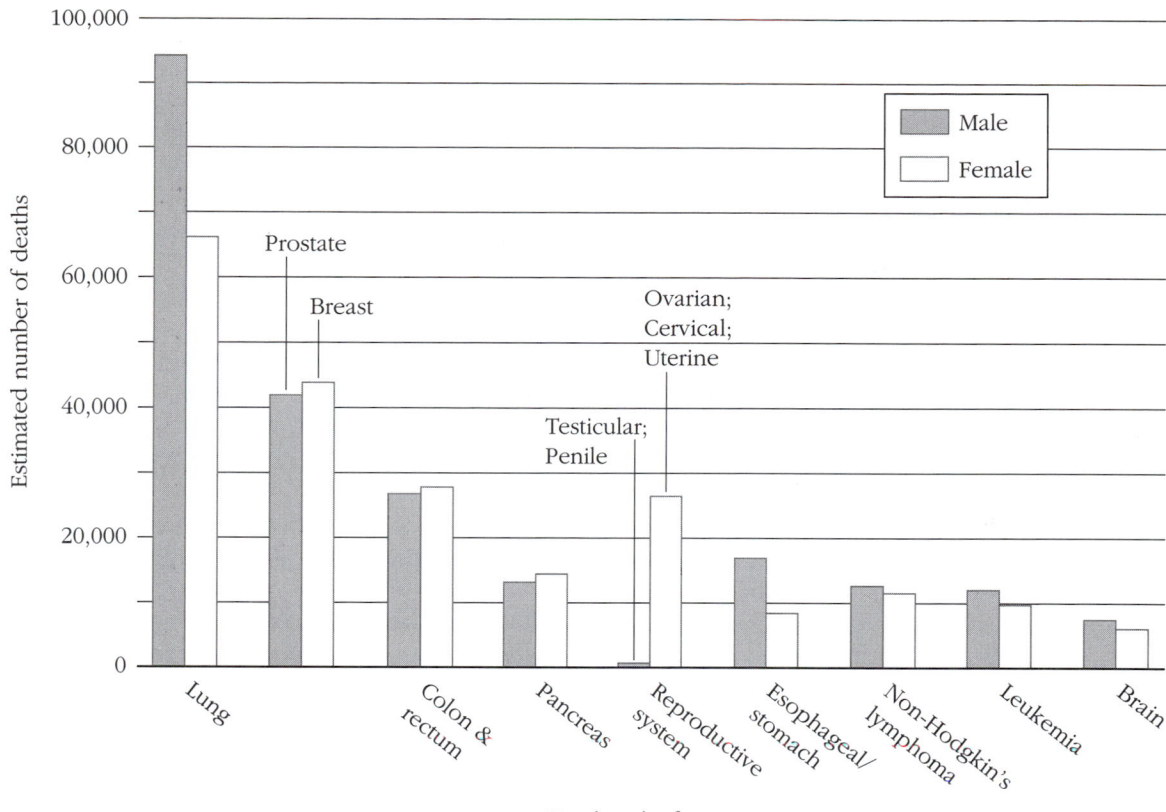

FIGURE 14.3   *The leading causes of cancer mortality are lung, breast, colon, and prostate cancer.*

Cancer Etiology: Biomedical Brief and Psychosocial Views

Cancer is not a unitary disease. It is a complex set of nearly 250 diseases with varied origins, pathologies, prognosis, and treatment regimens. To make this array manageable, we must condense what is known to common causes and important clinical categories. For this reason, only a brief outline of biomedical notions of cancer can be provided. There is good reason to believe that environmental stimuli and behavioral processes play an important role in triggering cancer. Further, there is some evidence that beliefs about and emotional responses to cancer

can influence the course and treatment of the disease. In the next few pages, then, we will discuss biomedical and psychosocial views of cancer.

Biomedical Views of Cancer: Mutations, Suppression, and Oncogenes

Cancer consists of renegade cells' reproducing explosively and then running wild. From conception to maturity, normal cells reproduce in a lawful controlled fashion to support growth of body structures. But at some point, body growth is finished, cells stop reproducing, and the body reaches a steady state. This tidy arrangement follows a simple rule: The number of cells produced in a given time equals the number of cells that die.

Cancer cells do not follow the rules. These cells begin to reproduce at an uncontrolled rate, and they grow into a larger mass called a tumor. Tumors may be benign or malignant. A **benign tumor** has the potential to crowd other cells (such as in the brain) and it may interfere with the function of adjacent structures or functions (such as choking off blood vessels). Yet benign tumors are not killers for the most part, and strictly speaking they are not cancers. They can usually be removed surgically and thrown away with little, if any, residual harm to the host. On the other hand, a **malignant tumor** attacks, invades, and destroys body tissue. If unchecked, it has the capacity to kill the host.

Tumors such as skin cancer in the early stages may be enclosed at a specific site. Malignant tumors may **metastasize;** that is, they may break out of their cages and spread throughout the body. When this happens, local treatments can no longer be used to cure the cancer, only to control growth and for symptomatic relief. At this point, treatments such as chemotherapy or immunotherapy that also can spread through the body must be used to track down and attack the runaway cells.

Types of cancer: carcinomas, lymphomas, and leukemias

Types of cancer: carcinomas, lymphomas, and leukemias   Although there are nearly 250 cancers, most can be grouped into one of four types: carcinomas, sarcomas, lymphomas, and leukemias. **Carcinomas** are cancers of the epidermis, dermis, and skin glands. Breast cancer, prostate cancer, colon cancer (adenocarcinoma), lung cancer, and pancreatic cancer belong in the general class of carcinomas. Basal-cell and squamous-cell skin cancers, possibly induced by prolonged exposure to ultraviolet rays, are the most frequent carcinomas to occur among white populations (Streilein, 1991). These skin cancers account for nearly 600,000 new cases each year, but fortunately only a small proportion result in death (Preston & Stern, 1992).

Sarcomas are cancers that develop from fat, muscle, bone, and other connective tissues. Technically, bone cancer is a sarcoma. The rapid onslaught of AIDS brought into the public eye another such cancer, Kaposi's sarcoma. This cancer is expressed as vascular nodules in the skin, but it may occur at multiple sites and invade the viscera as well (Haverkos, 1988).

Cancers of the lymph system are called **lymphomas.** Hodgkin's disease and non-Hodgkin's lymphoma are both conditions that involve the lymphatic system (Armitage, 1993). In Hodgkin's disease, cancer almost always occurs in single lymph nodes and then spreads to adjacent groups (Urba & Longo, 1992). In non-Hodgkin's lymphoma, the cancerous cells may be found at several different sites, but lymph nodes and bone marrow are among the possible sites. Finally, **leukemias** are cancers that attack the body's blood-forming system.

DNA, mutations, and oncogenes

DNA, mutations, and oncogenes   What causes cancer cells to begin their runaway destructive growth in the first place? There are several views of what happens to trigger cancer, but no single theory can explain all cancers. In fact, the range of cancers suggests that different theories, rather than being rivals, may be allies.

One readily available explanation is that cancer occurs because of some mutation to the cell's genetic code. One way a mutation may occur is through the cumulative effect of high doses of radiation in a short time, such as the X-rays that Franklin worked with or the ones used in medical X-ray procedures. At low doses or spread out over a long time, radiation may have few or no effects. In fact, exposure to clinically significant dosages of radiation is rare.

Another explanation is that cancer occurs because of a breakdown or impairment in the immune system. The immune system is responsible for *surveillance* of cells that exist naturally or that invade the body from other sources. The immune system has the capacity to recognize self and not-self (mutated cells, for example), and the responsibility to attack and kill cells that are not-self. It functions capably most of the time, killing cancer cells as they are produced.

Yet, immune system functioning may become weak or ineffective (immune suppression) under certain conditions.

We can illustrate this with smoking, lung cancer, and chronic stress. Under conditions of chronic stress, the anterior-pituitary adrenal-cortex system release corticosteroids, which lower the levels of circulating lymphocytes such as T cells. T-cells are the front-line defenders against cancer; they also attack cells from transplanted organs (Nossal, 1987). Smoking is related to more rapid growth by metastases and earlier metastases of tumors (Daniell, Tam, & Filice, 1993). Still, the notion of immune suppression is the subject of serious debate, and it appears to be much more complex than early simplistic suppression notions suggested (Dantzer & Kelley, 1989).

Yet another view of the origins of cancer is that an oncogene exists within the cell. Much like production controllers in factories, **oncogenes** regulate when and how rapidly new cells are produced. If something happens to the oncogene, the normally controlled process becomes uncontrolled. One way the oncogene can be altered is through exposure to **carcinogens,** or cancer-causing agents. Modern industrial societies produce a wide range of carcinogens. Still, it is not always clear that the carcinogen will lead to cancer except in the most extreme cases. We tread a narrow path between appropriate caution about potentially dangerous toxins and self-limiting obsessions that derive from fear.

The mutant p-53 oncogene has been linked to increased risk of certain cancers (Arbeit, 1990). Work on the oncogene has progressed to the point that several different oncogenes have been identified and correlated with various types of cancer. In breast cancer, for example, several oncogenes have been identified.

The two notions of mutations and oncogenes are not incompatible. To say that a mutation occurs may only be to say that the oncogene has been spontaneously altered from its regulating form to a nonregulated cancerous form. To say that a toxic waste triggered cancer may only be to say that the toxin has transformed the oncogene to produce uncontrolled growth.

Risk factors for cancer In addition to trying to find out what internal physical processes lead to cancer, research has tried to discover the risk factors for cancer. Genetic factors play a role in the etiology of leukemia, Hodgkin's lymphoma, kidney, bone, and brain tumors (Black, 1991). In some cases, such as non-Hodgkin's lymphoma, researchers have identified several different gene loci that correlate with different subtypes of lymphoma (Armitage, 1993). Environmental factors, such as radiation or chemical exposure, play a role in the etiology of leukemia, Hodgkin's, skin carcinomas, and certain sarcomas. Immunosuppression plays a role in non-Hodgkin's lymphoma. Viral infections contribute to leukemia, Hodgkin's, sarcomas, and cervical cancer (Dawes, 1992). In the case of cervical cancer, there is evidence that the virus (the human papilloma virus, or HPV) is sexually transmitted (Lambley, 1993). In addition, cervical cancer is predicted by the age of first intercourse and number of sexual partners.

Lifestyle can also influence risk. Obesity, for example, works indirectly through high dietary fat and low dietary fiber to increase risk for cancer. The link between smoking and cancer may involve a complex web of physical and behavioral factors. The by-products of smoking are carcinogenic and thus may have a direct effect on the oncogene. Smoking also is linked to lower intake of carotenoids and lower levels of beta-carotene, an effect that is more pronounced for female than for male smokers (Ziegler, 1988; Cade & Margetts, 1991). The body uses these compounds from natural food sources to convert to Vitamin A. Vitamin A itself is essential to the normal growth of lung tissue, but it also suppresses oncogenes involved in the early stages of carcinogenesis (Schapira, 1992). Lung cancer in smokers may be related to a combination of high-risk behaviors that alter several physical processes, resulting in cancer at the specific site.

We may be able to get a better perspective for risk factors by considering one cancer in more depth. In an extensive review of the data on breast cancer, Jay Harris and his colleagues found 11 risk factors that predict breast cancer (Harris et al., 1992a). These are listed in descending order with the nature of the relationship and the maximum relative risk (RR).

1. *Family history of breast cancer:* Relative risk increases with number of first-degree relatives affected (RR = 6.0).
2. *Benign breast disease:* The presence of any benign breast disease increases risk, but atypical hyperplasia is the most significant (RR = 4.0).
3. *Postmenopausal estrogen-replacement therapy:* Risk increases with age (RR = 2.1).
4. *Radiation exposure:* Increased exposure increases risk (RR = 2.0 for repeated fluoroscopy).
5. *Alcohol use:* Risk increases from one drink per day (RR = 1.4) to three drinks per day (RR = 2.0).
6. *Age at birth of first child:* Relative risk increases with age but remains essentially constant after age 30 (RR = 1.9).
7. *Oral contraceptive use:* Risk occurs only with current use (RR = 1.5).
8. *Age at menopause:* The older the woman is at menopause, the higher the risk (RR = 1.5).
9. *Height at or above the 90th percentile:* Increased risk also goes up slightly with age (RR = 1.4).
10. *Age at menarche:* The younger the age at menarche, the higher the risk (RR = 1.3).
11. *Obesity at or above the 90th percentile:* Risk interacts with age, such that obese women 49 years and younger have lower risk, but after age 50, risk goes up slightly (RR = 1.2).

The numerous factors and interactions involved suggest that simple unifactor causal connections will seldom explain the emergence of cancer. Harris's group noted that these identified factors are linked with only weak to moderate increases in risk. Further, even taking all these risk factors together does not "allow the identification of a small high-risk group that accounts for a large proportion of women" with cancer (1992a, p. 323).

Breast implants as a risk factor for cancer   Recently, risks associated with breast implants have been the subject of intense scrutiny. There are concerns that implants may be carcinogenic because of both construction and materials. Since nearly two million American women have received breast implants, the potential for harm is significant.

One Canadian study attempted to answer a basic health question about the safety of breast implants in general (Berkel, Birdsell, & Jenkins, 1992). In this study, the investigators compared 11,676 women who received implants between 1973 and 1986 to 13,557 cohorts who had a first primary breast cancer diagnosis. One significant factor had to be controlled. In the implant group, 86% were younger than 40 years, whereas nearly 92% of the cohort group were over 40 years of age. As noted earlier, breast cancer risk increases significantly with age. The investigators therefore used age-adjusted probability estimates to make their comparisons.

The investigators expected to find about 86 cancer cases among the breast implant group, but they found 41 cases, significantly fewer than expected. The average length of follow-up time was 10.5 years, and the average latency from implant to the diagnosis of breast cancer was 7.5 years. When the researchers excluded all cases with less than 10 years' follow-up, they found 11 actual cases of breast cancer compared to an estimated 68. Instead of leading to a higher risk, then, these findings suggested that breast implants may be a low risk factor for breast cancer.

Psychosocial Views of Cancer: Beliefs, Behaviors, and Personality

The psychosocial view of cancer looks at personality traits, cognitive styles, and high-risk behaviors. The social support system, both intimate and extended is viewed as important to the choices that people make about lifestyle, as well as to their adjustment to the emotional stress of coping with cancer (Cunningham, 1985; Levy & Wise, 1987).

No one questions that cancer is a clearly defined disease process with physical origins, identifiable pathophysiology, and necessary medical treatment. It is often difficult, however, to determine whether psychosocial correlates are antecedents or consequents of cancer. Therefore one must be very cautious about interpreting data on psychosocial processes in cancer.

With this caveat in mind, we may ask what the psychosocial view can add to cancer prevention and treatment. The issue of prevention is especially important, since numerous high-risk behaviors contribute to the incidence of cancer. Perhaps 20% of cancer deaths could be prevented by changing just one behavior—that is, smoking.[2] Emotional traits and coping styles have been linked to lower immunocompetence, survival, and recurrence of tumors.

Health beliefs, knowledge, and cancer
As we have seen previously, beliefs about personal risk and the costs of health behaviors can significantly affect the risks people take and the behaviors they are likely or not likely to carry out. This is no less true of cancer. Indeed, the great fear of cancer and inaccurate information about its curability can serve as important barriers to taking preventive steps.

Several studies have examined health beliefs and their relationship to health protective behaviors such as cancer screening. Both the Health Belief Model and the Theory of Reasoned Action have been tested in this context. Daniel Montano and Stephen Taplin (1991) wanted to find out which variables in an expanded TRA model best predicted participation in a breast cancer screening program. Four variables were identified, including two originally from TRA,

---

[2] Note that this is a global measure, not an individual measure. In other words, society in general would have to change its smoking pattern so that substantial numbers never start smoking to produce such a change. For people who have smoked heavily and long, quitting smoking will not lead to the same 20% reduction, though it would typically improve overall health status and prolong life.

social norms and attitudes. Attitudes included beliefs that the mammography would result in the desired outcome. Two variables were newly added, affect and facilitating conditions. Affect was defined as the person's emotional reaction to the thought of carrying out the behavior. Facilitating conditions were aspects of the person or environment (transportation and amount of time) that made it easier or harder to carry out the action. The TRA explained 39% of the variance in the intention to participate, but only 20% of the variance in actual behavior.

Susan Blalock and her colleagues examined the effect of risk perceptions on willingness to obtain colorectal screening (Blalock, De Vellis, Afifi, & Sandler, 1990). They used two groups of subjects, a high-risk group and an average risk group. The high-risk group consisted of siblings of patients recently diagnosed with colorectal cancer. Since heredity is believed to be one of the strongest risk factors for cancer, it was assumed that people in the high-risk group would be more inclined to seek screening to minimize personal risk through early detection.

In Blalock's study, high-risk siblings were more inclined to complete a Hemoccult test than average-risk subjects. Yet, high-risk subjects did not see themselves as at any greater risk than subjects in the average risk group. Blalock's team thought that this discrepancy might reflect an optimistic bias in processing information, but siblings in both groups showed an optimistic bias. The discrepancy may also reflect a not unusual mismatch between beliefs and behavior.

Finally, they found a race difference in that white siblings more often reported heredity as a risk-increasing factor than black siblings. One possible explanation of this finding is that nonminorities get much of their health information from the mass media and from family and friends (Newall, Gadd, & Priestman, 1987). Minority groups more often depend on their physicians. Since the information in this study did not come from primary care physicians, minority subjects may not have been disposed to accept it at face value.

Beliefs may differ between cultural groups as well. Nancy Bundek and her colleagues looked at health beliefs and health-related information in a group of elderly Hispanic women (Bundek, Marks, & Richardson, 1993). They were concerned about this group in particular because prior research suggested that Hispanic women are diagnosed with breast and cervical cancer at a more advanced stage than white women. Bundek's group found that women who had a stronger internal health locus of control were more likely to carry out breast self-examination. Also, an internal health locus of control was the only variable that predicted attention to health-related information. The investigators did not find that any change in health locus of control related to acculturation.

Cancer and personality

Learning that one has cancer leads to emotional upheaval for some time after the initial diagnosis (Lerman et al., 1991). Personal relationships and daily routines are disrupted. Pain may be recurrent or chronic, depending on the severity of the cancer and the relief provided by medicines. Medical treatments can be highly aversive, leading to fear and anticipatory anxiety. Anticipatory anxiety is more prominent in younger patients and those with higher trait anxiety (Jacobsen, Bovbjerg, & Redd, 1993).

Still, there is no reason to believe that all cancer victims will suffer chronic high levels of anxiety or depression. Some may cope with the disease extremely well. Indeed, estimates of cancer patients with depressive symptoms suggest that the rate is as little as 18% and no more than 58% (data cited in Given et al., 1993). It is possible, then, that personality traits relate primarily to the quality of adjustment to and recovery from cancer, not to the origins of cancer (Viney & Westbrook, 1982).

This argument may be carried one step further. To the extent that emotional upheaval continues over a long time—say, more than six months—the emotional state may have a negative impact on variables that predict response to treatment. For example, the person may not

sleep or eat well, which could affect physical stamina and healing resources. The HPA complex may be chronically activated, placing a further load on an already burdened immune system.

A second notion is that personality traits may be linked to the etiology of cancer, a more radical notion that requires critical analysis. Bernard Fox (1978) proposed two possible mechanisms that might link personality and cancer risk. He suggested, first, that a genetic trait could be linked both to a psychological trait and to increased cancer risk. A second possibility was that a genetic trait could produce a certain personality or proneness to stress, either of which could lead to increased risk for cancer. Neither of these ideas has been confirmed.

Some of this work is worthy of consideration, but much of it is flawed (Skrabanek, 1988). In an early review, Barofsky (1981) noted that design flaws included a lack of control groups, incorrect data analysis, and use of patients who knew their diagnosis as subjects. When patients know their diagnosis, it is impossible to distinguish psychological states that result from the illness and those that lead to the illness. Keeping these caveats in mind, we will look at some of the classic and recent work in this area.

Among the personality traits most frequently attributed to cancer patients are internalized anger and aggression. Morrison and Paffenbarger (1981) summarized the results of numerous studies showing that compared to noncancer controls, cancer patients tend to have higher levels of anxiety, anger, depression, hostility, denial, and repressed emotionality. Four of these emotional traits (depression, anxiety, anger, hostility), though, are linked to other diseases such as asthma, headaches, ulcers, coronary heart disease, and arthritis (Friedman & Booth-Kewley, 1987).

Greer and Morris (1975) carried out one of the better controlled studies using women who had breast cancer. They verified the pattern of suppressed anger and abnormal release of emotions in this group, but they could find no evidence for a distinct personality pattern. The conclusion is that emotional tones observed in cancer patients do not define in any sense a unique cancer-prone personality.

Still, there are numerous inconsistent findings. For example, one team found more repression and *less* depression in cancer patients relative to a control group (Dattore, Shontz, & Coyne, 1980). Paula Taylor's group used life events, repression-sensitization, and locus of control to predict presence of cancer (Taylor, Abrams, & Hewstone, 1988). This mix of variables, though, could explain no more than 8% of the variance in the development of cancer.

A prospective study by Barrie Cassileth and his colleagues may be noted as one that contradicts the idea that psychosocial factors influence survival (Cassileth, Lusk, Miller, Brown, & Miller, 1985). In this study, the research team measured seven variables suggested by previous research to be related to longevity. These variables included (1) social ties and marital history, (2) job satisfaction, (3) use of psychotropic drugs, (4) general life satisfaction, (5) subjective view of adult health, (6) hopelessness/helplessness,

and (7) perceived degree of adjustment to diagnosis. The results shown in Figure 14.4 are for the most serious cancer conditions. The results were similar in a second group of patients with malignant melanoma or breast cancer. In general, Cassileth's group found no evidence for the contention that psychosocial variables predict longer survival.

In spite of the inconsistent and contradictory findings, there is still a widespread belief that certain positive coping strategies and emotions, if not curative, may at least enable one to survive the threat of cancer. It is well known, if only quietly admitted, that the best medicine may be to no avail when given to someone who has already given up the struggle for life. On the other hand, hope, optimism, faith in a supreme power, and personal courage generally operate to marshal body defenses.

Michael Scheier and Charles Carver (1987) believe that optimism is one such important trait. They suggested that optimism has serious implications for stress coping and health status. **Optimism,** a generalized expectation that the

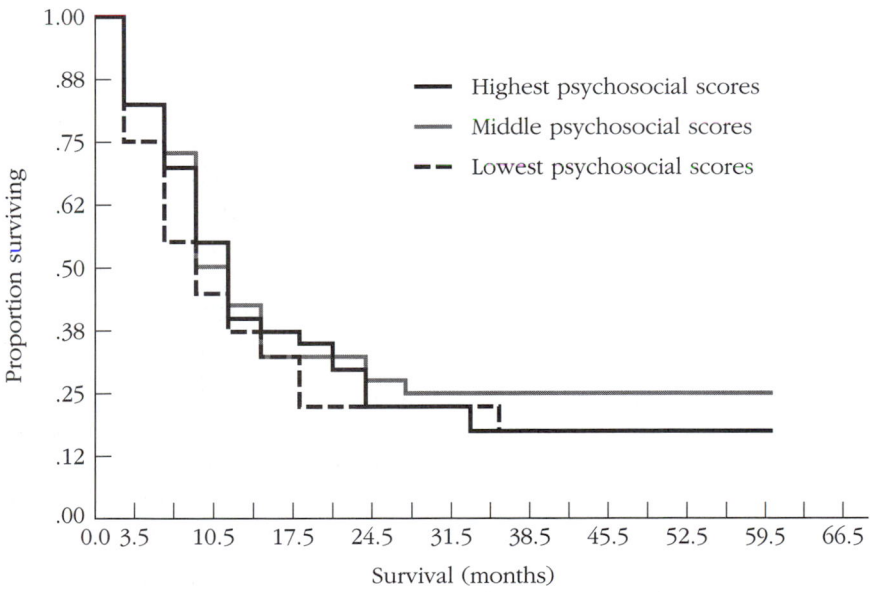

FIGURE 14.4 Length of survival of patients with advanced malignant conditions (from Cassileth et al., 1985).

future looks good, is a type of perceptual filter that colors a wide range of situations. **Pessimism** is a generalized expectation that the future looks bleak.

In one study, Carver and Scheier used women diagnosed in the early stages of breast cancer with good prognosis (Carver, Scheier, & Pozo, 1992). Some subjects were comparable to Cassileth's subjects who were in the second stage of breast cancer, but others were in the first stage. The patients were interviewed and measured for optimism the day before surgery, seven to ten days following surgery, and again at three months. Patients with higher levels of optimism used coping tactics at the time of the surgery that revolved around accepting reality, actively getting done what needed to be done, casting a positive light on the situation, and sometimes introducing humor to release tension. At three months' follow-up, optimism was still related to acceptance of the situation. Patients who had a pessimistic view used outright denial and engaged in behaviors that indicated a type of giving up. This link remained strong at three months' follow-up even though denial had declined.

Cancer and diet   Dietary habits presumably can increase or decrease risk for cancer. By one estimate, unhealthy dietary habits may account for 35% of all cancers (Schapira, 1992). Malnourished people are more prone to cancer. Eating certain types of foods has been associated with several different types of cancer (Boyd, 1993). The most common connection noted is that people whose diet consists of chronic high levels of fat are more disposed to cancer. Recent data suggest that colon cancer could be reduced by 50% with a 50% reduction in the consumption of animal fats (Henderson et al., 1991). Other risks come from alcohol consumption (Schatzkin et al., 1987), and the U.S. custom of overcooking and charcoal-grilling food, which deposits carcinogens on the food surface (Grunberg, 1988). Once again, though, note that these global estimates do not predict a specific individual's risk. Some people may eat a perfectly

healthy diet and yet be stricken by cancer for other reasons.

Evidence for the diet-cancer link comes not only by comparing people within a culture whose diets vary in fat intake, but also by comparing people across cultures. A comparison of Japanese women with Japanese American women showed that the women were more likely to develop cancer when they lived in the United States and ate an American diet (Wynder et al., 1963). As another example, the Hindi population has very low colon cancer attributed to a diet that is high in cellulose and fiber. Yet in the Bombay Paris community, whose diet is comparable to the Western diet, colon cancer rates rival those of the Western world (Schapira, 1992).

On the other hand, eating the right types of food is supposed to help prevent cancer. High-fiber foods typically help reduce fat deposits from rich foods. Certain vitamins, primarily the antioxidant vitamins, also may reduce cancer risk.[3] Vitamin C inhibits nitrosamines in the stomach, which reduces risk for stomach cancer. Lack of zinc in the diet can lead to lower immune system function. The benefits of these practices are sometimes oversold, though.

After an extensive review of data on antioxidant vitamins, Regina Ziegler (1988) summarized the major conclusions from both retrospective and prospective epidemiological studies. Low intake of vegetables and fruits has been linked to increased risk for lung cancer. Low levels of beta-carotene are associated with emergence of lung cancer.

Krinsky (1989) reported several studies using an animal model that tried to both verify this connection and uncover the mechanism of protection, if such a thing exists. Studies in cell cultures showed that carotenoids could prevent malignant transformation in the cell as well as damage to the nucleus. The bottom line from animal research, however, was that carotenoids

---

[3] Antioxidant vitamins work as scavengers to clear toxic debris from body cells (see Chapter 16).

work by interfering in the promotional phase of carcinogenesis. They prolong the latency to tumor formation but they do not reduce the number of animals with tumors.

To test this notion with humans, a research group headed by David Hunter conducted a long-term prospective large sample study of women (Hunter et al., 1993). The focus of the study was whether large supplements of anti-oxidant and carotenoid vitamins would reduce the risk of breast cancer. The results showed that supplements of C or E offered no protection against the risk of breast cancer, but that Vitamin A might bestow some protective benefit. Vitamin A appeared to be protective only when the woman's diet previously had been low in Vitamin A. When the woman's diet had provided adequate amounts of Vitamin A, increasing doses offered no additional protection. The benefit bestowed by Vitamin A, moreover, depends on carotenoids obtained from natural sources; Vitamin A supplements do not appear to confer the same benefit (Schapira, 1992). Therefore it is possible that something else in the natural vitamin source may be responsible for the protective effect, not just Vitamin A.

Cancer and social support   Because of the threat to survival associated with the disease, cancer is a severe stressor for both the patient and the family. In this context, it is certainly appropriate to consider how family members adjust to their loved one's condition and what means they use to cope with the situation. Lewis, Ellison, and Woods (1985) reported that cancer affects several areas of family life. Cancer places emotional strain on all family members, sometimes radically changes everyone's roles, disrupts intimate relations, and can seriously affect mental health—chiefly the primary caregiver's.

The first concern, though, is for the cancer victim and how the family may improve or worsen the patient's reaction to the diagnosis. Implicit in this concern is the notion that the family's reaction may influence the disease's course and the success of treatment. Borrowing a notion from stress theory, family and friends may provide a social support network that is either strong or weak, good or bad (Cobb, 1976). This social support presumably serves to buffer the effects of stress for the cancer patient and thus may improve the prognosis.

The most helpful behaviors seem to be providing emotional support, sympathy, and caring (Dakof & Taylor, 1990). Informational support is most helpful when provided by professional staff and less important within the family. The most harmful behaviors appear to be role models (other cancer patients) who behave badly or make rude and inappropriate remarks.

One surprising early finding indicates that social support might not bestow benefits on the cancer patient as predicted by support theory. In one study, patients who were not in chemotherapy or who were physically limited by their illness showed worse adjustment if they received more social support (Revenson, Wollman, & Felton, 1983). These patients showed more negative affect, lower self-esteem, and greater difficulty accepting their impending death than those who received less social support.

Attempts to explain this outcome have had to look in more detail at aspects of the relationship between husband and wife and other family members. Rosemary Lichtman headed a project that looked at numerous elements of the family network and marital adjustment after breast cancer (Lichtman, Taylor, & Wood, 1988). Lichtman's group found that the presence of positive and supportive family members had a positive effect on patient adjustment. Further, nearly 75% of their group reported that such positive support continued to exist in their social network after the diagnosis and treatment period. About 25% of the group reported some disturbance in family support, including some instances of isolation and even rejection. Finally, if there was a major change in social support following the diagnosis—even if that change was to increase support—it seemed to impair adjustment. How are we to explain this finding?

First, as the prognosis becomes more severe, more extensive family contacts seem to occur.

These contacts may make it more difficult for the patient to resolve personal fears. In addition, family fears and aversions may affect interpersonal transactions. The result may be feelings of conflict and ambivalence that further taint family relationships and perceived support (Dakof & Taylor, 1990). The continued presence of extended family members may only serve as a hurtful reminder of the disease, and negative emotions may be stirred over longer periods of time.

Social support appears to depend in part on how serious the situation is. Sandra Levy's research team followed a group of Stage I and Stage II breast cancer patients over a five-year period (Levy et al., 1992). The investigators' intent was to examine differences in psychosocial outcomes of breast surgery between a group of patients who had mastectomies and a group who had lumpectomies. On the positive side, indicators of emotional distress declined and functional status improved during a 15-month follow-up, regardless of the type of surgery.

The finding that most surprised the research team was the difference in emotional support that existed for the two groups, shown in Figure 14.5. At the time of surgery, no differences were apparent in emotional support. By three months afterward, however, the group that had elected breast-conserving surgery had much less emotional support than the group that chose mastectomies. This pattern was still apparent at 15 months' follow-up. In addition, the effect was more pronounced with younger patients. Further, although the lumpectomy group was rated more functional than the mastectomy group, they perceived that they were more fatigued and that they had less support than patients in the mastectomy group. Given the importance attached to social support as a buffer against stress, these findings were somewhat troubling. It suggests that the patients electing the less radical surgery may be better off physically in the sense that there is less damage to self-image, but they may be worse off emotionally because of lack of social support.

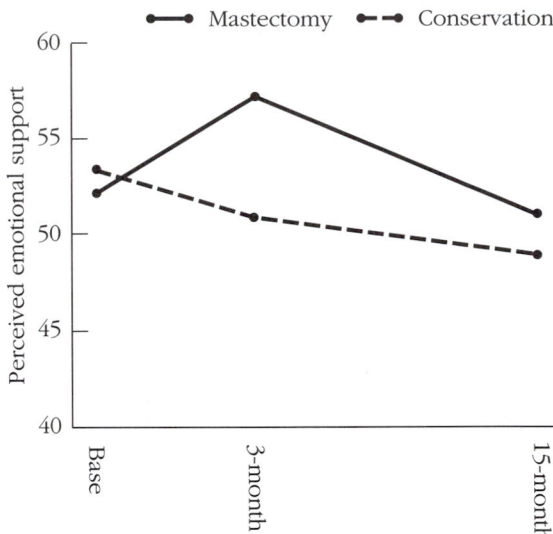

FIGURE 14.5   Perceived emotional support is higher for mastectomy patients than for lumpectomy patients at 3 months' and 15 months' follow-up (from Levy et al., 1992).

Finally, note that women without private health insurance are less likely to be screened for breast cancer than those who have private insurance (Ayanian, Kohler, Abe, & Epstein, 1993). Typically, uninsured women are diagnosed at a later stage in the disease process, receive lower quality care, and have shorter survival times than those with private insurance. All this adds up to a more pessimistic prognosis.

At the same time, the presence or absence of health insurance and the type of health insurance are not very helpful explanations for other differences that may exist among various socioeconomic or ethnic groups. There may be differences in health knowledge, preventive health behaviors, care-seeking intentions and behaviors, compliance behaviors, and social support systems that influence how early and how often a person seeks health care including screening. Educational programs that begin early to increase awareness of health issues and care opportunities may be equally as important as access to private health insurance, if not more so.

Cancer Treatment: Prevention and Intervention

Cancer treatment has become one of the most complex and costly treatments in modern medicine's arsenal of disease fighting weapons. New intervention methods and pain management techniques (Levy, 1996) continue to be investigated and put on-line even as older methods are refined. Psychosocial methods generally aim to help cancer patients adjust to life with a chronic condition, work toward better compliance with necessary medical regimens, and assist families in the grief process when a loved one has succumbed to cancer. Preventive efforts include increased recognition of the signs of cancer, more screening for early detection, and educational efforts aimed at altering lifestyle.

The search for a cure has led in all directions—to medicines, surgery, radiation therapy, vitamins, diet, carrot juice, Laetrile, and apricot pits. Many people, desperately seeking to cling to life and loved ones, grasp at any straw that seems to offer a ray of hope. Several alternative treatments have been investigated and found deficient in combating the progress of cancer. The next few pages will examine some basic approaches to intervening in cancer, first from a biomedical perspective, and then from a psychosocial perspective.

Medical Interventions: Surgery, Radiation, and Chemotherapy

Some measure of the success of medical technology can be gleaned from the rate of cure for various cancers. About 65% to 75% of patients with Hodgkin's disease can be cured with chemotherapy (Urba & Longo, 1992). Non-Hodgkin's lymphoma treated with chemotherapy approaches a 75% rate of cure (Armitage, 1993). The cure rates for breast carcinomas *in situ* treated with mastectomy are between 98% and 99% (Harris et al., 1992b).

The range of medical interventions now includes surgery, chemotherapy, radiation therapy, bone marrow transplants, and immunotherapy, each with its own highly technical subtypes. Surgical intervention in cancer may be used to obtain tissue specimens for biopsy, to determine the extent of the disease, to evaluate or remove a tumor, and to relieve symptoms (Dawes, 1992). At times, though, surgical interventions may do more harm than good, and watchful waiting or radiation therapy is the preferred course—as for example with prostate cancer in older men (Fleming, Wasson, Albertsen, Barry, & Wennberg, 1993). Skin cancer is often treated by surgical excision, but cryosurgery with liquid nitrogen, topical chemotherapy, and radiotherapy are also used (Preston & Stern, 1992).

Breast cancer is also treated surgically. At one time, the **radical mastectomy** was routinely prescribed, involving removal of the entire breast and some supporting muscle tissue resulting in large disfiguring scars. This method has profound psychological outcomes for the patient, which often spill over into intimate and family relations. Alternative less radical surgeries have been developed and tested with good success, although they may not confer the hoped-for psychological benefits. The **lumpectomy** removes the least amount of tissue necessary to ensure as much as possible that the breast is tumor-free. The **quadrantectomy** removes tissue both underlying and overlying the tumor. It preserves the essential structure of the breast, although the cosmetic effect is not always good.

It appears, though, that patients suffer anxiety with either procedure. With lumpectomy, the patient fears the possible return of cancer, since there is nearly a 40% recurrence of tumors in the same breast after five years. Further, because treatment often includes radiation, patients worry about more treatments, the pain and fatigue that goes with radiation, and what seems like a slow road to recovery. Mastectomy patients, on the other hand, worry more about interpersonal relations and personal appearance (Fallowfield, Baum, & Maguire, 1986).

Chemotherapy is used to disrupt the proliferation of cancer cells. It has side effects that many people find highly aversive. The side effects can lead to avoidance behaviors, such as missing treatments, and can thus reduce the success of treatment.

Radiation therapy is typically used in combination with surgery, chemotherapy, or both. About half of diagnosed cancer patients receive radiation treatments (Taylor, 1986). Radiation is used to destroy cancer cells, but success depends on numerous factors, including the type, size, and location of the tumor and the amount of radiation used. Radiation attacks the DNA of the cancerous cell, thus causing the cell itself to die.

Another treatment method is the bone marrow transplant. This method is used in leukemia, non-Hodgkin's lymphomas, and Hodgkin's disease among others (Urba & Longo, 1992). It is the therapy of choice for children with high-risk leukemias because then the physician can also provide high doses of chemotherapy and radiation that would otherwise be lethal. These treatments kill the malignant cells, and the bone marrow transplant reproduces nonmalignant cells from the donor bone marrow (Dawes, 1992).

One of the newer cancer treatment methods is **immunotherapy,** or treatment by stimulating the body's immune system to selectively target and destroy cancer cells. When the cell undergoes changes resulting in malignancy, it also acquires new antigens. Normally, the body's immune system recognizes these antigens as not-self and mounts a counterattack to destroy the tumor. Problems occur when the body's immune system is impaired or when the cancer spreads more rapidly than the immune system can handle. Because of the difficulty in treating malignant brain tumors, there is hope that one form of immunotherapy (using monoclonal antibodies) may offer some success (Black, 1991).

Cancer Screening: Exams, Mammograms, and Self-Exams

As knowledge of cancer continues to increase and treatments improve, it has become apparent that early diagnosis is crucial to successful treatment. Screening for colon cancer, for example, appears to lead to substantially reduced risk even if it is done only once every ten years (Selby, Friedman, Quesenberry, & Weiss, 1992). To this end, several screening programs have been proposed.

Currently, a great deal of emphasis is placed on screening for breast cancer. One goal of the National Cancer Institute is to increase screening for both breast and cervical cancer, which together account for 14% of all cancer deaths. Several methods of screening are possible including breast self-examination (BSE), mammography, thermography, and CT scans. The last two, although effective, are also very costly and are therefore not generally viewed as useful for large-scale preventive programs. According to Scanlon and Strax (1986), nearly 90% of breast tumors are discovered through BSE or by intimate partner, not from medical screening. Overall, screening may reduce cancer mortality by about 25% with early detection and appropriate medical intervention (Harris et al., 1992a). Harris's group estimated that screening 25% of the women between 40 and 75 years of age for ten years could save 4000 lives per year at a net cost of $1.3 billion per year.

Early in 1997, the American Cancer Society revised its recommendations for screening. They advise all women 40 years of age or older to have a mammogram (a detailed picture of breast tissue) done once each year. Little evidence suggests that more frequent screening or screening younger women will substantially alter risk. This advice has caused the number of women seeking a breast mammogram to increase substantially. Still, only 33% of U.S. women have mammograms taken on a regular basis (Rakowski, Fulton, & Feldman, 1993). As logical as screening may be, many factors enter into a woman's decision to use either BSE or mammography, and many barriers to completing the behaviors are involved as well.

According to the Health Belief Model, people are motivated to take health protective actions only if they perceive some vulnerability to disease. A meta-analysis of research on screening and breast cancer suggests that increased feelings of personal vulnerability led to increased likelihood of screening (McCaul, Branstetter, Schroeder, & Glasgow, 1996; this article appeared as part of a special section on cancer prevention in the November 1996 *Health Psychology*). Based on a study of about 850 women in Rhode Island, it appears that only about 25% perceived themselves at high risk for breast cancer (Fulton et al., 1991). Second, granted that one is at risk, the threat must be perceived as serious. In Fulton's study, only 30% of the sample perceived the seriousness of cancer risk as high. Third, one has to see any health protective actions as having some likelihood of success. About 50% of the women saw mammography as an effective tool. Finally, the person must perceive few barriers to taking action. A large percentage of the women in Fulton's sample perceived that mammography was both a safe (62%) and a comfortable (65%) procedure. Overall, the perceived benefits of mammography and the perceived barriers to mammography were more predictive of screening than either perceived vulnerability or seriousness of risk.

One cognitive factor that may determine whether a woman chooses to obtain a mammogram or not is decisional balance. This construct is derived from Prochaska and DiClemente's stage model of behavioral change, which we discussed in Chapter 8 (Velicer, DiClemente, Prochaska, & Brandenburg, 1985). Recall that this model proposes four stages people go through related to behavior change: precontemplation, contemplation, action, and maintenance.

Decisional balance combines the perceived positive and negative features of a target behav-ior. Having a mammogram done may be viewed as positive because it is a more reliable way to detect cancer early, it reduces uncertainty, and it may prevent the cancer from becoming a serious health threat. But a mammogram could also reveal the presence of cancer, leading to high levels of stress. In addition, mammography costs may not be covered by insurance, or the person may have to take time off from work to get the test done. Any of these factors could weight the decision to the negative side.

William Rakowski's research group looked at decisional balance in a large group of women in Rhode Island (Rakowski et al., 1993). They discovered several interesting aspects of the women's decisions about mammography. First, they found that women in the precontemplation stage had significantly more negative decisional balance than women in other stages. Women in the contemplation stage had more negative decisional balance than women in either the action or maintenance stage. Second, women with more education had more positive decisional balance compared to those with less education. Finally, a comparison across several ethnic and racial groups showed no differences in decisional balance.

Testicular cancer represents only about 1% of all cancer in men, but it is the most common cancer among 20- to 34-year-old American males. Several types of testicular cancer occur and malignancies occur in about 5,500 cases each year with about 400 deaths. About 50% of the cases are not diagnosed until the cancer has spread to adjacent regions, a fact that suggests the need for an early detection method. Although nearly 75% of the cases can be cured even when the condition is advanced, young men have been advised to engage in testicular self-examination to prevent potential problems such as metastasis. Still, efforts to persuade young men to engage in regular TSE encounter some of the same problems discovered with BSE (Sheley, Kinchen, Morgan, & Gordon, 1991; Brubaker & Wickersham, 1990). A large-scale study found that attempts to increase TSE outside the medical arena were largely ineffective (Sheley, Kinchen, Morgan, & Gordon, 1991).

Psychosocial Interventions: Cognitive Methods and Group Support

Psychosocial interventions may be educational and preventive. They may be directed to helping patients accept or better adjust to aspects of medical testing and interventions. They may be directed to the patient's emotional problems and family members' mental health. As such, a full range of psychological methods might be used at any given time to meet particular patient needs. In this section, we will discuss one cancer-preventive program intended to change attitudes toward suntanning, and later we will discuss intervention programs intended to help patients adjust to medical testing and interventions.

Prevention and education to reduce risk

Americans have been characterized as sun worshipers because of the widespread practice of tanning, presumably because being tan subjectively equates with health and good looks. Due to prolonged exposure to the sun's harmful rays, or to sunlamps in tanning salons, which are even more damaging, skin cancer is on the rise (Reif, 1981). Tanning slowly and staying tan may actually provide protection, but tanning cycles that alternate between pale skin, burns, and deep tans may present the most risk. The primary method of preventing skin cancer is to reduce amount of sun exposure. To counteract the tendency to remain in the sun longer than desirable, a variety of education programs have been developed.

Robin Mermelstein and Lee Riesenberg (1992) reported on one effort to increase knowledge and change tanning attitudes and behaviors among high school students. More than 1700 students from several Chicago schools participated in the study. The investigators measured perceived susceptibility to sun damage and skin cancer, perceived benefits of sun exposure, and awareness of changing social norms and adoption of sun-protective measures. They also grouped subjects into high- and low-risk groups based on the tendency for the skin to tan or burn. The one-day intervention changed knowledge about the dangers of prolonged exposure and increased perceived vulnerability. Yet it did not change behavioral intent.

Cognitive-behavioral interventions: dealing with pain, anxiety, and nausea

A number of different techniques have been used to help patients confront their struggle with cancer and the side effects of cancer treatments. Cancer patients often experience significant amounts of pain from the condition itself, but then they must also endure treatment procedures that can be uncomfortable if not also painful in their own right. Patients then become anxious about the procedures and may experience anticipatory anxiety that makes the treatment procedure even more difficult. To deal with these problems, psychologists have used several techniques including relaxation therapy, systematic desensitization, and cognitive-behavioral methods. Relaxation has been used as an adjunct to radiation therapy (Decker, Cline-Elsen, & Gallagher, 1992). The use of relaxation appears to reduce tension as expected, but it also appears to reduce anger and lessen the feeling of fatigue as well.

David Spiegel (1986) summarized his work on use of a group therapy and support treatment to reduce pain and anxiety in cancer patients. The group sessions included many elements, such as group support, confronting denial, extracting meaning from tragedy, information-seeking, and value clarification, to name a few. As measured on the POMS scale, the treatment group showed a significant reduction in both anxiety and self-reported pain compared to a nontreated control group. The frequency and duration of pain episodes did not decline, however. In addition, the differences between the two groups did not emerge for nearly nine months. Thus, even though the results may be viewed as positive, the costs for treatment and the amount of time for change to materialize suggest that the approach may be useful only in limited situations. Finally, it is impossible to determine which component or mix of components was the impetus for change.

One problem cancer patients confront is anxiety over painful tests or treatment procedures. Chemotherapy induces nausea and vomiting both in the situation and for some time after the treatment. Even with improved procedures, approximately 60% of patients continue to experience nausea and vomiting during treatment (Morrow et al., 1992). After just a few treatments, almost a third of all patients experience high levels of anticipatory anxiety about a scheduled treatment. When this happens, the patient may experience nausea and vomiting even before getting to the treatment. This phenomenon is viewed as a type of classically conditioned response. Many patients show a decline in anxiety between infusion sessions, however, suggesting that development of anticipatory anxiety depends on a number of variables and that the conditioning explanation may be oversimplified (Jacobsen et al., 1993).

Thomas Burish and Richard Jenkins (1992) compared biofeedback and relaxation training as a method to reduce the aversiveness of chemotherapy treatment. They used a classic factorial design (see Table 14.1) and several outcome measures of anxiety, depression, hostility, and nausea during chemotherapy. Burish and Jenkins found that relaxation training reduced the amount of patient-reported nausea. They also concluded that neither EMG or skin temperature biofeedback were effective in reducing the anxiety and nausea associated with chemotherapy.

Another method, systematic desensitization, has been shown effective in treating anticipatory nausea and vomiting. Typically, this method has been applied by trained clinical psychologists, but a variety of economic factors suggests that the demand for treatment in the oncology setting outstrips the availability of clinical psychologists. Therefore, Gary Morrow's group wanted to know whether systematic desensitization would be as effective when delivered by oncologists and oncology nurses. These investigators also wanted to know whether the procedure could provide some reduction in posttreatment nausea and vomiting.

As a first step, a group of oncologists and oncology nurses were trained to administer desensitization. Then 75 patients were randomly assigned to a control group or to two treatment groups, one conducted by a psychologist and one by the oncology staff. The data showed that desensitization significantly reduced anticipatory nausea, whoever provided the treatment. Although there were no differences in the numbers of patients reporting posttreatment nausea, there was a reduction in severity and in duration. The most pronounced effect occurred in the duration of nausea posttreatment. The group treated by psychologists declined by more than 28 hours and those treated by oncologists by 16 hours. In contrast, the control group *increased* in posttreatment nausea by more than 15 hours. These results suggest that desensitization can have beneficial effects on

TABLE 14.1 *Experimental design used by Burish and Jenkins (1992) to study the effects of biofeedback and relaxation training.*

| | BIOFEEDBACK TREATMENT CONDITIONS | | |
	EMG BFB	ST BFB	NO BFB
Relaxation Training	EMG + RT	ST + RT	RT only
No Relaxation Training	EMG only	ST only	Control

both anticipatory and posttreatment nausea and vomiting, whether delivered by psychologists or by oncology staff.

Arthritis: Etiology, Influences, and Interventions

As noted earlier, arthritis afflicts perhaps 37 million people in the United States. Sheer numbers make it the single most prevalent chronic disorder. Arthritis is a disease that some people may live with for much of their adult life, and the core feature is pain that can become excruciating as the disease progresses. Arthritic pain can lead to emotional distress, interfere with family and leisure activities, and impair the ability to function on a job. Space does not permit an extended treatment, but we will discuss the major points of etiology, psychosocial influences, and interventions to enable people to cope with arthritis. Additional information may be found in Chapter 13 and Chapter 16.

Origins of Arthritis: Definitions, Immunology, and Pathophysiology

Arthritis is a general term that refers to any inflammation or degeneration in the joints (Spence, 1989). It may occur as a reaction to certain infections such as Lyme disease, sexually transmitted diseases, and AIDS. Further, it may co-occur with other diseases such as hemophilia and cystic fibrosis. Before turning to the most common forms of arthritis, some basic information on joint anatomy may help to understand the pathophysiology of arthritis (Figure 14.6).

In simplified form, a joint has six major components: bone, cartilage, synovium and synovial fluid, joint capsule, tendon, and joint space. The ends of the two bones that meet at the joint are each covered with cartilage, a highly resilient but elastic capsule that can withstand tremendous pressure and sheer forces. The synovium is like a thin cap over the joint space, but it is held in place by the joint capsule. Outside the joint capsule are the strong ligaments that provide support to the structure and prevent extreme motion. In arthritis, damage usually involves the synovium, synovial fluid, cartilage, and bone. The synovium, joint capsule, and ligaments also have nerve fibers that send a steady stream of information, including pain signals, to the CNS.

Like cancer, arthritis is not a unitary disease but a group of conditions. The three major types are osteoarthritis, also commonly known as degenerative joint disease; rheumatoid arthritis; and gouty arthritis.

Osteoarthritis, which afflicts nearly 30 million Americans, may present in later stages as an inflammation of the joint, but it begins with minute cracks in the joint cartilage (Brewerton, 1992). As the cartilage becomes thinner, it provides less protection to the underlying bone structure, and the joint may itself become unstable. Lack of cartilage protection ultimately leads to defensive bone growth and bony spurs (Koopman, 1991). Movement becomes something like rubbing two pieces of bone together, which causes inflammation, swelling, and pain. Osteoarthritis may occur in the fingers causing disfigurement, but it more commonly occurs in the lower limbs and spinal column. When the condition exists in the spinal column, it may lead to spinal fusion (several vertebrae bond together), more limitations in movement, and more pain.

The disease process may begin with humoral factors that change cartilage cells (chondrocytes) into cells of destruction (Farrar, Kilian, Ruff, Hill, & Pert, 1988). Another hypothesis is that neuropeptides passing through the bone structure nourish the chrondrocytes and may help foster destruction of the cartilage (Brewerton, 1992).

Rheumatoid arthritis is an inflammation of the synovial membrane, which causes it to swell up producing pressure and severe pain in the joint. (Refer again to Figure 14.6.) Regarded as potentially the most serious and crippling type of arthritis, it afflicts about 1% of the population worldwide but is about three times more com-

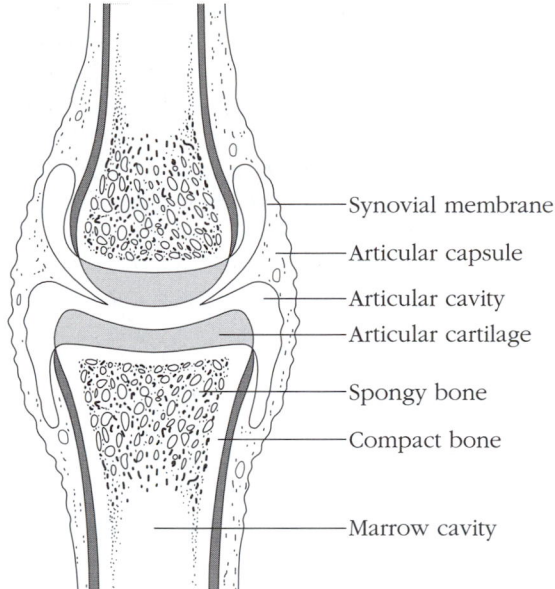

Synovial membrane
Articular capsule
Articular cavity
Articular cartilage
Spongy bone
Compact bone
Marrow cavity

FIGURE 14.6 Cross-section of free-moving joint showing components that are attacked in several aging conditions including arthritis (from Junqueira, Carneiro, & Long, 1986).

mon in women (Harris, 1990). The symptoms include peripheral joint inflammation, swelling, stiffness, and pain. A precise diagnosis usually involves a test for the so-called rheumatoid factor. Radiographic data also should show evidence of erosion in the joints.

As the disorder progresses, the person becomes more limited in movement in the afflicted limb. After prolonged inflammation, the membrane forms scar tissue and granular tissue, which then begins to destroy the articular cartilage and erode the bone beneath it. Biomedical science is still looking for the cause of rheumatoid arthritis, but several possible culprits are being examined. One popular theory is that rheumatoid arthritis is an autoimmune disease involving accumulation of neutrophils in the synovial fluid, followed by cartilage deterioration and bone erosion (Harris, 1990).

In spite of the evidence to support this view, the environmental triggers for this immune response are not well known. Several infectious

agents, such as bacteria or the Epstein-Barr virus, may be linked to rheumatoid arthritis. At this time, then, infections may explain the origins of the disease, and the autoimmune reaction may explain its process.

Gouty arthritis is considered an inherited condition in which excess uric acid builds up in the blood.[4] The uric acid then enters the joints, where some may be deposited in the synovium, and some in the synovial fluid. During an attack, crystals from the uric acid form in the synovial fluid, and the immune system rushes phagocytes to attack the crystals. The phagocytes swallow up the crystals but burst when they become engorged. This releases enzymes into the joint, which adds to the debris and inflammation. The symptoms, usually lasting no more than a few days, include severe pain usually localized in a single joint, such as the big toe. It may attack large joints with milder pain, and it may occur in the hands or wrist (Brewerton, 1992).

Psychosocial Influences in Arthritis

A number of cognitive and emotional traits are linked to the severity of pain in arthritis. These include helplessness and depression, social support (Fitzpatrick, Newman, Archer, & Shipley, 1991), cognitive distortions that increase the patient's tendency to depression, and pain coping strategies (see Chapter 13). Stress is also believed to play a significant role in the course and treatment of arthritis. Yet in a recent English study (cited in Creed, 1993), no more than 18% of recent onset arthritis patients had experienced a severe stressful event in the previous six months. Little evidence supports the notion of an arthritis personality (Lerman, 1987), and little evidence shows impaired mental health in arthritis patients.

Cognitive processes may play either a positive or a negative role in coping with arthritis.

[4] The term *gout* comes from the ancient humoral theory, which assumed that humors flowed into joints a drop at a time. The Latin word for *drop, gutta,* eventually became *gout.*

Some individuals may reinterpret information so that the situation does not seem as bleak. They may use distracting methods to help alleviate the perception of pain. They may engage in positive self-statements and remind themselves of the degree of control that they have over the situation and the pain. Conversely, some patients may find only the most dire significance in any change in pain or physical function and begin a sequence of catastrophizing thinking that only adds to their distress. There is also evidence that some people are hypervigilant to body symptoms, which may increase the perception of pain. Patients may also begin to feel helpless in the face of unremitting pain (Smith, Peck, & Ward, 1990). Keefe and colleagues provided evidence that pain catastrophizing increases reports of pain, depression, and disability (Keefe, Brown, Wallston, & Caldwell, 1989).

Craig Smith and Kenneth Wallston (1992) used cognitive-transactional theory to organize variables assumed to influence adaptation in arthritis patients. Smith and Wallston found evidence for two vicious cycles in adaptation to arthritis. First, the authors found that perceived competence, life satisfaction, and depression are related in a way that amplifies the loop. Stated in simple terms, lower life satisfaction decreases the person's perception of competence, which increases depression, which in turn lowers life satisfaction. Second, Smith and Wallston found that helplessness appraisals and passive coping tended to amplify this loop; that is, personal appraisals of helplessness tend to lead to passive coping methods, and passive coping methods tend to reinforce the perception of helplessness. The general conclusions support the notion that helplessness, passive coping, and psychosocial impairment promote maladaptive behaviors in adjusting to rheumatoid arthritis.

Glenn Affleck headed a study that investigated the relationship of neuroticism to the pain-mood connection in arthritis patients (Affleck, Tennen, Urrows, & Higgins, 1992). Affleck and his colleagues pointed out that neuroticism

is not the same as neurosis nor does it imply a psychopathology. It is a trait that is related to impulsiveness, vulnerability, and helplessness. High-N people report more body complaints, and they tend to be hypervigilant and more ruminative in cognitive style. In addition, people who are High-Ns are more prone to feel chronic distress and low self-esteem. If the cluster of mood-cognitions in neuroticism predicts the arthritic patient's response to the disease, then it might be possible to design programs to teach people more adaptive coping strategies.

Affleck's team used a prospective design that followed patients over 75 days. Patients were asked to record pertinent information in a diary each night, and they were paid a nominal sum for compliance. Of the possible 4050 days of diary records, the investigators collected 4031, for a 99.5% completion record. Information included visual analog pain ratings, joint-specific pain data, and daily mood reports using the POMS (Profile of Mood States). Further measures were taken of neuroticism, coping strategies, disability, catastrophizing, and depression.

The results showed that regardless of other variables, patients experienced significantly worse moods on days when pain was most severe. Further, those subjects who were high on neuroticism tended to experience more chronic distress, and their report of pain was mediated by their catastrophizing thoughts about pain.

According to recent studies of social support, the type of social network and support provided to the arthritic patient can be either bane or blessing. Positive support is defined as providing affection, personal affirmation, and needed help with daily chores. Problematic support is defined as attempting to provide assistance that is ill-timed or ill-conceived. For example, criticizing a person's coping method may be seen by the provider as helpful but by the recipient as not helpful. Receiving positive support is generally related to lower depression, whereas negative support is related to more depression

(Revenson, Schiaffino, Mjerovitz, & Gibofsky, 1991). In addition, those receiving more problematic support also reported the highest levels of pain symptoms. One interesting finding in this study was that some problematic support does not appear to cancel out the good effects from positive support. But low positive support combined with high problematic support had the strongest effect on depressive symptoms.

Coping with Arthritis: Biomedical and Psychosocial Strategies

Since we have already discussed several coping strategies to deal with pain in Chapter 13, we will consider only a few issues here. In addition, medical approaches to treatment of arthritis are largely confined to pain management, though new research shows promise of bringing more effective treatments before long.

Biomedical Treatment of Arthritis

One emerging possible treatment for arthritis is autoimmune therapy, which is being tested in human trials now. This technique, called oral antigen therapy, uses protein antigens of the type that triggered the abnormal reactions in the first place. Antigen feeding may activate a cell called the CD8 cell that can in turn suppress other immune cells. The method is considered to have some promise for both multiple sclerosis and rheumatoid arthritis.

Psychosocial Strategies: Cognitive, Behavioral, Coping

Ann O'Leary's group used a cognitive-behavioral intervention to help patients better manage stress, pain, and other symptoms of arthritis (O'Leary, Shoor, Lorig, Holman, 1988). They used a classic two-group design, with 15 subjects in an experimental group and 15 in a control group. The experimental group received training in several skills including relaxation, cognitive pain management, and goal setting. Subjects in the control group received an arthritis self-help book. O'Leary's group found that subjects in the experimental group increased their degree of perceived self-efficacy and also improved their psychosocial functioning. Further, this group reported lower pain and joint inflammation compared to the control group.

Summary

Chronic illnesses persist for long periods and are either incurable or result in pathological change that limits a person's functional ability. These illnesses often require long-term compliance with a medical regimen in order to control the disorder and slow potential progressive deterioration. Chronic illnesses often place patients under heavy emotional distress because they realize the medical regimen will be a lifelong burden and return to a normal life an apparently unreachable goal. The major issues addressed in this chapter are summarized below.

1. Chronic diseases have become more prominent in modern society, as medical technology has controlled epidemic diseases and preserved life for many who otherwise would have died at an early age.

2. Combining all chronic conditions, perhaps 50% of the U.S. population suffers from a chronic illness that requires medical intervention.

3. The most common chronic conditions are arthritis, asthma, cancer, coronary artery disease, chronic obstructive pulmonary disease, and diabetes.

4. The most deadly forms of cancer—lung, breast, colon, and prostate cancer—account for about 55% of cancer mortality.

5. Biomedical research has discovered several different causes of cancer, including mutation, immune suppression, and oncogenes. An oncogene regulates when and how fast new cells are produced. If the oncogene fails, regulation breaks down, and cells may be produced at a high uncontrolled rate.

6. Four general types of cancer are carcinomas, sarcomas, lymphomas, and leukemias. Carcinomas are cancers of the skin and skin glands. Sarcomas are cancers that develop from fat, muscle, bone, and other connective tissue. Lymphomas are cancers of the lymph system. Leukemias are cancers of the blood-forming system.

7. The most important risk factors for cancer are positive family history for cancer and lifestyle variables related to poor diet, heavy smoking, and excess alcohol consumption.

8. Cancer is a clearly defined physical disease that necessitates medical treatment. Still, investigators continue to look at psychosocial variables that could alter risk, disease course, or treatment success.

9. Most of the psychosocial focus has been on high-risk behaviors such as diet and drug addictions. Four cancer control goals are to reduce the percentage of smokers, to reduce fat and increase fiber in the diet, to increase screening for breast and cervical cancer, and to use the most advanced treatment.

10. Even when knowledge about cancer is adequate and the intention to engage in preventive programs is good, actual preventive behavior often occurs at a lower rate than desirable.

11. Cancer leads to varying degrees of anxiety, fear, and depression. These emotional states may interfere with medical test procedures, treatment, and slow the course of recovery.

12. Diets high in fat and low in fiber are correlated with increased prevalence of cancer. Antioxidant vitamins are supposed to reduce risk for cancer, but taking large quantities of antioxidants does not improve protection over that obtained from a diet that provides adequate amounts.

13. The connection between social support and reaction to cancer depends on the type of social support. With positive support that does not overwhelm the patient with reminders of change, the patient's adjustment is usually better. Support that changes social context dramatically—that makes the patient feel very different and helpless—typically leads to poor adjustment.

14. Biomedical treatment for cancer uses surgery, chemotherapy, radiation, bone marrow transplants, and immunotherapy.

15. One of the most important screening techniques is self-screening. Women can learn relatively simple examination techniques for breast cancer, and men can do the same for testicular cancer. Monthly self-examination can greatly improve the chances of early detection and successful treatment.

16. One effort in psychosocial treatment is to help patients deal with the anticipatory anxiety that grows with recurrent invasive and aversive test and treatment procedures. Relaxation therapy, desensitization, and cognitive-behavioral methods have been used with some success to this end.

17. Arthritis afflicts about 37 million people in the United States. It is a cluster of disorders with a core feature of pain and inflammation or degeneration of the joints.

18. Arthritis may be caused by an autoimmune process which causes neutrophils to accumulate in the synovial fluid followed by cartilage deterioration and bone erosion.

19. Psychological processes such as feelings of helplessness and depression can influence the severity of arthritic pain. Active coping tends to increase feelings of competence, which tends to contribute to overall better adjustment and less depression. Personal appraisals of helplessness tend to increase passive coping, which amplifies feelings of helplessness and leads to lower life satisfaction and more pain.

20. Biomedical science has been stymied in developing effective treatment methods for arthritis. A new approach called autoimmune therapy appears to suppress the process that leads to arthritis, but the technique depends on early identification and intervention. Autoimmune therapy does not appear to offer hope to older patients in whom the disease has progressed to an advanced stage.

21. Psychosocial methods focus on teaching patients coping skills and eliminating negative thoughts. This approach generally leads to better adjustment, lower subjective experience of pain, and reduced frequency of pain.

Key Words

arthritis	malignant tumor
benign tumor	metastasize
carcinogens	oncogenes
carcinomas	optimism
chronic illness	osteoarthritis
gouty arthritis	pessimism
immunotherapy	quadrantectomy
leukemias	radical mastectomy
lumpectomy	rheumatoid arthritis
lymphomas	sarcomas

Study Questions

1. What are the most commonly occurring chronic illnesses?

2. What are the special problems that chronic illnesses present from a psychosocial point of view?

3. What are the likely causes (etiologies) of cancer? Identify the different types of cancer (carcinomas, sarcomas, and so forth).

4. What are the risk factors for cancer in general? What are the risk factors for breast cancer in particular?

5. What psychosocial processes correlate with cancer (origins, treatment, or adjustment to cancer), and how?

6. What are the common biomedical treatments for cancer, and how successful are they?

7. How might psychosocial treatments be useful with cancer patients, and what treatments have proven most useful? Does current research support the notion that psychosocial treatments can cure cancer?

8. What is arthritis? What do we know about the likely causes of arthritis?

9. What is the typical focus of psychological treatment, and what treatments are generally most useful for arthritis patients?

Class Projects

1. Have a class debate on the pros and cons of psychosocial treatments for cancer patients.

2. Have interested class members present brief but focused reports on lifestyle (diet, smoking, alcohol, or stress) and risk for cancer.

3. View a film or have a detailed discussion of breast and testicular self-examination. Class discussion can use a variety of diagrams (available from the American Cancer Society or from other sources) to provide visual aids on the most effective techniques.

4. Have a round-table discussion on the newest theories and methods in treatment of arthritis. (There are signs of rapid change in this field.)

Suggested Readings

Beckham, J. C., Keefe, F. J., Caldwell, D. S., & Roodman, A. A. (1991). Pain coping strategies in rheumatoid arthritis: Relationships to pain, disability, depression and daily hassles. *Behavior Therapy, 22,* 113–124.

Brewerton, D. (1992). *All about arthritis: Past, present, future.* Cambridge, MA: Harvard University Press.

Carey, M. P., & Burish, T. G. (1988). Etiology and treatment of the psychological side effects associated with cancer chemotherapy: A critical review and discussion. *Psychological Bulletin, 104,* 307–325.

Holleb, A. I. (Ed.). (1986). *The American Cancer Society Cancer Book.* Garden City, NY: Doubleday.

Hunter, D. J., et al. (1993). A prospective study of the intake of vitamins C, E, and A and the risk of breast cancer. *The New England Journal of Medicine, 329,* 234–240.

Milan, A. R. (1980). *Breast self-examination.* New York: Liberty.

O'Leary, A., Shoor, S., Lorig, K., & Holman, H. R. (1988). A cognitive-behavioral treatment for rheumatoid arthritis. *Health Psychology, 7,* 527–544.

Spiegel, D., Kraemer, H. C., Bloom, J. R., & Gottheil, E. (1989). Effect of psychosocial treatment on survival of patients with metastatic breast cancer. *The Lancet, 2,* 888–891.

VandenBos, G. R., & Costa, P. T. Jr. (Eds.). (1990). *Psychological aspects of serious illness.* Washington, DC: American Psychological Association.

WEBSITES   *Chronic Illness, Cancer, Arthritis*

ADDRESS	DESCRIPTION
http://www.chronicillnet.org/	Chronic Illness Website covering several disorders
http://www.mdacc.tmc.edu/~acc/	Cancer Pain Page (also in Spanish)
http://www.arc.com/cancernet/cancernet.html	Link to National Cancer Institute (NCI) and other resources
http://www.ncl.ac.uk/~nchwww/guides/clinksl.htm	☆ Guide to Internet Resources for Cancer
http://www.cancer.med.umich.edu/prostcan/prostcan.html	☆ Prostate Cancer Home Page
http://www.microweb.com/clg/	☆ The Breast Cancer Compendium—a four-star site
http://nysernet.org/bcic/	☆ Breast Cancer Information Clearinghouse
http://www.oncolink.upenn.edu/	☆ A comprehensive information and link site for cancer patients, family, and professionals
http://www.aaaai.org	The American Academy of Allergy, Asthma and Immunology—offers a variety of links for information on immune system disorders
http://www.arthritis.org	Arthritis Foundation
http://www.aztec.co.za/	Arthritis Webpages

PART **6**

Promoting Health in Children and the Elderly

In this section, we take up issues of health at opposite ends of the age continuum. Both children and the elderly have special needs that differ markedly from the population of young and middle-aged adults. Although we have discussed issues pertaining to different populations throughout the book, it seems appropriate to end on this theme.

In Chapter 15, we will see how early socialization efforts in the home and school may serve to promote healthy habits that endure. There is evidence that many formative influences during this time can help or hurt the child's path to good hygiene, diet, exercise, or involvement in drugs. Schools may begin to play a more informative role in regard to both health and illness, including helping children to understand signs of illness, what medical professionals do, where they work, and how early detection and treatment can prevent many more serious problems later on.

Children also suffer from chronic illnesses that differ from adult chronic illness. Even when the illnesses are the same, the child's cognitive and emotional maturity presents many different and sometimes difficult problems for treatment teams. Three chronic illnesses that begin in childhood or afflict children more often than adults will be described: insulin-dependent diabetes, asthma, and cystic fibrosis. Biomedical and psychosocial theories will be presented followed by descriptions of common biomedical treatments and psychosocial interventions.

In Chapter 16, we will discuss how the aging process influences health. This will include a description of physical changes that may require monitoring. We will look at several theories of what controls the aging process. We will also consider the psychosocial context of aging and how it impacts on the mood and morale of the elderly. Finally, we will consider steps that aging citizens can take to preserve good health into the golden years.

CHAPTER 15

Pediatric Health Psychology: Promoting Health and Coping with Chronic Illness

Few events bring such joy as the birth of a child, especially a happy, healthy, and robust child. Most parents find it is a delightful challenge to teach the child, to foster social involvement, and to instill principles for a healthy lifestyle. Many parents also will acknowledge that the task of rearing a child carries the potential for great pain and heartbreak. Nowhere is this more evident than when a child suffers from a chronic disease or a life-threatening illness. Christine Eiser (1990, p. 1) calls this situation one that "sets the stage for a revolution in the way of life experienced by patient and family."

Gunnar's Fight for Life: Inhalers and Chest Massage

Norman and Cheryl Esiason know from personal experience what it means to run a household with a chronically ill child. Norman, nicknamed Boomer, was the strong-armed quarterback for the no-huddle offense of the Cincinnati Bengals. Cheryl tried to preserve some order in the chaotic glass house world of the professional athlete. Together, they worked to raise money for the Cincinnati Children's Hospital and the Arthritis Foundation.

They thought they were ready for anything. Then, in the heat of the football strike of 1987, a local radio station broadcast an untrue story. In short, the station alleged that Boomer had ordered the Bengals' wives to boycott a hospital fundraiser because of the strike. A fan called in with a vicious message: He hoped the

Esiasons would someday have a child with something wrong and the hospital would turn them away. Boomer and Cheryl blocked this cruelty from their minds, never dreaming that it was a portent of the living nightmare they would endure later.

Gunnar, or "G Man" as Boomer affectionately calls him, was born about four years later. A blond-haired Adonis, Gunnar was as beautiful a child as any parents could ask for. He had been home only a short while, however, when unmistakable signs of some serious illness began to appear. Gunnar repeatedly battled colds and pneumonia, and he coughed constantly. He had earaches, stomach problems, diarrhea, and lost his appetite (Smith, 1993).

At first, the doctors said it was asthma. The first test for cystic fibrosis (CF) came back negative. But he kept coughing. They kept feeding Gunnar cough suppressants to soothe his irritated throat. Little did they realize that he was coughing for his life, coughing to rid his lungs of the drowning mucous of CF. In their many visits to cheer up children in the hospital, they met patients with CF. They wondered that Gunnar's symptoms, his look and smell, were so similar to CF children. Still, the doctors continued to believe that Gunnar had asthma.

Two years after he was born, though, doctors confirmed that it was CF. Boomer and Cheryl must have felt the same anguish, even guilt, that many parents seem to feel at times like this. They repeatedly cried, "We're sorry," over their son's bed (Smith, 1993, p. 24), as though they were personally responsible for the genetic lottery that led to Gunnar's condition. But they also pledged to make whatever changes were needed to make his life count.

Gunnar's days follow a certain rhythm now. Twice each day, he goes through a routine of physical therapy. First, he puts on an inhaler mask for about 15 minutes. The inhaler vaporizes two drugs that are supposed to clear his breathing passages. Then, Gunnar stretches out with his head down on a sloping board. Next, Boomer pounds Gunnar's chest and back to force out the mucous that clogs his lungs (Smith, 1993). Somewhere along the way, Gunnar may get his licks in on Boomer's chest, perhaps to signal that what's good for him must be good for his dad.

Now, however, Gunnar and his parents have hope that the illness can be controlled. New discoveries on the cause of CF and more effective treatments make it more likely that Gunnar can do the things that children and adolescents do. Finally, there is increasing awareness of the need to help patients and their families cope with the many stressors, that occur in families with chronic illness.

Battles with Chronic Illness: Fear and Frustration

For many parents with chronically ill children, life can be a constant battle with anxiety. These parents must make crucial decisions about whether to allow painful, even risky, medical procedures. They feel anxious when insurance providers give mixed messages about coverage,

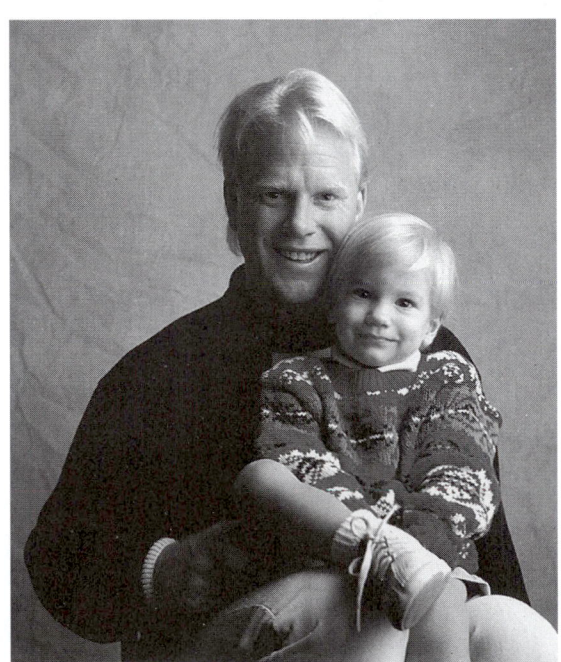

FIGURE 15.1   Gunnar and Boomer Esiason.

and frustrated when insurance payments are delayed. They have problems meeting household expenses, and may lack energy to meet the needs of their spouse and other children.

When life-threatening illness occurs, parents bear the pain of thinking about life without their beloved child. Folk wisdom suggests that children bury their parents; parents should never have to bury their child. The following lines from the pen of Gerard Manley Hopkins (*Spring and Death,* 1967, pp. 13, 14) captured the essence of sorrow over a life cut off before the chance to bloom.

> *And the flowers that he [Death] had tied,*
> *As I mark'd, not always died*
> *Sooner than their mates; and yet*
> *Their fall was fuller of regret:*
> *It seem'd so hard and dismal thing,*
> *Death, to mark them in the Spring.*

If fate should deal the mortal blow, parents confront more anxiety as they consider the wisdom of bringing more children into the world.

The child struggles to understand the pain, the illness, and the threat of death all with a cognitive system that is still immature. Children invariably raise questions: "Why me?" "Why can't I just be like everyone else?" Some illnesses may be less serious but still require lifelong monitoring and controlling tactics. The child may come to feel that he or she is somehow different. This sense of difference may pose a threat to the core of the child's identity, emotional stability, and social adjustment. Also, children may experience guilt when they realize how much their illness influences family interactions and how it strains finances. If faced with the prospect of death, they must try to integrate a notion that is beyond words and that still troubles and sometimes even terrifies adults.

Chronic illness in the child, or any family member, creates a ripple effect that engulfs the entire family system (Drotar & Crawford, 1985). The family must strengthen old or learn new coping skills (Shapiro, 1983). It is not just a matter of helping the ill child, but of helping all family members adjust, siblings included. The

noted English author C. S. Lewis (1955) wrote about his grief as a child when he lost his mother: "If I may trust my own experience, the sight of adult misery and adult terror has an effect on children which is merely paralyzing and alienating" (p. 19).

This chapter takes up issues of health and illness in childhood and adolescence. As professionals continue to think about how psychosocial factors influence health, it has become clear that prevention should begin early.[1] Society can do much to encourage good health habits in children. Only rarely do adult models of prevention serve the needs of children, though. The chapter outlines several programs designed to address these issues and reviews related research.

Then we discuss the impact the chronically ill child has on the family. We will consider coping techniques that may be useful to families confronting this problem. Later, we will discuss how the chronic illnesses that youths experience differ from the chronic illnesses adults encounter. We will consider how the child experiences pain, comprehends medical procedures, and understands death. Finally, we will look at three major childhood illnesses: asthma, cystic fibrosis, and diabetes. In each case, I will outline the pathophysiology and describe clinical interventions devised to help patients deal with their illness.

The Healthy Child: Healthy Lifestyles and Prevention

During the sensitive developmental years from early childhood to adolescence, parents speak volumes, for good or bad, about lifestyle. They do so not just through what they say, but more

---

[1] The growing interest in this area is reflected in the increasing number of journal articles, conferences, and specialized journals devoted to these issues. The *Journal of Pediatric Psychology* and the *Journal of Developmental and Behavioral Pediatrics* are among the recent publications to emerge with this focus.

so through what they do. Parents set many expectations for what to eat, how often to eat, and when to eat. They may model good habits of exercise or set standards of an idle existence. Through their silence, parents may lend support to high-risk behaviors.

The child needs to develop knowledge and skills early in six important health-related areas. We discussed two, drug addiction and high-risk sexual behavior, in earlier chapters. Three issues—nutrition, exercise, and personal hygiene—require some added attention because children build a foundation for these health habits in their early years. The sixth area is a broad category that combines knowledge of the body, notions of illness and disease, and experience with the medical people and systems.

The Eating Habit: Diet and Heart Health

Children require the same balance of carbohydrates, fats and proteins that adults do, but they require fewer calories. Between 2 and 10 years of age, caloric needs nearly double, from about 1300 to 2400 calories. Still, the child's daily energy intake can vary widely. In a study of 2- to 5-year-old children, total daily energy intake ranged from 1100 to 1800 kcal (Birch, Johnson, Andresen, Peters, & Schulte, 1991). Children probably can balance their energy needs with little parental intervention. The same thing is not necessarily true of nutritional balance.

Adolescents reach their peak calorie needs when they are about 16 to 18 years of age. After this, calorie needs begin to decline. This peak and decline pattern probably depends largely on physical changes. Yet, caloric intake also shows a socialization effect. The recommended caloric allowance for 15- to 18-year-old males is about 3000 calories per day. For a female of the same age, the recommended allowance is about 2200 calories. Data reported by Rolls, Fedoroff, and Guthrie (1991) reveal that males eat close to the recommended allowance (3048 kcal/day), but

females tend to eat much less than the recommended allowance (1687 kcal/day). This discrepancy may be explained in part by social pressures on the female to be slim.

One practice commonly used by parents may spur problem eating behavior later. This is when parents use food rewards to influence other behaviors including eating behaviors. Most often, the parents' intent is simple. They want the child to eat some food the child sees as unappetizing but the parents define as "good for you." The parents' strategy is something like this: "If you eat your cauliflower, you can have a piece of apple pie."[2]

Striegel-Moore and Rodin (1985) reviewed this reward strategy and found that more often than not, the child develops a more intense disliking of the unappetizing food. Conversely, the child probably will come to prefer the food used as a reward even more (Birch, Zimmerman, & Hind, 1980). Food rewards are often sweet and high in calories. Thus, the child may be pushed toward weaker preferences for distasteful but healthy foods and stronger preferences for desirable but less healthy food. The best strategy may be for parents to model eating healthy foods without resorting to pressuring or explicit reward maneuvers.

Additional evidence for the negative effect of coercive tactics in feeding comes from studies of problem feeders. Problem feeders are children who frequently refuse food and complain about food. They also play with food and engage in a variety of disruptive and oppositional behaviors during meals. These behaviors usually are very stressful to parents. Most important, the behaviors may deprive the child of proper nutrition. In certain cases, this can lead to malnutrition and medical problems.

Matthew Sanders and his colleagues studied a group of parents with toddlers or preschool-aged children with eating problems (Sanders, Patel, Le Grice, & Shepherd, 1993). Compared to

---

[2] I am trying to avoid White House disputes on broccoli and peas.

nonproblem eaters, parents of problem eaters used more coercive tactics and negative instructions to goad their children to eat. These parents may have used positive techniques without success when the child was younger, and the coercive tactics represent an attempt later to find some more successful method. Sanders's group made a different argument, though. They suggested that when parents use coercive tactics with their toddler, it is more likely that these tactics contribute causally to problem feeding.

Another major influence on the child's eating habits is television (Jeffrey & Lemnitzer, 1981; Story & Faulkner, 1990). Current estimates indicate that children watch between 6 to 7 hours of TV each day. Assuming this estimate is accurate, the average child will see perhaps 10,000 commercials just for food in one year of viewing. One study revealed that 51% of the advertising is for cereals, 22% is for candy and gum, and 11% is for cookies. These foods are not high in nutritional value. For example, many cereals targeted to the child contain as much as 40% sugar (Wadden & Brownell, 1984). Besides the commercials, children will see another five references to food, mostly unhealthy foods, each half hour (Story & Faulkner, 1990). These

brief comments suggest a complex interplay of forces that mold the child's eating habits and food preferences from home, school, and mass media.

Early dietary practices may also significantly influence heart health in adult years. In the 1 to 19 age group, 25% have total cholesterol levels above 170 mg/dL, which is the current definition of borderline hypercholesterolemia (National Cholesterol Education Program, 1992). In the same age group, 5% have total cholesterol levels above 200 mg/dL, which is clinically high hypercholesterolemia. Although numerous factors contribute to hypercholesterolemia, diet is one of the most important.

Exercise Among Youths: Patterns, Influences, and Benefits

We often see the child as a bundle of energy, a whirlwind in constant motion. As tempting as this image may be, some data suggest that fewer youths are exercising (66%) than targeted by the 1990 health goals (90%). Further, the average American youth is exercising less and keeping less fit than desirable (Dishman & Dunn, 1988). Children begin to lose their active habits during the age range from 10 to 17.

One sketch of this trend came from a study done by Gilliam and his colleagues. This group compared the pattern of activity in young children to that of older children (Gilliam, Freedson, Geenen, & Shahraray, 1981). In children 6 to 7 years old, activity was vigorous enough for about 45 minutes to elevate heart rates to the 160 bpm needed for aerobic improvement. The group of 11- to 13-year-olds only had about 30 minutes of activity during which they reached this target level. In the group of 16- to 17-year-olds, only about 15 minutes of aerobic activity took place.

There are only slight differences between adults and children in the standards of effective exercise. Children need three to four exercise sessions per week just as adults do, but the child's sessions need only be about 20 minutes

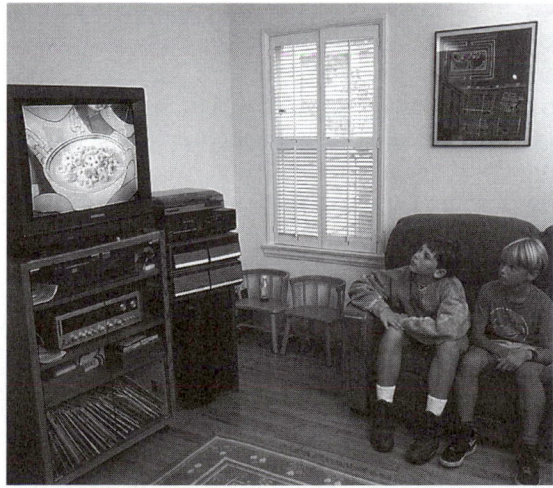

FIGURE 15.2   Commercials target children with a wide array of foods that are not healthy.

or more at aerobic levels compared to the adult's 30 minutes or more (Dishman & Dunn, 1988). The more obvious differences pertain to performance standards. Because the child's body is still growing, the child should not expect to reach (or be encouraged to emulate) adult standards for speed, endurance, and strength. At the same time, load-bearing exercise before bone growth stops appears to increase bone density. Denser bones may reduce or prevent problems with osteoporosis in later life (Nilsson, Anderson, Havdrup, & Westlin, 1978).

Children should have the opportunity to experience a broad range of different exercise activities, not just to learn new skills but for motivational reasons as well. Regular switching between different exercise routines, called cross-training, has become something of a sport itself. Cross-training combats boredom through variety and thus helps maintain higher motivation. Children may then find exercise more fun and they may keep at it more consistently. As one study suggests, having fun is still a major motivation for participating in exercise or sports (Gould, Feltz, & Weiss, 1985).

There is evidence that school recreation programs can have a positive effect on health, fitness, and exercise outside school hours (MacConnie, Gilliam, Geenen, & Pels, 1982; Brownell & Kaye, 1982). Still, it is not clear what specific program factors increase the likelihood of continuing to exercise. In addition, school programs may increase exercise generally, but investigators are not sure how school exercise generalizes to specific activities or settings.

Finally, schools seem to invest a disproportionate amount of time and money in a small group of skilled competitive athletes who prop up the school's ego. Simultaneously, schools seem to ignore the vast majority of students who could learn much from a varied exercise program. A near-obsessive tendency to make physical education classes competitive instead of teaching children to compete against a personal standard is one reason, among many, for an increase in the numbers of youths dropping out

of sports activities (Gould & Horn, 1984). Another factor cited is the incessant pressure from parents and peers to win at any cost.

Personal Hygiene and Safety: Flossing and Seat Belts

There are many more aspects of personal hygiene and safety than can be discussed here. Still, several research programs reveal how one might work to change high-risk behaviors and promote health in childhood. Two approaches will be reviewed here: promoting dental hygiene with regular flossing and reducing risk for injury or death by use of seat belts.

Dental hygiene: flossing, plaque, and health

Dental hygiene is a topic that probably generates little excitement, yet there are several benefits of proper dental care. First, it helps to keep the teeth healthy, which is important in its own right. Further, it has aesthetic, personal appearance benefits. Dental hygiene also preserves an important function in digestion—the ability to chew food efficiently. This permits the person to enjoy nutritious and appetizing meals. Finally, it has the potential to reduce dental care costs for both the family and the insurance provider.

Lynnda Dahlquist and Karen Gil (1986) used an intervention program of prompts, self-monitoring, and rewards for plaque reduction to increase dental flossing in children. They used a multiple baseline design with four children. The investigators trained the children's parents to implement and monitor the program. The results showed a significant reduction in plaque from baseline (75 to 94% plaque) to the end of the intervention (22 to 33%). Over the course of a three to four months' follow-up, three of the four subjects maintained lower levels of plaque (20% to 44%) compared to their baseline levels. Dahlquist and Gil noted that training the parents appeared to be important to maintaining the flossing habit.

Personal injury: helmets and seat belts

Injuries are the cause of more deaths in children than the next six causes of death combined (Christophersen, 1989). One accidental death occurs every six minutes (National Safety Council, 1986), leading to more than 1,500 fatalities and 125,000 injuries in children under 14. Approximately 317,700 children suffer moderate to severe injuries from assault, physical abuse, neglect, or sexual abuse (Finkelhor & Dziuba-Leatherman, 1994). For preschoolers, most accidental deaths result from injuries in the home. For adolescents, the three primary causes of death are auto accidents, homicide, and suicide (Millstein, 1989).

Attempts to reduce the numbers of accidental injuries and fatalities often start with public policy. At the local level, educational programs, safety reminders, prompts, and other behavioral techniques may effectively change high-risk behaviors. Among the targeted high-risk behaviors are speeding, failure to use seat belts, or failure to wear protective helmets while bicycling or riding a motorcycle.

Karen Sowers-Hoag and her associates used a multidimensional approach to increase children's use of seat belts (Sowers-Hoag, Thyer, & Bailey, 1987). The program used a combination of small-group education, role-playing, behavioral rehearsal, and prizes for the group with the highest ratio of buckling-up. They targeted children in the 5 to 7 year age range because these children are above the mandatory child restraint age. The school always had teachers' aids escort children to their parents' cars after school. This enabled the investigators to obtain data on seat-belt use unobtrusively.

The results, shown in Figure 15.4, reveal that the intervention dramatically changed the children's seat-belt use compared to baseline. Seat belt use went from 0% in both groups to an average 95% use in the first group and 81% in the second group. The prizes stopped being given out on the 34th day but probes continued for the next three months. Even after the intervention program ended, the children continued to use

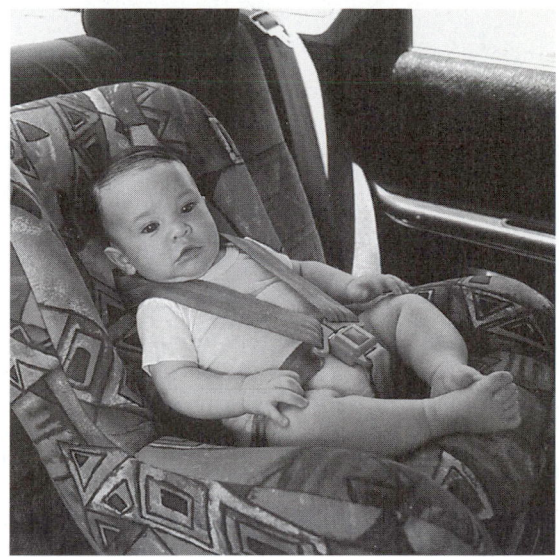

FIGURE 15.3 *Many states now require use of restraint seats and seat belts because many lives can be saved through their proper use.*

their seat belts at a much higher rate than they did prior to the program.

Teaching About the Body and Illness

Parents face the challenge of teaching their children basic principles of body structure and function. They must also help their child comprehend what the body's distress signals mean for health or illness. This task can be difficult at best when dealing with a normally healthy child. It can become torture when the child is suffering with chronic illness.

Teaching about the body and illness depends, first, on parents' basic knowledge and, second, on their judgment about how and when to convey important information to the child. Then, parents must try to adjust the information to fit the child's cognitive level, which changes rapidly, continuously, and dramatically during these formative years. Many notions, including ideas about health and illness, evolve from primitive and concrete to refined and abstract. During adolescence, there is still a great deal of

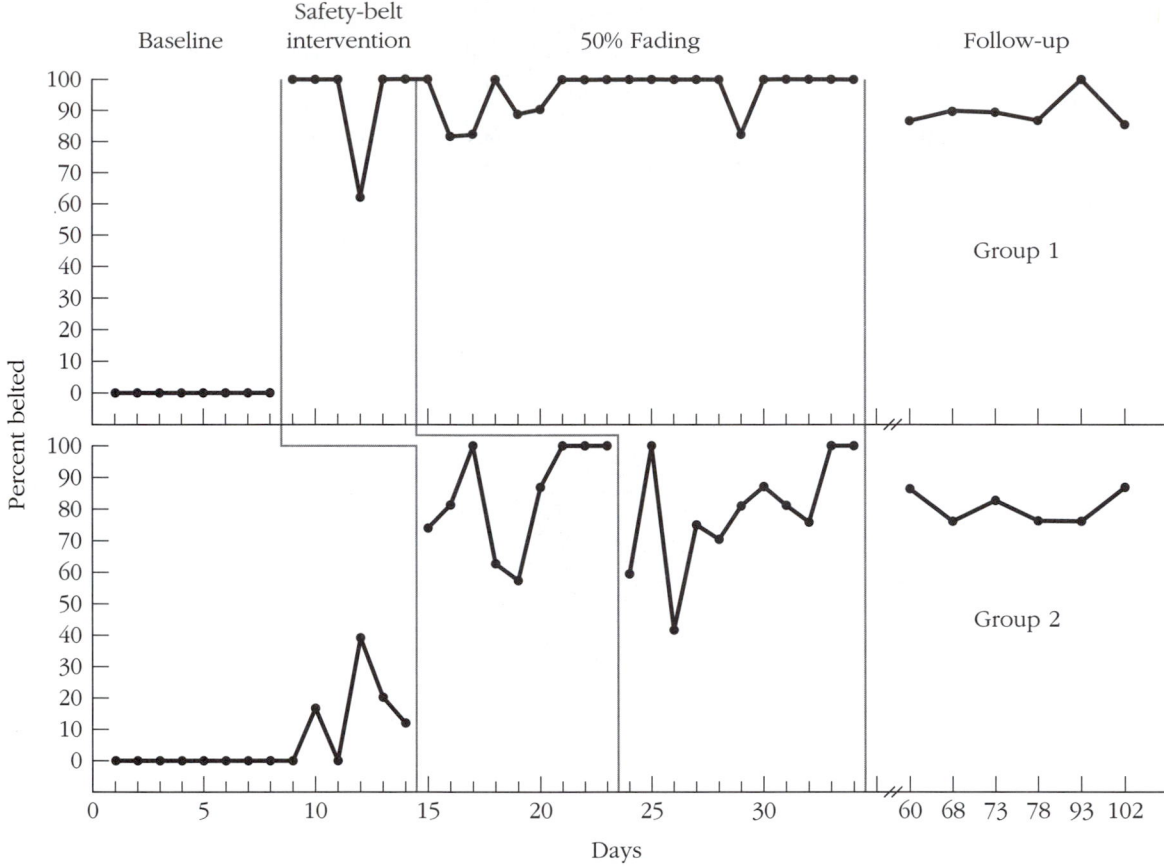

FIGURE 15.4 *Change in the percentage of children using seat belts. A multiple baseline design with follow-up shows the positive effect of the intervention and the persistence of the behavior after the intervention stopped (from Sowers-Hoag et al., 1987).*

variability in understanding of medical terms (Hastrup, Phillips, Vullo, Kang, & Slomka, 1992). Adolescents can verbalize illness definitions much better than health definitions (Millstein & Irwin, 1987). Adolescents express their illness ideas largely in terms of somatic feelings. As their health concepts evolve, they connect these ideas to preventive behaviors. Later, there is less reliance on the notion of the absence of illness to define health.

Siegal (1988) presented evidence that young children have a better idea of contagion and contamination than previously thought. They seem to understand, for example, that a dirty spoon can cause illness. Colds are often con-

tracted because people do not wash their hands after blowing or touching their nose. Then, they touch someone and pass the virus on. Getting children to understand this may not be as difficult if they already understand an idea like the dirty spoon–illness connection. Finally, teaching children the habit of washing their hands regularly, just as they know it is important to wash dishes, is an important preventive hygiene behavior.

Several programs now in process intend to measure the potential impact of health education on health behaviors. Two such programs are the School Health Curriculum Project and the Minnesota Heart Health Program.

The U.S. Public Health Service developed the School Health Curriculum Project in 1970. The program was designed to impact high-risk behaviors such as smoking, alcohol consumption, and drug addiction. The program also provided instruction in four body systems (digestive, respiratory, cardiovascular, and CNS) spaced respectively across four levels from fourth to seventh grades. Teaching methods included peer discussion groups, films, experiments, and plays.

A three-year study compared this program to schools with no systematic program and to health-education programs in Ohio, Oregon, and Georgia (Connell, Turner, & Mason, 1985). The research team collected data on health knowledge and health behaviors from more than 30,000 students in 20 states. One outcome was obvious: the more extensive the intervention, the better the results. Yet, the complete results were not very encouraging. Although the children learned a great deal about health, they did not change their attitudes or behaviors as hoped. One can only guess whether the knowledge, like a dormant seed once planted, might nonetheless later blossom under more supportive conditions.

The Minnesota Heart Health Program was a community-based health education program designed primarily to reduce cardiovascular risk (Perry, Klepp, & Sillers, 1989; Perry, Kelder, Murray, & Klepp, 1992). Under the direction of Cheryl Perry, the program ran over a ten-year period beginning in 1980 with assessments beginning in 1983. Table 15.1 shows the structure of this program. The results showed a reduction in smoking behavior from 22.7% in the control group to 13.1% in the experimental group. Additional analyses showed that duration and intensity of physical activity rose significantly in the intervention communities during the follow-up period (Kelder, Perry, & Klepp, 1993).

Finally, children's conceptions of doctors, hospitals, and illness are often not accurate. For example, some children have a basic fear that if they go into a hospital, they will not come out (Eiser, 1990). They look at the hospital as a place where bad things happen, where people go to die. Thus, they may not view the hospital as a place to go to get well.

To deal with this issue, school activities may incorporate some discussion about the people who work in hospitals and what goes on in

TABLE 15.1   *The education and survey plan for the Minnesota Heart Program (from Perry et al., 1989).*

	EDUCATED COMMUNITY	REFERENCE COMMUNITY
Sixth grade 1982–1983	Baseline survey I	Baseline survey I
	The Lunch Bag Program	
Seventh grade 1983–1984	The Minnesota Smoking Prevention Program (Keep It Clean)[a]	
	Survey II	Survey II
	Health Olympics greeting card I[a]	
Eighth grade 1984–1985	Health Olympics greeting card II	
	Survey III	Survey III
	FM 250 physical activity challenge	
Ninth grade 1985–1986	Shifting gears[a]	
	Survey IV	Survey IV
Tenth grade 1986–1987	Slice of life	
	Survey V	Survey V

[a]Denotes smoking interventions.

hospitals. Another approach where medical community support exists is to take children on a hospital tour. Children may learn about the types of equipment found in a hospital, the types of procedures used, and the typical benefits that come from use of medical services. Schools may provide demonstrations, and set up pretend hospitals that provide a type of play education (Eiser, 1990). The combination of parental and school teaching should help children come to better understand their own bodies and the valuable resources available in the medical community to help maintain health.

Chronically Ill Children: Habits, Lifestyle, and Prevention

Chronic illness is an uncurable or physically limiting condition that lasts for more than three months. The person's physical limitations require special procedures or assistance to manage daily living tasks. Certain chronic illnesses—such as asthma, hemophilia, and epilepsy—can be managed but not cured with present medical knowledge.

The incidence of chronic illness among children is approximately 10 per 1000 live births (Eiser, 1990). Estimates of prevalence, as tenuous as they are, suggest a combined rate of about 22 cases per 1000. This rate has remained nearly constant over the past 20 years or more (Gortmaker, 1985).

Happily, major changes in medical technology have been occurring very rapidly. Thus, illnesses thought incurable just a short while ago have become curable. Improved medical technology and treatment have extended life expectancy and quality of life for several chronic illnesses. One notable example is cystic fibrosis. One outcome of this improved care is an increase in the percentage of chronically ill children in the pediatric population (Jackson, 1992).

The chronic illnesses commonly found among children differ from the chronic illnesses that typically afflict adults. The top ten chronic illnesses for children, shown rank ordered in Table 15.2, include asthma, congenital heart disease, chronic kidney disease, spina bifida, cystic fibrosis, juvenile diabetes (an insulin-dependent diabetes), cleft palate, sickle-cell anemia, muscular dystrophy, and hemophilia.

TABLE 15.2   *Age of onset, incidence, prevalence, and survival estimates for the ten leading chronic illnesses in children (data from Eiser, 1990, and Gortmaker, 1985).*

DISEASE	AGE OF ONSET	INCIDENCE PER 1,000 BIRTHS	MAXIUM PREVALENCE PER 1000	SURVIVAL ESTIMATES TO AGE 20
Asthma	1 to 2; variable	10.00	10.20	98%
Congenital heart disease	1 year	8.00	9.33	65%
Chronic kidney disease	1 to 15; variable	2.00	1.89	25%
Spina bifida	birth	1.00	.67	50%
Cystic fibrosis	before 1; variable	.50	.26	60%
Diabetes mellitus	before 12	.40	1.89	95%
Cleft palate		.40	1.62	92%
Sickle-cell anemia		.36	.29	90%
Muscular dystrophy		.14	.14	25%
Hemophilia		.13	.16	90%

In the next few pages, we will discuss several common features of chronic illness including special issues concerning pain in children. Then, we will consider the essential features—epidemiology, etiology, and interventions—of a select group of chronic illnesses, specifically asthma, cystic fibrosis, and diabetes.

Common Features of Chronic Illness: Pain, Distress, and Isolation

A common denominator of many illnesses is discomfort ranging from mildly distressing symptoms to excruciating and unremitting pain. Children experience pain just as surely as adults do. Unfortunately, some medical practice still treats children as though they do not suffer from pain to the same degree as adults. This practice has led to serious concerns that children are not treated for pain in the same way as adults (Langreth, 1991). Here we will briefly review the child's experience of pain and the techniques recommended to treat it.

Two factors in particular appear to increase the child's pain experience. First, lack of control and predictability tend to increase the children's anxiety and their experience of pain tends to increase as anxiety increases. According to McGrath (1990), about 30% of children suffer from recurrent headache or abdominal pain. The more unpredictable the pain episodes are, the more likely the child is to suffer psychologically and socially. Second, an inability to understand how serious the injury is or to comprehend the nature of the medical procedure also adds to the perception of pain.

Children's ideas of pain: punishment and hurt

The child's idea of pain is most succinctly stated: "Pain is what hurts" (McGrath, 1990, p. 8). Gaffney and Dunn (1986, 1987) have probably carried out the most extensive work on children's notions of pain. They argued, as others have (Bush, 1987; Harbeck & Peterson, 1992), that the child's ideas of pain can be profitably viewed within a cognitive development stage model. Two general findings are of interest. First, Gaffney and Dunn found that many children view pain as a punishment for some type of transgression. Second, they found that children use increasingly objective yet abstract notions to explain pain as they mature cognitively.

To illustrate, in the preoperational stage, children seem to attend primarily to the location and the feeling of pain: "Pain is . . . something in my belly." In the concrete operational period, children may discuss pain in more abstract terms: "Pain is . . . a hurting sensation." They may provide analogies for pain and they may point to the subjective side effects of pain. In the formal operations stage, children define pain in more extended terms including references to physical and psychosocial aspects of pain: "Pain is something that hurts a person . . . suffering mentally or physically." (Examples are from Gaffney & Dunn, 1986, p. 109.)

Treating children's pain: medical, behavioral, and cognitive

As noted earlier, there is concern that children are not treated for pain in the same way as adults. Low or no pain medication for children is usually justified with the notion that children do not feel pain as keenly as adults. This notion may be backed up by an appeal to differences in physiology—in other words, the claim that some part of the nervous system crucial to pain perception is not mature in infants and children. Another justification is that children are more resilient and recover better than adults (Eland & Anderson, 1977). Emerging research on children's pain, however, makes these justifications suspect in whole or in part.

Further, more detailed guidelines on pain management accord the child the same right to pain management that is accorded the adult. Children's pain may be managed through a blend of pharmacological, physical, behavioral, and cognitive therapies (Agency of Health Care Policy and Research, 1992). Most of these methods were reviewed in Chapter 14; only one qualifying comment is necessary here. Many of the cognitive-behavioral pain control methods described in Chapter 14 may be used with children, but instructions, timing and sequencing usually must be altered to suit the child's age and cognitive level.

Patricia McGrath (1990) presented a comprehensive pain management program that emphasizes understanding and control in working with children's pains. Her guidelines indicate that pharmacological therapy or physical therapy should be the primary intervention for moderate to severe pain that is due to disease, injury, or surgery. Behavioral-cognitive methods can serve as allies to the primary therapy to improve pain management, but they should not be considered the first line of defense in such situations. When the pain is recurrent or chronic with identified psychosocial factors involved, then the primary therapy should be psychological, but analgesics may still be used to help control pain.

Children's views of death: temporary versus permanent separation

Several years ago, the mass media reported on a tragic case of a little boy who became angry because his mother refused him cookies just before supper. He grabbed a knife and stabbed her to death. Later, his comments revealed the thought processes behind his act: it never occurred to him that his mother would not be back to take care of him later. He had formed his notions about the temporary nature of death from TV soaps with the constant cycles of stars dying only to return in another role the next day.

Very young children do seem to have difficulty fully comprehending the permanence of death. Still, it is clear that already at an early age, children observe various forms of death (including deaths of pets and wild animals), that they begin to think and ask questions about death in serious terms, and that their conception of death follows a more or less predictable path of increasing abstractness as their cognitive system develops.

Maria Nagy (1948), for example, interviewed Hungarian children 3 to 10 years old. She found evidence of three stages in children's under-

standing of death. In the first stage, up to about 5 years of age, children saw death as a separation not unlike sleep. There was an underlying expectation that the person would return. In the second stage, up to about 9 years of age, the children saw death as final but not universal. It was something that did not necessarily have personal relevance. In the third and final stage, the children's ideas approximated that of adults. They saw death as permanent and irreversible, but they also came to understand that death was personally inevitable.

Children in families with a terminally ill member (whether parent or sibling) must confront the anguish that comes with impending or actual death. In this situation, they appear to experience greater depression, heightened anxiety, lower self-esteem, lower social competence, and more behavioral problems than children in homes without a terminally ill member (Siegel et al., 1992).

For the terminally ill child, the issue is how they will understand and cope with their own mortality. In spite of the extreme stress the child's illness places on all family members, it does not necessarily result in psychopathology in the child or dysfunctionality in the family. A study by Brown and his colleagues found that children and their parents apparently cope with the child's illness through problem solving, keeping a positive outlook on life, and maintaining good communication (Brown et al., 1992). Children still apparently go through grieving stages similar to those described by Kubler-Ross based on her work with adults (1969). Further, children need support in working through the bereavement process at least as much as, if not more than, adults do. Programs have been developed to help children deal with the death of a parent or to confront their own mortality.

Karolynn Siegel and her colleagues described an early intervention psychoeducational program designed to help children cope with the impending death of a parent (Siegel, Mesagno, & Christ, 1990). The program was based on a parent guidance model that assumes healthy parents are in the best position to foster their children's healthy grief work. The program then tried to provide healthy parents with the necessary support, knowledge, and insight to help their children. Siegel's group typically began their work about six months prior to the expected death, and they follow up after death about the same amount of time. Although only subjective evidence was available, it appeared that both parents and children benefited from the program.

From the work of Myra Bluebond-Langner (1997), children seem to go through five stages in comprehending their own illness and the prospect of dying. In the first stage, they are aware of the seriousness of the illness, but they are most concerned with the discomfort the illness brings. In the second stage, they come to a more sophisticated knowledge of their illness, the recommended treatments, and the potential outcomes. They see themselves as sick, but they are very optimistic about getting better. In the third stage, they come to even better understanding of the illness, but they also begin to integrate knowledge that their illness is going to be a long-term part of their life and identity. Still, they retain some optimism for getting better even if it is going to take longer. In the fourth stage, their view begins to take on a pessimistic complexion with the realization that they will never get better. Finally, as the illness progresses and they feel the steady decline in their condition, they come to view themselves as dying.

At each step, parents and health care personnel must make crucial decisions about what to reveal and how to help the child cope. It appears that even when medical staff and parents withhold the frightful truth about the illness, children seem to be well aware of their condition and reveal this in both word and action (Katz, Kellerman, & Siegel, 1980). Parents play an important role in helping their child come to grips with the stark reality. They need to be keen observers of changes in their child's physical or emotional condition. Further, there needs to be good communication among the family members on a continual basis, strong emotional support for each member, and every effort expended to maintain as high a quality of life as disease conditions permit. Programs similar to those described above as well as hospice programs for terminally ill children also provide the parent with needed resources to cope with this situation and to provide the type of support and information the child needs.

Coping with Chronic Illness: Barriers, Influences, and Strategies

The American Academy of Pediatrics (AAP Special Report, 1989) identified three barriers commonly encountered by families faced with chronic illness. These are financial barriers, system barriers, and knowledge barriers. Financial barriers often occur because the family has inadequate or no health insurance coverage. One group is especially vulnerable, the uninsured poor who cannot afford health insurance themselves but who also do not qualify for Medicaid (Jackson, 1992). System barriers include an often complex maze of local, state, and federal agencies and service centers each with its own peculiar set of rules.

Knowledge barriers influence both the practitioner and the family. The practitioner may be limited in the technical competency and quality of care that can be provided. This difficulty occurs most often with illnesses that are on the leading edge of medical science. Parents may not fully understand the nature of the illness, or the subtleties involved in dietary, exercise, or medication regimens required for their child. Further, parents' committment to help manage the illness may be undermined in the face of complex dietary, exercise, or medication requirements.

Parents' knowledge, skills and ability to identify and report children's illness can be improved through role playing (Delgado & Lutzker, 1988) or community-wide health education programs (Chamberlin, 1984). Role-playing programs are labor intensive, expensive on a mass scale, and thus impractical. Conversely, community programs seem to return dividends in proportion to the amount spent (Connell et al., 1985).

Eiser (1990) noted three influences on the child's response to a chronic illness. First, diseases can be benign or they can be life-threatening, disabling, restricting, and extended. As any illness reaches the extreme on one or more of these dimensions, it will more likely evoke negative reactions in the child.

Personal traits and coping skills form the second influence. The older, more mature, and informed the child, the more likely the child will take the disorder in stride. In addition, the quality of the child's coping skills will influence the response (see the review by Rudolph, Dennig, & Weisz, 1995).

The third influence reflects the unique traits of the patient's family. A close-knit family with good organization, communication, and problem-solving skills will benefit both the healthy members and the patient. When parents model effective coping skills, their children also tend to be less distressed when confronted with medical procedures (Shapiro, 1983). The emotional response to a disorder can influence treatment success.

Many children with chronic illnesses will be admitted to a hospital, if not for extended treatment, at least for diagnostic tests and observations. Hospital admission presents a challenge to parents and hospital staff, especially with very young children. A child's anxiety may be heightened because of the dramatic changes encountered in the strange hospital environment. To ease the child's anxiety, many hospitals have children's wards designed to house parents who wish to stay with their children. Under these conditions, Taylor and O'Connor (1989) found that children got out of the hospital 31% sooner than children whose parents did not stay.

Anxiety in hospitalized children is linked to several factors, such as degree of trait anxiety and perceived maternal anxiety (Teichman, Rafael, & Lerman, 1986). Children with higher levels of trait anxiety reported higher levels of anxiety no matter what medical procedure was

planned. Children who believed their mothers had higher anxiety also had higher levels of anxiety.

Still, the exact outcomes probably depend on subtle interactions between traits of the child and parents and contextual cues in the situation. Mark Lumley headed a study that described two groups of children, approachers and avoiders. Approachers are interested in and seek out novel stimuli, whereas avoiders are more passive and resistant to change (Lumley, Abeles, Melamed, Pistone, & Johnson, 1990). Lumley's group classified mothers based on whether they used distracting means to help their child cope with medical procedures or they provided information. Mothers who gave information lowered distress most when their children were approachers. Mothers who used a distracting tactic lowered distress most when their children were avoiders. Although the findings are provocative, their clinical significance is not clear at this time.

Barbara Melamed and her colleagues began an interesting line of research at Case Western Reserve. This work suggested that a peer narrated film could help to lower anxiety and promote compliance with diagnostic procedures (Melamed & Siegel, 1975). This early work led numerous hospitals and dental clinics to adopt modeling films in their routine. However, a recent meta-analysis of modeling procedures revealed that treatment strength depended on use of the blind control procedure to eliminate bias. That is, treatment effects nearly disappeared in experiments using adequate blind procedures. Treatment effects remained strong (almost three times the effect size) only in experiments that did not use blind control procedures (Saile, Burgmeier, & Schmidt, 1988).

Effects on the Family: Siblings, Parents, and Marital Stress

Chronically ill children certainly deserve all the research and clinical attention given over the past years. Still, other members of the family, siblings included, may be touched by chronic

Phase 3: anesthesia induction

● Children with low distracting, high informing mothers

○ Children with high distracting, low informing mothers

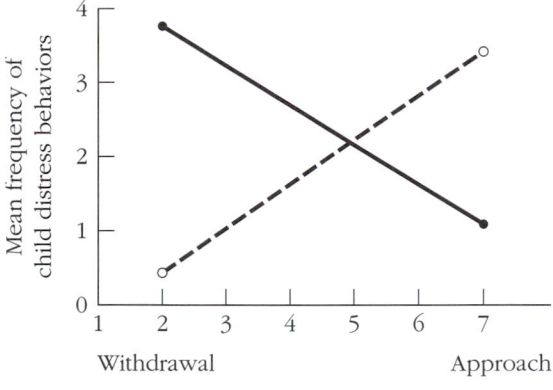

FIGURE 15.5   *Mean frequency of child's operating room distress as a function of the child's approach or withdrawal temperament and mother's distracting or information behavior (from Lumley et al., 1990).*

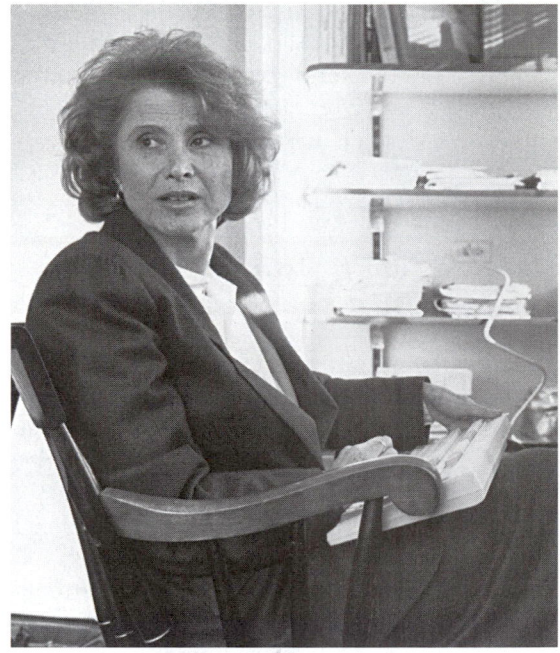

FIGURE 15.6   *Barbara Melamed, former president of APA Division of Health Psychology, has worked extensively on modeling to reduce anxiety in surgical procedures.*

illness in various ways. Drotar and Crawford (1985) reviewed numerous issues in the psychological adaptation of siblings living with a chronically ill child. They concluded that siblings of a chronically ill child do suffer some negative outcomes, but not to the degree previously believed. Negative psychological effects include lower self-concept, negative emotional responses to disease and pain, and higher stress scores. Some siblings display headaches, irritability, worry about contracting the same illness, depression, abdominal pain, and enuresis. They report feeling jealous of their sick brother or sister during treatment. Finally, social withdrawal and poorer school performance may occur. These outcomes are nowhere near universal. They vary by type of illness, age, spacing, and sex of siblings. Younger and more closely spaced males appear to suffer most. Most important, some studies show that severe adjust-

ment problems may be notably absent among siblings of chronically ill children compared to control groups.

There is concern, though, that these conclusions come from studies with methodological problems (Lobato, Faust, & Spirito, 1988). To counter criticisms, some investigators have developed special scales to assess psychosocial functioning in homes with a chronically ill member (Walker, Stein, Perrin, & Jessop, 1990). Still, the assessment strategies and instruments used vary widely, making it difficult to compare studies directly.

On the positive side, Drotar and Crawford (1985) suggested that chronic illness may have worthwhile outcomes for personal and family resilience. Support for this view comes from studies of marital adjustment. The extra care required for the chronically ill child certainly creates the potential for marital strain. Yet, the risk for divorce appears to decline in families with a chronically ill child. Further, there may be increased bonding and cohesion because of the struggle the family endures together (Barbarin, Hughes, & Chesler, 1985).

Children with Asthma: Risks, Origins, and Intervention

Asthma (technically bronchial asthma) is the most common chronic ailment among children. It is one of a group of diseases known as chronic obstructive lung diseases that also includes bronchitis and emphysema. Asthma is not a modern disease. Medical lore recognized asthma as early as the time of Hippocrates (400 B.C.E.), and medical literature described asthma in detail by the second century C.E.

Prevalence and incidence figures are not very reliable. Asthma occurs in about 10 cases per 1000 births, but it accounts for about 50% of chronic conditions. Based on estimates that are admittedly crude, possibly 12 million Americans suffer from asthma, and asthma handicaps about 9 million in this group (Weiss, Gergen, & Hodgson, 1992). In both prevalence and incidence, perhaps 50% of asthma sufferers are under 15 years of age. The best estimate is that approximately 10% of children have had symptoms of asthma (Goldenhersh & Rachelefsky, 1989a). The annual cost of direct medical care for children under 17 years of age is more than $465 million in 1985 dollars (Weiss et al., 1992).

Asthma is more frequent in males than females under 5 and again after 60. Between 5 and 9, the incidence is approximately the same for both males and females. After 9, there is slightly higher incidence among females until age 60. Contrary to what some believe, there is evidence that people do not really outgrow asthma. They may be symptom free for a long time, but there are still signs of change in the pulmonary tract.

Asthma is rarely a life-threatening illness. Compared to a normal cohort surviving to 20 years of age, about 98% of asthmatic children survive (Gortmaker, 1985). Nonetheless, there is concern because asthma deaths increased by

TABLE 15.3   *Costs of asthma in 1985 in children and adults (from Weiss, Gergen, & Hodgson, 1992).*

CATEGORY	17 OR UNDER	18 OR OVER	ALL
Direct Medical Costs	(*millions of dollars*)		
Hospital care			
Inpatient	250.3	808.4	1,058.8
Emergency room	90.4	109.9	200.3
Outpatient	37.1	92.1	129.2
Physicians' services			
Inpatient	20.2	61.2	81.3
Outpatient	67.1	126.2	193.3
Medications	—	—	712.7
All direct costs	465.1	1,197.8	2,375.6
Indirect Costs			
School days lost	726.1	—	726.1
Loss of work			
Outside employment	—	284.7	284.7
Housekeeping	—	406.0	406.0
Mortality	99.0	577.3	676.2
All indirect costs	825.1	1,268.0	2,093.0
All Costs	1,290.2	2,465.8	4,468.7

31% between 1980 and 1987 (Friday & Fireman, 1988; McFadden & Gilbert, 1992). The reason for this increase is unknown, but it may be linked to inadequate treatment or access to treatment. One statistic that supports these conclusions is that the mortality rate is much higher in nonwhites than whites.

The Symptoms of Asthma: Wheezing, Phases, and Triggers

The symptoms of asthma are difficult breathing, a persistent cough related to bronchoconstriction and mucus, noisy respiration typically called wheezing, tightness in the chest, and the sensation of choking. Night awakening is so common that its absence leads to doubt about a diagnosis of asthma (McFadden & Gilbert, 1992). Diagnosis and treatment require tests to rule out illnesses that also produce a wheezing cough such as viral respiratory infections or cystic fibrosis.

Following some trigger, an asthmatic attack generally goes through two response phases. In the early phase, smooth muscle contraction and bronchospasms occur in the airways. This response may be triggered by immunoglobulin-E[3] in response to the release of histamines (Dolovich, 1988). The late phase occurs about 2 to 4 hours after the trigger. It peaks between 6 to 12 hours, and finally disappears about 12 to 24 hours after the trigger.

There are many triggers for an asthma attack.[4] One common trigger is an upper respiratory

infection (URI). Other triggers include airborne irritants (for example, smoke, pollens, and air pollution) and allergens. Allergic triggers may come from foods (especially fresh foods) treated with sulfites to make them look fresh. Animal dander or dust mites also may bring on an attack. Finally, exercise stress and psychosocial stressors can trigger asthmatic attacks (Leffert, 1985). Still, the stressors encountered in asthmatic children are not unique, but occur in most families coping with chronic disease.

Etiology of Asthma: Biomedical and Psychosocial Aspects

Medical science once defined asthma as an intermittent, reversible obstruction of the bronchial airways caused by bronchial constriction. One known agent of airway hyperreactivity and obstruction is a respiratory infection, which can trigger an asthma attack (Frick & Busse, 1988). Yet this does not adequately explain the etiology of asthma.

As biomedical science learned more about the disorder, it became evident that other factors (inflammation and mucus secretion, for example) were important (Larter & Kieckhefer, 1992). One hypothesis—still intensely debated—suggests that asthma occurs because of allergic reactions with increased levels of immunoglobulin-E (IgE) (Larsen, 1992). In a large-scale study of children in New Zealand, one team found no diagnosed cases of asthma when IgE levels were low (less than 32 IU/ml). Conversely, they found 36% of the cases had asthma when IgE levels were high (more than 1000 IU/ml). Further, airway hyperreactivity and IgE levels were highly associated even when controlling for the presence of asthma (Sears et al., 1991). This suggests that asthma may be linked to an allergic process although the disorder does not strictly fit the allergic profile.

Psychological processes may play a role at least in the expression of asthma. From a behavioral point of view, an asthma attack may bring immediate attention from parents or

---

[3] You may recall from Chapter 3 that the body defends itself against foreign agents through humoral immunity. The immune system produces various antibodies, also called immunoglobulins, that attack and destroy germs. One is IgE, which is involved in allergic reactions.

[4] The notion of triggers helps to keep distinct the physical origins of asthma itself and some event that prompts a single episode of asthma. In this context, then, a trigger should not be considered the cause of asthma, and an asthma attack should be regarded as a single isolated episode. By way of analogy, a person may have battled depression for years, but a new bout of depression might be triggered by the death of a loved one.

friends. The condition may permit children to escape responsibility from household chores, unwanted exercise, or social events. It may provide an excuse for absence from school. In this way, asthma attacks may provide secondary gains and thus occur more often than predicted from physical pathology.

Another view links emotional states of fear and panic to the onset of an attack. Richard Carr and his colleagues tested the theory that fear of dyspnea (the inability to breathe) increases the chances of an attack (Carr, Lehrer, & Hochron, 1992). They compared a group of asthmatic patients to panic disorder patients and normal subjects. They found support for a link between dyspnea and panic in the asthma group but not in the panic group. More will be said of the behavioral view and fear idea later in this chapter.

Finally, some believe that the home environment may contribute to asthma attacks. Home environment is typically defined in terms of parental style of control, reactions to the child's illness symptoms, problem-solving skills, stress coping skills, and knowledge specific to the child's illness. Several studies have tried to identify family factors that may be related to asthma. One research group found three major dysfunctional family actions linked to increased asthma attacks (Weinstein, Faust, McKee, & Padman, 1992). These were chain-smoking in the home; inadequate parental supervision of the child while taking prescribed medicines; and ineffective disciplinary practices.

Two studies conducted in Germany showed that asthmatic children had more frequent asthmatic attacks when confronted with hostile criticism from their mothers and when they had less face-to-face contact with their fathers (Hermanns, Florin, Dietrich, Rieger, & Hahlweg, 1989; Schobinger, Florin, Zimmer, Lindemann, & Winter, 1992). It should be noted, though, that the methods used in these studies do not allow one to draw causal conclusions. Most investigators suggest that family environment does not play a causal role in the initiation of asthma, only that family factors serve as triggers to attacks.

Interventions for Asthma: Biomedical and Psychosocial Plans

Treatment and management of asthma symptoms typically require medicines combined with educational strategies aimed at self-management and environmental control. Other techniques, such as relaxation, may be useful to prevent the occurrence of symptoms or to reduce their intensity.

Management with medications   The medications used to treat asthma are most conveniently grouped as bronchodilators, anti-inflammatory drugs, and anticholinergic drugs. The annual costs of medications for asthma treatment exceeded $1.5 billion in 1990 (Weiss et al., 1992). Because of the potentially dangerous side effects of some of these drugs, parents need to instruct their children carefully and maintain close supervision of asthma medications.

The drugs most commonly used to treat chronic mild asthma, in emergency treatment of asthma, and to relieve exercise-induced asthma are bronchodilators (Barnes, 1989). These drugs act to reduce the constriction that occurs in an asthma attack. One such drug, albuterol, has been linked to some undesirable side effects including hyperactivity, sleeplessness, increased heart rate, elevated blood pressure, hand tremors, and irritability (Larsen, 1992).

A second group includes the newer anti-inflammatory agents such as Intal (cromolyn sodium), an aerosol inhalant, or corticosteroids such as prednisone. Intal is rapidly becoming the first choice medication for chronic moderate asthma. Intal has few side effects and it appears to act on both the early and late phase responses (Goldenhersh & Rachelefsky, 1989b). The corticosteroids act only on the late phase response. The corticosteroids have several problems as well, including weight gain, delayed growth, hypertension, cataracts, and delayed sexual development. These problems can be managed by medicating every other day or morning only.

Finally, anticholinergic agents, such as Atrovent (ipratropium bromide), work on the cholinergic reflex that brings about broncho-constriction. They do not act in late phase response, and they do not help when the trigger is an allergen.

Educational programs

A primary treatment approach targets parents and young asthma sufferers with educational programs. The American Lung Association; the National Heart, Blood, and Lung Institute; and the Asthma and Allergy Foundation produce self-management curricular guides for this purpose. The programs' goals are to prevent asthma attacks from occurring if possible, and to minimize the intensity of episodes when they cannot be prevented. Reaching these goals depends on the family's learning to work together as a team. The family also learns how to modify the environment to eliminate or reduce contacts with likely asthma triggers. Family members learn how to anticipate when attacks are likely to occur and how to implement appropriate treatments when needed.

Recall that Weinstein's group identified three dysfunctional parental activities in the home (Weinstein et al., 1992). Because of severe asthmatic symptoms, the children involved in this study were admitted to a hospital. During this time, the study group carried out an intervention with parents that focused on behavior methods to deal with acute attacks, improving supervision of medical regimens, behavior contracting with their children for better compliance, and family therapy in some cases. After this intervention, hospitalizations among the group dropped by 91% and emergency room visits dropped by 81%.

A major goal is to get the children to take more responsibility for self-monitoring and self-management of their own treatment. Children need to develop a sense of mastery over the disease and confidence in their ability to manage personal care (Lewis, Rachelefsky, Lewis, de la Suta, & Kaplan, 1984). Since most school-aged children know little about their illness, they do not know how to avoid the most likely triggers (Eiser, Town, & Tripp, 1988). Parents need to learn how to share information with their children on an age appropriate basis. Still, information alone will not get children involved or guarantee functional independence.

One major effect of asthma is to reduce physical activity and to isolate the child from social activities and peers. Having the chance to participate in normal childhood activities is essential to the child's psychological and physical health. Without them, self-esteem, a sense of mastery, and feelings of personal control may decrease, and conversely, anxiety and dependency are likely to increase.

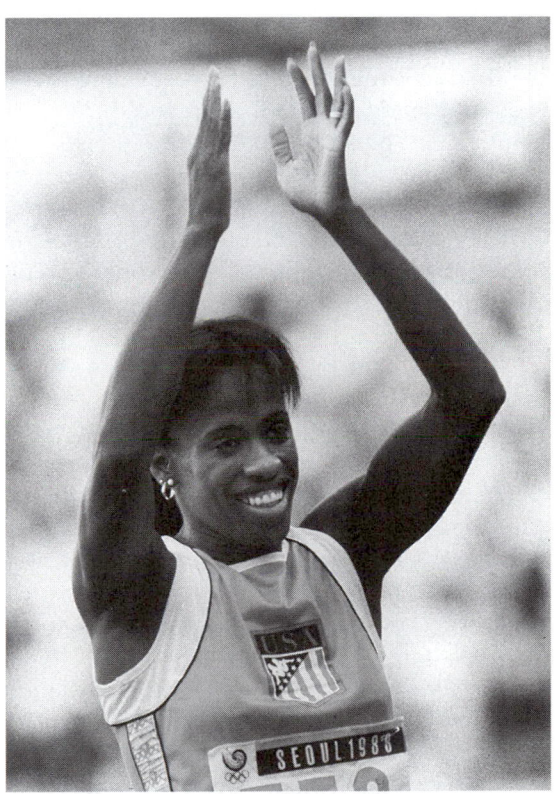

FIGURE 15.7 *Jackie Joyner-Kersee has overcome many barriers, including asthma, in order to become a world-class athlete with gold medals from two Olympic games. She continues to run even though she cannot take some asthma medicines because they are barred by Olympic rules.*

Barriers to a normal lifestyle may depend more on beliefs about asthma than about actual incapacity. If an activity triggers an asthmatic attack, parents should not assume that the child must never engage in that activity again. Instead, parents need to look for likely triggers in the activity, and guide their child through the discovery process as well. If they discover a trigger that can be controlled, the child may resume the activity. Most importantly, the discovery process should become a crucial part of environmental control. Finally, parents may need to help their child identify other activities that can be carried out with little chance of an attack.

Other family members may have to make lifestyle changes, especially when family members are habitual smokers. It may require changing house cleaning routines to reduce airborne irritants, changing food shopping habits, or getting rid of pets. One interesting study looked at changing life styles in families with an asthmatic child. The results showed that only 20% of parents were willing to give up smoking for their asthmatic child, but 85% would give up the family pet (Donnelly, Donnelly, & Thong, 1987).

Behavioral, relaxation, and family therapy approaches Behavioral treatment strategies assume that the appearance of asthma symptoms is under the control of environmental stimuli and thus may be modified through relearning models. Classical and instrumental conditioning models are most often used to explain how asthma may be triggered through learned connections.

The Pavlovian model assumes that certain stimuli (CS) become classically conditioned to elicit an attack. As noted earlier, fear or anxiety may be a crucial element that serves to trigger an attack (Stein, 1982). According to this view, past episodes of asthma probably produced pain because of severe coughing and wheezing. When shortness of breath occurs, it can be very frightening. Then, when the person feels another attack coming on, these stimuli serve to trigger anticipatory anxiety. This anxiety, unfortunately, only serves to increase the likelihood that the attack will occur.

The operant model assumes that reinforcing stimuli serve to maintain or intensify an attack. Some reinforcers may occur as secondary gains. These are unexpected benefits of being sick. Secondary gains seem to be involved most with children who are extremely dependent.

Based on this reasoning, clinicians developed several strategies to control or alleviate the symptoms of asthma. Three techniques have received attention: desensitization, relaxation aided by biofeedback, and operant reinforcement approaches. Clinical outcome studies with these interventions have been only marginally positive. Several studies have shown statistically significant improved forced respiratory volume, but the changes have been clinically meaningless (Rainwater & Alexander, 1982). These methods still may reduce the level of anxiety that could trigger episodes or alter the person's satisfaction with life.

Gustafsson, Kjellman, and Cederblad (1986) used a family therapy approach. The therapy lasted for eight sessions and dealt with what the child's symptoms did to the functioning of the family system. The researchers also focused on emotional components of the family's efforts to cope with the child's symptoms. Over the course of 3½ years, the research team took measures of several aspects of functioning in the child. A pediatric allergist (blind to the treatment conditions) collected the data. Gustafsson's group found evidence that breathing volume and air flow improved, days without impairment increased, and medication use decreased.

Operant techniques may prove helpful when used primarily to help the young child learn and maintain a strict medical regimen. Parents may provide small rewards for cooperating with treatment and when the child takes small steps toward self-treatment. Although each of these clinical methods adds small improvements, the most effective interventions are pharmacotherapy and environmental control to reduce contact with known triggers.

Children with Cystic Fibrosis: Pathology, Care, and Prognosis

At the beginning of this chapter, we met Gunnar, Boomer and Cheryl Esiason's little boy who has cystic fibrosis. CF is a frightening disease for parents to deal with, and it is difficult to manage because of the daily care required. It is also frightening because most CF patients will die before reaching 30. Still, several significant recent developments offer more hope than ever before.

CF is a genetically transmitted disease that follows an **autosomal recessive** mode of inheritance (The Cystic Fibrosis Genotype-Phenotype Consortium, 1993). An autosomal transmission means that the trait is determined by one of the 22 chromosome pairs (autosomes) not involved in sex determination. A recessive trait is latent unless both parents are carriers. A simple laboratory test used to confirm a CF diagnosis detects high concentrations of sodium and chloride in sweat (Lewiston, 1985) but more extensive testing may be necessary in some cases (Stern, 1997). CF has an uncertain course in symptom development, but most patients receive the diagnosis by two years of age. Approximately 10% of CF patients are not diagnosed until adolescence.

CF occurs about once in every 2500 births in the white population. In the black population, it occurs only 1 time in 17,000 live births. CF rarely occurs in Asians or Native Americans (McMullen, 1992).

In 1940, life expectancy for a CF child was less than 2 years. Improvements in life expectancy were slow to come until about 1959 when major improvements were made (see Figure 15.8). Entering the decade of the 1990s, the median survival age was 28 years, meaning that of all CF children born in 1963, about half were still alive in 1990 (Office of Technology Assessment, 1992). Although opinion is divided on what is realistic without further major advances in treating CF, some hold out hope that life expectancy may rise to about 40. Clinicians now encourage CF patients to plan and live life as close to normal as possible including physical activity, college, and marriage.

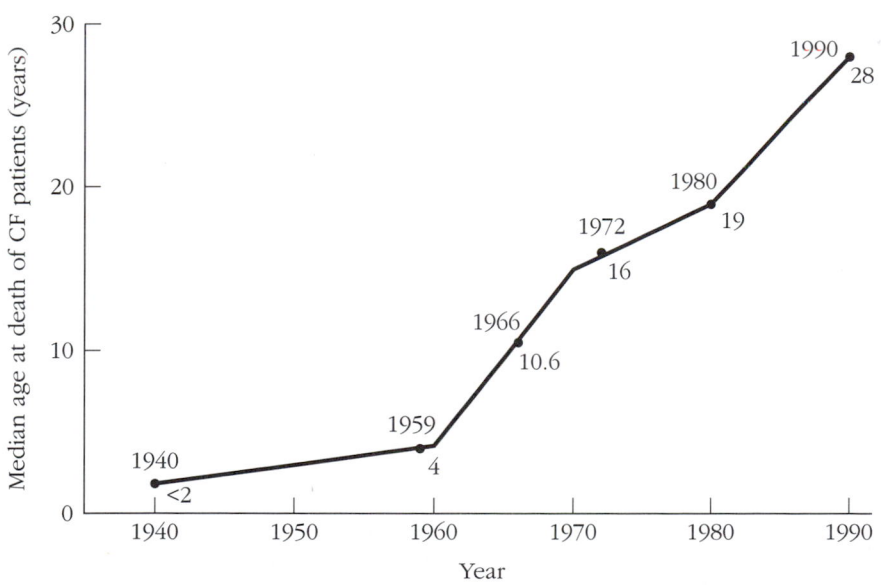

FIGURE 15.8   *Changes in the median survival age for individuals with cystic fibrosis (from Office of Technology Assessment, 1992).*

Origins of Cystic Fibrosis: Pathology and Genetics

A Swiss children's song from the 18th century said: "The child will soon die, Whose brow tastes salty when kissed" (cited in Lewiston, 1985). Now, medical research shows that CF is an extensive systemic disorder beginning with obstruction of the pancreatic ducts with abnormal electrolytes. Symptoms of these changes include disturbed digestive processes that can lead to bulky smelly stools, and disturbed absorption of fats including fat-soluble vitamins. The sweat glands do not function properly leading to high sodium and chloride concentrations in the sweat. Changes in the reproductive system can lead to sterility in the male and lowered fertility in the female. If not managed properly, then, the patient may suffer from pancreatitis, failure to thrive, and delayed maturation.

Still, the most serious pathology is pulmonary deterioration, which leads to more than 90% of patient deaths. Thick bronchial mucus hinders normal cleansing of the lungs. This leads to build up of mucous material and obstruction of the airways. The dangerous sequel is an inability to expel bacteria, which increases the risk for respiratory infections. Sooner or later, irreversible lung damage occurs with hypoxia, respiratory failure, and death.

Medical research has been looking for the cause of this wholesale systemic corruption for years. Finally, in 1989, a group of investigators found the cystic fibrosis gene on chromosome 7 (Rommens et al., 1989). In addition, investigators identified the crucial mechanism that translates the abnormal gene into physical illness. In brief, the CF gene produces a protein called cystic fibrosis transmembrane regulator (CFTR). This appears to interfere with sodium and, most important, chloride ion transport across the cell membrane (Quinton, 1989).

Working in an artificial environment, molecular geneticists recently inserted normal copies of the CFTR protein into CF epithelial cells. The effect of this insertion was to repair the chloride transport defect. This accomplishment raises the hope that doctors will not have to rely on mere symptom management and that genetic therapy may provide a cure for CF (The Cystic Fibrosis Genotype-Phenotype Consortium, 1993).

Treatment for Cystic Fibrosis: Biomedical and Psychosocial Aspects

Treatment of CF requires a complex, time-consuming set of medical procedures that involves parents and patients in symptom management. Still, the methods now in use have the potential to increase both quality and length of life for CF patients.

Elements of home-managed medical treatment The primary medical treatment is oral enzyme replacement therapy. Digestive disturbances often require antacids. Oral antibiotics combat respiratory infections. Aerosols and bronchodilators clear the airways for more comfortable breathing, but the mist tents once widely used are now mostly medical relics (Lewiston, 1985). At the same time, since CF children suffer from pulmonary distress, either active or passive tobacco smoke is especially irritating and harmful (Rubin, 1990). It makes little sense to launch an intensive medical intervention program to clear the lungs on the one hand while putting irritants back in the air that can aggravate the condition.

The most prominent feature of CF treatment is chest physical therapy, a method of draining bronchial mucus through palpation or clapping on the chest and back. A sloping board adjusts posture to help gravity drainage. Just as Boomer and Cheryl do for Gunnar, parents usually give chest physical therapy two to four times daily. Occasionally, CF patients may be hospitalized to help clean out lung mucus and restore nutritional deficiencies (McMullen, 1992).

CF adolescents ask for more medical information about their condition, and they show more interest in self-care (Strube, Smith, Rothbaum, & Sotelo, 1991). These changes probably are related to their cognitive maturation, but wide individual differences are still apparent. Strube's group found that potentially troublesome mismatches may occur between the amount of involvement and information the person desires and the amount of involvement and information the treatment requires.

Susan Geiss and her associates observed that compliance with medical routines increases with maternal involvement (Geiss, Hobbs, Hammersley-Maercklein, Kramer, & Henley, 1992). In turn, maternal involvement tends to increase with less satisfactory marital adjustment. There are several possible interpretations of this outcome, but this research group suggested that the need for high parental involvement may put too much strain on marital relationships. If this is correct, then parents may need help to minimize the chances of negative impact on the marriage.

The child may resent the frequent intrusions called for by the medical regimen. This situation seems to get worse as adolescence approaches and social involvements become more important. Then, CF children may notice differences between sexual development in peers and their own delayed sexual maturation. Some speculate that this may be behind the emotional problems experienced by CF children (Landon et al., 1980). To compensate, the CF child may put more effort into school activities and try to excel in this way. During these times, both parents and the child may need counseling support to deal with many related issues.

At times, the patient may be overwhelmed by the gravity of the situation and psychological counseling is appropriate. Parents also may need counseling or support groups to help cope with the stress and emotional upheaval that often goes with caring for a CF child. They often feel guilt, just as Boomer and Cheryl Esiason did, because CF is genetically transmitted. Counseling can help parents deal with these feelings as well.

Home-managed dietary and behavioral interventions Beyond medical controls and chest therapy, diet and exercise are important components of the CF patient's treatment. First, because of digestive absorption abnormalities, calorie and protein needs generally increase. Energy requirements may be 25% to 50% higher than in the non-CF population. Because of fat malabsorption and reported fat-soluble vitamin deficiencies, many treatment centers recommend doubling daily doses of fat-soluble vitamins. The aversive side effect of digestive difficulties include indigestion, nausea, cramping, and gas. Several problems result from this situation including food avoidance (which only compounds the problem of increased nutritional needs), behavioral problems at mealtime, and increased stress for the parents (Crist et al., 1994).

Numerous programs have been developed to offset these problems (Singer et al., 1991; Stark et al., 1994). For example, Lori Stark and her colleagues provided training in behavioral management techniques to parents, videotaped mealtime interactions with parents, and provided practice in management techniques. One focus was to reduce parents' attention to disruptive behavior and increase attention to appropriate behavior. Results showed that the parents had benefited from the training, as evidenced by their shift in attentional rewards. Most important, the children showed a significant shift from disruptive to appropriate mealtime behavior, increased food intake, and improved weight.

Patterson (1985) studied 72 families with a CF child to discover what factors led to compliance with the treatment procedures. Through telephone interviews, Patterson assessed the family environment, coping styles, stressors, and health of the child. Patterson found six variables that accounted for more than half the variance in compliance. Compliance was higher when caring for a younger child, when the child was female, when there was more emphasis on maintaining family integration, when the family was more openly expressive, when the mother did not work outside the home, and when the family was less active and involved recreationally. Exercise can have positive effects on cardiopulmonary function and airway clearance, though, suggesting that recreational activities should be managed in a way to complement the overall treatment program instead of competing with it.

Preventive Programs: Carrier Screening

The primary means for prevention is carrier screening, which is technically possible now. This method is reliable for siblings and family members of a CF patient (Beaudet, Feldman, Fernbach, Buffone, & O'Brien, 1989). In the general population, though, it allows identification of only 70% of carrier couples (Beaudet, Fenwick, Fernbach, & O'Brien, 1990).

Children with Diabetes Mellitus: Origins and Interventions

With nearly 48,000 deaths each year, diabetes mellitus is now the seventh leading cause of death in the U.S. (U.S. Bureau of the Census, 1993). It is the number one cause of acquired blindness, and one of the most common causes of kidney damage. The life expectancy for a child with diabetes at age 10 is just 44 years compared to an age-mate without diabetes, whose life expectancy is 62 (Raskin & Rosenstock, 1987).

Estimates of the prevalence of diabetes vary but one survey suggests a rate of about 6.6% of the population between 20 and 74 years (Warram, Rich, & Krolewski, 1994). Under 20 years, the estimate is about 2% to 5% of the U.S. population, or about 150,000 children. Prevalence is about the same in boys and girls.

There is some evidence that the incidence of diabetes is on the rise (Warram et al., 1994). Recent data show that there is wide variation in incidence related to age and race. In white children under the age of 20, the incidence of insulin-dependent diabetes is about 6.5 per 100,000 through 9 years of age, but 12.5 in the

10 to 19 year range. In black children, the incidence is about 10 per 100,000. Hispanic children have incidence rates in the 4.6 to 9.7 range. Yet, incidence is much different for non-insulin-dependent diabetes. For example, Pima Indians (55+%), Mexican Americans (14%), and blacks (11%) have higher incidence rates than whites (8%).

Types of Diabetes: Insulin- and Non-Insulin-Dependent Diabetes

Diabetes is not a single disease but a small group of diseases (Bennett, 1994). The National Diabetes Data Group (NDDG) devised a classification system that is now the world standard. This system recognizes two major forms of diabetes, plus diabetes that stems from malnutrition or disease syndromes. The first major group is insulin-dependent diabetes mellitus (IDDM), the type that will most concern us. The second is noninsulin-dependent diabetes mellitus (NIDDM). For the most part, the names are self-explanatory. People with IDDM must have insulin regularly so the body's cells can convert food to energy. People with NIDDM do not need insulin daily. Yet, there is more to it, as we shall soon see.

Two further points on terminology are relevant. Prior to the NDDG standard, a diagnostic category existed called juvenile onset diabetes (JOD). JOD is an insulin-dependent diabetes in the current NDDG system. Also, until recently, medical science commonly used a different set of terms: Type I and Type II diabetes. Roughly speaking, IDDM and Type I refer to the same syndrome, and NIDDM and Type II refer to the same syndrome. NDDG prefers the IDDM/NIDDM terminology and discourages use of the older terms.

There are other correlates that help to distinguish insulin-dependent from non-insulin-dependent diabetes. IDDM typically is marked by an early onset. It is a disease with a strong genetic factor (diathesis), but it depends on an environmental trigger (stressor) for it to appear. Cardiovascular problems are not uncommon in people with IDDM. About 45% of IDDM diabetics suffer from hypertension, and they are at increased risk of mortality from atherosclerosis. This latter finding is of great interest because the gene for lipid formation control and the gene implicated in diabetes are close together on chromosome 6. IDDM diabetics also are susceptible to small-blood-vessel disease, a condition that may lead to several related disorders (Nathan, 1993).

One such disorder is **retinopathy,** or damage to the retina with possible impaired vision or blindness. Among patients who have survived with diabetes for seven years, about 50% suffer from retinopathy. Annually, about 5000 diabetes patients will become blind from retinopathy (Merimee, 1990). Research with dogs suggests that the condition can be prevented only when glycemic control begins within two months of onset. Laser therapy may arrest the condition, but it cannot reverse existing vision loss.

A second related disorder is **neuropathy,** or damage to peripheral neurons. This condition can lead to severe pain and loss of tactile sensation as the disorder advances. A third is **nephropathy,** or damage to the kidneys, which can lead to renal failure and death. After 15 years, about 40% of IDDM patients but less than 20% of NIDDM patients will develop this disorder. Children seem to be protected from most of these complications by growth. Still, recent work by the Diabetes Control and Complications Trial (DCCT) Research Group (1993) suggests that intensive early treatment delays onset and slows the progression of all three conditions.

NIDDM has a later onset, typically 30 years or older. It accounts for more than 85% of diabetes cases worldwide (Weir & Leahy, 1994). The body's flaw in insulin production differs from the flaw in IDDM. In NIDDM, the pancreas produces too much insulin, or it fails to regulate the timing of insulin release. Further, NIDDM shows peripheral resistance to the action of insulin (Drash & Berlin, 1985).

Symptoms of Diabetes: Polydipsia, Polyuria, and Polyphagia

In IDDM, three classic symptoms, called the clinical triad, signal the presence of the disease. These three symptoms are polydipsia, polyuria, and polyphagia. **Polyuria** is excessive urination. **Polydipsia** is frequent drinking to replenish fluids loss from excessive urination. **Polyphagia** is increased food (caloric) intake to compensate for loss of energy. This often occurs, though, with paradoxical weight loss.

Etiology of Diabetes: Biomedical and Psychosocial Aspects

Diabetes is a systemic disease caused by the inability of the pancreas to manufacture and release insulin. Insulin is a polypeptide hormone that is crucial to the cell's use of glucose. The primary cause of diabetes is a long-term progressive destruction of beta cells (or β cells) that occurs over a period of about 2 to 10 years.

The mechanism has only recently come to light. IDDM is viewed as a genetic disease, but what the person inherits is vulnerability to damage of beta cells. Whether damage occurs or not depends on environmental events (Eisenbarth et al., 1994).[5] This view is supported by twin concordance studies that show only 50% of identical twins are concordant.

The genetic defect seems to be with Human Lymphocyte Antigen (HLA) located on chromosome 6. Comparisons of NIDDM with IDDM people shows that NIDDM people have the same HLA arrangement on chromosome 6 that exists in the normal population, but about 85% of IDDM patients have a different pattern of HLA. The genesis of IDDM appears to be an autoimmune process in which an inherited trait

---

[5] Several theoretical models suggest probable environmental factors as well including how viruses might trigger the disease. Detailed discussion of these models can be found in the Eisenbarth group's study.

of the pancreatic tissue leads to increased risk for infections. When the infection occurs (environmental), the pancreatic tissue suffers damage from the autoimmune process that sees only the necessity to fight the infection.

When enough cells have been destroyed, the pancreas can no longer produce and release enough insulin. Without insulin, serious disturbances occur in metabolism of the three essential nutrients: carbohydrates, proteins, and fats. David Leaf (1991) suggested a simple lock-and-key analogy: insulin is the key that opens the receptor lock and allows glucose to enter the cells. With progressive metabolic disturbance, the clinical triad of symptoms appears, and a diagnosis will likely follow within a matter of two to three weeks (Drash & Berlin, 1985).

When insulin production falls, three general changes occur. First, the amount of glucose that enters the cells drops leaving glucose to build up in the bloodstream. The liver senses the reduced cell absorption and acts as it normally does by stepping up production. Sooner or later, the unused glucose builds to a level that creates **hyperglycemia.** This causes increased urination (polyuria), dehydration, and thirst (polydipsia). Second, carbohydrates—the body's prime energy source—are no longer available. This unavailability triggers increased caloric intake (polyphagia). Third, the body compensates for its energy shortage by metabolizing fatty acids and amino acids (Grey, 1992). This reverses the normal process, in which insulin synthesizes fat and protein from excess calories and stores them in cells.

Patients who fail to stick with insulin injections for even two or three days may quickly learn some tough lessons. When the body turns to fatty acids for energy, it produces toxic byproducts or ketones (for example, acetone). Without insulin, ketones build up, and the blood gradually becomes more acidic. This condition is **diabetic ketoacidosis** (DKA). If untreated, DKA can lead to a diabetic coma and eventually death (Drash & Berlin, 1985). Further, stress hormones reduce insulin and increase blood glucose. Thus, patients are more vulnerable to increased levels of glucose and free fatty acids in the blood following stress (Surwit & Feinglos, 1988). This process, starting with insulin deficiency, is shown in Figure 15.9.

Interventions for Diabetes: Biomedical and Psychosocial Techniques

Short of a transplant, diabetes is uncurable. Immunotherapy using a drug called Cyclosporin A increases the rate and length of remission in recent onset cases of IDDM, but it has adverse effects on the kidneys (Eisenbarth et al., 1994).

Medical science has focused primarily on ways to manage diabetes, with two major objectives. First, seek treatment to return blood glucose to near normal levels, specifically between 60 and 120 mg/dl. Second, management seeks to prevent such complications as retinopathy and neuropathy, among others (American Diabetes Association, 1989). To accomplish these objectives, patients must monitor glucose daily, adjust insulin dosage accordingly, and then inject themselves with insulin. Even then, they may fear that one miscue could produce a diabetic crisis such as hypoglycemia or ketoacidosis (Irvine, Cox, & Gonder-Frederick, 1992). Finally, because weight complicates management of diabetes, patients must work to obtain and then maintain normal body weight.

Still, the adequacy of management depends on knowing how to carry out self-monitoring. In one study, investigators asked children over the age of 8 to show their self-monitoring skills and provide a value for blood glucose from the test. Only 58% of the children gave values that were even close to the actual values (Wing et al., 1985). Now, newer equipment seems to be making accurate measurement much easier.

There are several types of insulin ranging from short-acting, to intermediate, to long-acting insulin. Dosage has to be adjusted to individual cases and to monitored information on the level of blood glucose. Most children receive two injections daily, one in the morning and one in the evening (Grey, 1992).

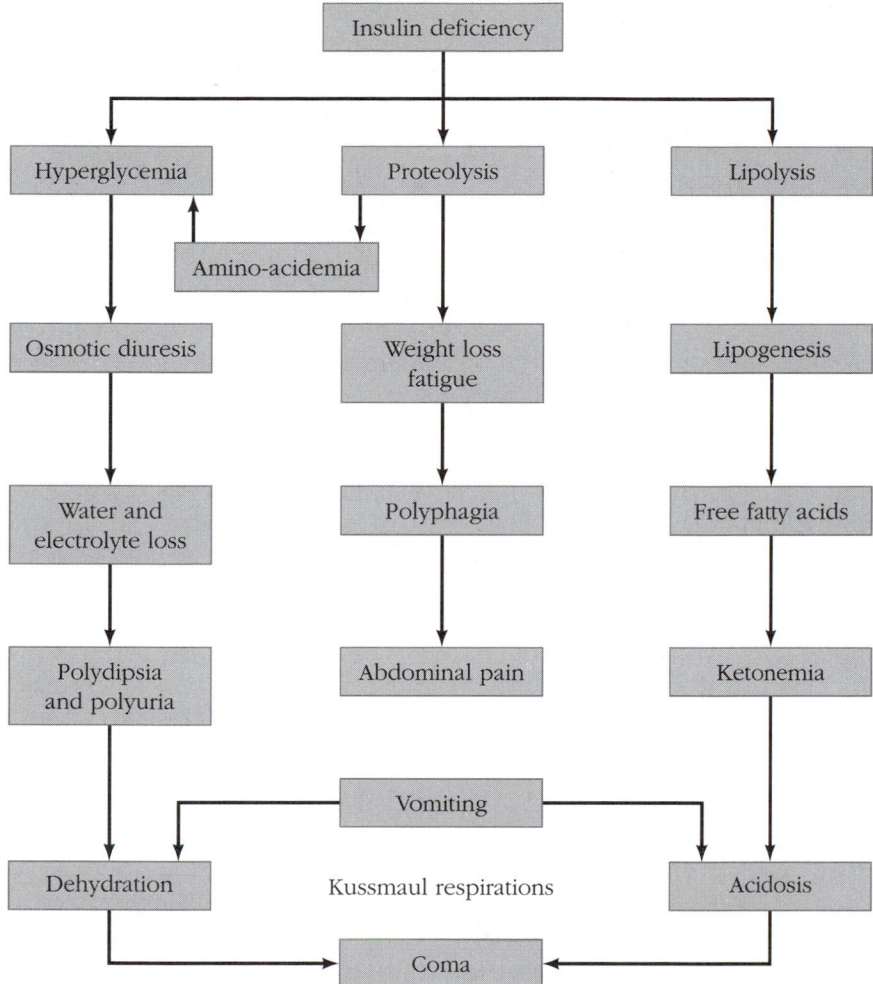

FIGURE 15.9 *The steps from insulin deficiency to several symptoms of diabetes are shown in this diagram. The most dangerous condition is diabetic ketoacidosis (from Grey, 1992).*

After the initial diagnosis of diabetes occurs and the child begins insulin treatment, there are dramatic reversals in symptoms. There is, first, a so-called honeymoon effect that lasts no more than six months when the body does not seem to require as much insulin as it first did (Grey, 1992). After this time, the child needs daily insulin. This honeymoon period can be very difficult for the child because they form the unrealistic expectation that their diabetes is cured. Primary care personnel and parents must find a way then to explain what happened. The child's level of cognitive development affects how easy or difficult this task may be. Further, parents may not understand the disease very well themselves, and they may harbor their own false hopes. It may be helpful also to assess the parents' level of comprehension.

Most children can learn how to carry out self-monitoring and insulin self-injection. Even so, they may not comply perfectly with the medical prescription. Health care personnel including health psychologists try to design programs that increase total compliance and reduce risks. Wysocki and his colleagues used a behavioral contract with IDDM adolescents (Wysocki, Green, & Huxtable, 1989). All the subjects received blood glucose meters with computer memory banks to record glucose levels. Half the subjects also agreed to a behavior contract that paid a monetary reward for sticking to a monitoring schedule. The group with the meter and the contract had a higher level of compliance over the 16 weeks of the study.

One recurring concern is that parent-child relationships may become more strained with a diabetic child. Shari Miller-Johnson and her coworkers found that several measures— parental warmth, discipline, and behavioral support—did not predict diabetes management (Miller-Johnson et al., 1994). Conflict was significantly related to both adherence and metabolic control, however. Stated in other terms, the more conflict, the less likely the adolescent was to comply with medically prescribed management procedures. Then as adherence went down, metabolic control also became worse.

Diet and exercise in the management of diabetes

One encouraging finding is that diet and exercise are very helpful in diabetes management, especially with NIDDM. In the absence of well-controlled diet and adequate exercise, blood glucose levels show more extreme swings, which can be potentially dangerous. Too much exercise, however, can result in **hypoglycemia,** a drop in blood glucose. Hypoglycemia can be very dangerous since it can occur up to 12 hours after the exercise.

With a proper diet in place and carefully planned exercise routines, blood glucose typically stabilizes, thus making it easier to manage. In addition, proper management of diet and exercise can greatly reduce the person's need for insulin. Drash and Berlin (1985) pointed out that a fit person uses energy more efficiently and thus has less need for insulin. It is important to emphasize that the need is only lessened; diet

and exercise do not eliminate insulin dependence totally.[6]

Meals must provide sufficient calories frequently enough so that the diabetic can sustain energy, avoid hyperglycemia, and keep the metabolism balanced as much as possible (Brink, 1988). For the young child, this usually means three regular meals plus two snacks between meals. Total calories should be about 1,000 calories, increasing by 100 calories per year to between 10 and 12 years. The percentage of carbohydrates needs to be raised to between 50 and 65% to provide quick energy sources.[7] Protein content should be between 12 and 20%.

Unfortunately, diet and exercise may fall prey to the same traps that catch normal people. Forbidden foods taste too good to pass up, and exercise is not always convenient or pleasant. In addition, stress may alter the person's perceptual processes and affect diabetes control strategies. Betty Kirkley found that 26% of dietary violations occurred when the person experienced negative emotions and conflicts related to stressful events (Fisher, Delamater, Bertelson, & Kirkley, 1982).

A recent study among diabetic girls and young women also found one major negative outcome from loss of dietary control—that is, poor glucose control (Balfour, White, Schiffrin, Dougherty, & Dufresne, 1993). In this study, age and stress were positively correlated with loss of dietary control as follows. Older girls were more likely to report stress and more likely to experience loss of dietary control. When the girls experienced both high stress and loss of dietary control, glucose control was very poor. Figure 15.10 shows this outcome. These results suggest that extra steps may be needed to teach diabetics how to cope with stress. One likely strategy is

---

[6] For obese patients with NIDDM, dietary control is important throughout life.

[7] Recall that the current recommendation for the general population is to have about 50% carbohydrates, 20% fats, and 30% proteins.

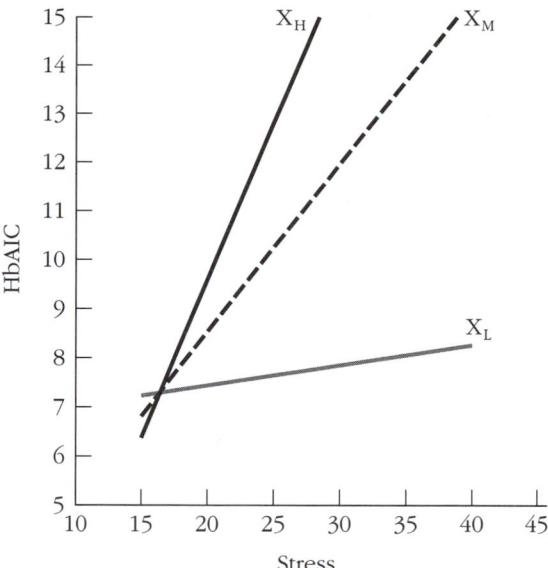

FIGURE 15.10 Relationship between stress, loss of dietary control, and blood glucose control. HbAlC is a common measure of blood glucose levels. X_H is a high disinhibitor of diet control; X_M is an average disinhibitor; and X_L is a low inhibitor (from Balfour et al., 1993).

cognitive restructuring to reduce the tendency for the person to flee to food when stress occurs.

Coping with Diabetes: Knowledge, Control, and Efficacy

Children with diabetes confront many emotional battles. They already face an uncertain future and prospects for debilitating complications. They must cope with delayed sexual development and comparisons to peers whose lives are much less regimented. It should not be surprising, then, that emotional problems surface in the diabetic, including depression, withdrawal, isolation, and hostility (Drash & Berlin, 1985). These problems have generated attempts to understand the emotional needs of the diabetic patient and family.

Eve Band and John Weisz (1990) studied children with diabetes to discover whether differences in coping are related to level of cognitive development. Band and Weisz reasoned that perceptions of control and efficacy might impact adjustment differently for children in the late concrete operations period compared to those in the formal operations stage. They classified 64 subjects into two groups, preformal or formal operations, based on a Piagetian task. They found that the two groups differed in coping approaches, on factual knowledge, and in medical adjustment. For pre-formal children, perceived control was the best predictor of adjustment. Children with greater perceived control had fewer psychosomatic complaints. Band and Weisz suggested that this result is consistent with the pre-formal child's very concrete concerns over pains such as headaches and stomachaches. If children have persistent somatic difficulties, they could conclude that their self-care efforts were ineffective and feel less in control.

With formal operations children, though, a very different picture emerged. More knowledge about their condition predicted better adjustment. Band and Weisz suggested that the adolescent looks for and expects more independence. In the context of diabetes, knowledge is important to manage one's disorder and to have a sense of personal freedom as well. Knowledge would not be as important to younger children since they have less autonomy in making medical decisions and following a medical routine.

A second variable that predicted adjustment in the formal operations group was somewhat surprising: Primary coping methods predicted better adjustment than secondary coping methods. Primary coping involves taking direct actions to alleviate stress. In diabetes management, primary coping is an action that could immediately change a physiological state. Band and Weisz defined secondary coping as a strategy that seeks to alter the impact of a stressor by managing subjective states such as mood, emotions, and expectations. Band and Weisz argued that the secondary coping strategies could undermine adjustment. One example is the diabetic youth who believes the medical regimen does not matter. Finally, Band and Weisz found evidence that lack of efficacy might be related to behavioral problems in the adolescent diabetic patient. As the perception of coping efficacy went up, there were fewer conduct problems.

A final element of coping with diabetes is home-school communication. School personnel need to know when a child with diabetes enrolls. They may then more effectively plan so that the child's needs for time and a place to self-monitor and inject if necessary can be met.

Summary

Children present many unique health problems. They are at a crucial formative stage for learning health habits that may last a lifetime. Socialization and educational experiences that occur at home and in the school should work to consolidate good health habits. Further, children may be born with or acquire diseases that require special attention. Children with chronic illnesses can place great emotional strain on family and health care personnel. Several points were made during the course of this chapter that address these issues.

1. Because the cognitive system is still maturing, children often do not understand the nature of disease, the necessity of treatment, and the pain that accompanies treatment.

2. Children need to develop knowledge and skills in six health-related areas including nutrition, exercise, personal hygiene, notions of disease and medical systems, drugs, and high-risk sexual behavior.

3. Children require the same basic combination of foods as adults—that is, a high-fiber, low-fat diet.

4. High calorie intake during infancy is a risk factor for obesity later, as is bottle feeding and an irregular meal schedule.

5. One negative influence in contemporary American culture is that both TV commercials and programs targeted to children tend to promote and portray unhealthy foods.

6. Children should exercise 3 to 4 times per week for 20 to 30 minutes. Exercise should elevate heart rate to 60% of cardiorespiratory capacity. Exercise should be fun, focus less on competitive standards, and encourage children to strive to meet personal goals.

7. Programs designed to encourage children to use seat belts suggest that educational procedures can reduce risk.

8. Several community-based intervention programs have been successful in changing children and adolescents' lifestyle to reduce risk (persuading them to avoid drugs and reduce smoking, for example).

9. The incidence of chronic illness among children is about 1 in 10,000 births. The most common chronic illnesses among children are asthma, congenital heart disease, chronic kidney disease, spina bifida, cystic fibrosis, and diabetes.

10. Children feel pain just as adults do, but there is concern that children may not receive the same consideration for pain when undergoing medical tests or treatments.

11. Families typically encounter three barriers in dealing with chronic illness. They have financial barriers because of no or poor health insurance. They encounter system barriers because of the complex maze of local, state, and federal agencies that operate in health care delivery. There are knowledge barriers for parents related to understanding the disease and treatment, and for the physician related to keeping up to date on the best method of treatment.

12. Families seem to be extremely resilient when dealing with a chronically ill member. Still, there is some evidence of negative effects on siblings, stress for the marriage, and various pressures related to time and money.

13. Asthma is a chronic obstructive lung disease that occurs in about 10 cases per 1,000 births. It is more frequent in males than females.

14. Asthma attacks may be triggered by various stimuli including a respiratory infection, airborne irritants, allergens, animal dander, and even foods.

15. Biomedical knowledge of asthma suggests that it is an allergic reaction.

16. Psychological states may work to precipitate, intensify, or prolong an attack, but they do not appear to explain asthma.

17. Management of asthma typically is accomplished through use of bronchodilators and dilator drugs.

18. A primary focus of behavioral education research has been to help parents and patient identify the triggers for attacks and then to reduce the chances of encountering a known trigger.

19. Cystic fibrosis is a systemic disorder with a core feature of pulmonary deterioration and build up of lung mucus.

20. Recent identification of a CF gene on chromosome 7 may bring new treatment methods to prevent the appearance of CF.

21. Treatment of CF includes chest and back palpation, bronchodilators, diet changes, dietary supplements, and enzyme replacement therapy, among other techniques.

22. Families with a CF child seem to cope well with the disruption in routines. The need for high parental involvement can put a strain on the marriage.

23. Insulin dependent diabetes mellitus (IDDM) typically has an early onset. IDDM is associated with retinopathy, neuropathy, and nephropathy.

24. The symptoms of diabetes are polydipsia (frequent drinking), polyuria (frequent urination), and polyphagia (increased food intake).

25. Diabetic patients run the risk of hyperglycemia, a build-up of glucose in the blood stream. Without insulin, patients may suffer from diabetic ketoacidosis and go into a diabetic coma.

26. Medical management of diabetes focuses on holding glucose levels at normal levels and preventing complications such as retinopathy or neuropathy.

27. Behavioral methods usually focus on helping the diabetic comply with the program, but they may also focus on better management of diet and exercise, both of which have positive effects by stabilizing glucose levels.

28. Psychological processes such as self-efficacy, control, and knowledge can influence the diabetic's adjustment, but these variables are sensitive to age progression and level of cognitive maturation.

Key Words

autosomal recessive disease
chronic illness
diabetic ketoacidosis
hyperglycemia
hypoglycemia
nephropathy
neuropathy
polydipsia
polyphagia
polyuria
retinopathy

Study Questions

1. What are the major health issues for children? How may the family and school system influence the child to develop skills and knowledge in these areas?

2. What impact do chronic illnesses in children have on their families? What are the psychological consequences for the patient, siblings, and parents? Is the outcome generally negative or positive?

3. Describe the basic symptoms of the three disorders presented. What biomedical explanations are available for the causes of these disorders?

4. Are psychological processes important to the origin, course, or prognosis of any of these three disorders?

5. What biomedical treatments are available for these disorders? What problems exist in implementing treatments for children with these illnesses?

6. What role do cognitive-behavioral treatments play in managing any of these disorders?

Class Projects

1. Survey community specialists who may be most experienced with the disorders described. If possible, have one or more address the class on current developments in understanding etiology and treatment.

Suggested Readings

Branson, S. M., & Craig, K. D. (1988). Children's spontaneous strategies for coping with pain: A review of the literature [Special issue: Child and adolescent health]. *Canadian Journal of Behavioural Science, 20,* 402–412.

Donnelly, J. E., Donnelly, W. J., & Thong, Y. H. (1987). Parental perceptions and attitudes toward asthma and its treatment: A controlled study. *Social Science and Medicine, 24,* 431–437.

Eiser, C. (1990). *Chronic childhood disease: An introduction to psychological theory and research.* Cambridge: Cambridge University Press.

Hobbs, N., & Perrin, J. M., (Gen. Eds.). (1985). *Issues in the care of children with chronic illness.* San Francisco: Jossey-Bass.

Larsen, G. L (1992). Asthma in children. *The New England Journal of Medicine, 326,* 1540–1545.

Saile, H., Burgmeier, R., & Schmidt, L. R. (1988). A meta-analysis of studies on psychological preparation of children facing medical procedures. *Psychology and Health, 2,* 107–132.

Siegal, M. (1988). Children's knowledge of contagion and contamination as causes of illness. *Child Development, 59,* 1353–1359.

WEBSITES   *Children's Health, Diabetes, Asthma, Cystic Fibrosis*

ADDRESS	DESCRIPTION
http://www.starbright.org/people/index.html	☆ A partnership of high-tech companies and entertainment industry with pediatric health care to help sick children while hospitalized
http://www.diabetes.org	☆ American Diabetes Association—extensive resources with guide to Internet sites
http://www.cdc.gov/nccdphp/ddt/ddthome.htm	Center for Disease Control's Diabetes Home Page
http://www.castleweb.com/diabetes/index.html	On-line Community for Children with Diabetes
http://www.mdcc.com/fourstar.htm	☆ Diabetes Monitor—Provides links to fourstar sites for diabetes
http://129.171.43.143/SPP/	Society of Pediatric Psychology, Section V of Division 12 of the APA—Clinical Psychology
http://www.phd.msu.edu/cf/fam.html	A family centered guide to genetic testing for cystic fibrosis
http://web.idirect.com/~cprprog/diabetes/services.htm	Diabetes International Services, FAQs and links
http://www.ginasthma.com	Global Initiative for Asthma
http://www.pslgroup.com/ASTHMA.HTM	Doctors Guide to Asthma Information & Resources

CHAPTER 16

Aging and Health: Myths, Realities, and Actions

The fantasies that children play out in their minds seldom may be realized. No matter. They are only the fuel of hope, matches that ignite an inner flame and drive the youthful heart on. They are straws that stir the mind to think of the impossible, goads to try.

For me, those fantasies often revolved around the romantic legends of the Wild West: Dodge City, Boot Hill, Wyatt Earp. Yes, I admit, my first heroes were the cowboys who rode through the black and white television movies of the early 1950s. The settings were often wilderness areas where pioneers worked to carve out an existence, usually against formidable odds, often succeeding in spite of the worst that both nature and humanity could throw at them. A recent movie, *Far and Away,* tells such a story, evokes kindred feelings, and has some uncanny parallels to the true story I want to tell.

I outgrew my romantic fantasies, as most children do. Still, as the press of classes, committees, writing, and the bustle of city life weigh on me, a certain feeling surges inside me. I long then for the solitude granted by those vast western plains. I long for a place just down the road from Dodge City, where my only companion is a lone hawk circling a sentinel cottonwood standing tall over an old homestead.

I do not know what H. D. and Anna Weikal's dreams were when they were growing up. Even as my fantasies took root, I was just getting to know them. They lived at a time, in a place, that required hardiness of body and soul to survive. As I look back, it seems they wrote a living pioneer script. Now I know their story, and I know so many stories they could tell. Only later have I come to realize that they had become my living heroes.

I suspect H. D. and Anna had no pretensions to fame or status, yet they lived their lives with a certain nobility of purpose and clarity of vision. Through their many years together, no matter the toil or hardship, their wit helped them laugh at adversity, even smile at calamity. And always, they seemed to find ways to seize life's full measure of happiness.

In the early 1800s, H. D. and Anna's great-grandparents were part of a great migration from the eastern seaboard to what was then the rugged territory of western Pennsylvania. The homestead acts that drew many to this frontier, though, were already calling thousands to the great western plains. The blue haze of gunpow-

der had barely cleared from the civil war when Anna's family settled in Miami County south of Kansas City. In 1881, H.D.'s family left Pennsylvania for Kansas where they homesteaded southeast of Dodge City.

When she was barely a teenager, Anna went with her father and two brothers to Enid in the panhandle of Oklahoma. That was as far as the train could take them. There, they bought wagons and supplies and headed farther west in pursuit of land for a family farm. They slept in tents, and Anna cooked off the back of a wagon for the crew. They were there only a short while before harsh conditions conspired to doom their efforts. Taking their few belongings, they found their way to a beautiful valley in the south central hills of Kansas, and a meeting that joined H. D. and Anna as husband and wife in 1915.

His given name was Harry David, his family called him Hal, and his friends always knew him as H. D. To me, he was always and only Grandpa. He was the man who set me at a very tender age on top of Romeo, a tall, sometimes rank palamino gelding, and kindled in me an abiding love of horses.

At the turn of the century and only a teenager, Grandpa became enchanted with the new technology of cameras and film development. Later, he worked hard to get the first phone lines into the valley. When the terrible dust bowl years hit, he found ways to manage the land so that it would not blow away. When rains were plentiful and flash floods threatened to wash the soil away, he followed his intuition and a good eye for slopes. Then, he terraced the land to prevent erosion.

Together, Grandpa and Grandma raised five children (my mother their third), and they swelled with pride as grandchildren and great-grandchildren arrived. They survived the unpredictable, sometimes wild, erratic cycles of good and bad weather. They endured fickle cycles of modest to poor crop prices. Throughout their lives, they were avid readers and travelers. They watched with interest the dawn of the motor age. Already nearing normal retirement age, they were no less excited to see the first step on the moon.

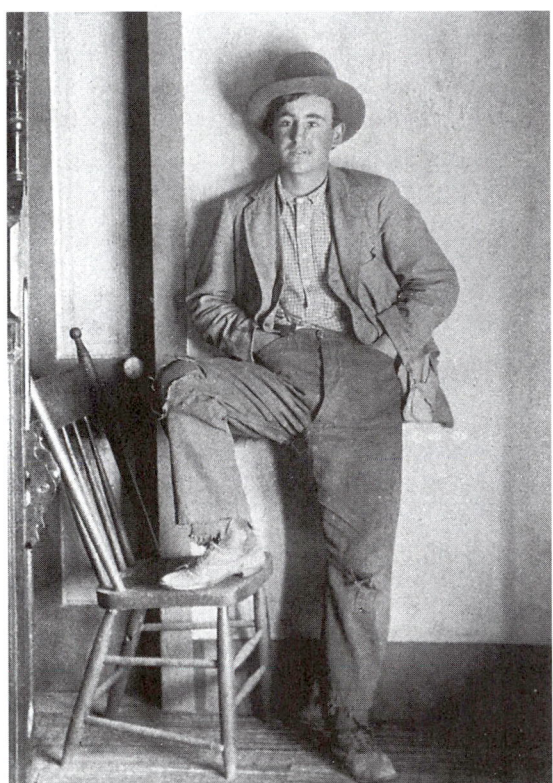

FIGURE 16.1   H. D. Weikal, Grandpa, as a teenager near the turn of the century, in a photographic self-portrait.

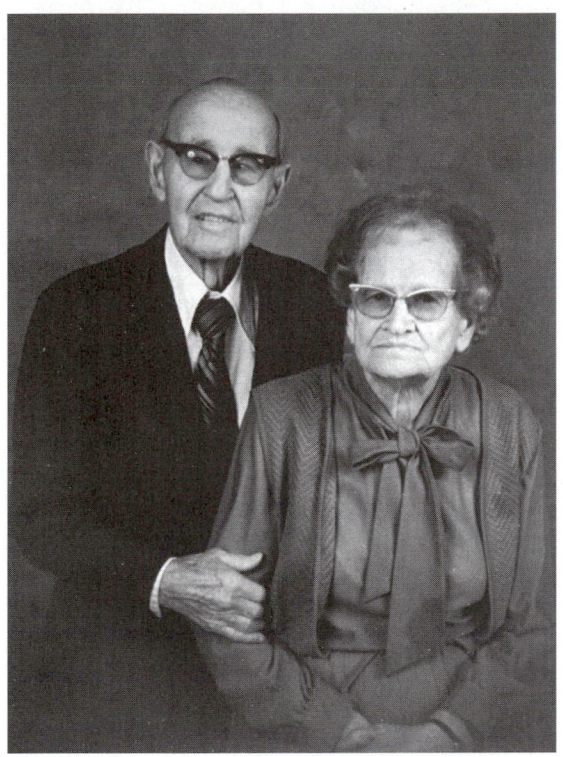

FIGURE 16.2   H. D. and Anna Weikal near the time of Grandpa's 100th birthday.

Far beyond the time when many people position themselves in rockers to wait the inevitable, they were still working and living independently on their homestead. Even into their mid to late 80s, Grandma tended her garden, and Grandpa still turned the soil or racked hay bales. With his son, Willis, he shared oversight of the cattle operation into his 90s. At 92, he still drove his old yellow Buick into town, often at 80 miles an hour, to get supplies or parts to repair a piece of broken machinery.

As I watched Grandpa and Grandma grow older, they provided many object lessons in aging. Their steps were nearly always sure even as age made them more frail. Their minds remained alert and inquisitive, their wit sharpened from years of activity, even as memories became more troublesome to retrieve. And their spirit, their indomitable spirit, clothed them with an aura of timeless energy, even as it was apparent that time had tempered their pace. But

always, above all, I remember how they aged with grace, never complaining of time's tracings on their brows. Perhaps Robert Browning had people like them in mind when he wrote, "Grow old along with me! The best is yet to be, the last of life for which the first was made."

Grandma died at 94 years just shortly after suffering a second broken hip. She had survived to this time in spite of a broken hip years earlier, then breast cancer and chemotherapy at the age of 87. I visited Grandma when she was still on chemotherapy. She had lost a lot of weight, could take only tea and toast because most other foods made her sick. Yet, she was delighted to see me. Even as she sank into the couch in exhaustion, worried that another bout of nausea might overtake her, she could still smile and somehow crack a small joke that had just crossed her mind.

Later, on the morning Grandma died, we gathered to help with funeral details. Grandpa spoke quietly, deliberately, always assuredly still head of the family, of the great good fortune that had been theirs to share. He revealed one fact that, to my knowledge, if some had noted, no one had spoken before: From the time he and Grandma married in 1915 until that day in 1987, not a single child or grandchild or great-grandchild had died.

Grandpa suffered from typhoid fever as a child, and for all his remaining years, his heart kept a measured pace of 45 beats per minute. When he was fitted with a pacemaker at 99, he became something of a medical legend as one of the oldest people to ever have such a procedure. Approaching 103, he needed a part-time house-keeper. His son's family looked in on him daily to help with his needs and make sure he was all right. And he did need help with one chore in particular. That was when he had to dial into the medical center and, through a modem, put his heart on line so the medical staff could monitor his vital signs. Still, he tended to many of his own needs and lived in his own home until just weeks before his death.

I was not there when Grandpa died. In some ways, I am thankful I was not, because it is his life, his and Grandma's, that we remember and celebrate, and to whose memory I have dedicated this book. Even now in my mind's eye, I often see that lonely hawk circling the sentinel cottonwood east of their homestead. Then I imagine it is bearing up with exquisite grace the spirit of the man and woman who walked that land for nearly a century.

Aging: Definitions, Issues, and Perspectives

America's pop culture has demythologized many cherished customs and institutions. Still, the emphasis on staying young has created unfortunate myths about growing old. For one, it has made growing old something to be feared. Most aging myths seem to be spawned by extreme examples, should we say horror stories of physical disability, sexual incapacity, and mental senility that can occur among a few aged individuals. At times, it seems these myths created a lower caste of the elderly, second-class citizens to be looked down on. Jensen and Oakley (1982–83) call this negative stereotyping ageism, and they suggested that it "has a significantly detrimental effect on the quality of life, morbidity, and premature death" (p. 20).

Parallel to my experience with my grandparents, society now sees many examples of the high quality of life the elderly achieve. They enjoy freedom to pursue avocations, hobbies, and travels that perhaps could not be done during their early adult life. This is not to ignore or minimize the plight of many elderly who live on fixed incomes with minimal housing, food, and medical care. It is only a heightened awareness of the important and special place older people have in modern society.

The Science of Aging: Terms, Research, and Vocations

Parallel to heightened social awareness, there is increased emphasis on research in aging with a rapid, now exponential increase in the rate of published work (Woodruff-Pak, 1988). This work has spawned a small technical vocabulary that needs definition.

To begin, **aging** is the process of growing old. It is not something that happens just to the old; it is a lifelong process. Further, aging is not a unitary process. Diane Woodruff-Pak (1988) pointed out that three forces—biological, psychological, and sociological—interact to determine aging. The body may begin to deteriorate. This is biological aging. Still, the person may continue to mature cognitively and creatively. This is psychological aging. In the social arena, the person may continue to extend their network of friends and civic involvements. This is sociological aging. The process of aging does not follow the same trajectory in all three domains.

Senescence describes the decline in efficient function and deterioration in structure that leads to accelerated mortality. **Biological senescence** is the upper limit of life if it runs its full course without premature damage. If all causes of heart disease were brought under control, for example, life expectancy would be raised by 11 years. **Senility** is a severe loss of physical and mental ability that may (but does not inevitably) occur among the elderly.

Life expectancy is technically the age at which 50 per cent of a group of cohorts still survive. Currently, life expectancy in the United States is about 75 years. A related term, **life span,** refers to the maximum age attained by the last surviving member of the cohort group. Human life span is in the 110 to 113 year range (Cunningham & Brookbank, 1988), although there are claims of longevity in the 120 (Mazess & Forman, 1979) to 160 age range (Benet, 1974). The longest-living person with a valid birth record was a Japanese man who died in 1986 at the age of 120 years 7 months.

Gerontology, a word that goes back to the Greek *geronto* or *geron* (meaning an old man), is the scientific study of the process of aging. Gerontology focuses as much on the triumphs as it does the struggles of older people. Several disciplines have vested interest in the study of aging. A psychologist interested in aging could receive training in a special doctoral program and become a **geropsychologist** (Reid & Willis, 1991). Health psychology has a branch called **geriatric health psychology** devoted to understanding and developing treatment strategies for the special needs of older people.

The Aging Boom: Culture, Gender, and Centenarians

Entering the 21st century, the world's population has a much different look than it did entering the 20th century. At the beginning of this century, life expectancy for U.S. citizens was a little over 47 years (Barsky, 1988; U.S. Bureau of the Census, 1991). Now, life-expectancy is 75 years but with notable variation.[1] The shortest life-expectancy is 65 years for African American

males, and the longest is 79 years for white women. In Israel, life expectancy for men is about 73, and for women 77 (Shuval, 1990). Nearly 50 years ago in Shanghai, a citizen might live to 35 years. Life expectancy there rose to 75 years by 1989.

In some developing countries, life expectancy is still relatively short. In most of India and Africa, for example, life expectancy at birth is from 48 to 54 years for men, and 53 to 61 years for women (Caldwell, 1993; Wahlqvist & Kouris, 1990). In Ethiopia, a man might expect to live to 38 years, a woman to 41 years. This is currently the shortest life expectancy among the world's nations. Notably, it is even shorter than life expectancy in the United States in 1840.

At the turn of the century, the number of people over 65 years of age made up about 4% of the population. As we enter the 21st century, the number of people over 65 will make up more than 13% of the total population. The population over 65, elderly ethnic minorities in particular, is among the fastest growing groups in the United States (Wray, 1992). There are now more than 32,000 centenarians in the United

---

[1] This nearly 30-year increase in life expectancy in less than 90 years is noteworthy. In the previous 125 years, there had been only a 12-year increase in life expectancy based on a life expectancy of 35 years in 1776.

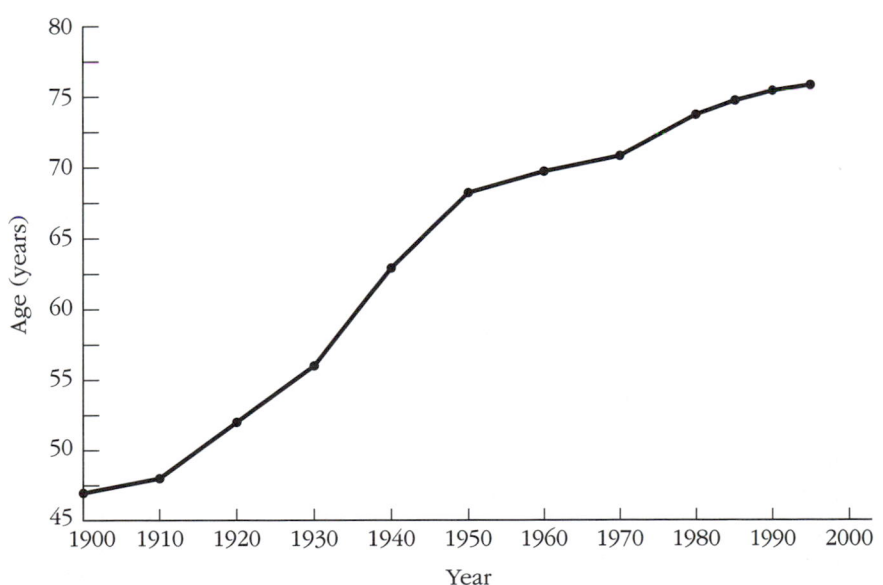

FIGURE 16.3   Life expectancy at birth, 1900–1995 (Source: U.S. Census data).

TABLE 16.1   Estimates and projections of the total population in the United States and the percentage of elderly, 1900–2030 (from Spence, 1989).

YEAR	TOTAL POPULATION	OVER 65	%
1900	75,600,000	3,100,000	4.1
1940	132,300,000	9,000,000	6.8
1960	181,000,000	16,600,000	9.2
1970	203,100,000	20,300,000	10.0
1980	228,000,000	25,600,000	11.2
2000	268,500,000	34,900,000	13.0
2030	304,700,000	64,600,000	21.2

States (Spence, 1989). Estimates suggest that the percentage of elderly Americans may grow to about 21% by 2030. (See Table 16.1.) Socially, this situation has the potential to create significant pressures on any welfare or health system.

Much of the aging boom is due to declining birth rates, reduced infant mortality, control if not eradication of communicable diseases, improvements in nutrition, and reductions in malnutrition (Gordon, 1987). Geriatric specialists believe society will continue to eliminate the causes of premature death until death will be purely natural—in other words, due to biological senescence. Fries (1980) estimated the upper limit of natural life expectancy at about 85 years, a figure that several countries (Japan, for example) are already approaching.

Biology of Aging: Structural and Functional Change

Aging is a part of the lifelong process of maturation. Some believe it is a program genetically set at conception that marches to an inevitable end with biological senescence unless interrupted by premature death. This idea, of course, assumes that a biological definition of aging is sufficient. The changes that occur in aging typically become noticeable at about 40, but they may appear in some people who are only in their early thirties. Others may not show signs of aging until into their fifties. The emphasis here is on biological changes. Yet it is important to make a key point: Even when biological changes appear, they do not necessarily mean dramatic changes in lifestyle or the quality of life that many older people enjoy.

Biological changes in aging typically reflect both changes in structure and function. The following discussion emphasizes structural changes sometimes and functional changes at other times. In reality, though, most structural changes lead to functional changes as well.

Structural Changes: Skin, Strength, and Vital Capacity

Structural changes include changes in skin, height, weight, muscles, and thorax. The skin becomes thinner and less elastic due to cross-linking of collagen.[2] Cutaneous pain sensitivity declines about 12%, probably because of a change in the skin's pain receptors and greater heat dispersion in aged skin (Cunningham & Brookbank, 1988).

Another age-related skeletal problem, osteoporosis, results from losing bone calcium. **Osteoporosis** is characterized by decreased skeletal mass and increased bone fragility (Malasanos, Barkauskas, & Stoltenberg-Allen, 1990). Women, especially postmenopausal women, suffer more from this condition than men. By age 65, one-third of women will have suffered a bone fracture due to osteoporosis. A 70-year-old woman has only about 70% of her normal bone calcium. By age 81, one-third of women and one-sixth of men will have suffered a hip fracture, an event that is often terminal (Rowe & Kahn, 1987). Osteoporosis can be partially

---

[2] Collagen is an intercellular body material that provides support to body structures such as skin tissue, muscles, and brain cells. A crude analogy may help explain collagen cross-linking. Imagine several strands of human hair laying on a table. Each by itself is very flexible. Spray the strands with a lacquer hair spray and they stick together. The more strands that bond together, the more rigid the cluster is.

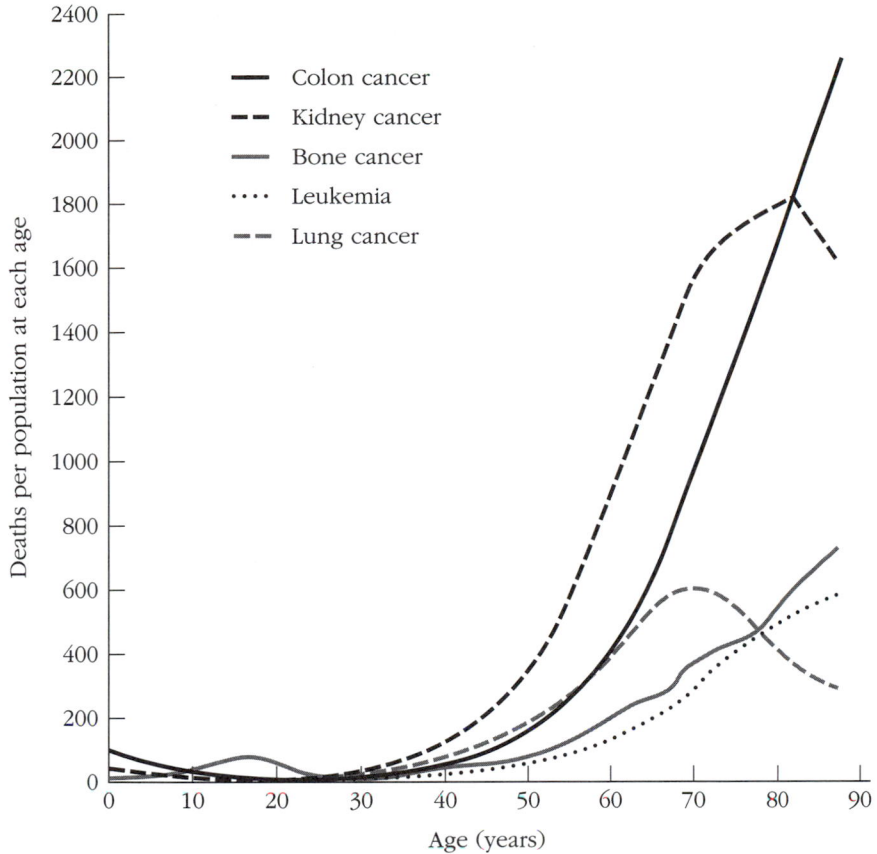

FIGURE 16.4   *Age-specific death rates for various types of cancer. Deaths are plotted with age on the abscissa and the rate of deaths per million population on the ordinate (from Kohn, 1978).*

reversed with calcium supplements. Yet women must begin thinking about it around 30 years of age in order to prevent significant problems later (Klohn & Rogers, 1991).

Body composition changes because of increasing fat deposits and lower total body water. Muscles gradually deteriorate losing both tone and strength. Muscle mass declines primarily due to atrophy. Total fiber mass loss may reach 30% between ages 30 and 80, but up to 70 years, loss in strength may be no more than 10% to 20%.

Occupation and lifestyle both influence strength. People who work in physically demanding jobs or exercise regularly can maintain tone and strength until late in life. Even formerly sedentary 60- and 70-year-old people can increase strength by beginning a regular exercise program. Also, they can significantly increase **maximum oxygen consumption,** which is the capacity to deliver oxygen to the muscles.

The lungs lose elasticity (a structural change) but the effect is to make breathing harder (a functional change). This leads to an increase in the size of the thorax. Loss of lung elasticity has a negative effect on **maximum breathing capacity,** the amount of air that can be moved into and out of the lungs in a given period. Loss of lung elasticity also lowers vital capacity, the amount of air that can be taken in with forced deep inhalation and move out with forced expiration. Between 40 and 70, vital capacity may drop to 60% of original volume (Spence, 1989). Practically speaking, these changes reduce the oxygen reaching the lungs, lowering the older person's capacity for work.

Functional Changes: Brain, Sight, and Hearing

Functional changes occur, with few exceptions, in almost every body system. We probably worry most about the heart and the brain. The brain atrophies in size and loses about 10% weight (up to 90 years) with a related increase in the fluid-filled cavities. The number of neurons decreases but the loss is not equal throughout the brain. The cerebellum loses about 25% of its cells. This may contribute to the older person's difficulties with fine motor movement and coordination (Spence, 1989). One distressing age-related CNS disease is **Parkinson's disease,** a chronic, progressive disorder that reveals itself in muscle tremors and rigidity.

In the hippocampus, neural tangles appear from collagen cross-linking. For most people,

this means only a gradual decline in memory power. But in extreme cases, such as senile dementia and Alzheimer's disease, memory loss is severe. More will be said of Alzheimer's disease later.

Information processing, cataracts, and hearing loss   Ocular problems, such as cataracts and glaucoma, also increase. A **cataract** is a cloudy or opaque lens caused by continuing production of fibers that make up the lens. This interferes with light transmission to the retina, a situation that can be partly corrected through surgery. The prevalence of cataracts in the U.S. population jumps dramatically with age. Approximately 400,000 people develop cataracts each year. About 50% of people aged 65 to 74 have a cataract, but among those aged 75 to 85, the prevalence jumps to nearly 70% (Special Committee on Aging, 1993).

Glaucoma is an increase in fluid pressure in the eye. The increased pressure shuts off the eye's blood vessels, causing degeneration of the retina. The first sign of glaucoma is a loss of peripheral vision. Glaucoma rarely occurs in people under 40, but becomes more common

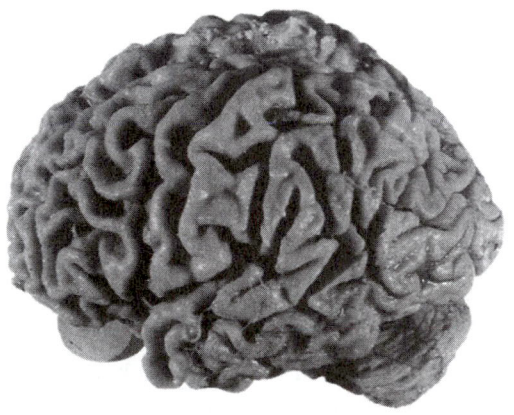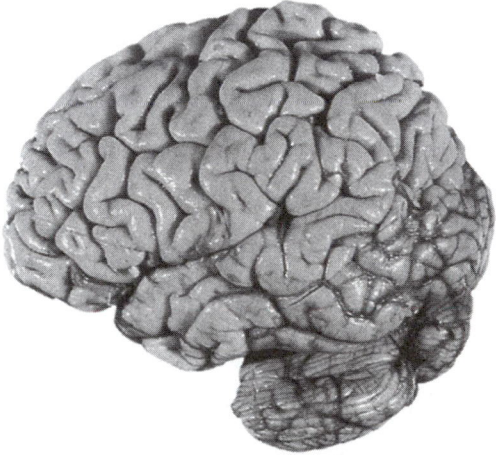

FIGURE 16.5   *The brain on the left shows marked atrophy characteristic of Alzheimer's disease, while the brain on the right is that of a normal person.*

with aging. It occurs about six times more often and begins about 10 years earlier among African Americans than among whites (Sommer et al., 1991). Although glaucoma cannot be cured, it is manageable through stepped treatment consisting of first eye drops, then oral medication, laser treatment, and surgery.

Another blow to information processing is physiological decay in the auditory system and hearing loss, a condition called **presbycusis.** Hearing loss is due mostly to changes in the inner ear related to decreased nutrient supply to the cochlea and degeneration of inner cells. Hearing problems are most disturbing when the person can no longer follow normal conversation. Speech often becomes garbled when distracting background noise or variations in pitch or loudness of the speaker's voice cause dropouts. Some elderly people may show signs of paranoia, revealed in comments that ongoing conversations, not directed to them, are about them.

Sleep disturbances, dream sleep, and apnea

Sleep disturbances can be a serious problem for older people (Prinz, Vitiello, Raskind, & Thorpy, 1990). Insomnia occurs in about 5 to 6% of the population and sleep apnea occurs in about 1 to 4% of the population (Jamieson & Becker, 1992). Older people typically spend more time in bed, but they spend significantly less time in deep sleep.

Sleep apnea leads to disturbed sleep for the sufferer, but it may also produce distress in the sleep partner as well. Imagine what it might be like to hear your sleep partner stop breathing completely, possibly for 45 seconds several times each night. This recurrent cessation in breathing is **sleep apnea.** Typically, the person resumes breathing through a motor struggle and gasping reaction. Sleep apnea is more prevalent in obese males, and prevalence increases with age (Prinz et al., 1990). Presumably, the disorder is caused by functional control problems in nerves that regulate the respiratory process. Another explanation suggests that sleep apnea is related to glottal tissue folds at the opening of the windpipe.

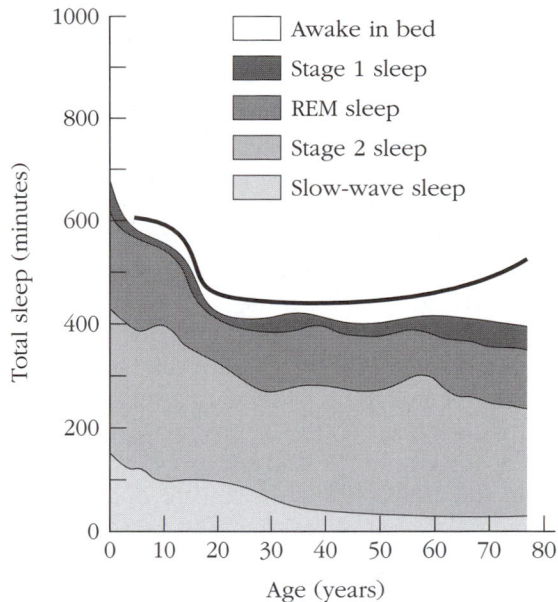

FIGURE 16.6 *The typical pattern of change in sleep stages across the life span. Notice the drop in slow-wave sleep and the increased time awake in bed that typifies sleep in the older population (from Prinz et al., 1990).*

Toileting, incontinence, and control

Among the more embarrassing problems for older people is control over toilet functions. The elderly lose these functions through no lack of willpower but through failure of the body to follow the mind's bidding. Incontinence can be a major blow to the person's pride, mobility, independence, and socializing. The primary control problems are urinary and fecal incontinence.

Urinary incontinence is involuntary loss of urine usually due to the inability to keep the urethral sphincter closed. Loss of control may occur because of defective organs, weakened muscles, or a descending bladder. A recent study revealed that urinary incontinence occurs in 37.7% of older women and 18.9% of older men (Herzog, Brown, Diokno, Normolle, & Brock, 1990). The total number of American adults with urinary control problems may be close to 10 million. By comparison, about 10% to 15% of 5-year-old children suffer from enuresis, but this percentage drops to no more than 1% to 2% by about 16 years.

Fecal incontinence is the diminished capacity to control bowel movements voluntarily. It may be caused by loss of neural control over the anal sphincter, or it may result from cancer of the lower bowel. Fecal incontinence is more a problem in long-term patients for whom the incidence may be as high as 60% (Spence, 1989).

Behavioral treatment methods include charting, EMG biofeedback, environmental redesign, and operant retraining. Charting may be used to discover elimination patterns that permit scheduling timely trips to the bathroom, reducing the chances for untimely and embarrassing elimination. Biofeedback may help to reeducate neuromuscular control and thus restore some control over elimination.

Theories of Aging: Programs, Genetics, and Damage

Scientists have devised several theories of aging that in part follow our knowledge of three structural parts of the body.[3] First, the body has cells that divide and reproduce as long as the person lives, but there may be limits to the cells' ability to reproduce. These limits suggest one theory of aging. Second, cells called **postmitotic cells** divide in the embryonic stage, but they cannot divide after birth. Nerve and muscle cells fit in this group. These cells are subject to wear and tear. The second theory proposes the body loses these cells through deterioration and injury. Since these cells cannot be replaced, the older body cannot function as effectively. After a certain point, death occurs. Third, the body has a significant amount of tissue, dubbed noncellular tissue, located between the cells. One major intercellular material is **collagen.** Collagen supports the skin, bones, tendons, and cartilage, but it also becomes cross-linked. According to the third theory, cross-linking causes problems in multiple body systems that signify aging.

Biomedical Aspects of Aging: Genes, Cells, and Progeria

At the core of biological aging theories is the notion that the genetic code controls body processes that influence longevity. There are several arguments for genetic aging control.

Family studies show that longevity tends to run in families. In monozygotic twins, death ages are more similar than among dizygotic twins (McGue, Vaupel, Holm, & Harvald, 1993). McGue and his colleagues estimated the heritability of life span at 0.333. This estimate suggests that genetics contributes only moderately to longevity and that other factors contribute substantially to longevity.

A second argument for genetic control of aging comes from work on cellular aging. The assumption is that damage to DNA, errors in transcription of DNA, or errors in protein synthesis contribute to aging of the cell. Observations of laboratory cultures show that most cells have a small number (perhaps 50 to 60) of divisions possible. This is called the **Hayflick phenomenon,** named after the person who discovered it (Hayflick, 1976). To oversimplify, the older the cell, the fewer divisions remain. There is one notable exception to this rule: Cancer cells appear to be immortal.

Exchanging nuclei between different age cells reveals that the nucleus controls the aging process. A young nucleus transplanted to old cytoplasm rejuvenates the cell, but an old nucleus placed in young cytoplasm does not rejuvenate the cell.

An extreme example of aging and genetics is a rare disease known as **progeria,** a disorder that produces rapid aging. Progeria patients usually die of heart attacks at a median age of 12 years. Progeria appears in just 1 of about 8 million live births. Patients look normal for a

---

[3] In actuality, there are many theories of aging, too numerous to describe in this work. Rather than being exhaustive, then, this scheme is a convenient way of condensing the wide array of aging theories to a representative sample.

short time after birth, but then profound changes begin to appear. Growth slows dramatically, and dramatic hair loss occurs. Height and weight both decline, and subcutaneous fat is lost, allowing veins to protrude.

In summary, it seems indisputable that genetic factors influence the aging process. Still, scientists do not completely understand how the genotype works its way through body systems to produce aging.

Nongenetic Aging Theories: Free Radicals, Scavengers, and Vitamins

Some theories choose to focus on body chemistry or tissues that might be involved in aging.

One theory suggests that free radicals alter cells and lead to death. **Free radicals** are cellular chemicals with unpaired electrons formed during cell processes that depend on oxygen (Spence, 1989). They react chemically with other cell substances, especially unsaturated fats.

Certain chemicals act as scavengers to pick up free radicals almost as fast as they form. The primary scavenger is an enzyme called superoxide dismutase (SOD). Other cell scavengers include the antioxidant vitamins C and E. Taking daily doses of these vitamins presumably retards build-up of free radicals and slows aging. Balin (1982) reviewed the free radical theory, though, and concluded that it is not possible to determine whether free radicals are the cause or the result of aging.

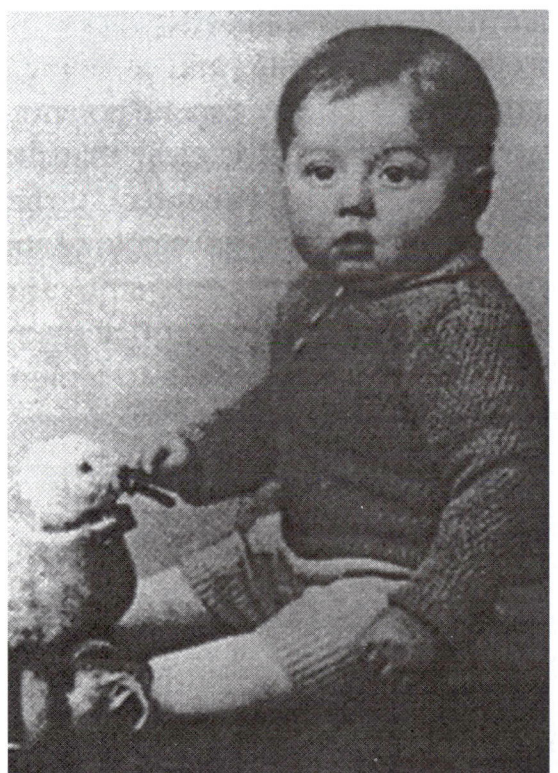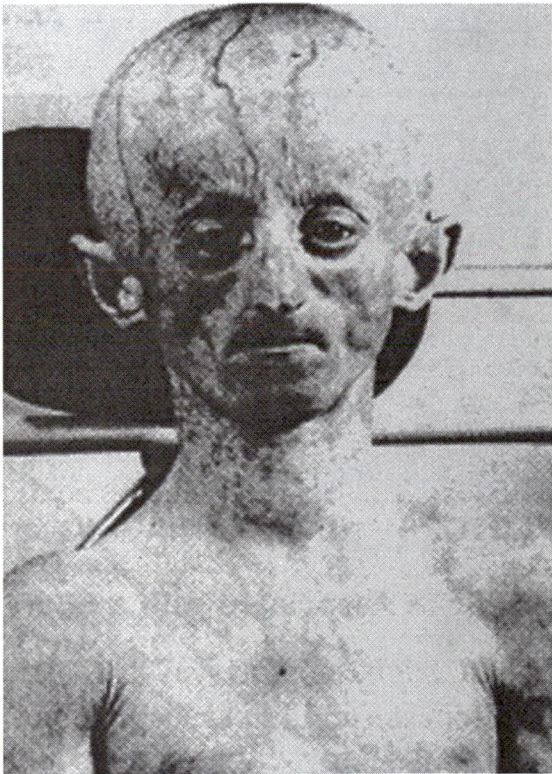

FIGURE 16.7   *A patient with progeria, or accelerated aging: On the left at 10 months of age, the boy appears normal; shown on the right at age 14.5 years, the same boy has baldness, protruding veins, and the appearance of a very aged person (from DeBusk, 1972).*

Psychosocial Theories of Aging: Life Crises and Tasks

As we have just seen, biomedical scientists constructed theories of aging using various physical models. Yet another group of theories comes from behavioral scientists who think about aging as a psychosocial process. Their theories embrace the idea that older people experience tremendous pressures while aging. Such pressures come from role changes and crucial losses. Elderly people may lose jobs, income, pride, health, and companionship.

Perhaps the best known psychosocial theory of aging comes from the work of psychoanalyst Erik Erikson. Erikson (1968) believed that all people pass through eight developmental stages in their quest for identity. Further, he believed that each stage has a "developmental crisis evoked by the necessity to manage new encounters within a given time allowance" (p. 103). Table 16.2 shows these stages, their approximate age range, and the related crisis. Erikson's last two stages deal specifically with aging.

The seventh stage in Erikson's scheme is middle adulthood. The developmental crisis is a

TABLE 16.2   *Erikson's eight stages in the life cycle and the development crisis to be resolved.*

AGE (IN YEARS)	LIFE STAGE	DEVELOPMENTAL CRISIS
0–2	trust vs. mistrust	Infants learn to trust people if their needs are met or to be distrustful if their needs are not met.
2–4	autonomy vs. shame and doubt	Toddlers learn independence if they are able to control their bodies, but they experience shame and doubt if they fail.
5–7	initiative vs. guilt	In the process of learning many new skills, preschoolers must also learn to control their impulses without becoming overly inhibited and guilt ridden.
8–12	competence vs. inferiority	As children learn many new skills, they should also come to view themselves as competent persons, but they may suffer from low self-esteem instead if they are compared negatively to others.
13–22	identity vs. role confusion	Adolescents struggle to integrate various roles. If successful, they emerge with a consistent self-identity. Otherwise, they have role confusion.
23–30	intimacy vs. isolation	During early adulthood, people must learn how to form and manage deep and intimate relationships, else they become isolated.
31–50	generativity vs. stagnation	In middle adulthood, people assume both family and social duties. These duties include helping children to become responsible citizens. Failing this, people become self-absorbed and stagnant.
51 plus	integrity vs. despair	In late adulthood, people review their lives, seeking answers to basic questions of meaning and worth. With positive answers, people face the future, including death, with integrity; otherwise, with despair.

generativity or stagnation crisis. During this time, adults typically peak in productivity, creativity, and social-mindedness. Some people may withdraw from job, family, and social challenges, while some may become completely self-absorbed in personal needs and activities. If unchecked, these tendencies lead to stagnation.

The eighth and final stage Erikson called later adulthood. This period brings major changes in lifestyle and quality of life. There is retirement, loss of income, declining physical ability, death of siblings and peers, and preparation for one's own death. Typically, people take stock of life's achievements and weigh them against failures and missed opportunities. They may ask basic questions about the meaning of life in general and the impact of their lives in particular. The crisis to be resolved is to maintain integrity in the face of change and the prospect of death, or to fall into despair. The person's unique experiences with aging, personal beliefs about death, and methods of coping with crises in previous stages will push the person to either integrity or despair.

Psychosocial Changes in Aging: Perception, Memory, and Mastery

The age-related biological changes described earlier may alter basic psychological processes such as perceptual-motor speed and memory, among others. Even when the biological change does not have a direct effect on cognitive processes, it may alter the person's self-concept and influence mood. Imagine elderly people who can no longer move freely in their community because of physical incapacity. Perhaps they cannot drive because of failing eyesight, or they cannot walk because of frailty. Many elderly people have difficulty accepting these limitations. Sensing these growing limits, they may suffer short periods of mild to moderate depression. This section will briefly describe several age-related psychosocial changes, as

well as one frightening disorder that afflicts some elderly people, Alzheimer's disease.

Sensory-Perceptual Changes

Earlier we noted that visual and auditory sensory processes decline in the elderly. Some of these changes may increase the risk of accidents and injury, both at home and while moving about the person's locale.

Another change is slower **reaction time,** the speed with which a motor movement can be made after the onset of an external signal. Consider the traffic signal that turns yellow as you approach. In a split second, you make several calculations before deciding to stop or go through. In the elderly, the amount of time required to make the judgment and carry out the response takes longer, which also tends to increase the risk of accidents. The elderly typically compensate by driving more cautiously. Differences in reaction time between older and younger people depend on task complexity. With simple tasks, there are few if any differences. As the task becomes more complex, differences are more noticeable and always favor the younger person (Cerella, 1985).

Self-management and behavior modification of sleep apnea   In retirement communities, self-management techniques may prove useful to increase participation in health promoting behaviors. For elderly people living at home, self-management techniques appear to enable them to manage aspects of chronic diseases more efficiently (Clark et al., 1991). These models often use a social-cognitive learning framework and incorporate behavioral, cognitive, and educational components.

Insomnia and sleep apnea may respond to behavior modification (Engle-Friedman et al., 1992).[4] For insomnia, drug therapy produces a more immediate effect (see Kupfer & Reynolds,

---

[4] See Chapter 6 for a more detailed discussion of treatment for sleep disturbances.

1997, for a review of medical/behavioral management of insomnia). Still, stimulus control and relaxation training have greater long-term positive effects (McClusky et al., 1991) and sleep restriction therapy may have the most positive effects (Bliwise, Friedman, Nekich, & Yesavage, 1995). Therapists often combine behavioral techniques with cognitive methods to alter dysfunctional beliefs about sleeplessness (Morin, Kowatch, Barry, & Walton, 1993). This approach also can reduce sleep latency and waking after sleep onset. The goal in treating sleep apnea is to change habits from sleeping on the back to sleeping on the side. This reduces the chances that sleep apnea episodes will occur.

Alzheimer's Disease: Memory, Movement, and Management

Among the more terrifying diseases is Alzheimer's, a neurological disorder that reveals itself only gradually. The recent announcement that former president Ronald Reagan now suffers from Alzheimer's brought the disorder again into the national spotlight. A primary feature is the increasing decay of several mental functions, most notably memory. To diagnose Alzheimer's, the physician must exclude all other causes of senile dementia. Even then, the presence of Alzheimer's remains a guess since it can be confirmed only by autopsy.

As the disease progresses, the person not only loses memory, but cannot carry out simple functions. Tasks that once were routine such as dressing, using a phone, and toileting now become major problems. Alzheimer's patients lose memory for motor movements needed to do basic daily tasks, a condition called **apraxia.** They may go into the bathroom only to forget why they went there in the first place. They may forget names of family members including their spouse. They also show semantic memory disturbances in dealing with concepts (Nebes, 1989).

Alzheimer's patients appear to go through three stages beginning with impairment of

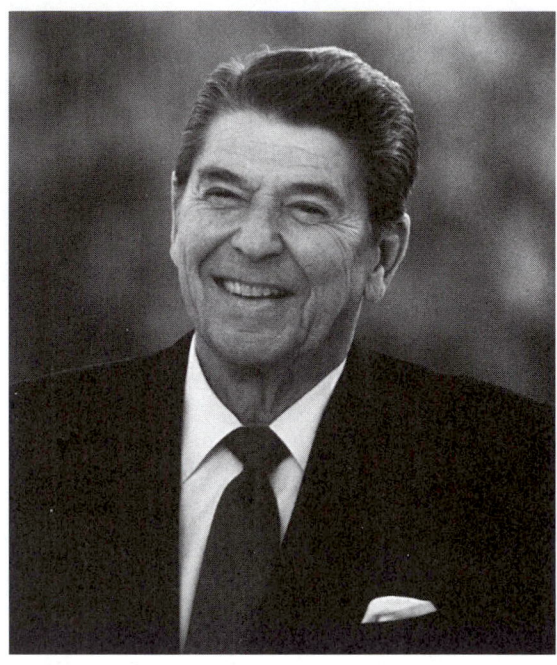

FIGURE 16.8   *Former president Ronald Reagan recently announced that he has Alzheimer's.*

recent memory. In the second stage, they lose several higher cognitive functions such as the ability to read, write (agraphia), and carry out simple calculations. In the third stage, seizures begin, and they lose their ability to speak **(aphasia).** Speech in Alzheimer's patients shows a distinct word-finding problem. Their speech lacks content words even though their grammar is basically correct (Nebes, 1989). The presence of aphasia and apraxia are core diagnostic symptoms of Alzheimer's disease.

Most Alzheimer's patients show the first symptoms in their 50s or 60s. This is typical of early onset Alzheimer's. As aging progresses, more at-risk individuals will show symptoms. Current estimates indicate that 11% of the population over 85 has Alzheimer's.

The pathophysiology of Alzheimer's involves marked degeneration in the function of cholinergic neurons in the brain (Davis et al., 1992). The neurons become tangled because of cross-linking that leaves long threadlike strands made

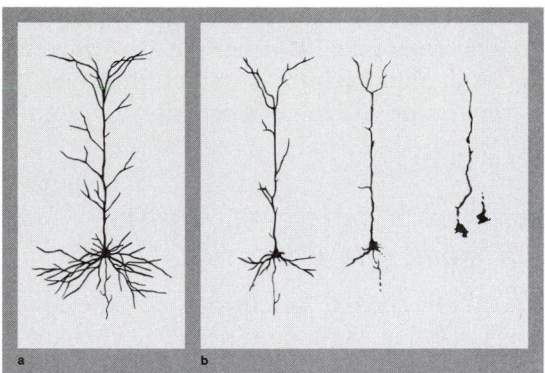

FIGURE 16.9   A view of an Alzheimer's brain showing the large numbers of neurofibrillary tangles or clusters of threadlike proteins (from Kolata, 1986, p. 449).

of amyloid-beta peptides (Yan et al., 1996). This effect can be seen in Figure 16.9. Clusters of degenerating neurons appear unevenly throughout the cerebral cortex. They are especially prominent in the hippocampus, an important region for memory consolidation.

Based on studies of families with histories of Alzheimer's, scientists believe the inheritance pattern is autosomal dominant and not sex-linked (Davies, 1986). The likely culprit is chromosome 21. From Chapter 2, you may recall that Down's syndrome results from a trisomy (three chromosomes) of chromosome 21. Scientists consider this fact significant because Down's patients who live past 40 have almost a 100% chance of developing Alzheimer's. Still, Davies cautions that Alzheimer's may reflect genetic heterogeneity. It could, in other words, result from more than one genetic defect. This is not a minor problem because heterogeneity complicates efforts to track down genetic markers. Finally, heterogeneity could seriously hinder work on treatments to minimize damage or reduce the number of victims.

Investigators estimate that first degree relatives of Alzheimer's patients have a 50% chance of getting the disease, but only if they live to 90 years (Mohs, Breitner, Silverman, & Davis, 1987). This estimate seems to put a seal of doom on family members, but the other side of the coin is more optimistic; that is, most people will die of other causes before Alzheimer's reveals itself. Thus, the individual risk is closer to 17% among siblings, a figure that is close to the rate of senile dementia (25%) in the general population at 90 years. Twin studies show a higher concordance for monozygotic twins, but the age of onset can differ from 6 to 10 years between twins. This finding suggests that nongenetic factors determine the age of onset.

There is no cure for Alzheimer's, but medical research is now conducting trials with drugs (Tacrine, for example) to slow the rate of decline. The strategy is to compensate for the loss of cholinergic neurons by selectively increasing the activity of remaining cells (Davis et al., 1992). Early results show that Tacrine may slow both the decline of mental function and the decline of functional living skills. Unfortunately, Davis's group could detect the slower decline statistically but not clinically, an outcome that must temper enthusiasm at this time.

Alzheimer's families have several counseling needs. Most work with Alzheimer's patients and families has focused on providing support in the face of loss. It may be useful, at least in the earlier stages, to look at ways to get around some memory problems, such as list making. Some investigators have considered ways to retrain memory, but these efforts are not encouraging (Zarit, Zarit, & Reever, 1982).

One serious problem is that Alzheimer's patients reveal a strong pattern of comorbidity for depression (Teri & Wagner, 1992). This tendency has profound effects on both patients and caregivers. Depression appears to have added negative effects on functional skills, behavioral problems, and cognitive impairment. Counseling directed to reduce the impact of depression may be beneficial for all concerned.

One patient behavior that causes great distress for the caregiver is **sundowning.** This is the onset or intensification of delirium typically around sunset or during the night (Prinz et al., 1990).

Numerous pressures of this nature make the primary caregiver vulnerable to serious emotional distress, and the physical pressure of daily caregiving takes its toll. A project led by Jason Dura showed that caregivers for Alzheimer's were as distressed and depressed as caregivers for Parkinson's patients (Dura, Haywood-Niler, & Kiecolt-Glaser, 1990). Both groups of caregivers were more distressed than a matched control group. Either brief psychodynamic psychotherapy or cognitive-behavioral therapy appears to be equally effective in reducing caregiver depression (Gallagher-Thompson & Steffen, 1994). The longer the person has functioned as caregiver, though, the more the cognitive-behavioral approach emerges as a more effective strategy.

Another option is the family support group. These groups provide a sympathetic forum where caregivers can ventilate pent-up frustrations and emotions. Also, people may exchange practical solutions to common problems in caring for the Alzheimer's patient.

Personality and Aging: Mastery, Paranoia, and Depression

Based on certain stereotypes, it is easy to conclude that profound personality changes must occur among the elderly. In fact, such a conclusion would be in gross error. Bluntly stated, there are few meaningful changes in personality among the elderly. Here, I will comment on just three issues.

First, one gender difference appears consistently; that is, men show a decline in masculinity, the tendency to espouse views and express

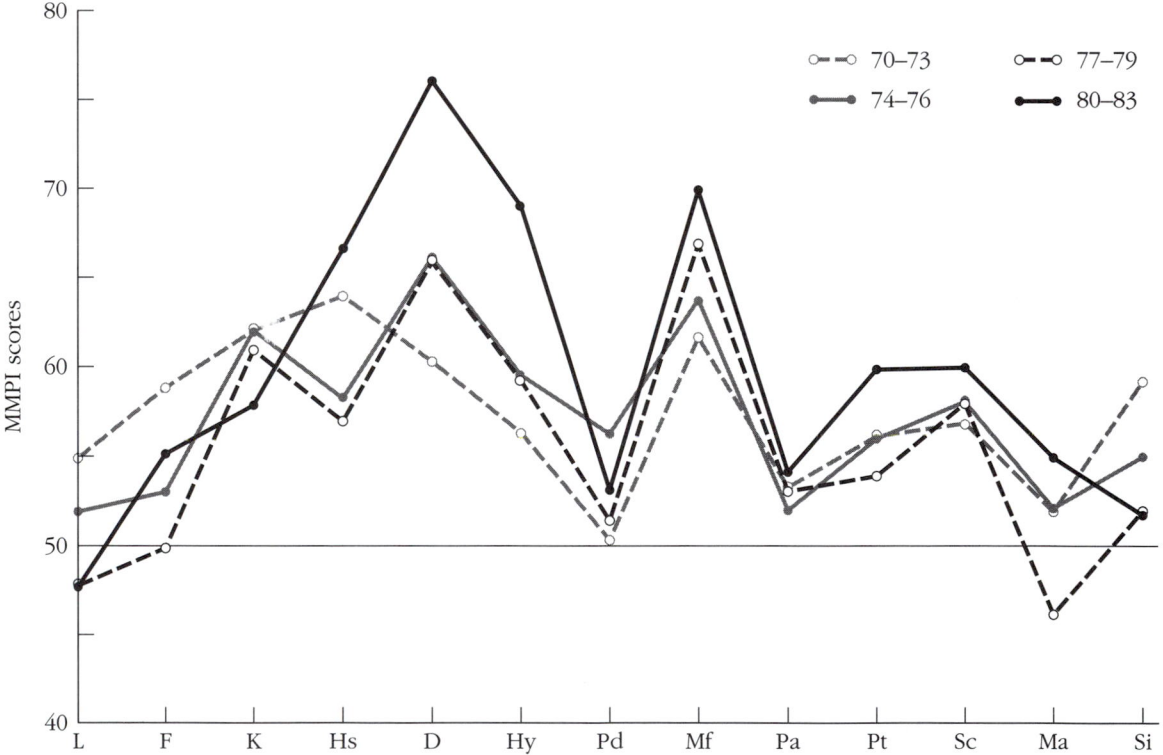

FIGURE 16.10   *Comparison of MMPI scores for 70- to 80-year-old subjects from the Terman study. The depression scale is designated "D" (from Shneidman, 1989).*

emotions in a culturally defined male fashion. Women, on the other hand, tend to show significant increases in their sense of active mastery.

Second, the elderly have slightly increased tendencies to mild paranoia, depression, and hypochondriasis. Paranoia does not typically reach clinical proportions, but depression can be severe including bouts of major depression. When Shneidman (1989) looked at the gifted subjects from the Terman study, he found that MMPI scores were similar for all the 70-year-old subjects. But the 80-year-old group differed markedly on just one scale, the depression scale, as shown in Figure 16.10. A secondary effect with critical repercussions is that depression can confuse diagnostic and assessment procedures, and complicate treatment (Teri & Wagner, 1992).

Finally, it is refreshing to note that the young do not have a monopoly on thrill seeking. In October 1993, national TV reported on a man who decided to bungee jump off a 300-foot tower to celebrate his birthday. He timed it so that during the jump he left his 100th and entered his 101st year (see Figure 16.11).

Social Aspects of Aging: Work, Family, and Service

One of the major changes of aging is retirement. Retirement and several other changes related to aging are involuntary. Most people face forced retirement around 65 years of age, a tradition that goes back to an arbitrary decision made by Otto von Bismarck when very few people lived beyond 65 years. For many people, the end of a career is a blow to their sense of identity, and they may feel bewildered about what direction life should take. Now, however, society has taken steps to ensure that competency, not age, is the criterion for retirement so more people may choose to prolong their careers if they so desire. Margaret Mead, the noted anthropologist, commented, "I expect to die, but I don't plan to retire" (quoted in Howard, 1984, p. 392).

Poverty, health insurance, and health care One customary outcome of retirement is a change in financial status. Living on a limited, fixed income entails cutting back or dropping various healthful activities and security plans.

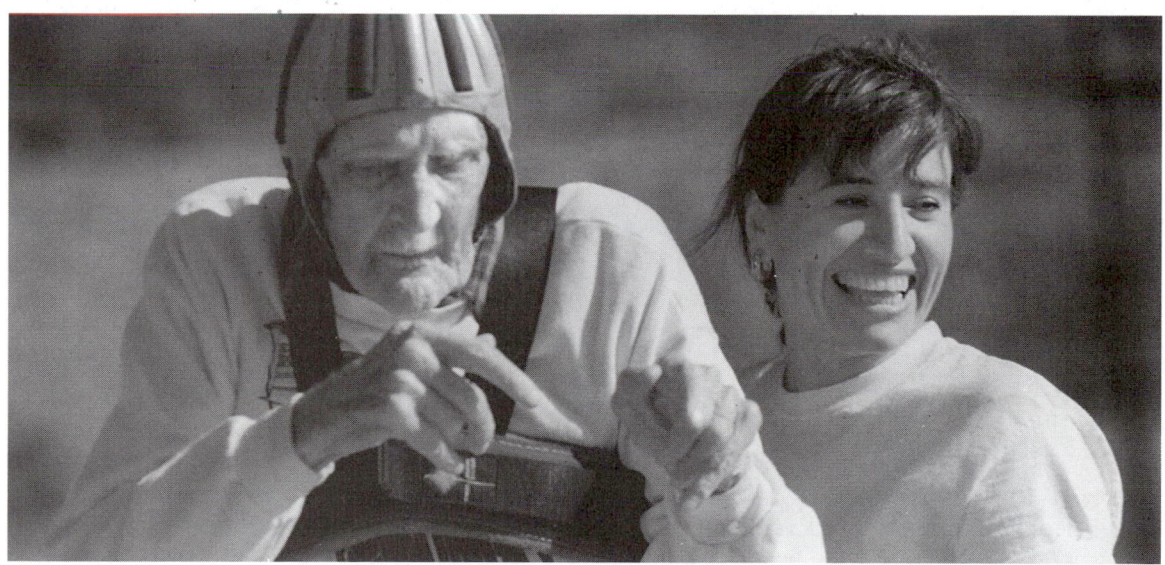

FIGURE 16.11   *This elderly gentleman demonstrates that adventure, even thrill-seeking, knows no age limit.*

These include adequate nutrition, access to health clubs, and adequate health insurance. Reduced health insurance usually results in fewer visits to the doctor and reduced likelihood that early detection may prevent more serious physical problems.

When we consider the socioeconomic status of older Americans, gender and ethnic differences have important implications. In simple terms, older women experience more economic problems than older men, and minority groups experience more economic problems than the white population. The usual marker is the federally defined poverty level. The percentage of white males below the poverty level is about 11% for those over 65 years, but 19% for white women of comparable age. In the same 65+ age group, about 27% of Mexican American males live in poverty, but about 34% of Mexican American women live in poverty. For black males, the percentage below poverty is more than 31%, but for black women it is about 43%. Thus, minorities make up a larger percentage of the lower socioeconomic group. As a result, they usually have less adequate health insurance, and they use health services less often. These statistics suggest that ethnic minorities are still disadvantaged when it comes to access to health care (Wray, 1992).

Friendships, intimacy, and role reversals Aging also brings many changes in social relationships with work associates, family members, and spouse. Older men tend to have more friends, but they depend on their spouse for emotional support. They also have fewer contacts when ill. Older women tend to have more intimate and diverse friends, and they have more contacts when ill (McDaniel & McKinnon, 1993). Women tend to deal with the empty nest better than men do, and they tend to be involved more in keeping family ties strong.

Not too long ago, the person who lived long enough to retire from a job was rare. Now, because of the extended life expectancy, many people live 10 to 20 years following retirement.

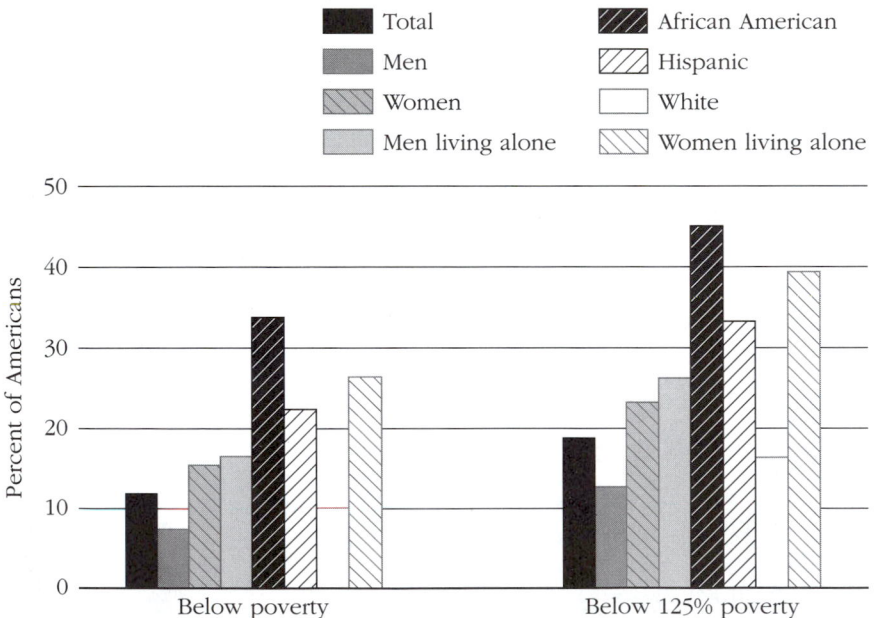

FIGURE 16.12   *The percentage of persons 65 years or older living on incomes below the poverty line is shown by sex, by racial or ethnic group, and by whether they live alone (from Wray, 1992).*

Given the shorter life expectancy for males, though, the living situation is often very different for women. Women tend to marry men who are older. This increases the likelihood that a woman will outlive her husband by several years. Men more often remarry when their mates die, whereas women more often remain single (Burch, 1990). The average older woman, then, is a widow living alone, but the average older male is married and living with his spouse.

Finally, many older adults face a second parenting role. This occurs when they become caregivers to their parents whose health has begun to decline. Typically, it is very hard for adult children to watch their parents' health deteriorate. This caregiver role also entails a form of role reversal; the parent is now the dependent child and the child is now the provider. This change may put great stress on the younger adult. The same stresses occur again when a spouse begins to deteriorate physically and requires increased attention and care.

Retirement communities, nursing homes, and home Popular images of living arrangements for the elderly typically center around the retirement village or the nursing home. Yet a surprisingly large percentage of the elderly live in family settings either independently or with members of their extended family. Estimates vary, but recent survey data suggest that between 75% and 80% of the elderly still receive their primary care at home from family members (Malonebeach & Zarit, 1991). This arrangement may offer a healthy environment, both psychologically and physically (Zheng et al., 1993). Conversely, less than 5% of people over 65 require a hospital or nursing home (Moritz & Ostfeld, 1990).

Still, retirement villages may have some advantages (Sherman, 1975). Data from Sherman's project suggests that people living in retirement communities surrounded by peers of like mind and ability are very satisfied with the quality of their life. They also reported being happier than those who did not have this type of arrangement.

On the other hand, there are continuing concerns about problems with institutional care for the elderly. Residents typically complain about a lack of the privacy needed for intimacy and loss of human dignity. They worry about poor nutrition and lack of exercise or other engaging activities. Finally, they cite staff negligence, use of restraints, and excessive use of drugs as problems (Avorn et al., 1992).

Many studies have looked at ways to improve quality of life and health in nursing homes. Langer and Rodin (1976), for example, used a simple experimental design with profound implications. Residents on one floor listened to a lecture designed to increase their degree of perceived control. Residents on another floor heard a lecture on how staff could deal with the same issues. Residents in the personal control group were much happier and more active in the three weeks following the lecture compared to the staff-controlled group.

Perceived control is also important to elderly caregivers. Margaret Wallhagen (1993) studied 60 elderly caregivers ranging in age from 60 to 84 years. She observed that life satisfaction increased as perceived control increased. Further, caregivers reported lower levels of depression as perceived control increased. Finally, when caregivers perceived more control, they also reported fewer symptoms of stress.

Lifestyle and Aging: Stress, Nutrition, and Exercise

I first met the Delany sisters, Sadie and Bessie, through a TV news magazine. Their story so fascinated me that I tracked down their book, *Having Our Say*. At the time of the book's publication, Sadie was 103, and Bessie, 101.[5] Their coauthor, Amy Hearth, described them as vivacious and playful people who "seemed to have conquered old age" (Delany & Delany with Hearth, 1993, p. xi). In reflecting on their

---

[5] Bessie Delaney died on September 25, 1995.

longevity, Sadie noted that the hardest part was to have buried so many loved ones.

Their remarkable story began in North Carolina in 1889 and 1891, respectively. Their father, Henry Delany, was born into slavery. Yet, he had the good fortune, against Georgia law, to learn to read and write. After the war, a white Episcopal priest encouraged him to go to college. He jumped at the chance and later rose through the ranks of the Episcopal Church, U.S.A., to become its first black elected bishop. Just as he valued his education, he saw to it that his ten children all became college-educated professionals.

Sadie went to Columbia and earned a B.S degree in 1920, and a master's degree in 1925. She became the first black woman to teach science in the public schools of New York City. Bessie went to school at Boardman where, among her many memories, she recalled the poor, fatty diet and a large weight gain. Later, she enrolled in dentistry at Columbia University, the only black woman in her class. She became just the second black woman to be licensed to practice dentistry in New York. She recalls that her position still could not protect her from sexual harassment and racism. Sadie's consolation comes from the fact that she has outlived most of those who mistreated her.

By most standards, Sadie and Bessie lived a high quality of life. They owned a home and did their own housekeeping, shopping, and banking. They bore a distrust of doctors and hospitals, though, believing that hospitals overtreat and that doctors treat the elderly like exhibits.

Sadie and Bessie's health habits have been a model for the elderly. Bessie credited Sadie for this: "Sadie has taken on this business of getting old like it's a big *project*. She has it all figured out, about diet and exercise" (p. 207). They boil their tap water before drinking it. They changed their diet to less fatty foods with more fruits and about seven different vegetables each day. They took antioxidant vitamins daily, plus minerals, raw cloves of garlic, and a teaspoon of cod liver oil for the heart. Also, once a week they washed their teeth with their own homemade soap, a formula that enabled them to keep healthy teeth. For exercise, they did an hour of yoga exercises each day, Monday through Friday. Sadie got into yoga about 40 years ago to help her mother loosen her joints and muscles.

Aging and Stress: Coping, Reframing, and Avoidance

Given the large number of involuntary transitions the older person must make, it would not be at all surprising to find a high level of stress among the elderly. Instead, a 1985 national survey of stress suggests the opposite (Silverman, Eichler, & Williams, 1987). Men and women over the age of 65 report much less stress than their younger peers.[6] A large percentage report that they experience almost no stress at all. (See Table 16.3.) This relative absence of stress may be due partly to the coping skills people learn through the course of life. It may be due in part to changes in attitudes and expectations that produce less catastrophic appraisals. Lower stress may be due to lower emotional reactivity.

Folkman and her colleagues found that older people are more likely to use cognitive reappraisals and avoidance strategies to manage stress compared to younger people (Folkman, Lazarus, Pimley, & Novacek, 1987). Cognitive reappraisals usually reframe an event in benign terms or possibly transform the event to a positive. In spite of their increased use of cognitive reappraisals, older people are less likely to use direct problem-solving strategies. Instead of confrontation and expression of hostility or emotionality, they tend to prefer avoidance strategies such as distancing or escape (Costa, Zonderman, & McCrae, 1991). Further, the elderly are less likely to seek social support as a coping strategy. This tendency is in

---

[6] These data were obtained in a cross-sectional design, so historical factors, which may differ substantively between older and younger groups, cannot be eliminated as possible factors contributing to differences in stress reports.

TABLE 16.3   *Percentage distribution of stress for total group and by age, based on the 1985 Health Promotion and Disease Prevention Survey (adapted from Silverman et al., 1987).*

	MEN'S REPORTED STRESS				WOMEN'S REPORTED STRESS			
	A LOT	MODERATE	LITTLE	NONE	A LOT	MODERATE	LITTLE	NONE
Total	*18*	*32*	*23*	*28*	*23*	*31*	*23*	*24*
18–29	20	34	24	22	23	32	25	20
30–44	22	37	22	19	27	35	22	16
45–64	17	31	22	30	23	31	22	25
65+	7	15	22	56	14	20	22	43

most respects undesirable since social networks presumably provide a buffer against stress.

Within the family, though, strong positive support increases the use of approach coping as opposed to avoidance coping (Holahan & Moos, 1987). Manne and Zautra (1989) demonstrated this pattern in an interesting study. Subjects were husband and wife dyads where the woman suffered from rheumatoid arthritis. When the husband was critical of the wife's coping, the woman more often coped by using wishful thinking, which usually led to poorer adjustment. When the husband was very supportive, however, the woman used more cognitive restructuring. She also sought more information to help in the management of her condition. Both these strategies are positive and active methods of coping.

Aging and Nutrition: Taste, Smell, and Culinary Delights

We have noted throughout this book that high-risk behaviors may lead to lower health status while avoiding these risks can improve health. As age advances, high-risk behaviors may hasten aging, but keeping a healthy lifestyle may allow one to age closer to biological senescence. John Rowe and Robert Kahn (1987) believe that the biological model overstates the case for loss and underestimates the positive influence of diet, exercise, and good personal habits.

Nutrition is an important part of a healthy lifestyle for the elderly, but sticking to good dietary habits is often difficult. Physical and psychosocial changes conspire to change both appetite and taste. The decline in body mass, lowered activity, and lowered basal metabolic rate reduce the absolute amount of energy required. Loss of teeth or ill-fitting dentures make chewing difficult. There may be some loss of taste sensitivity and the sense of smell gradually fades, which has a detrimental effect on taste. The esophageal sphincter does not close properly, which permits digestive gases to leak up the throat, sometimes causing heartburn and belching. The stomach's mucosal lining may atrophy, which may lead to chronic gastritis and an unhealthy dependence on drug store antacids.

Older people may substitute softer foods to compensate for poor teeth or lose interest in eating altogether. They may modify their diet to avoid healthy foods they blame for gastritis. In the process, the elderly may unwittingly change the balance in essential food groups needed to maintain a healthy body.

The only change that elderly need to make is a modest reduction in the amount of food eaten. The primary energy sources are fat and carbohydrate calories. These two sources can be reduced slightly without harm, but all other nutritional requirements remain roughly the same as any adult. Water is vital to all metabolic processes and to prevent dehydration. The elderly are prone to dehydration, and they must be careful to maintain adequate fluid intake. A comparison of food requirements across the lifespan is shown in Table 16.4 based on data from Gershoff (1990).

One problem that both diet and exercise may help control is blood triglyceride and cholesterol levels, both of which tend to increase with age. Older people may need to monitor diet more closely to ensure that they keep fats to a minimum. Still, they should not cut fats severely because fats help the body absorb the fat-soluble vitamins A, D, E, and K. Further, the elderly have some decrease in absorption of calcium and vitamins B_6 and B_{12}: one area where supplements may be appropriate.

There has been great excitement, mostly in the popular press, about the benefits of Vitamin E for sexual prowess, cardiovascular health, and longevity. Little credible research evidence supports these claims. A recent large-scale prospective epidemiologic study (published in

two gender-specific parts) provided some evidence that Vitamin E might reduce risk for coronary disease (Stampfer et al., 1993; Rimm et al., 1993). In the first study, women who were in the top 20% on daily Vitamin E consumption had a relative risk for major coronary of 0.66 after adjusting for age and smoking. This lower risk was not observed in part-time vitamin users. Reduction in risk occurred above 100 IU per day, but taking more than 250 IU of Vitamin E provided no further reduction. In the second study, men in the top 20% of daily Vitamin E consumption had a relative risk of 0.59.

Aging and Exercise: Energy, Strength, and Health

Cicero, the Roman statesman-orator, gave a famous speech on old age in which he noted, "It is possible for a man by exercise and self-

TABLE 16.4   *Recommended dietary allowances at four points in the lifespan (data from Gershoff, 1990).*

NUTRIENT GROUPS	AGE GROUPS ACROSS THE LIFESPAN						
	4 TO 6 CHILDREN	19 TO 24 YEARS MALE	FEMALE	25 TO 50 YEARS MALE	FEMALE	51 PLUS MALE	FEMALE
Vitamins							
Fat-Soluble							
A	500 µg	1 mg	800 µg	1 mg	800 µg	1 mg	800 µg
D	10 µg	10 µg	10 µg	5 µg	5 µg	5 µg	5 µg
E	7 mg	10 mg	8 mg	10 mg	8 mg	10 mg	8 mg
K	20 µg	70 µg	60 µg	80 µg	65 µg	80 µg	65 µg
Water-Soluble							
C	45.0 mg	60.0 mg	60.0 mg	60.0 mg	60.0 mg	60.0 mg	60.0 mg
Thiamine	0.9 µg	1.5 µg	1.1 mg	1.5 µg	1.1 mg	1.2 µg	1.0 mg
Riboflavin	1.1 mg	1.7 mg	1.3 mg	1.7 mg	1.3 mg	1.4 mg	1.2 mg
Niacin	12.0 mg	19.0 mg	15.0 mg	19.0 mg	15.0 mg	15.0 mg	13.0 mg
B_6	1.1 mg	2.0 mg	1.6 mg	2.0 mg	1.6 mg	2.0 mg	1.6 mg
Folacin	75.0 µg	200.0 µg	180.0 µg	200.0 µg	180.0 µg	200.0 µg	180.0 µg
B_{12}	1.0 µg	2.0 µg	2.0 µg	2.0 µg	2.0 µg	2.0 µg	2.0 µg
Minerals							
Calcium	800 mg	1200 mg	1200 mg	800 mg	800 mg	800 mg	800 mg
Iron	10 mg	10 mg	15 mg	10 mg	15 mg	10 mg	10 mg
Protein	24 g	53 g	46 g	63 g	50 g	63 g	50 g

control, even in old age, to preserve some of his original vigor." In the elderly, the heart's capacity for work decreases even with physical conditioning. Yet, the decline would be even greater without the benefit of exercise. The elderly also may offset frailty and enhance mobility through resistance training (Nautilus-type exercise).

Maria Fiatarone and her coworkers demonstrated this effect in a randomized placebo-controlled experiment comparing resistance training to a diet enriched with a multinutrient supplement (Fiatarone et al., 1994). A third group received both the resistance training and the diet supplement. Yet a fourth group, the placebo group, could engage in three activities of their choice (including aerobic exercise), but they could not engage in resistance training. The 100 subjects who enrolled in the study averaged 87 years of age. Muscle strength increased 113% in the resistance groups compared to 3% in the nonexercising subjects. In the group that received both exercise training and diet supplement, the supplement did not bestow any statistically significant increase in muscle strength. Gait velocity and stair climbing also improved significantly. Finally, the two resistance exercise groups increased spontaneous physical activity nearly 35% while the other two groups declined about 3%.

Some other physiological functions improve with exercise even in the elderly: Exercise promoted cardiac efficiency, lowered systolic blood pressure, enhanced respiratory function, and lowered loss of bone calcium. Exercise improves morale in elderly people. Also, it may help the elderly retain cognitive functions longer, although it does not appear to improve cognitive functions (Hill, Storandt, & Malley, 1993).

Emery, Pinder, and Blumenthal (1989) reviewed the literature on exercise effects among elderly cardiac patients. They noted that the findings are often inconsistent and plagued by methodological problems. Still, exercise may restore the cardiac patient's capacity to enjoy normal, even moderately stressful, pursuits including sexual activity.

Aging and Drug Use: Polypharmacy, Alcohol, and Compliance

Health care officials consider drug use and abuse among the elderly a major health risk. The elderly do not so much abuse illegal drugs, but prescription and over-the-counter drugs. People over 65 comprise just 12% of the population in the United States, but they consume about 33% of the 1.5 billion prescriptions written each year (Eng & Emlet, 1990). More than 80% of the elderly report using at least one prescription drug. Approximately 20% of the elderly use some type of psychotropic drug that carries risk for harmful effects (Ried, Christensen, & Stergachis, 1990).

Even more important than the amount of drugs the elderly consume is the mixture of drugs they take. Kathryn Eng and Charles Emlet (1990) found that the average person over 65 uses from 2 to 7 prescriptions daily and more than 13 prescriptions during the year. This **polypharmacy**—taking a large number of different drugs simultaneously—can prove very dangerous if not lethal. For example, one study revealed that 19% of an elderly sample bought OTC pain relief medications and then drank alcohol with the painkiller (Forster, Pollow, & Stoller, 1993). No one knows how the countless potential drug combinations interact. The risk for adverse reactions from drug interactions is roughly 17% (Smyer, 1989).

One physical change, declining liver function, magnifies the problem of drug use in the elderly. As liver function drops, so does the ability to process drugs. Some drugs (for example, barbiturates, benzodiazepines, antidepressants, and tranquilizers) then may build up in the body and produce negative effects that do not occur in younger people.

Alcohol use is serious problem among the elderly. The good news is that about 43% of the elderly abstain from alcohol use completely (Forster et al., 1993). The bad news is that those who do consume alcohol tend to increase intake after age 60. About 33% of the elderly with alcohol problems began drinking excessively after age 60 (Tufts University, 1993).

Efforts are under way to try to remedy misuse and compliance problems. One approach is to try to match types of caregivers to the special medication schedules and needs of elderly patients. Barbara Kail and Eugene Litwak (1989) devised a theoretical framework based on three factors: the technical knowledge required to dispense medications, types of caregivers, and potential caregiver activities. Within this framework, Kail and Litwak suggested that a spouse is most helpful for chronic illnesses when the prescription requires a complex schedule. Relief could be provided in close-knit or extended families that live nearby. Relatives may be helpful with chronic illness when the medication schedule is simple. Neighbors may help to purchase medication for an acute illness or in an emergency, but they cannot typically make a long-term commitment. Friends are also helpful to spot subtle changes in the patient that family members may not have observed because they are living so closely with the patient.

Death and Dying: Grief and Preparation

Aging brings direct confrontations with mortality in two ways. First, the elderly suffer the loss of parents, siblings, spouse, and friends. Second, they confront the specter of personal mortality, the realization that death is fast approaching for them. Research on death and dying has provided certain insights into the stages that people go through in these conditions.

A spouse's death is one of the most traumatic losses an elderly person will ever suffer. Even as the person tries to support the spouse in preparation for death, the person also must prepare himself or herself. After death, there appear to be four stages to mourning. The first reaction may be shock and panic. The person may feel overwhelmed by the thought of adjusting to life without the soulmate and helpmate. The second stage is extreme grief when the person experiences the most intense sadness

and despair. This period may go on for months or years, even wearing down younger family members. In the third stage, the person begins to accept reality: The beloved partner is gone. Finally, the person reaches a point of more complete reality orientation. The person makes more deliberate and successful efforts to resume normal tasks and social pursuits.

Following a spouse's death, there is concern not only for psychosocial functioning but also for physical functioning. This concern stems from observations that many bereaved elderly dramatically change their lifestyles following death of a spouse. They may not eat as they should, exercise properly, or sleep as much as before. These changes can have a cumulative effect potentially more serious in the elderly than in a younger person.

Another observation suggests there may be crucial times when the surviving partner could be vulnerable to death. This is the so-called anniversary reaction (Dlin, 1985). The **anniversary reaction** is the survivor's death on some day that has special significance related to the lost partner. It typically means death of the survivor on the anniversary day of the partner's death, such as a month later, or a year later. Several theories try to explain this reaction. One suggests that death is a type of conditioned emotional reaction, while another suggests conditioned suppression of the immune system. The immune suppression notion suggests that bereavement triggers a response in the survivor sufficient to produce a decline in health and ultimately death.[7]

Confronting Personal Mortality: The Final Developmental Task

Themes of personal death have replayed in literary works over the years. Some paint a picture of the explorer facing the unknown. Some admonish the traveler to face impending death with courage and grace. William Cullen

---

[7] Research bearing on this theory was presented in Chapter 7.

Bryant's Thanatopsis took this view, as did a short poem from the Sufi tradition: "So live, that sinking in thy last long sleep, Calm thou may'st smile while all around thee weep" (cited in Shah, 1970, p. 41). Clinical efforts with terminally ill patients provide slightly different portraits of what the dying person may experience. Among the most insightful work is that of Elizabeth Kübler-Ross (1969). Drawing on many observations of people confronting death, Kübler-Ross suggested that preparing for personal death proceeds through five stages: denial, anger, bargaining, depression, and acceptance.

In the denial stage, the person refuses to believe that this (impending death) is happening to them. This stage does not last very long, though, before the person becomes angry, even combative. They see the illness as unfair and demand explanations: "Why me?" In the third stage, anger gives way to bargaining, most often bargaining with a superior being whom the person apprehends as God. They pray for a reprieve trading offers for charitable work or promises to change personal behavior. Typically, depression follows bargaining, an overwhelming sadness that comes to grips with the grimness of the message, the finality of the process. Finally, the person concedes that death is inevitable and begins preparing for the end. This preparation usually includes putting personal and family affairs in order, saying farewell to friends, and spending every available minute with family. During any of this time, the psychologist might be called to provide support to the patient or to family members.

Kübler-Ross's model has been criticized. Some do not see the linear progression in the stages suggested by the model. All people do not experience all the stages, and the course people follow among the stages often varies. In spite of these criticisms, Kübler-Ross's observations serve as an invaluable guide to those who work with the terminally ill.

The hospice program A program designed to help families confronting death of a family member is the hospice program, which began in England in the mid 1960s (Saunders, 1976) and spread to the United States about 1975. The United States now has more than 1200 hospices. The hospice is not an agency but a philosophy implemented in a special environment designed to meet the needs of dying patients and their families. The hospice program emphasizes (1) control and alleviation of pain, (2) care given in the home or a homelike environment, (3) patient autonomy in care decisions, and (4) attention to the patient's emotional, social, and spiritual needs (Osterweis, Solomon, & Green, 1984). The hospice does not treat the patient to the exclusion of the family, but looks for ways to deal with the needs of the entire family. The staff is typically a multidisciplinary team trained to deal with the patient's pain as well as the family's grief.

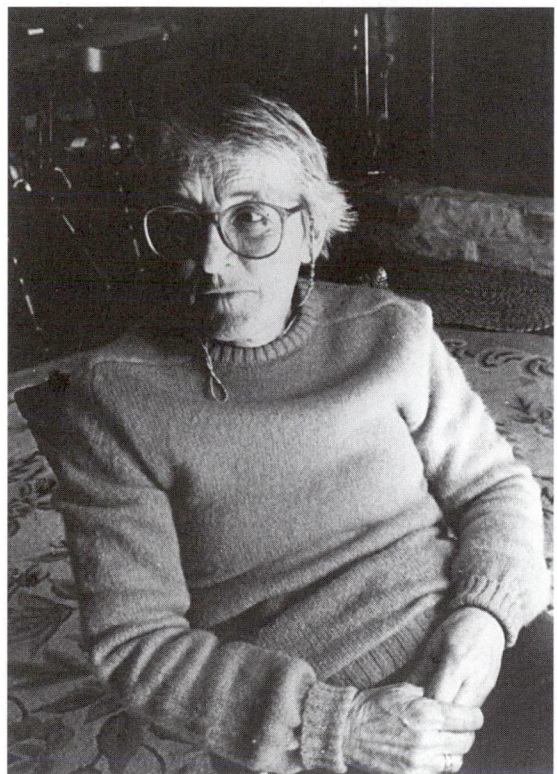

FIGURE 16.13   Elizabeth Kübler-Ross has spent much of her career tending to the needs of the dying and writing about life's final growth stage.

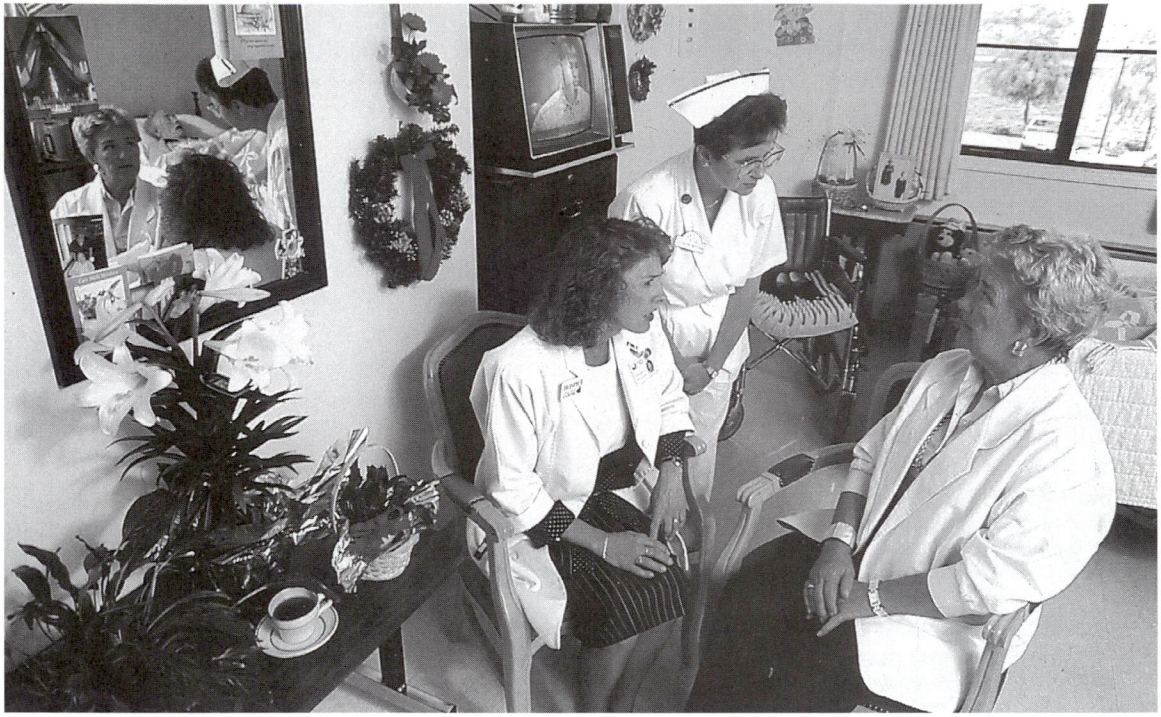

FIGURE 16.14   Patients living in a hospice meet their family and friends in a more normal setting than the hospital's sterile environment.

The focus of the hospice has much less to do with the high-tech life-saving methods used in the modern hospital than with the emotional, social, and spiritual needs of the patient and family. The primary purpose is to ensure a high quality of life for the patient in the last days or weeks of life. This means creating a climate that fosters a sense of time well spent with family in an open expression of love and respect. In the process, the hospice works to help survivors make the transition to life without their loved one with less pain and in celebration of the life that was lived.

Summary

Although aging is associated with declining health, we have seen that aging still can be linked to vitality and a high quality of life. Adopting a positive lifestyle can preserve quality of life among the elderly and increase resistance to illness. The major points made in the chapter are summarized here.

1. American culture tends to emphasize youthfulness, but many cultures hold their elders in high esteem, provide them a special position, and encourage their continued active involvement in society.

2. Aging is a lifelong process of growing old. Aging includes biological, psychological, and social changes.

3. Biological senescence is the upper limit of life when the organism is not afflicted by debilitating disease or damage.

4. The population of elderly citizens is growing rapidly due to declining birth rates, reduced infant mortality, medical technology that delivers better health care, and improved nutrition.

5. Physical changes during aging affect nearly every component of the body, but at differing rates. Changes in vital capacity, muscle strength, and bones impact on mobility and the capacity for work. Changes in sensory capacity may interfere with normal activities such as driving, going to the theater, and so forth.

6. Changes in mental ability may occur due to physical ailments such as hardening of the arteries and Alzheimer's disease. Yet, mental processes tend to deteriorate somewhat with aging even in the absence of severe illnesses.

7. Biomedical theories of aging may focus on genetics, since longevity tends to run in families. Another view is that the cell contains some type of code or program that allows it to divide only a finite number of times. Cells may also become loaded with free radicals that alter cell function and lead to death.

8. Psychosocial theories of aging usually focus on such things as emotional distress that accompanies aging, loss of position, power, financial stability, limitation in activities, and loss of social support with the death of family members and friends.

9. Alzheimer's disease is a neurological disorder that impairs recent memory, then progressively attacks higher mental functions such as the ability to read, write, and speak.

10. It is believed that Alzheimer's is an inherited disorder that results in cross-linking of neurons, especially neurons in the hippocampus, an area that is very important to memory function.

11. The major personality changes that occur with aging include a decline in masculinity in men, and increased tendencies to mild paranoia, depression, and hypochondriasis in both genders.

12. In spite of the image of retirement villages and nursing homes as the last accommodation for the elderly, a surprisingly high percentage of elderly (75 to 80%) still live on their own or with family.

13. Elderly men and women report less stress than their younger peers—perhaps because older people have learned to use more coping methods, such as cognitive reappraisals, compared to younger adults.

14. The elderly still need a balanced diet, but changes in taste, smell, and energy level may reduce the desire for food. A modest reduction in food intake is appropriate. Two crucial needs are water intake to avoid dehydration and calcium intake to avoid bone deterioration.

15. Exercise is beneficial to the elderly in various ways. Exercise maintains strength and agility, and it tends to improve morale.

16. One problem among the elderly is polypharmacy, or taking a large number of drugs at the same time.

17. The elderly person suffers increasing emotional distress as more of their circle of family and friends dies. Awareness of impending personal death and confronting the last of life's stages is a major daunting task.

18. The hospice program was designed to help patients and family members confronting death. It is intended to provide for a high quality of life, social exchange, and intimacy within the family during the patient's last days.

Key Words

aging	maximum breathing
anniversary reaction	capacity
aphasia	maximum oxygen
apraxia	consumption
biological senescence	osteoporosis
cataracts	Parkinson's disease
collagen	polypharmacy
free radicals	postmitotic cells
geriatric health	presbycusis
psychology	progeria
gerontology	reaction time
geropsychologist	senescence
glaucoma	senility
Hayflick phenomenon	sleep apnea
life expectancy	sundowning
life-span	vital capacity

Study Questions

1. Identify major physical and psychological changes that occur with aging. How do these changes relate to functional capacity in the elderly? How do these changes impact on the quality of life that the elderly may enjoy?

2. What are the major biological theories of aging? Are these theories mutually exclusive or might some combination of the theories be needed to explain physical aging?

3. What are the principal psychosocial theories of aging? How do these theories differ from biological theories?

4. What are the symptoms of Alzheimer's disease? What is known of the cause and course of Alzheimer's? What are some problems confronted by an Alzheimer's caregiver?

5. Do personality traits change substantially with aging? What traits, if any, change, and how?

6. What are the major social losses suffered by the elderly? How do these impact on the morale of the elderly?

7. Are there gender differences in confronting the stress of aging? If so, describe how they operate.

8. What problems may arise in diet and nutrition for the elderly? What guidelines are recommended for dietary practice?

9. How does exercise benefit the elderly?

10. What is the hospice program?

Class Projects

1. Have interested class members research the latest status of longitudinal investigations among elderly populations.

2. Invite community professionals from retirement centers and nursing homes to talk about the programs offered at their centers. Have them address core issues such as independence, responsibility, privacy, and polypharmacy.

3. Have a roundtable discussion on cross-cultural practices and issues in aging.

Suggested Readings

Adelman, R. C., & Roth, G. S. (Eds.). (1982). *Testing the theories of aging*. Boca Raton: CRC Press.

Clark, N. M., Becker, M. H., Janz, N. K., Lorig, K., Rakowski, W., & Anderson, L. (1991). Self-management of chronic disease by older adults: A review and questions for research. *Journal of Aging and Health, 3,* 3–27.

Davies, P. (1986). The genetics of Alzheimer's disease: A review and a discussion of the implications. *Neurobiology of Aging, 7,* 459–466.

Folkman, S., Lazarus, R. S., Pimley, S., & Novacek, J. (1987). Age differences in stress and coping processes. *Psychology and Aging, 2,* 171–184.

Hazzard, W. R., Andres, R., Bierman, E. L., & Blass, J. P. (Eds.). (1990). *Principles of geriatric medicine and gerontology* (2nd ed.). New York: McGraw-Hill.

McDaniel, S. A., & McKinnon, A. L. (1993). Gender differences in informal support and coping among elders: Findings from Canada's 1985 and 1990 general social surveys. *Journal of Women and Aging, 5,* 79–98.

Moritz, D. J., & Ostfeld, A. M. (1990). The epidemiology and demography of aging. In W. R. Hazzard, et al. (Eds.), *Principles of geriatric medicine and gerontology* (2nd ed., pp. 146–156). New York: McGraw-Hill.

Prinz, P. N., Vitiello, M. V., Raskind, M. A., & Thorpy, M. J. (1990). Geriatrics: Sleep disorders and aging. *The New England Journal of Medicine, 323,* 520–526.

Spence, A. P. (1989). *Biology of human aging*. Englewood Cliffs, NJ.: Prentice-Hall.

Woodruff-Pak, D. S. (1988). *Psychology and aging*. Englewood Cliffs, NJ.: Prentice-Hall.

WEBSITES   *Aging and Health, Alzheimer's*

ADDRESS	DESCRIPTION
http://www.alz.org/frames/main.html	Alzheimer's Association Web Page
http://www.cais.net/adear/	Alzheimer's Disease Education & Referral Center—service of National Institute on Aging
http://www.iog.wayne.edu/APADIV20/APADIV20.HTM	Division 20 of the APA—Adult Development and Aging
http://www2.dgsys.com/~tgolden/	☆ Crisis, Grief & Healing—support, information, and links to web resources for grief and healing from loss
http://www.aoa.dhhs.gov/aoa/webres/craig.htm	Directory of WEB and Gopher Aging Sites—an excellent starting point to locate resources
http://med-amsa.bu.edu/Alzheimer/Cgivers.htm	Resources for the Family and Caregiver—includes link to Today's Caregiver Magazine
http://web.aimnet.com/~hyperion/meno/menotimes.index.html	Quarterly publication on menopause and osteoporosis—table of contents
http://www-leland.stanford.edu/~dement	The Sleep Well—extensive resources for sleep disorders and links to web sites

References

Ackerknecht, E. H. (1982). The history of psychosomatic medicine. *Psychological Medicine, 12,* 17–24.

ADAMHA NEWS. (1989, August). U.S. Department of Health and Human Services, Public Health Service, Alcohol, Drug Abuse, and Mental Health Administration. *XV,* 1 & 13.

Adams, E. R., & McGuire, F. A. (1986). Is laughter the best medicine? A study of the effects of humor on perceived pain and affect. *Activities, Adaptation and Aging, 8,* 157–175.

Adelman, R. C., & Roth, G. S. (Eds.). (1982). *Testing the theories of aging.* Boca Raton: CRC Press.

Ader, R. (1983). Developmental psychoneuroimmunology. *Developmental Psychobiology, 16,* 251–267.

Ader, R., Cohen, N., & Felten, D. L. (1987). Brain, behavior, and immunity. *Brain, Behavior, and Immunity, 1,* 1–16.

Affleck, G., Tennen, H., Urrows, S., & Higgins, P. (1992). Neuroticism and the pain-mood relation in rheumatoid arthritis: Insights from a prospective daily study. *Journal of Consulting and Clinical Psychology, 60,* 119–126.

Agency for Health Care Policy and Research (ACPR). (1992). Acute pain management in infants, children and adolescents: Operative and medical procedures. *American Family Physician, 46,* 469–479.

Agnew, R., & White, H. R. (1992). An empirical test of general strain theory. *Criminology, 30,* 475–499.

Agras, W. S. (1984). The behavioral treatment of somatic disorders. In W. D. Gentry (Ed.), *Handbook of behavioral medicine* (pp. 479–530). New York: Guilford.

Aiken, L. S., West, S. G., Sechrest, L., Reno, R. R., Roediger, H. L., Scarr, S., Kazdin, A. E., & Sherman, S. J. (1990). Graduate training in statistics, methodology, and measurement in psychology: A survey of PhD programs in North America. *American Psychologist, 45,* 721–734.

Ajzen, I., & Fishbein, M. (1970). The prediction of behavior from attitudinal and normative variables. *Journal of Experimental Social Psychology, 6,* 466–487.

Ajzen, I., & Fishbein, M. (1980). *Understanding attitudes and predicting social behavior.* Englewood Cliffs, NJ: Prentice-Hall.

Alexander, F. (1950). *Psychosomatic medicine: Its principles and applications.* New York: Norton.

Allport, G. W. (1961). *Pattern and growth in personality.* New York: Holt, Rinehart & Winston.

Allred, K., & Smith, T. W. (1989). The hardy personality: Cognitive and physiological responses to evaluative threat. *Journal of Personality and Social Psychology, 56,* 257–266.

Alpert, J. S. (1993). Chronic ischemic heart disease. In R. P. Lewis (Ed.), *Adult clinical cardiology self-assessment program* (Section 3), Bethesda, MD: American College of Cardiology.

Alterman, A. I., & Tarter, R. E. (1983). The transmission of psychological vulnerability: Implications for alcoholism etiology. *The Journal of Nervous and Mental Disease, 171,* 147–154.

Altmaier, E. M., & Meyer, M. E. (1985). *Applied specialties in psychology.* New York: Random House.

Amaro, H. (1995). Love, sex, and power: Considering women's realities in HIV prevention. *American Psychologist, 50,* 437–447.

Amaro, H., Beckman, L. J., & Mays, V. M. (1987). A comparison of black and white women entering alcoholism treatment. *Journal of Studies on Alcohol, 48,* 220–228.

American Academy of Pediatrics. (1989). Newborn screening fact sheets. *Pediatrics, 83,* 449–464.

American Diabetes Association. (1989). Standards of medical care for patients with diabetes mellitus. *Diabetes Care, 12,* 365–368.

American Psychiatric Association. (1987). *Diagnostic and statistical manual of mental disorders* (3rd ed., rev.). Washington, DC: Author.

American Psychiatric Association. (1994). *Diagnostic and statistical manual of mental disorders* (4th ed.). Washington, DC: Author.

Anastasi, A. (1988). *Psychological testing* (6th ed.). New York: Macmillan.

Antoni, M. H. (1987). Neuroendocrine influences in psychoimmunology and neoplasia: A review. *Psychology and Health, 1,* 3–24.

Antonovsky, A. (1989). Islands rather than bridgeheads: The problematic status of the biopsychosocial model. *Family Systems Medicine, 7,* 243–253.

Apao, W. K., & Damon, A. M. (1982). Locus of control and the quantity-frequency index of alcohol use. *Journal of Studies on Alcohol, 43,* 233–239.

Arbeit, J. M. (1990). Molecules, cancer, and the surgeon. *Annals of Surgery, 212,* 3–13.

Arias, I. M. (1989). Training basic scientists to bridge the gap between basic science and its application to human disease. *The New England Journal of Medicine, 321,* 972–974.

Armitage, J. O. (1993). Treatment of non-Hodgkin's lymphoma. *The New England Journal of Medicine, 328,* 1023–1030.

Aronoff, G. M., Wagner, J. M., & Spangler, A. S. (1986). Chemical interventions for pain. *Journal of Consulting and Clinical Psychology, 54,* 769–775.

Ashe, A. (1988). *A hard road to glory* (3 vols.). New York: Warner.

Ashe, A., & Rampersad, A. (1993). *Days of grace.* New York: Knopf.

Aslan, S., Nelson, L., Carruthers, M., & Lader, M. (1981). Stress and age effects on catecholamines in normal subjects. *Journal of Psychosomatic Research, 25,* 33–41.

Atkinson, J. M. (1993). The patient as sufferer. *British Journal of Medical Psychology, 66,* 113–120.

Austin, M. A., & Newman, B. (1993). Genetic influence on smoking. *The New England Journal of Medicine, 328,* 353.

Avorn, J., Soumerai, S. B., Everitt, D. E., Ross-Degnan, D., Beers, M. H., Sherman, D., Salem-Schatz, S. R., & Fields, D. (1992). A randomized trial of a program to reduce the use of psychoactive drugs in nursing homes. *The New England Journal of Medicine, 327,* 168–173.

Ayanian, J. Z., & Epstein, A. M. (1991). Differences in the use of procedures between women and men hospitalized for coronary heart disease. *The New England Journal of Medicine, 325,* 221–225.

Ayanian, J. Z., Kohler, B. A., Abe, T., & Epstein, A. M. (1993). The relation between health insurance coverage and clinical outcomes among women with breast cancer. *The New England Journal of Medicine, 329,* 326–331.

Bachman, J. G., Wallace, J. M., O'Malley, P. M.,

Johnston, L. D., Kurth, C. L., & Neighbors, H. W. (1991). Racial/ethnic differences in smoking, drinking, and illicit drug use among American high school seniors, 1976–89. *American Journal of Public Health, 81,* 372–377.

Baer, H. A. (Ed.). (1987). *Encounters with biomedicine: Case studies in medical anthropology.* New York: Gordon & Breach.

Baer, J. S., Marlatt, G. A., Kivlahan, D. R., Fromme, K., Larimer, M. E., & Williams, E. (1992). An experimental test of three methods of alcohol risk reduction with young adults. *Journal of Consulting and Clinical Psychology, 60,* 974–979.

Bakeman, R., Lumb, J. R., Jackson, R. E., & Smith, D. W. (1986). AIDS risk-group profiles in whites and members of minority groups. *The New England Journal of Medicine, 315,* 191–192.

Baker, G. H. B. (1987). Invited review: Psychological factors and immunity. *Journal of Psychosomatic Research, 31,* 1–10.

Balfour, L., White, D. R., Schiffrin, A., Dougherty, G., & Dufresne, J. (1993). Dietary disinhibition, perceived stress, and glucose control in young, Type I diabetic women. *Health Psychology, 12,* 33–38.

Balin, A. K. (1982). Testing the free radical theory of aging. In R. C. Adelman & G. S. Roth (Eds.), *Testing the theories of aging* (pp. 137–182). Boca Raton: CRC Press.

Ball, R. (1984). Chronic pain. *The Jefferson Journal of Psychiatry, 2,* 11–24.

Band, E. B., & Weisz, J. R. (1990). Developmental differences in primary and secondary control coping and adjustment to juvenile diabetes. *Journal of Clinical Child Psychology, 19,* 150–158.

Bandura, A. (1977). Self-efficacy: Toward a unifying theory of behavioral change. *Psychological Review, 84,* 191–215.

Bandura, A. (1989). Human agency in social cognitive theory. *American Psychologist, 44,* 1175–1184.

Bandura, A., O'Leary, A., Taylor, C. B., Gauthier, J., & Gossard, D. (1987). Perceived self-efficacy and pain control: Opioid and nonopioid mechanisms. *Journal of Personality and Social Psychology, 53,* 563–571.

Banks, S. M., & Kerns, R. D. (1996). Explaining high rates of depression in chronic pain: A diathesis-stress framework. *Psychological Bulletin, 119,* 95–110.

Barbarin, O. A., Hughes, D., & Chesler, M. A. (1985). Stress, coping, and marital functioning among parents of children with cancer. *Journal of Marriage and the Family, 47,* 473–480.

Barber, B. L., & Eccles, J. S. (1992). Long-term influence of divorce and single parenting on adolescent family- and work-related values, behaviors, and aspirations. *Psychological Bulletin, 111,* 108–126.

Barlow, D. H., & Durand, V. M. (1995). *Abnormal psychology: An integrative approach.* Pacific Grove, CA: Brooks/Cole.

Barnes, D. M. (1988). The biological tangle of drug addiction. *Science, 241,* 415–417.

Barnes, P. J. (1989). A new approach to the treatment of asthma. *The New England Journal of Medicine, 321,* 1517–1527.

Barnett, R. C., Davidson, H., & Marshall, N. L. (1991). Physical symptoms and the interplay of work and family roles. *Health Psychology, 10,* 94–101.

Barofsky, I. (1981). Issues and approaches to the psychosocial assessment of the cancer patient. In C. K. Prokop & L. A. Bradley (Eds.), *Medical psychology: Contributions to behavioral medicine* (pp. 55–65). New York: Academic Press.

Baron, R. A. (1992). *Psychology* (2nd ed.). Boston: Allyn & Bacon.

Baron, R. S., Logan, H., & Hoppe, S. (1993). Emotional and sensory focus as mediators of dental pain among patients differing in desired and felt dental control. *Health Psychology, 12,* 381–389.

Barr, H. M., Streissguth, A. P., Darby, B. L., & Sampson, P. D. (1990). Prenatal exposure to alcohol, caffeine, tobacco, and aspirin: Effects on fine and gross motor performance in 4-year-old children. *Developmental Psychology, 26,* 339–348.

Barsky, A. J. (1988). The paradox of health. *The New England Journal of Medicine, 318,* 414–418.

Bartlett, E. E., & Windsor, R. A. (1985). Health education and medicine: Competition or cooperation? *Health Education Quarterly, 12,* 219–229.

Bartlett, S. J., Wadden, T. A., & Vogt, R. A. (1996). Psychosocial consequences of weight cycling. *Journal of Consulting and Clinical Psychology, 64,* 587–592.

Bartrop, R. W., Lazarus, L., Luckhurst, E., Kiloh, L. G., & Penny, R. (1977). Depressed lymphocyte function after bereavement. *Lancet, 1,* 834–836.

Basbaum, A. I., & Field, H. L. (1978). Endogenous pain control mechanisms: Review and hypothesis. *Annals of Neurology, 4,* 451–462.

Batchelor, W. F. (1984). AIDS: A public health and psychological emergency. *American Psychologist, 39,* 1279–1284.

Batchelor, W. F. (1988). AIDS 1988: The science and limits of science. *American Psychologist, 43,* 853–858.

Bates, M. S. (1990). A critical perspective on coronary artery disease and coronary bypass surgery. *Social Science & Medicine, 30,* 249–260.

Baum, A., & Fleming, I. (1993). Implications of psychological research on stress and technological accidents. *American Psychologist, 48,* 665–672.

Baum, A., Fleming, R., & Singer, J. (1983). Coping with victimization by technological disaster. *Journal of Social Issues, 39,* 117–138.

Baumeister, R. F., Kahn, J., & Tice, D. M. (1990). Obesity as a self-handicapping strategy: Personality, selective attribution of problems, and weight loss. *Journal of Social Psychology, 130,* 121–123.

Beaudet, A. L., Feldman, G. L., Fernbach, S. D., Buffone, G. J., & O'Brien, W. E. (1989). Linkage disequilibrium, cystic fibrosis, and genetic counseling. *American Journal of Human Genetics, 44,* 319–326.

Beaudet, A. L., Fenwick, R. G., Fernbach, S. D., & O'Brien, W. E. (1990). Genetic diagnosis using mutation analysis. In G. Polgar (Ed.), *Pediatric pulmonology: Program and papers of Fourth Annual North American and 1990 International Cystic Fibrosis Conference* (Suppl. 5), 116–117.

Becker, L. B., Han, B. H., Meyer, P. M., Wright, F. A., Rhodes, K. V., Smith, D. W., Barrett, J., & the Chicago CPR Project. (1993). Racial differences in the incidence of cardiac arrest and subsequent survival. *The New England Journal of Medicine, 329,* 600–606.

Becker, M. H., & Maiman, L. A. (1975). Sociobehavioral determinants of compliance with health and medical care recommendations. *Medical Care, 13,* 10–24.

Beckham, J. C., Keefe, F. J., Caldwell, D. S., & Roodman, A. A. (1991). Pain coping strategies in rheumatoid arthritis: Relationships to pain, disability, depression and daily hassles. *Behavior Therapy, 22,* 113–124.

Beecher, H. K. (1956). Relationship of significance of wound to the pain experienced. *The Journal of the American Medical Association, 161,* 1609–1613.

Begleiter, H., Porjesz, B., Bihari, B., & Kissin, B. (1984). Event-related brain potentials in boys at risk for alcoholism. *Science, 225,* 1493–1496.

Belar, C. D., Wilson, E., & Hughes, H. (1982). Health psychology training in doctoral programs. *Health Psychology, 1,* 289–299.

Belar, C. D. (1990). Issues in training clinical health psychologists. *Psychology and Health, 4,* 31–37.

Belar, C. D., Deardorff, W. W., & Kelly, K. E. (1987). *The practice of clinical health psychology*. New York: Pergamon.

Bellack, A. S., & Hersen, M. (Eds.). (1988). *Behavioral assessment: A practical handbook* (3rd ed.). New York: Pergamon.

Benet, S. (1974). *Abkhasians: The long-living people of the Caucasus*. New York: Holt, Rinehart & Winston.

Bennett, J. C. (1993). Inclusion of women in clinical trials—policies for population subgroups. *The New England Journal of Medicine, 329,* 288–292.

Bennett, P. H. (1994). Definition, diagnosis, and classification of diabetes mellitus and impaired glucose tolerance. In C. R. Kahn & G. C. Weir (Eds.), *Joslin's diabetes mellitus—13th* (pp. 193–200). Malvern, PA: Lea & Febiger.

Benowitz, N. L., Jacob, P., Kozlowski, L. T., & Yu, L. (1986). Influence of smoking fewer cigarettes on exposure to tar, nicotine, and carbon monoxide. *The New England Journal of Medicine, 315,* 1310–1313.

Benson, H. (1975). *The relaxation response.* New York: Avon Books.

Berenson, G. S. (1993). Epidemiology and prevention. In R. P. Lewis (Ed.), *Adult clinical cardiology self-assessment program* (Section 1). Bethesda, MD: American College of Cardiology.

Bergin, A. E., & Lambert, M. J. (1978). The evaluation of therapeutic outcomes. In S. L. Garfield & A. E. Bergin (Eds.), *Handbook of psychotherapy and behavior change* (pp. 139–189). New York: Wiley.

Berkel, H., Birdsell, D. C., & Jenkins, H. (1992). Breast augmentation: A risk factor for breast cancer? *The New England Journal of Medicine, 326,* 1649–1653.

Bernstein, D. A., & Borkovec, T. D. (1978). *Progressive relaxation training: A manual for the helping professions.* Champaign, IL: Research Press.

Berntson, G. G., Cacioppo, J. T., & Quigley, K. A. (1991). Autonomic determinism: The modes of autonomic control, the doctrine of autonomic space, and the laws of autonomic constraint. *Psychological Review, 98,* 459–487.

Beutler, L. E. (1979). Toward specific psychological therapies for specific conditions. *Journal of Consulting and Clinical Psychology, 47,* 882–892.

Biener, L., & Abrams, D. B. (1991). The contemplation ladder: Validation of a measure of readiness to consider smoking cessation. *Health Psychology, 10,* 360–365.

Binkley, S. (1979). A timekeeping enzyme in the pineal gland. *Scientific American, 240,* 66–71.

Birch, L. L., Johnson, S. L., Andresen, G., Peters, J. C., & Schulte, M. C. (1991). The variability of young children's energy intake. *The New England Journal of Medicine, 324,* 232–235.

Birch, L. L., Zimmerman, S. I., & Hind, H. (1980). The influence of social-affective context on the formation of children's food preferences. *Child Development, 55,* 431–439.

Birk, L. (Ed.). (1973). *Biofeedback: Behavioral medicine.* New York: Grune & Stratton.

Björntorp, P. (1986). Fat cells and obesity. In K. D. Brownell & J. P. Foreyt (Eds.), *Handbook of eating disorders: Physiology, psychology, and treatment of obesity, anorexia, and bulimia* (pp. 88–98). New York: Basic Books.

Black, P. M. (1991). Brain tumors (second of two parts). *The New England Journal of Medicine, 324,* 1555–1564.

Blackburn, G. L., Lynch, M. E., & Wong, S. L. (1986). The very-low-calorie diet: A weight-reduction technique. In K. D. Brownell & J. P. Foreyt (Eds.), *Handbook of eating disorders: Physiology, psychology, and treatment of obesity, anorexia, and bulimia* (pp. 198–212). New York: Basic Books.

Blalock, S. J., DeVellis, B. M., Afifi, R. A., & Sandler, R. S. (1990). Risk perceptions and participation in colorectal cancer screening. *Health Psychology, 9,* 792–806.

Blanchard, E. B., Andrasik, F., Neff, D. F., Arena, J. G., Ahles, T. A., Jurish, S. E., Pallmeyer, T. P., Saunders, N. L., Teders, S. J., Barron, K. D., & Rodichok, L. D. (1982). Biofeedback and relaxation training with three kinds of headache: Treatment effects and their prediction. *Journal of Consulting and Clinical Psychology, 50,* 562–575.

Blanchard, E. B., McCoy, G. C., Berger, M., Musso, A., Pallmeyer, T. P., Gerardi, R., Gerardi, M. A., & Pangburn, L. (1989). A controlled comparison of thermal biofeedback and relaxation training in the treatment of essential hypertension IV: Prediction of short-term clinical outcome. *Behavior Therapy, 20,* 405–415.

Blanchard, E. B., McCoy, G. C., Musso, A., Gerardi, M. A., Pallmeyer, T. P., Gerardi, R. J., Cotch, P. A., Siracusa, K., & Andrasik, F. (1986). A controlled comparison of thermal biofeedback and relaxation training in the treatment of essential hypertension: I. Short-term and long-term outcome. *Behavior Therapy, 17,* 563–579.

Blechman, E. A., & Brownell, K. D. (Eds.). (1988). *Handbook of behavioral medicine for women*. New York: Pergamon.

Bliwise, D. L., Friedman, L., Nekich, J. C., & Yesavage, J. A. (1995). Prediction of outcome in behaviorally based insomnia treatments. *Journal of Behavior Therapy and Experimental Psychiatry, 26,* 17–23.

Bloom, F. E., & Herd, J. A. (1983). Physiologic and neurobiologic mechanisms in arteriosclerosis. In J. A. Herd & S. M. Weiss (Eds.), *Behavior and arteriosclerosis* (33–43). New York: Plenum.

Bluebond-Langner, M. (1997). Meanings of death to children. In H. Feifel (Ed.), *New meanings of death* (pp. 47–66). New York: McGraw-Hill.

Blum, K., & Trachtenberg, M. C. (1988). Alcoholism: Scientific basis of a neuropsychogenetic disease. *The International Journal of the Addictions, 23,* 781–796.

Blum, K., Noble, E. P., Sheridan, P. J., & Finley, O. (1991). Association of the A1 allele of the D-sub-2 dopamine receptor gene with severe alcoholism. *Alcohol, 8,* 409–416.

Blumenthal, J. A., Barefoot, J., Burg, M. M., & Williams, R. B. (1987). Psychological correlates of hostility among patients undergoing coronary angiography. *British Journal of Medical Psychology, 60,* 349–355.

Boakes, R. (1984). *From Darwin to behaviorism: Psychology and the minds of animals*. Cambridge: Cambridge University Press.

Bochner, B. S., & Lichtenstein, L. M. (1991). Anaphylaxis. *The New England Journal of Medicine, 324,* 1785–1790.

Bohart, A. C., & Todd, J. (1988). *Foundations of clinical and counseling psychology*. New York: Harper & Row.

Booth-Kewley, S., & Friedman, H. S. (1987). Psychological predictors of heart disease: A quantitative review. *Psychological Bulletin, 101,* 343–362.

Bootzin, R. R., & Ruggill, J. S. (1988). Training issues in behavior therapy. *Journal of Consulting and Clinical Psychology, 56,* 703–709.

Bootzin, R. R., Engle-Friedman, M., & Hazelwood, L. (1983). Insomnia. In P. M. Lewinsohn & L. Teri (Eds.), *Clinical geropsychology: New directions in assessment and treatment* (pp. 81–115). New York: Pergamon.

Borland, R., Owen, N., Hill, D., & Schofield, P. (1991). Predicting attempts and sustained cessation of smoking after the introduction of workplace smoking bans. *Health Psychology, 10,* 336–342.

Boskind-White, M., & White, W. C. (1986). Bulimarexia: A historical-sociocultural perspective. In K. D. Brownell & J. P. Foreyt (Eds.), *Handbook of eating disorders: Physiology, psychology, and treatment of obesity, anorexia, and bulimia* (pp. 353–366). New York: Basic Books.

Bosse, R., Garvey, A. J., & Costa, P. T. (1980). Predictors of weight change following smoking cessation. *International Journal of Addictive Behavior, 15,* 969–991.

Botvin, G., Eng, A., & Williams, C. L. (1980). Preventing the onset of cigarette smoking through life skill training. *Preventative Medicine, 9,* 135–143.

Bouchard C. (1991). Is weight fluctuation a risk factor? *The New England Journal of Medicine, 324,* 1887–1889.

Bouchard, C. Bray, G. A., & Hubbard, V. S. (1990). Basic and clinical aspects of regional fat distribution. *American Journal of Clinical Nutrition, 52,* 946–950.

Bouchard, C., Tremblay, A., Després, J. P., Nadeau, A., Lupien, P. J., Thériault, G., Dussault, J., Moorjani, S., Pinault, S., & Fournier, G. (1990). The response to long-term overfeeding in identical twins. *The New England Journal of Medicine, 322,* 1477–1482.

Bovbjerg, D., Cohen, N., & Ader, R. (1987). Behaviorally conditioned enhancement of delayed-type hypersensitivity in the mouse. *Brain, Behavior, and Immunity, 1,* 64–71.

Bower, B. (1996). New pitch for placebo power. *Science News, 150,* 123.

Bowser, M. S. (1991). Giving up the ghost: A review of phantom limb phenomena. *The Journal of Rehabilitation, 57,* 55–62.

Boyd, N. F. (1993). Nutrition and breast cancer. *Journal of the National Cancer Institute, 85,* 6–7.

Boyd, D. P., & Begley, T. M. (1987). Assessing the Type A behavior pattern with the Jenkins Activity Survey. *British Journal of Medical Psychology, 60,* 155–161.

Boyer, W. F., & Blumhardt, C. L. (1992). The safety profile of paroxetine. *Journal of Clinical Psychiatry, 53,* 61–66.

Boyko, E. J., Koepsell, T. D., Perera, D. R., & Inui, T. S. (1987). Risk of ulcerative colitis among former and current cigarette smokers. *The New England Journal of Medicine, 316,* 707–710.

Bradley, L. A., Prokop, C. K., & Clayman, D. A. (1981). Medical psychology and behavioral medicine: Summary and future concerns. In C. K. Prokop,

& L. A. Bradley (Eds.). (1981). *Medical psychology: Contributions to behavioral medicine* (pp. 497–502). New York: Academic Press.

Brady, J. V., Porter, R. W., Conrad, D. G., & Mason, J. W. (1958). Avoidance behavior and the development of gastroduodenal ulcers. *Journal of the Experimental Analysis of Behavior, 1,* 69–72.

Branson, S. M., & Craig, K. D. (1988). Children's spontaneous strategies for coping with pain: A review of the literature [Special issue: Child and adolescent health]. *Canadian Journal of Behavioural Science, 20,* 402–412.

Bray, G. A. (1978). Definitions, measurements and classification of the syndromes of obesity. *International Journal of Obesity, 2,* 99–112.

Bray, G. A. (1986). Effects of obesity on health and happiness. In K. D. Brownell & J. P. Foreyt (Eds.), *Handbook of eating disorders: Physiology, psychology, and treatment of obesity, anorexia, and bulimia* (pp. 3–44). New York: Basic Books.

Brennan, T. A., Leape, L. L., Laird, N. M., Hebert, L., Localio, A. R., Lawthers, A. G., Newhouse, J. P., Weiler, P. C., & Hiatt, H. H. (1991). Incidence of adverse events and negligence in hospitalized patients: Results of the Harvard medical practice study I. *The New England Journal of Medicine, 324,* 370–376.

Brett, J. F., Brief, A. P., Burke, M. J., George, J. M., & Webster, J. (1990). Negative affectivity and the reporting of stressful life events. *Health Psychology, 9,* 57–68.

Brewerton, D. (1992). *All about arthritis: Past, present, future.* Cambridge, MA: Harvard University Press.

Bridge, T. P. (1988). AIDS and HIV CNS disease: A neuropsychiatric disorder. In T. P. Bridge, A. F. Mirsky, & F. K. Goodwin (Eds.), *Psychological, neuropsychiatric, and substance abuse aspects of AIDS* (pp. 1–13). New York: Raven Press.

Brink, S. J. (1988). Pediatric, adolescent, and young-adult nutrition issues in IDDM. *Diabetes Care, 11,* 192–200.

Brown, R. T., Kaslow, N. J., Hazzard, A. P., Madan-Swain, A., Sexson, S. B., Lambert, R., & Baldwin, K. (1992). Psychiatric and family functioning in children with leukemia and their parents. *Journal of the American Academy of Child and Adolescent Psychiatry, 31,* 495–502.

Brown, S. A., & Munson, E. (1987). Extroversion, anxiety and the perceived effects of alcohol. *Journal of Studies on Alcohol, 48,* 272–276.

Brown, T. M. (1989). Cartesian dualism and psychosomatics. *Psychosomatics, 30,* 322–331.

Brownell, K. D., & Kaye, F. S. (1982). A school-based behavior modification, nutrition education, and physical activity program for obese children. *The American Journal of Clinical Nutrition, 35,* 277–283.

Brownell, K. D., & Foreyt, J. P. (Eds.). (1986). *Handbook of eating disorders: Physiology, psychology, and treatment of obesity, anorexia, and bulimia.* New York: Basic Books.

Brownell, K. D., & Wadden, T. A. (1986). Behavior therapy for obesity: Modern approaches and better results. In K. D. Brownell & J. P. Foreyt (Eds.), *Handbook of eating disorders: Physiology, psychology, and treatment of obesity, anorexia, and bulimia* (pp. 180–197). New York: Basic Books.

Brubaker, R. G., & Wickersham, D. (1990). Encouraging the practice of testicular self-examination: A field application of the theory of reasoned action. *Health Psychology, 9,* 154–163.

Bruch, H. (1973). *Eating disorders: Obesity, anorexia nervosa, and the person within.* New York: Basic Books.

Buckley, R. H., & Schiff, R. I. (1991). The use of intravenous immune globulin in immunodeficiency diseases. *The New England Journal of Medicine, 325,* 110–117.

Budzynski, T., Stoyva, J., & Adler, C. (1970). Feedback-induced muscle relaxation: Application to tension headache. *Journal of Behavior Therapy and Experimental Psychiatry, 1,* 205–211.

Bundek, N. I., Marks, G., & Richardson, J. L. (1993). Role of health locus of control beliefs in cancer screening of elderly Hispanic women. *Health Psychology, 12,* 193–199.

Bunge, M. (1980). *The mind-body problem.* New York: Pergamon.

Burch, T. K. (1990). Remarriage of older Canadians: Description and interpretation. *Research on Aging, 12,* 546–559.

Burd, S. (1994). NIH issues rules requiring women and minorities in clinical trials. *The Chronicle of Higher Education, 40,* A50.

Burish, T. G., & Jenkins, R. A. (1992). Effectiveness of biofeedback and relaxation training in reducing the side effects of cancer chemotherapy. *Health Psychology, 11,* 17–23.

Burish, T. G., Vasterling, J. J., Carey, M. P., Matt, D. A., & Krozely, M. G. (1988). Posttreatment use of relaxation training by cancer patients. *The Hospice Journal, 4,* 1–8.

Burny, A. (1986). More and better trans-activation. *Nature, 321,* 378.

Bush, J. P. (1987). Pain in children: A review of the literature from a developmental perspective. *Psychology and Health, 1,* 215–236.

Cade, J. E., & Margetts, B. M. (1991). Relationship between diet and smoking—Is the diet of smokers different? *Journal of Epidemiology and Community Health, 45,* 270–272.

Calabrese, L. H., & Gopalakrishna, K. V. (1986). Transmission of HTLV-III infection from man to woman to man. *The New England Journal of Medicine, 314,* 987.

Caldwell, J. C. (1993). Health transition: The cultural, social and behavioural determinants of health in the Third World. *Social Science and Medicine, 36,* 125–135.

Callaway, C. W., Foreyt, J. P., Nuckolls, J. G., & VanItallie, T. B. (1992). Obesity: A quartet of approaches. *Patient Care, 26,* 157–199.

Calnan, M. W., & Moss, S. (1984). The Health Belief Model and compliance with education given at a class in breast self-examination. *Journal of Health and Social Behavior, 25,* 198–210.

Camp, D. E., Klesges, R. C., & Relyea, G. (1993). The relationship between body weight concerns and adolescent smoking. *Health Psychology, 12,* 24–32.

Campbell, D. T., & Fiske, D. W. (1959). Convergent and discriminant validation by the multitrait-multimethod matrix. *Psychological Bulletin, 56,* 8–105.

Cannon, W. (1942). "Voodoo" death. *American Anthropologist, 44,* 169–181.

Cannon, W. B. (1932). *The wisdom of the body.* New York: Norton.

Caplan, G. (1964). *Principles of preventive psychiatry.* New York: Basic.

Caporael, L. R. (1976). Ergotism: The Satan loosed in Salem? *Science, 192,* 21–26.

Carey, M. P., & Burish, T. G. (1988). Etiology and treatment of the psychological side effects associated with cancer chemotherapy: A critical review and discussion. *Psychological Bulletin, 104,* 307–325.

Caris, T. N. (1985). *A clinical guide to hypertension.* Littleton, MA: PSG Publishing.

Carmelli, D., Swan, G. E., Robinette, D., & Fabsitz, R. (1992). Genetic influence on smoking—A study of male twins. *The New England Journal of Medicine, 327,* 829–833.

Carmody, T. P., Fey, S. G., Pierce, D. K., Connor, W. E., & Matarazzo, J. D. (1982). Behavioral treatment of hyperlipidemia: Techniques, results, and future directions. *Journal of Behavioral Medicine, 5,* 91–116.

Carr, J. E. (1987). Federal impact on psychology in medical schools. *American Psychologist, 42,* 869–872.

Carr, R. E., Lehrer, P. M., & Hochron, S. M. (1992). Panic symptoms in asthma and panic disorder: A preliminary test of the dyspnea-fear theory. *Behaviour Research and Therapy, 30,* 251–260.

Carver, C. S., Scheier, M. F., & Pozo, C. (1992). Conceptualizing the process of coping with health problems. In H. S. Friedman (Ed.), *Hostility, coping, and health* (pp. 167–187). Washington, DC: American Psychological Association.

Cassileth, B. B., Lusk, E. J., Miller, D. S., Brown, L. L., & Miller, C. (1985). Psychosocial correlates of survival in advanced malignant disease. *The New England Journal of Medicine, 312,* 1551–1555.

Castiglioni, A. (1947). *A history of medicine* (E. B. Krumbhaar, Trans., 2nd ed.). New York: Knopf.

Castro, K. G., & Hardy, A. M. (1984). Acquired immunodeficiency syndrome (AIDS): An epidemiologic and clinical overview. *Journal of Medical Association of Georgia, 73,* 537–542.

Catania, J. A., Coates, T. J., Stall, R., Turner, H., Peterson, J., Hearst, N., Dolcini, M. M., Hudes, E., Gagnon, J., Wiley, J., & Groves, R. (1992). Prevalence of AIDS-related risk factors and condom use in the United States. *Science, 258,* 1101–1106.

Catania, J. A., Gibson, D. R., Chitwood, D. D., & Coates, T. J. (1990). Methodological problems in AIDS behavioral research: Influences on measurement error and participation bias in studies of sexual behavior. *Psychological Bulletin, 108,* 339–362.

Cattanach, L., & Rodin, J. (1988). Psychosocial components of the stress process in bulimia. *International Journal of Eating Disorders, 7,* 75–88.

Cautela, J. R. (1977). The use of covert conditioning in modifying pain behavior. *Journal of Behavior Therapy and Experimental Psychiatry, 8,* 45–52.

Celermajer, D. S., Adams, M. R., Clarkson, P., Robinson, J., McCredie, R., Donald, A., & Deanfield, J. E. (1996). Passive smoking and impaired endothelium-dependent arterial dilatation in healthy young adults. *The New England Journal of Medicine, 334,* 150–154.

Centers for Disease Control. (1989). Chronic obstructive pulmonary disease mortality—United States, 1986. *Mortality and Morbidity Weekly Reports, 38,* 549–552.

Centers for Disease Control. (1992, September 18). Tobacco, alcohol, and other drug use among high school students—United States, 1991. *Mortality and Morbidity Weekly Reports, 41,* 698–703.

Centers for Disease Control. (1992, December 18). 1993 Revised classification system for HIV infection and expanded surveillance case definition for AIDS among adolescents and adults. *Mortality and Morbidity Weekly Reports, 41,* 1–19.

Centers for Disease Control. (1992, December 25). 1993 Revised classification system for HIV infection and expanded surveillance case definition for AIDS among adolescents and adults. *Mortality and Morbidity Weekly Reports, 41,* 961–962.

Centers for Disease Control. (1992, March 13). Publication of 1992 Surgeon General's Report on smoking and health. *Mortality and Morbidity Weekly Reports, 41,* 183.

Centers for Disease Control. (1992, March 20). Quarterly table reporting alcohol involvement in fatal motor vehicle crashes. *Mortality and Morbidity Weekly Reports, 41,* 199.

Centers for Disease Control. (1992, May 22). Discomfort from environmental tobacco smoke among employees at worksites with minimal smoking restrictions—United States, 1988. *Mortality and Morbidity Weekly Reports, 41,* 351–354.

Centers for Disease Control. (1993, January 8). Deaths and hospitalizations from chronic liver disease and cirrhosis—United States, 1980–1989. *Mortality and Morbidity Weekly Reports, 41,* 969–973.

Centers for Disease Control. (1996). *HIV/AIDS surveillance report, 8*(2).

Centers for Disease Control. (1993, May 7). Fetal alcohol syndrome—United States, 1979–1992. *Morbidity and Mortality Weekly Report, 42*(17), 339–341.

Cepeda-Benito, A. (1993). Meta-analytical review of the efficacy of nicotine chewing gum in smoking treatment programs. *Journal of Consulting and Clinical Psychology, 61,* 822–830.

Cerella, J. (1985). Information processing rates in the elderly. *Psychological Bulletin, 95,* 67–83.

Chamberlin, R. W. (1984). Strategies for disease prevention and health promotion in maternal and child health: The "Ecologic" versus the "high risk" approach. *Journal of Public Health Policy, 74,* 185–197.

Chaplin, J. P., & Krawiec, T. S. (1979). *Systems and theories of psychology* (4th ed.). New York: Holt, Rinehart & Winston.

Chapman, S. L. (1986). A review and clinical perspective on the use of EMG and thermal biofeedback for chronic headaches. *Pain, 27,* 1–43.

Charness, M. E., Simon, R. P., & Greenberg, D. A. (1989). Medical progress: Ethanol and the nervous system. *The New England Journal of Medicine, 321,* 442–451.

Chase, M. (1992, July 21). AIDS gender gap is seen closing fast. *The Wall Street Journal,* B4.

Chase, W. G., & Simon, H. A. (1973). The mind's eye in chess. In W. G. Chase (Ed.), *Visual information processing.* New York: Academic Press.

Chaves, J. F. (1993). Hypnosis in pain management. In J. W. Rhue, S. J. Lynn, & I. Kirsch (Eds.), *Handbook of clinical hypnosis* (pp. 511–553). Washington, DC: American Psychological Association.

Chesney, M. A. (1993). Health Psychology in the 21st century: Acquired immunodeficiency syndrome as a harbinger of things to come. *Health Psychology, 12,* 259–268.

Chesney, M. A., & Coates, T. J. (1990). Health promotion and disease prevention: AIDS put the models to the test. In S. Petro, P. Franks, & T. R. Wolfred (Eds.), *Ending the HIV epidemic: Community strategies in disease prevention and health promotion* (pp. 48–62). Santa Cruz, CA: ETR Associates.

Chilmonczyk, B. A., Salumn, L. M., Megathlin, K. N., Neveux, L. M., Palomaki, G. E., Knight, G. J., Pulkkinen, A. J., & Haddow, J. E. (1993). Association between exposure to environmental tobacco smoke and exacerbations of asthma in children. *The New England Journal of Medicine, 328,* 1665–1669.

Christophersen, E. R. (1989). Injury control. *American Psychologist, 44,* 237–241.

Churchland, P. S. (1986). *Neurophilosophy: Toward a unified science of the mind-brain.* Cambridge, MA: MIT Press.

Clark, D. C., & Zeldow, P. B. (1988). Vicissitudes of depressed mood during four years of medical school. *Journal of the American Medical Association, 260,* 2521–2529.

Clark, J. M., & Paivio, A. (1989). Observational and theoretical terms in psychology: A cognitive perspective on scientific language. *American Psychologist, 44,* 500–512.

Clark, N. M., Becker, M. H., Janz, N. K., Lorig, K., Rakowski, W., & Anderson, L. (1991). Self-management of chronic disease by older adults: A review and questions for research. *Journal of Aging and Health, 3,* 3–27.

Clayson, D., & Mensh, I. N. (1987). Psychologists in medical schools: The trials of emerging political activism. *American Psychologist, 42,* 859–862.

Cloninger, C. R. (1991). D_2 dopamine receptor gene is associated but not linked with alcoholism. *Journal of the American Medical Association, 266,* 1833–1834.

Cloninger, C. R., Bohman, M., & Sigvardsson, S. (1981). Inheritance of alcohol abuse. *Archives of General Psychiatry, 38,* 861–868.

Coates, T. J. (1990). Strategies for modifying sexual behavior for primary and secondary prevention of HIV disease. *Journal of Consulting and Clinical Psychology, 58,* 57–69.

Coates, T. J., Stall, R. D., Catania, J. A., & Kegeles, S. (1988). Behavioral factors in HIV infection. *AIDS 1988, 2*(Suppl. 1), S239–S246.

Cobb, S. (1976). Social support as a moderator of life stress. *Psychosomatic Medicine, 38,* 300–314.

Cockerham, W. C. (1982). *Medical sociology* (2nd ed.). Englewood Cliffs, NJ: Prentice-Hall.

Cody, R. J. (1993). Myocardial disease and congestive heart failure. In R. P. Lewis (Ed.), *Adult clinical cardiology self-assessment program* (Section 4). Bethesda, MD: American College of Cardiology.

Coffin, J., Haase, A., Levy, J. A., Mautagnier, L., Oroszlan, S., Teich, N., Temin, H., Toyoshima, K., Varmus, H., Vogt, P., & Weiss, R. (1986). What to call the AIDS virus? *Nature, 321,* 10.

Cohen, R. A., Williamson, D. A., Monguillot, J. E., Hutchinson, P. C., Gottlieb, J., & Waters, W. F. (1983). Psychophysiological response patterns in vascular and muscle-contraction headaches. *Journal of Behavioral Medicine, 6,* 93–107.

Cohen, S. (1988). Psychosocial models of the role of social support in the etiology of physical disease. *Health Psychology, 7,* 269–297.

Cohen, S., & Syme, S. L. (Eds.). (1985). *Social support and health.* New York: Academic.

Cohen, S., & Wills, T. A. (1985). Stress, social support, and the buffering hypothesis. *Psychological Bulletin, 98,* 310–357.

Cohen, S., Lichtenstein, E., Prochaska, J. O., Rossi, J. S., Gritz, E. R., Carr, C. R., Orleans, C. T., Schoen-bach, V. J., Biener, L., Abrams, D., DiClemente, C. C., Curry, S. Marlatt, G. A., Cummings, K. M., Emont, S. L., Giovino, G., & Ossip-Klein, D. (1989). Debunking myths about self quitting: Evidence from 10 prospective studies of persons who attempt to quit smoking by themselves. *American Psychologist, 44,* 1355–1365.

Cohen, S., Tyrrell, D. A. J., & Smith, A. P. (1991). Psychological stress and susceptibility to the common cold. *The New England Journal of Medicine, 325,* 606–612.

Coile, D. C., & Miller, N. (1984). How radical animal activists try to mislead humane people. *American Psychologist, 39,* 700–701.

Colditz, G. A. (1992). Economic costs of obesity. *American Journal of Clinical Nutrition, 55,* 503S–507S.

Collins, C., & Garcia, M. E. (1989). Position of the American Dietetic Association: Nutrition intervention in the treatment of human immunodeficiency virus infection. *Journal of the American Dietetic Association, 89,* 839–841.

Comings, D. E., Comings, B. G., Muhleman, D., Dietz, G., Shahbahrami, B., Tast, D., Knell, E., Kocsis, P., Baumgarten, R., Kovacs, B. W., Levy, D. L., Smith, M., Borison, R. L., Evans, D., Klein, D. N., MacMurray, J., Tosk, J. M., Sverd, J., Gysin, R., & Flanagan, S. D. (1991). The dopamine D_2 receptor locus as a modifying gene in neuropsychiatric disorders. *Journal of the American Medical Association, 266,* 1793–1800.

Connell, D., Turner, R., & Mason, E. (1985). Summary of findings of the school health education evaluation: Health promotion effectiveness, implementation, and costs. *Journal of School Health, 55,* 316–321.

Conroy, R. W. (1988). The many facets of adolescent drinking. *Bulletin of the Menninger Clinic, 52,* 229–245.

Consensus Conference. (1987). Newborn screening for sickle cell disease and other hemoglobinopathies. *Journal of the American Medical Association, 258,* 1205–1209.

Contrada, R. J. (1989). Type A behavior, personality hardiness, and cardiovascular responses to stress. *Journal of Personality and Social Psychology, 57,* 895–903.

Cook, D. G., Shaper, A. G., Pocock, S. J., & Kussick, S. J. (1986). Giving up smoking and the risk of heart attacks: A report from the British Regional Study. *Lancet, 2,* 1376–1379.

Cook, T. D., & Campbell, D. T. (1979). *Quasi-experimentation: Design & analysis issues for field settings*. Chicago: Rand McNally.

Cooper, M. L. (1992, Winter). Alcohol and increased behavioral risk for AIDS. *Alcohol Health & Research World, 16,* 64–72.

Cornes, C. (1990). Interpersonal psychotherapy of depression (IPT). In R. A. Wells & V. J. Giannetti (Eds.), *Handbook of the brief psychotherapies* (pp. 261–276). New York: Plenum.

Costa, P. T., Zonderman, A. B., & McCrae, R. R. (1991). Personality, defense, coping, and adaptation in older adulthood. In E. M. Cummings, A. L. Greene, & K. K. Karraker (Eds.), *Life span developmental psychology: Perspectives on stress and coping* (pp. 277–293). Hillsdale, NJ: Erlbaum.

Cousins, N. (1979). *Anatomy of an illness*. New York: Norton.

Cousins, N. (1983). *The healing heart*. New York: Norton.

Cox, W. M., & Klinger, E. (1988). A motivational model of alcohol use [Special issue: Models of addiction]. *Journal of Abnormal Psychology, 97,* 168–180.

Coyne, J. C., & Holroyd, K. (1982). Stress, coping, and illness: A transactional perspective. In T. Millon, C. Green, & R. Meagher, *Handbook of clinical health psychology* (pp. 103–127). New York: Plenum.

Crabbe, J. C., Belknap, J. K., & Buck, K. J. (1995). Genetic animal models of alcohol and drug abuse. *Science, 264,* 1715–1723.

Crawford, A. M. (1996). Stigma associated with AIDS: A meta-analysis. *Journal of Applied Social Psychology, 26,* 398–416.

Creed, F. (1993). Stress and psychosomatic disorders. In L. Goldberger & S. Breznitz (Eds.), *Handbook of stress: Theoretical and clinical aspects* (2nd ed., pp. 496–510). New York: Free Press.

Crisp, A. H., Hall, A., & Holland, A. J. (1985). Nature and nurture in anorexia nervosa: A study of 34 pairs of twins, one pair of triplets, and an adoptive family. *International Journal of Eating Disorders, 4,* 5–27.

Crist, W., McDonnell, P., Beck, M., Gillespie, C. T., et al. (1994). Behavior at mealtimes and the young child with cystic fibrosis. *Journal of Developmental and Behavioral Pediatrics, 15,* 157–161.

Cross, D. G., Sheehan, P. W., & Khan, J. A. (1980). Alternative advice and counsel in psychotherapy. *Journal of Consulting and Clinical Psychology, 48,* 615–625.

Crowley, T. J., & Andrews, A. E. (1987). Alcoholic-like drinking in simian social groups. *Psychopharmacology, 92,* 196–205.

Cullen, M. R., Cherniack, M. G., & Rosenstock, L. (1990a). Occupational medicine (First of two parts). *The New England Journal of Medicine, 322,* 594–601.

Cullen, M. R., Cherniack, M. G., & Rosenstock, L. (1990b). Occupational medicine (Second of two parts). *The New England Journal of Medicine, 322,* 675–683.

Cunningham, A. J. (1985). The influence of mind on cancer. *Canadian Psychology, 26,* 13–29.

Cunningham, F. G., & Lindheimer, M. D. (1992). Hypertension in pregnancy. *The New England Journal of Medicine, 326,* 927–932.

Cunningham, W. R., & Brookbank, J. W. (1988). *Gerontology*. New York: Harper & Row.

Cystic Fibrosis Genotype-Phenotype Consortium (The). (1993). Correlation between genotype and phenotype in patients with Cystic Fibrosis. *The New England Journal of Medicine, 329,* 1308–1313.

D'Alton, M. E., & DeCherney, A. H. (1993). Prenatal diagnosis. *The New England Journal of Medicine, 328,* 114–120.

Dackis, C. A., Gold, M. S., & Pottash, A. L. (1986). Central stimulant abuse: Neurochemistry and pharmacotherapy. *Advances in Alcohol and Substance Abuse, 6,* 7–21.

Dahlquist, L. M., & Gil, K. M. (1986). Using parents to maintain improved dental flossing skills in children. *Journal of Applied Behavior Analysis, 19,* 255–260.

Dakof, G. A., & Taylor, S. E. (1990). Victims' perceptions of social support: What is helpful from whom? *Journal of Personality and Social Psychology, 58,* 80–89.

Dana, R. H., & May, W. T. (Eds.). (1987). *Internship training in professional psychology*. Washington: Hemisphere Publishing Cooperation.

Daniell, H. W., Tam, E., & Filice, A. (1993). Larger axillary metastases in obese women and smokers with breast cancer—an influence by host factors on early tumor behavior. *Breast Cancer Research and Treatment, 25,* 193–201.

Dantzer, R., & Kelley, K. W. (1989). Stress and immunity: An integrated view of relationships between the brain and the immune system. *Life Sciences, 44,* 1995–2008.

Dattore, P. J., Shontz, F. C., & Coyne, L. (1980). Premorbid personality differentiation of cancer and noncancer groups: A test of the hypothesis of cancer proneness. *Journal of Consulting and Clinical Psychology, 48,* 388–394.

Davies, P. (1986). The genetics of Alzheimer's disease: A review and a discussion of the implications. *Neurobiology of Aging, 7,* 459–466.

Davis, H. P., Rosenzweig, M. R., Becker, L. A., & Sather, K. J. (1988). Biological psychology's relationships to psychology and neuroscience. *American Psychologist, 43,* 359–371.

Davis, R. M. (1987). Current trends in cigarette advertising and marketing. *The New England Journal of Medicine, 316,* 725–732.

Davis, R. M., Boyd, G. M., & Schoenborn, C. A. (1990). "Common courtesy" and the elimination of passive smoking: Results of the 1987 National Health Interview Survey. *Journal of the American Medical Association, 263,* 2208–2210.

Davis, K. L., Thal, L. J., Gamzu, E. R., Davis, C. S., Woolson, R. F., Gracon, S. I., Drachman, D. A., Schneider, L. S., Whitehouse, P. J., Hoover, T. M., Morris, J. C., Kawas, C. H., Knopman, D. S., Earl, N. L., Kumar, V., Doody, R. S., & the Tacrine Collaborative Study Group. (1992). A double-blind, placebo-controlled multicenter study of tacrine for Alzheimer's disease. *The New England Journal of Medicine, 327,* 1253–1259.

Dawes, E. S. (1992). Cancer. In P. L. Jackson & J. A. Vessey (Eds.), *Primary care of the child with a chronic condition* (pp. 117–147). St. Louis: Mosby.

DeBusk, F. L. (1972). The Hutchinson-Gilford progeria syndrome. *Journal of Pediatrics, 80,* 697–724.

Decker, T. W., Cline-Elsen, J., & Gallagher, M. (1992). Relaxation therapy as an adjunct in radiation oncology. *Journal of Clinical Psychology, 48,* 388–393.

Deeks, S. G., Smith, M., Holodniy, M., & Kahn, J. O. (1997). HIV-1 protease inhibitors: A review for clinicians. *Journal of the American Medical Association, 277,* 145–153.

Deitch, E. A. (1990). The management of burns. *The New England Journal of Medicine, 323,* 1249–1253.

DeJong, W., & Kleck, R. E. (1986). The social psychological effects of overweight. In C. P. Herman, M. P. Zanna, & E. T. Higgins (Eds.), *Physical appearance, stigma, and social behavior: The Ontario Symposium* (Vol. 3, pp. 65–87). Hillsdale, NJ: Erlbaum.

De Kruif, P. H. (1926). *Microbe hunters.* New York, NY: Harcourt, Brace.

Delany, S., & Delany, A. E., with Hearth, A. H. (1993). *Having our say.* New York: Kodansha International.

DeLeon, P. H., Fox, R. E., & Graham, S. R. (1991). Prescription privileges: Psychology's next frontier? *American Psychologist, 46,* 384–393.

Delgado, L. E., & Lutzker, J. R. (1988). Training young parents to identify and report their children's illnesses. *Journal of Applied Behavior Analysis, 21,* 311–319.

Deltito, J. A., Argyle, N., Psych, M. R. C., & Klerman, G. L. (1991). Patients with panic disorder unaccompanied by depression improve with alprazolam and imipramine treatment. *Journal of Clinical Psychiatry, 52,* 121–127.

Demaret, K. (1984a, Oct. 29). David's story. *People Weekly, 22,* 120–131.

Demaret, K. (1984b, Nov. 5). The bubble boy (Part two). *People Weekly, 22,* 107–116.

Dembroski, T. M., & Costa, P. (1987). Coronary prone behavior: Components of the Type A pattern and hostility. *Journal of Personality, 55,* 211–235.

Dembroski, T. M., MacDougall, J. M., Williams, R. B., Jr., Haney, T. L., & Blumenthal, J. A. (1985). Components of Type A, hostility and anger-in: Relationship to angiographic findings. *Psychosomatic Medicine, 247,* 219–233.

Dennett, D. C. (1991). *Consciousness explained.* Boston: Little, Brown.

Des Jarlais, D. C., & Friedman, S. R. (1988). The psychology of preventing AIDS among intravenous drug users: A social learning conceptualization. *American Psychologist, 43,* 865–870.

Deyo, R. A. (1991). Fads in the treatment of low back pain. *The New England Journal of Medicine, 325,* 1039–1040.

Deyo, R. A., Walsh, N. E., Martin, D. C., Schoenfeld, L. S., & Ramamurthy, S. (1990). A controlled trial of transcutaneous electrical nerve stimulation (TENS) and exercise for chronic low back pain. *The New England Journal of Medicine, 322,* 1627–1634.

Diabetes Control and Complications Trial Research Group. (1993). The effect of intensive treatment of diabetes on the development and progression of long-term complications in insulin-dependent diabetes mellitus. *The New England Journal of Medicine, 329,* 977–986.

DiClemente, C. C., Prochaska, J. O., Fairhurst, S. D., Velicer, W. F., Valesquez, M. M., & Rossi, J. S. (1991). The processes of smoking cessation: An analysis of precontemplation, contemplation, and preparation stages of change. *Journal of Consulting and Clinical Psychology, 59,* 295–304.

DiClemente, R. J., Lanier, M. M., Horan, P. F., & Lodico, M. (1991). Comparison of AIDS knowledge, attitudes, and behaviors among incarcerated adolescents and a public school sample in San Francisco. *American Journal of Public Health, 81,* 628–630.

Dienstbier, R. A. (1989). Arousal and physiological toughness: Implications for mental and physical health. *Psychological Review, 96,* 84–100.

Dietz, W. H., Jr., & Gortmaker, S. L. (1985). Do we fatten our children at the television set? Obesity and television viewing in children and adolescents. *Pediatrics, 75,* 807–812.

Dijkstra, A., deVries, H., & Bakker, M. (1996). Pros and cons of quitting, self-efficacy, and the stages of change in smoking cessation. *Journal of Consulting and Clinical Psychology, 64,* 758–763.

Diliberto, G. (1985, May 13). Karen Carpenter was killed by an over-the-counter drug some doctors say may be killing many others. *People Weekly, 23,* 67–70.

Dilley, J. W., Ochitill, H. N., Perl, M., & Volberding, P. A. (1985). Findings in psychiatric consultations with patients with acquired immune deficiency syndrome. *American Journal of Psychiatry, 142,* 82–85.

Dimsdale, J. E. (1988). A perspective on Type A behavior and coronary disease. *The New England Journal of Medicine, 318,* 110–112.

Dinwiddie, S. H., & Cloninger, C. R. (1991). Family and adoption studies in alcoholism and drug addiction. *Psychiatric Annals, 21,* 206–214.

Dion, D., & Blalock, J. E. (1988). Neuroendocrine properties of the immune system. In T. P. Bridge, A. F. Mirsky, & F. K. Goodwin (Eds.), *Psychological, neuropsychiatric, and substance abuse aspects of AIDS* (pp. 15–20). New York: Raven Press.

Dishman, R. K., & Dunn, A. L. (1988). Exercise adherence in children and youth: Implications for adulthood. In R. K. Dishman (Ed.), *Exercise adherence: Its impact on public health* (pp. 155–200). Champaign, IL: Human Kinetics.

Dlin, B. (1985). Psychobiology and treatment of anniversary reactions. *Psychosomatics, 26,* 505–520.

Dobson, K. S. (Ed.). (1988). *Handbook of cognitive-behavioral therapies.* New York: Guilford Press.

Dobson, K. S., & Shaw, B. F. (1988). The use of treatment manuals in cognitive therapy: Experience and issues. *Journal of Consulting and Clinical Psychology, 56,* 673–680.

Dohrenwend, B. S., & Dohrenwend, B. P. (1982). Some issues in research on stressful life events. In T. Millon, C. Green, & R. Meagher (Eds.), *Handbook of clinical health psychology* (pp. 91–102). New York: Plenum.

Dolan, C. A., Sherwood, A., & Light, K. C. (1992). Cognitive coping strategies and blood pressure responses to real-life stress in healthy young men. *Health Psychology, 11,* 233–240.

Doleys, D. M., Meredith, R. L., & Ciminero, A. R. (Eds.). (1982). *Behavioral medicine: Assessment and treatment strategies.* Plenum Press: New York.

Dolovich, J. (1988). Early/late response model: Implications for control of asthma and chronic cough in children. *Pediatric Clinics of North America, 35,* 969–979.

Donnelly, J. E., Donnelly, W. J., & Thong, Y. H. (1987). Parental perceptions and attitudes toward asthma and its treatment: A controlled study. *Social Science & Medicine, 24,* 431–437.

Drash, A. L., & Berlin, N. (1985). Juvenile diabetes. In N. Hobbs & J. M. Perrin (Gen. Eds.), *Issues in the care of children with chronic illness* (pp. 155–182). San Francisco: Jossey-Bass.

Drotar, P., & Crawford, P. (1985). Psychological adaption of siblings of chronically ill children. *Journal of Developmental and Behavioral Pediatrics, 6,* 355–362.

DuBois, P. H. (1970). *A history of psychological testing.* Boston: Allyn & Bacon.

Dunbar, G. C., Cohn, J. B., Fabre, L. F., Feighner, J. P., Fieve, R. R., Mendels, J., & Shrivastava, R. K. (1991). A comparison of paroxetine, imipramine and placebo in depressed outpatients. *British Journal of Psychiatry, 159,* 394–398.

Dunbar, H. F. (1947). *Mind and body: Psychosomatic medicine.* New York: Random House.

Dunkel, L. D., & Glaros, A. G. (1978). Comparison of self-instructional and stimulus control treatments for obesity. *Cognitive Therapy and Research, 2,* 75–78.

Dura, J. R., Haywood-Niler, E., & Kiecolt-Glaser, J. K. (1990). Spousal caregivers of persons with Alzheimer's and Parkinson's disease dementia: A preliminary comparison. *The Gerontologist, 30,* 332–336.

Dutton, D. B. (1988). *Worse than the disease: Pitfalls of medical progress.* Cambridge: Cambridge University Press.

Earls, F., Robins, L. N., Stiffman, A. R., & Powell, J. (1989). Comprehensive health care for high-risk adolescents: An evaluation study. *American Journal of Public Health, 79,* 999–1005.

Ehrensvard, G. (1965). *Man on another world* (L. Roden & K. Roden, Trans.). Chicago: University of Chicago Press.

Eimas, P. D., & Galaburda, A. M. (1989). Some agenda items for a neurobiology of cognition: An introduction. *Cognition, 33,* 1–23.

Eisenbarth, G. S., Ziegler, A. G., & Colman, P. A. (1994). Pathogenesis of insulin-dependent (Type I) diabetes mellitus. In C. R. Kahn & G. C. Weir (Eds.), *Joslin's diabetes mellitus—13th.* (pp. 216–239). Malvern, PA: Lea & Febiger.

Eisenberg, D. M., Kessler, R. C., Foster, C., Norlock, F. E., Calkins, D. R., Delbanco, T. L. (1993). Unconventional medicine in the United States: Prevalence, costs, and patterns of use. *The New England Journal of Medicine, 328,* 246–252.

Eiser, C. (1990). *Chronic childhood disease: An introduction to psychological theory and research.* Cambridge: Cambridge University Press.

Eiser, C., Town, C., & Tripp, J. H. (1988). Knowledge and understanding of asthma. *Child: Care, Health and Development, 14,* 11–24.

Ekstrand, M. L., & Coates, T. J. (1990). Maintenance of safer sexual behaviors and predictors of risky sex: The San Francisco Men's Health Study. *American Journal of Public Health, 90,* 973–977.

Eland, J. M., & Anderson, J. E. (1977). The experience of pain in children. In A. K. Jacox (Ed.), *Pain: A source book for nurses and other health professionals* (pp. 453–471). Boston: Little, Brown.

Eley, J. W., Hill, H. A., Chen, V. W., Austin, D. F., Wesley, M. N., Muss, H. B., Greenberg, R. S., Coates, R. J., Correa, P., Redmond, C. K., Hunter, C. P., Herman, A. A., Kurman, R., Blacklow, R., Shapiro, S., & Edwards, B. K. (1994). Racial differences in survival from breast cancer: Results of the National Cancer Institute Black/White Cancer Survival Study. *Journal of the American Medical Association, 272,* 947–954.

Ellerbrock, T. V., Lieb, S., Harrington, P. E., Bush, T. J., Schoenfisch, S. A., Oxtoby, M. J., Howell, J. T., Rogers, M. F., & Witte, J. J. (1992). Heterosexually transmitted human immunodeficiency virus infection among pregnant women in a rural Florida community. *The New England Journal of Medicine, 327,* 1704–1709.

Ellickson, P. L., & Hays, R. D. (1992). On becoming involved with drugs: Modeling adolescent drug use over time. *Health Psychology, 11,* 377–385.

Elliott, T. R., & Gramling, S. E. (1990). Psychologists and rehabilitation: New roles and old training models. *American Psychologist, 45,* 762–765.

Emery, C. F., Pinder, S. L., & Blumenthal, J. A. (1989). Psychological effects of exercise among elderly cardiac patients. *Journal of Cardiopulmonary Rehabilitation, 9,* 46–53.

Emery, R. E. (1989). Family violence. *American Psychologist, 44,* 321–328.

Emmelkamp, P. M. G., & Mersch, P. P. (1982). Cognition and exposure in vivo in the treatment of agoraphobia: Short-term and delayed effects. *Cognitive Therapy and Research, 6,* 77–90.

Emmelkamp, P. M. P. (1986). Behavior therapy with adults. In S. L. Garfield & A. E. Bergin (Eds.). *Handbook of psychotherapy and behavior change* (3rd ed., pp. 385–442). New York: Wiley.

Eng, K., & Emlet, C. A. (1990). SRx: A regional approach to geriatric medication education. *The Gerontologist, 30,* 408–482.

Engel, B. T., Glasgow, M. S., & Gaarder, K. R. (1983). Behavioral treatment of high blood pressure: III. Follow-up results and treatment recommendations. *Psychosomatic Medicine, 45,* 23–29.

Engel, G. L. (1977). The need for a new medical model: A challenge for biomedicine. *Science, 196,* 129–136.

Engel, G. L. (1987). Physician-scientists and scientific physicians: Resolving the humanism-science dichotomy. *American Journal of Medicine, 82,* 107–111.

Engle-Friedman, M., Bootzin, R. R., Hazlewood, L., & Tsao, C. (1992). An evaluation of behavioral treatments for insomnia in the older adult. *Journal of Clinical Psychology, 48,* 77–90.

Epstein, L. H. (1984). The direct effects of compliance on health outcome. *Health Psychology, 3,* 385–393.

Epstein, L. H. (1986). Treatment of childhood obesity. In K. D. Brownell & J. P. Foreyt (Eds.), *Handbook of eating disorders: Physiology, psychology, and treatment of obesity, anorexia, and bulimia* (pp. 159–179). New York: Basic Books.

Erikson, E. H. (1968). *Identity, youth and crisis.* New York: Norton.

Evans, A. S. (1978). Causation and disease: A chronological journey. *American Journal of Epidemiology, 108,* 249–258.

Evans, R. I., Smith, C. K., & Raines, B. E. (1984). Deterring cigarette smoking in adolescents: A psychosocial-behavioral analysis of an intervention strategy. In A. Baum, S. E. Taylor, & J. E. Singer

(Eds.), *Handbook of psychology and health. Vol. 4: Social psychological aspects of health* (pp. 301–318). Hillsdale, NJ: Erlbaum.

Evans, R. I., Henderson, A. H., Hill, P. C., & Raines, B. E. (1979). Current psychological, social, and educational programs in control and prevention of smoking: A critical methodological review. *Atherosclerosis Reviews, 6,* 203–245.

Everall, I. P., Luthert, P. J., & Lantos, P. L. (1991). Neuronal loss in the frontal cortex in HIV infection. *The Lancet, 337,* 1119–1121.

Ewart, C. K., Taylor, C. B., Kraemer, H. C., & Agras, W. S. (1991). High blood pressure and marital discord: Not being nasty matters more than being nice. *Health Psychology, 10,* 155–163.

Ewing, C. P. (1990). Crisis intervention as brief psychotherapy. In R. A. Wells & V. J. Giannetti (Eds.), *Handbook of the brief psychotherapies* (pp. 277–294). New York: Plenum.

Eysenck, H. J. (1952). The effects of psychotherapy: An evaluation. *Journal of Consulting Psychology, 16,* 319–324.

FDA chief urges curbs. (1995, March 16). *Facts on File, 55,* 192.

Fairburn, C. G., & Beglin, S. J. (1990). Studies of the epidemiology of bulimia nervosa. *The American Journal of Psychiatry, 147,* 401–408.

Fairburn, C. G., Kirk, J., O'Connor, M. E., & Cooper, P. J. (1986). A comparison of two psychological treatments for bulimia nervosa. *Behaviour Research and Therapy, 24,* 629–643.

Fairburn, C. G., Peveler, R. C., Jones, R., Hope, R. A., & Doll, H. A. (1993). Predictors of 12-month outcome to bulimia nervosa and the influence of attitudes to shape and weight. *Journal of Consulting and Clinical Psychology, 61,* 696–698.

Fallowfield, L. J., Baum, M., & Maguire, G. P. (1986). Effects of breast conservation on psychological morbidity associated with diagnosis and treatment of early breast cancer. *British Medical Journal, 293,* 1331–1334.

Farrar, W. L., Kilian, P. L., Ruff, M. R., Hill, J. M., & Pert, C. B. (1988). Characterization of interleukin 1 receptors in brain. In T. P. Bridge, A. F. Mirsky, & F. K. Goodwin (Eds.), *Psychological, neuropsychiatric, and substance abuse aspects of AIDS* (pp. 35–44). New York: Raven Press.

Fauci, A. S., Pantaleo, G., Stanley, S., & Weissman, D. (1996). Immunopathologenic mechanisms of HIV infection. *Annals of Internal Medicine, 124,* 654–663.

Fava, M., Copeland, P. M., Schweiger, U., & Herzog, D. B. (1989). Neurochemical abnormalities of anorexia nervosa and bulimia nervosa. *American Journal of Psychiatry, 146,* 963–969.

FDA Consumer. (1995, October). *Updates.*

Fernandez, E., & Turk, D. C. (1989). The utility of cognitive coping strategies for altering pain perception: A meta-analysis. *Pain, 38,* 123–135.

Fernandez, E., & Turk, D. C. (1992). Sensory and affective components of pain: Separation and synthesis. *Psychological Bulletin, 112,* 205–217.

Fiatarone, M. A., O'Neill, E. F., Ryan, N. D., Clements, K. M., Solares, G. R., Nelson, M. E., Roberts, S. B., Kehayias, J. J., Lipsitz, L. A., & Evans, W. J. (1994). Exercise training and nutritional supplementation for physical frailty in very elderly people. *The New England Journal of Medicine, 330,* 1769–1775.

Fielding, J. E., & Phenow, K. J. (1988). Health effects of involuntary smoking. *The New England Journal of Medicine, 319,* 1452–1460.

Filice, G. A., & Pomeroy, C. (1991). Preventing secondary infections among HIV-positive persons. *Public Health Reports, 106,* 503–517.

Finkelhor, D., & Dziuba-Leatherman, J. (1994). Victimization of children. *American Psychologist, 49,* 178–183.

Finkelstein, J. S., McCully, W. F., MacLaughlin, D. T., Godine, J. E., & Crowley, W. F. (1988). The mortician's mystery: Gynecomastia and reversible hypogonadotroic hypogonadism in an embalmer. *The New England Journal of Medicine, 318,* 961–965.

Finney, J. W., & Moos, R. H. (1992). The long-term course of treated alcoholism: II. Predictors and correlates of 10-year functioning and mortality. *Journal of Studies on Alcohol, 53,* 142–153.

Fischl, M. A., Parker, C. B., Pettinelli, C., Wulfsohn, M., Hirsch, M. S., Collier, A. C., Antoniskis, D., Ho, M., Richman, D. D., Fuchs, E., Merigan, T. C., Reichman, R. C., Gold, J., Steigbigel, N., Leoung, G. S., Rasheed, S., Tsiatis, A., & the AIDS Clinical Trials Group. (1990). A randomized controlled trial of a reduced daily dose of zidovudine in patients with the acquired immunodeficiency syndrome. *The New England Journal of Medicine, 323,* 1009–1014.

Fisher, E. B., Delamater, A. M., Bertelson, A. D., & Kirkley, B. G. (1982). Psychological factors in diabetes and its treatment. *Journal of Consulting and Clinical Psychology, 50,* 993–1003.

Fisher, J. D., & Fisher, W. A. (1992). Changing AIDS-risk behavior. *Psychological Bulletin, 111,* 455–474.

Fiske, M. (1993). Challenge and defeat: Stability and change in adulthood. In L. Goldberger & S. Breznitz (Eds.), *Handbook of stress: Theoretical and clinical aspects* (2nd ed., pp. 413–426). New York: Free Press.

Fitzgerald, J. L., & Mulford, H. A. (1987). Self-report validity issues. *Journal of Studies on Alcohol, 48,* 207–211.

FitzGibbon, C. (1987). *The life of Dylan Thomas.* London: Plantin.

Fitzpatrick, R., Newman, S., Archer, R., & Shipley, M. (1991). Social support, disability, and depression: A longitudinal study of rheumatoid arthritis. *Social Science & Medicine, 33,* 605–611.

Fleming, C., Wasson, J. H., Albertsen, P. C., Barry, M. J., & Wennberg, J. E. (1993). A decision analysis of alternative treatment strategies for clinically localized prostate cancer. *Journal of the American Medical Association, 269,* 2650–2658.

Fletcher, A. E., & Bulpitt, C. J. (1992). How far should blood pressure be lowered? *The New England Journal of Medicine, 326,* 251–254.

Flor, H., & Birbaumer, N. (1993). Comparison of the efficacy of electromyographic biofeedback, cognitive-behavioral therapy, and conservative medical interventions in the treatment of chronic musculoskeletal pain. *Journal of Consulting and Clinical Psychology, 61,* 653–658.

Flor, H., & Turk, D. C. (1989). Psychophysiology of chronic pain: Do chronic pain patients exhibit symptom-specific psychophysiological responses? *Psychological Bulletin, 105,* 215–259.

Folkman, S. (1993). Psychosocial effects of HIV infection. In L. Goldberger & S. Breznitz (Eds.), *Handbook of stress: Theoretical and clinical aspects* (2nd ed., pp. 658–681). New York: Free Press.

Folkman, S., & Lazarus, R. S. (1980). An analysis of coping in a middle-aged community sample. *Journal of Health and Social Behavior, 21,* 219–239.

Folkman, S., Chesney, M. A., Pollack, L., & Phillips, C. (1992). Stress, coping, and high-risk sexual behavior. *Health Psychology, 11,* 218–222.

Folkman, S., Lazarus, R. S., Pimley, S., & Novacek, J. (1987). Age differences in stress and coping processes. *Psychology and Aging, 2,* 171–184.

Fontana, B. L., & Schaefer, J. P. (1979). *Tarahumara:*

Where night is the day of the moon. Flagstaff, AZ: Northland.

Fordyce, W. E. (1976). *Behavioral methods for chronic pain and illness.* St. Louis, MO: Mosby.

Fordyce, W. E. (1988). Pain and suffering: A reappraisal. *American Psychologist, 43,* 276–283.

Forster, L. E., Pollow, R., & Stoller, E. P. (1993). Alcohol use and potential risk for alcohol-related adverse drug reactions among community-based elderly. *Journal of Community Health, 18,* 225–239.

Foster, G. D., Wadden, T. A., Kendall, P. C., Stunkard, A. J., & Vogt, R. A. (1996). Psychological effects of weight loss and regain: A prospective evaluation. *Journal of Consulting and Clinical Psychology, 64,* 752–757.

Foster, G. M., & Anderson, B. G. (1978). *Medical anthropology.* New York: Wiley.

Fowles, D. C. (1992). Schizophrenia: Diathesis-stress revisited. *Annual Review of Psychology, 43,* 303–336.

Fox, B. H. (1978). Premorbid psychological factors as related to cancer incidence. *Journal of Behavioral Medicine, 1,* 45–133.

Frank, A. L. (1990). Occupational medicine. *Journal of American Medical Association, 263,* 2665–2666.

Frank, R. G. (1993). Health-care reform: An introduction. *American Psychologist, 48,* 258–260.

Frankenhaeuser, M. (1986). A psychological framework for research on human stress and coping. In M. H. Appley & R. Trumbull (Eds.), *Dynamics of stress: Physiological, psychological, and social perspectives* (pp. 101–116). New York: Plenum.

Franks, C. M. (1969). Introduction: Behavior therapy and its Pavlovian origins: Review and perspectives. In C. M. Franks (Ed.). *Behavior therapy: Appraisal and status* (pp. 1–26). New York: McGraw-Hill.

Frasure-Smith, N., Lespérance, F., & Talajic, M. (1995). The impact of negative emotions on prognosis following myocardial infarction: Is it more than depression? *Health Psychology, 14,* 388–398.

Freedman, D. G. (1979). *Human sociobiology: A holistic approach.* New York: The Free Press.

Freeman, L. J., Nixon, P. G. F., Sallabank, P., & Reaveley, D. (1987). Psychological stress and silent myocardial ischemia. *American Heart Journal, 114,* 477–482.

Freud, S. (1885/1974). *Cocaine papers* (edited and introduction by R. Byck; notes by A. Freud). New York: Stonehill.

Frezza, M., di Padova, C., Pozzato, G., Terpin, M.,

Baraona, E., & Lieber, C. S. (1990). High blood alcohol levels in women: The role of decreased gastric alcohol dehydrogenase activity and first-pass metabolism. *The New England Journal of Medicine, 322,* 95–99.

Frick, M. H., Elo, O., Haapa, K., Heinonen, O. P., Heinsalmi, P., Helo, P., Huttunen, J. K., Kaitaniemi, P., Koskinen, P., Manninen, V., Mäenpää, H., Mälkönen, M., Mänttäri, M., Norola, S., Pasternack, A., Pikkarainen, J., Romo, M., Sjöblom, T., & Nikkilä, E. A. (1987). Helsinki heart study: Primary-prevention trial with gemfibrozil in middle-aged men with dyslipidemia. *The New England Journal of Medicine, 317,* 1237–1245.

Frick, W., & Busse, W. (1988). Respiratory infections: Their role in airway responsiveness and pathogenesis of asthma. *Clinical Chest Medicine, 9,* 539–549.

Friday, G., & Fireman, P. (1988). Morbidity and mortality of asthma. *Pediatric Clinics of North America, 35,* 1149–1162.

Friedland, G. H., & Klein, R. S. (1987). Transmission of the human immunodeficiency virus. *The New England Journal of Medicine, 317,* 1125–1135.

Friedland, G. H., Saltzman, B. R., Rogers, M. F., Kahl, P. A., Lesser, M. L., Mayers, M. M., & Klein, R. S. (1986). Lack of transmission of HTLV-III/LAV infection to household contacts of patients with AIDS or AIDS-related complex with oral candidiasis. *The New England Journal of Medicine, 314,* 344–349.

Friedman, H. S., & Booth-Kewley, S. (1987). The "disease-prone personality:" A meta-analytic view of the construct. *American Psychologist, 42,* 539–555.

Friedman, L., Bliwise, D. L., Yesavage, J. A., & Salom, S. R. (1991). A preliminary study comparing sleep restriction and relaxation treatments for insomnia in older adults. *Journal of Gerontology, 46,* 1–8.

Friedman, M., & Rosenman, R. H. (1974). *Type A behavior and your heart.* New York: Knopf.

Fries, J. F. (1980). Aging, natural death, and the comparison of morbidity. *The New England Journal of Medicine, 303,* 130–135.

Frohlich, E. D. (1993). Hypertension. In R. P. Lewis (Ed.) *Adult clinical cardiology self-assessment program* (Section 6), Bethesda, MD: American College of Cardiology.

Frohlich, E. D., Apstein, C., Chobanian, A. V., Devereux, R. B., Dustan, H. P., Dzau, V., Fauad-Tarazi, F., Horan, M. J., Marcus, M., Massie, B.,

Pfeffer, M. A., Re, R. N., Roccella, E. J., Savage, D., & Shub, C. (1992). The heart in hypertension. *The New England Journal of Medicine, 327,* 998–1008.

Fulton, J. P., Buechner, J. S., Scott, H. D., DeBuono, B. A., Feldman, J. P., Smith, R. A., & Kovenock, D. (1991). A study guided by the Health Belief Model of the predictors of breast cancer screening of women ages 40 and older. *Public Health Reports, 106,* 410–420.

Furnham, A., & Hume-Wright, A. (1992). Lay theories of anorexia nervosa. *Journal of Clinical Psychology, 48,* 20–36.

Fuster, V., Badimon, L., Badimon, J. J., & Chesebro, J. H. (1992a). The pathogenesis of coronary artery disease and the acute coronary syndromes (First of two parts). *The New England Journal of Medicine, 326,* 242–250.

Fuster, V., Badimon, L., Badimon, J. J., & Chesebro, J. H. (1992b). The pathogenesis of coronary artery disease and the acute coronary syndromes (Second of two parts). *The New England Journal of Medicine, 326,* 310–318.

Gaffney, A., & Dunn, E. G. (1986). Developmental aspects of children's definition of pain. *Pain, 26,* 105–117.

Gaffney, A., & Dunn, E. G. (1987). Children's understanding of the causality of pain. *Pain, 29,* 91–104.

Gallagher-Thompson, D., & Steffen, A. M. (1994). Comparative effects of cognitive-behavioral and brief psychodynamic psychotherapies for depressed family caregivers. *Journal of Consulting and Clinical Psychology, 62,* 543–549.

Gallistel, C. R., Shizgal, P., & Yeomans, J. S. (1981). A portrait of the substrate for self-stimulation. *Psychological Review, 88,* 228–273.

Gallup, G., Jr. (1984). *The Gallup poll: Public opinion 1984.* Wilmington, DE: Scholarly Resources.

Garcia, J., & Koelling, R. A. (1966). Relation of cue to consequence in avoidance learning. *Psychonomic Science, 4,* 123–124.

Garfield, S. L. (1986). Research on client variables in psychotherapy. In S. L. Garfield & A. E. Bergin (Eds.). *Handbook of psychotherapy and behavior change* (3rd ed., pp. 213–256). New York: Wiley.

Garfield, S. L. (1989). *The practice of brief psychotherapy.* New York: Pergamon.

Garfield, S. L., & Bergin, A. E. (Eds.). (1986). *Handbook of psychotherapy and behavior change* (3rd ed.). New York: Wiley.

Garrow, J. S. (1992). Treatment of obesity. *The Lancet, 340,* 409–413.

Gay, P. (1988). *Freud: A life for our time*. New York: Norton.

Gayle, H. D., Keeling, R. P., Garcia-Tunon, M., Kilbourne, B. W., Narkunas, J. P., Ingram, F. R., Rogers, M. F., & Curran, J. W. (1990). Prevalence of the human immunodeficiency virus among university students. *The New England Journal of Medicine, 323,* 1538–1541.

Gaziano, J. M., Buring, J. E., Breslow, J. L., Goldhaber, S. Z., Rosner, B., VanDenburgh, M., Willett, W., & Hennekens, C. H. (1993). Moderate alcohol intake, increased levels of high-density lipoprotein and its subfractions, and decreased risk of myocardial infarction. *The New England Journal of Medicine, 329,* 1829–1834.

Geer, B. W., McKechnie, S. W., Heinstra, P. W. H., & Pyka, M. J. (1991). Heritable variation in ethanol tolerance and its association with biochemical traits in Drosophila melanogaster. *Evolution, 45,* 1107–1119.

Geiss, S. K., Hobbs, S. A., Hammersley-Maercklein, G., Kramer, J. C., & Henley, M. (1992). Psychosocial factors related to perceived compliance with cystic fibrosis treatment. *Journal of Clinical Psychology, 48,* 99–103.

Geist, C. R., & Herrman, S. M. (1990). A comparison of the psychological characteristics of smokers, ex-smokers, and nonsmokers. *Journal of Clinical Psychology, 46,* 102–105.

Gelehrter, T. D., & Collins, F. S. (1990). *Principles of medical genetics*. Baltimore, MD: Williams & Wilkins.

Gelernter, J., O'Malley, S., Risch, N., Kranzier, H. R., Krystal, J., Merikangas, K., Kennedy, J. L., & Kidd, K. K. (1991). No association between an allele at the D_2 dopamine receptor gene (DRD2) and alcoholism. *Journal of the American Medical Association, 266,* 1801–1807.

Gentry, W. D., & Matarazzo, J. D. (1981). Medical psychology: Three decades of growth and development. In C. K. Prokop, & L. A. Bradley (Eds.). (1981). *Medical psychology: Contributions to behavioral medicine* (pp. 5–15). New York: Academic Press.

George, F. R. (1987). Genetic and environmental factors in ethanol self-administration. *Pharmacology, Biochemistry and Behavior, 27,* 379–384.

George, F. R. (1990). Genetic approaches to studying drug abuse: Correlates of drug self-administration. *Alcohol, 7,* 207–211.

George, F. R. (1988). Genetic tools in the study of drug self-administration. *Alcoholism: Clinical and Experimental Research, 12,* 586–590.

Geronimus, A. T., Andersen, H. F., & Bound, J. (1991). Differences in hypertension prevalence among U.S. black and white women of childbearing age. *Public Health Reports, 106,* 393–399.

Geronimus, A. T., Bound, J., Waidman, T. A., Hillemeier, M. M., & Burns, P. (1996). Excess mortality among blacks and whites in the United States. *The New England Journal of Medicine, 335,* 1552–1558.

Gerrard, M., Gibbons, F. X., & Bushman, B. J. (1996). Relation between perceived vulnerability to HIV and precautionary sexual behavior. *Psychological Bulletin, 119,* 390–409.

Gershman, H., & Steeper, J. (1991). Rate of clearance of ethanol from the blood of intoxicated patients in the emergency department. *Journal of Emergency Medicine, 9,* 307–311.

Gershoff, S. (1990). *The Tufts University guide to total nutrition*. New York: Harper & Row.

Gershon, E. S., Schreiber, J. L., Hamovit, J. R., Dibble, E. D., Kaye, W. H., Nurnberger, J. I., Andersen, A., & Ebert, M. H. (1983). Anorexia nervosa and major affective disorders associated in families: A preliminary report. In S. B. Guze, F. J. Earls, & J. E. Barrett (Eds.), *Childhood psychopathology and development* (pp. 279–284). New York: Raven Press.

Giannini, A. J., & Miller, N. S. (1989). Drug abuse: A biopsychiatric model. *American Family Physician, 40,* 173–182.

Gigerenzer, G., Hoffrage, U., & Kleinbölting, H. (1991). Probabilistic mental models: A Brunswikian theory of confidence. *Psychological Review, 98,* 506–528.

Gil, K. M., Williams, D. A., Keefe, F. J., & Beckham, J. C. (1990). The relationship of negative thoughts to pain and psychological distress. *Behavior Therapy, 21,* 349–362.

Gilada, I. S. (1991). AIDS in Asia. *AIDS Care, 3,* 391–394.

Gilliam, T. B., Freedson, P. S., Geenen, D. L., & Shahraray, B. (1981). Physical activity patterns determined by heart rate monitoring in 6–7 year old children. *Medicine and Science in Sports and Exercise, 13,* 65–67.

Gillin, J. C. (1991). The long and short of sleeping pills. *The New England Journal of Medicine, 324,* 1735–1737.

Given, C. W., Stommel, M., Given, B., Osuch, J., Kurtz, M. E., & Kurtz, J. C. (1993). The influence of cancer patients' symptoms and functional states on patients's depression and family caregivers' reactions and depression. *Health Psychology, 12,* 277–285.

Glass, G. V. (1976). Primary, secondary, and meta-analysis of research. *Educational Researchers, 5,* 3–8.

Glassman, J. N., Rich, C. L., Darko, D., & Clarkin, A. (1991). Menstrual dysfunction in bulimia. *Annals of Clinical Psychiatry, 3,* 161–165.

Glenn, S. W., & Parsons, O. A. (1989). Alcohol abuse and familial alcoholism: Psychosocial correlates in men and women. *Journal of Studies on Alcohol, 50,* 116–127.

Gold, D. A., Wang, X., Wypij, D., Speizer, F. E., Ware, J. H., & Dockery, D. W. (1996). Effects of cigarette smoking on lung function in adolescent boys and girls. *The New England Journal of Medicine, 335,* 931–937.

Gold, M. (1977). A crisis of identity: The case of medical sociology. *Journal of Health and Social Behavior, 18,* 160–168.

Gold, P. W., Goodwin, F. K., & Chrousos, G. P. (1988). Clinical and biochemical manifestations of depression: Relation to the neurobiology of stress (Second of two parts). *The New England Journal of Medicine, 319,* 413–420.

Goldband, S. (1980). Stimulus specificity of physiological response to stress and the Type A coronary-prone behavior pattern. *Journal of Personality and Social Psychology, 39,* 670–679.

Goldenhersh, M., & Rachelefsky, G. (1989a). Childhood asthma: Overview. *Pediatric Review, 10,* 227–233.

Goldenhersh, M., & Rachelefsky, G. (1989b). Childhood asthma: Management. *Pediatric Review, 10,* 259–267.

Goldstein, D. S. (1994). Stress and science. In O. G. Cameron (Ed.), *Adrenergic dysfunction and psychobiology* (pp. 179–236). Washington, DC: American Psychiatric Press.

Goldstein, E. B. (1994). *Psychology.* Pacific Grove, CA: Brooks/Cole.

Goodgame, R. W. (1990). AIDS in Uganda—Clinical and social features. *The New England Journal of Medicine, 323,* 383–388.

Goodwin, D. W., Schulsinger, F., Moller, N., Hermansen, L., Winokur, L., & Guze, S. B. (1974). Drinking problems in adopted and non-adopted sons of alcoholics. *Archives of General Psychiatry, 31,* 164–169.

Goodwin, D. W. (1988). Genetic factors in the development of alcoholism. *Psychiatric Clinics of North America, 9,* 427–433.

Gordon, T. J. (1987). Medical breakthroughs: Cutting the toll of killer diseases. *The Futurist, January-February,* 15–17.

Gornick, M. E., Eggers, P. W., Reilly, T. W., Mentnech, R. M., Fitterman, L. K., Kucken, L. E., & Vladeck, B. C. (1996). Effects of race and income on mortality and use of services among medicare beneficiaries. *The New England Journal of Medicine, 335,* 791–799.

Gortmaker, S. L. (1985). Demography of chronic childhood diseases. In N. Hobbs & J. M. Perrin (Gen. Eds.), *Issues in the care of children with chronic illness* (pp. 135–154). San Francisco: Jossey-Bass.

Gortmaker, S. L., Must, A., Perrin, J. M., Sobol, A. M., & Dietz, W. H. (1993). Social and economic consequences of overweight in adolescence and young adulthood. *The New England Journal of Medicine, 329,* 1008–1012.

Gould, D., & Horn, T. (1984). Participation motivation in young athletes. In J. M. Silva & R. S. Weinberg (Eds.), *Psychological foundations of sport* (pp. 359–370). Champaign, IL: Human Kinetics.

Gould, D., Feltz, D. L., & Weiss, M. (1985). Motives for participating in competitive youth swimming. *International Journal of Sport Psychology, 16,* 126–140.

Graham, N. M. H., Zeger, S. L., Park, L. P., Vermund, S. H., Detels, R., Rinaldo, C. R., & Phair, J. P. (1992). The effects on survival of early treatment of human immunodeficiency virus infection. *The New England Journal of Medicine, 326,* 1037–1042.

Green, R. G. (1985). Stress and accidents. *Aviation, Space, and Environmental Medicine, 56,* 638–641.

Greenberg, E. R., Baron, J. A., Stukel, T. A., Stevens, M. M., Mandel, J. S., Spencer, S. K., Elias, P. M., Lowe, N., Nierenberg, D. W., Bayrd, G., Vance, J. C., Freeman, D. H., Jr., Clendenning, W. E., Kwan, T., & the Skin Cancer Prevention Study Group. (1990). A clinical trial of beta carotene to prevent basal-cell and squamous-cell cancers of the skin. *The New England Journal of Medicine, 323,* 789–795.

Greenberg, L. S., & Goldman, R. L. (1988). Training in experiential therapy. *Journal of Consulting and Clinical Psychology, 56,* 696–702.

Greene, W. C. (1991). The molecular biology of human immunodeficiency virus type 1 infection.

The New England Journal of Medicine, 324, 308–317.

Greer, S., & Morris, T. (1975). Psychological attributes of women who develop breast cancer: A controlled study. *Journal of Psychosomatic Research, 19,* 147–153.

Grey, M. (1992). Diabetes mellitus (Type I). In P. L. Jackson & J. A. Vessey (Eds.), *Primary care of the child with a chronic condition* (pp. 229–244). St. Louis: Mosby.

Grilo, C. M., & Pogue-Geile, M. F. (1991). The nature of environmental influences on weight and obesity: A behavior gentic analysis. *Psychological Bulletin, 110,* 520–537.

Grinspoon, S. K., & Bilezikian, J. P. (1992). HIV disease and the endocrine system. *The New England Journal of Medicine, 327,* 1360–1365.

Grissett, N. I., & Norvell, N. K. (1992). Perceived social support, social skills, and quality of relationships in bulimic women. *Journal of Consulting and Clinical Psychology, 60,* 293–299.

Gritz, E. R., & Crane, L. A. (1991). Use of diet pills and amphetamines to lose weight among smoking and nonsmoking high school seniors. *Health Psychology, 10,* 330–335.

Grobbee, D. E., Rimm, E. B., Giovannucci, E., Colditz, G., Stampfer, M., & Willett, W. (1990). Coffee, caffeine, and cardiovascular disease in men. *The New England Journal of Medicine, 323,* 1026–1032.

Grodstein, F., Stampfer, M. J., Manson, J. E., Colditz, G. A., Willett, W. C., Rosner, B., Speizer, F. E., & Hennekens, C. H. (1996). Postmenopausal estrogen and progestin use and the risk of cardiovascular disease. *The New England Journal of Medicine, 335,* 453–461.

Groër, M. W., & Shekleton, M. E. (1983). *Basic pathophysiology: A conceptual approach* (2nd ed.). St. Louis: C. V. Mosby.

Gruder, C. L., Mermelstein, R. J., Kirkendol, S., Hedeker, D., Wong, S. C., Schreckengost, J., Warnecke, R. B., Burzette, R., & Miller, T. Q. (1993). Effects of social support and relapse prevention training as adjuncts to a televised smoking-cessation intervention. *Journal of Consulting and Clinical Psychology, 61,* 113–120.

Grünbaum, A. (1985). Explication and implications of the placebo concept. In L. White, B. Tursky, & G. E. Schwartz (Eds.), *Placebo: Theory, research, and mechanisms* (pp. 9–36). New York: Guilford Press.

Grunberg, N. E., Bowen, D. J., & Morse, D. E. (1984). Effects of nicotine on body weight and food consumption in rats. *Psychopharmacology, 83,* 93–98.

Grunberg, N. E. (1988). Behavioral factors in preventive medicine and health promotion. In W. Gordon, A. Herd, & A. Baum (Eds.), *Perspectives on behavioral medicine* (Vol. 3, pp. 1–41). New York: Academic Press.

Grunberg, N. E., Greenwood, M. R. C., Collins, F., Epstein, L. H., Hatsukami, D., Niaura, R., O'Connell, K., Pomerleau, O. F., Ravussin, E., Rolls, B. J., Audrain, J., & Coday, M. (1992). Task Force 1: Mechanisms relevant to the relations between cigarette smoking and body weight. *Health Psychology, 11* (Suppl.), 4–9.

Grych, J. H., & Fincham, F. D. (1990). Marital conflict and children's adjustment: A cognitive-contextual framework. *Psychological Bulletin, 108,* 267–290.

Gunby, P. (1987). Nation's expenditures for alcohol, other drugs, in terms of therapy, prevention, now exceed $1.6 billion. *Journal of the American Medical Association, 258,* 2023.

Gustafsson, P. A., Kjellman, N. I. M., & Cederblad, M. (1986). Family therapy in the treatment of severe childhood asthma. *Journal of Psychosomatic Research, 30,* 369–374.

Gutlin, B., & Kessler, G. (1983). *The high energy factor.* New York: Random House.

Guyton, A. C. (1977). *Basic human physiology: Normal function and mechanisms of disease.* Philadelphia: W. B. Saunders.

Hall, A. (1987). The place of family therapy in the treatment of anorexia nervosa. *Australian and New Zealand Journal of Psychiatry, 21,* 568–574.

Hall, R. C. W., & Beresford, T. P. (1983). The psychosocial aspect of medicine. *Psychiatric Medicine, 1,* 111–119.

Hamilton, J. D., Hartigan, P. M., Simberkoff, M. S., Day, P. L., Giamond, G. R., Dickinson, G. M., Drusano, G. L., Egorin, M. J., George, W. L., Gordin, F. M., Hawkes, C. A., Jensen, P. C., Klimas, N. G., Labriola, A. M., Lahart, C. J., O'Brien, W. A., Oster, C. N., Weinhold, K. J., Wray, N. P., Zolla-Pazner, S. B., & the Veterans Affairs Cooperative Study Group on AIDS Treatment. (1992). A controlled trial of early versus late treatment with zidovudine in symptomatic human immunodeficiency virus infection. *The New England Journal of Medicine, 326,* 437–443.

Harbeck, C., & Peterson, L. (1992). Elephants dancing in my head: A developmental approach to children's concepts of specific pains. *Child Development, 63,* 138–149.

Harbin, T. J. (1989). The relationship between Type A behavior pattern and physiological responsivity: A quantitative review. *Psychophysiology, 26,* 110–119.

Hare-Mustin, R. T. (1983). An appraisal of the relationship between women and psychotherapy: 80 years after the case of Dora. *American Psychologist, 38,* 593–601.

Harris, E. D. (1990). Rheumatoid arthritis: Pathophysiology and implications for therapy. *The New England Journal of Medicine, 322,* 1277–1289.

Harris, J. R., Lippman, M. E., Veronesi, U., & Willett, W. (1992a). Breast cancer (First of three parts). *The New England Journal of Medicine, 327,* 319–328.

Harris, J. R., Lippman, M. E., Veronesi, U., & Willett, W. (1992b). Breast cancer (Second of three parts). *The New England Journal of Medicine, 327,* 390–398.

Hastrup, J. L., Phillips, S. M., Vullo, K., Kang, G., & Slomka, L. (1992). Adolescents' knowledge of medical terminology and family health history. *Health Psychology, 11,* 41–47.

Hatton, D. C., Scrogin, K. E., Levine, D., Feller, D., & McCarron, D. A. (1993). Dietary calcium modulates blood pressure through alpha1-adrenergic receptors. *The American Journal of Physiology, 264,* F234–F238.

Haverkos, H. W. (1988). Kaposi's sarcoma and nitrite inhalants. In T. P. Bridge, A. F. Mirsky, & F. K. Goodwin (Eds.), *Psychological, neuropsychiatric, and substance abuse aspects of AIDS* (pp. 165–172). New York: Raven.

Hawking, S. W. (1988). *A brief history of time.* New York: Bantam.

Hayashida, M., Alterman, A. I., McLellan, A. T., O'Brien, C. P., Purtill, J. J., Volpicelli, J. R., Raphaelson, A. H., & Hall, C. P. (1989). Comparative effectiveness and costs of inpatient and outpatient detoxification of patients with mild-to-moderate alcohol withdrawal syndrome. *The New England Journal of Medicine, 320,* 358–365.

Hayflick, L. (1976). The cell biology of human aging. *The New England Journal of Medicine, 295,* 1302–1308.

Hays, R. B., Turner, H., & Coates, T. J. (1992). Social support, AIDS-related symptoms, and depression among gay men. *Journal of Consulting and Clinical Psychology, 60,* 463–469.

Hazzard, W. R., Andres, R., Bierman, E. L., & Blass, J. P. (Eds.). (1990). *Principles of geriatric medicine and gerontology* (2nd ed.). New York: McGraw-Hill.

Health Care Finance Administration. (1997, January 27). *National health care expenditures for 1995.* HCFA Press Office.

Health Psychology, 10. (1991). Special issue on gender and health.

Heatherton, T. F., & Baumeister, R. F. (1991). Binge eating as escape from self-awareness. *Psychological Bulletin, 110,* 86–108.

Hegel, M. T., Abel, G. G., Etscheidt, M., Cohen-Cole, S., & Wilmer, C. I. (1989). Behavioral treatment of angina-like chest pain in patients with hyperventilation syndrome. *Journal of Behavior Therapy and Experimental Psychiatry, 20,* 31–39.

Heller, D. A., de Faire, U., Pedersen, N. L., Dahlén, G., & McClearn, G. E. (1993). Genetic and environmental influences on serum lipid levels in twins. *The New England Journal of Medicine, 328,* 1150–1156.

Heller, K. W., Alberto, P. A., Forney, P. E., & Schwartzman, M. N. (1996). *Understanding physical, sensory, and health impairments: Characteristics and educational implications.* Pacific Grove, CA: Brooks/Cole.

Helmers, K. F., Krantz, D. S., Merz, C. N. B., Klein, J., Kop, W. J., Gottdiener, J. S., & Rozanski, A. (1995). Defensive hostility: Relationship to multiple markers of cardiac ischemia in patients with coronary disease. *Health Psychology, 14,* 202–209.

Helps, A. (1859). *Worry.* In the Oxford Dictionary of Quotations (3rd ed.) (p. 244). Oxford: Oxford University Press.

Henderson, B. E., Ross, R. K., & Pike, M. C. (1991). Toward the primary prevention of cancer. *Science, 254,* 1131–1138.

Henningfield, J. E., & Woodson, P. P. (1989). Dose-related actions of nicotine on behavior and physiology: Review and implications for replacement therapy for nicotine dependence. *Journal of Substance Abuse, 1,* 301–317.

Herbert, L., & Teague, M. L. (1989). Exercise adherence and older adults: A theoretical perspective. *Activities, Adaptation, & Aging, 13,* 91–105.

Herek, G. M., & Glunt, E. K. (1988). An epidemic of stigma: Public reactions to AIDS. *American Psychologist, 43,* 886–891.

Hergenhahn, B. R. (1986). *An introduction to the history of psychology.* Belmont, CA: Wadsworth.

Herink, R. (Ed.). (1980). *The psychotherapy handbook*. New York: New American Library.

Herman, C. P., & Polivy, J. (1975). Anxiety, restraint and eating behavior. *Journal of Abnormal Psychology, 84,* 666–672.

Hermanns, J., Florin, I., Dietrich, M., Rieger, C., & Hahlweg, K. (1989). Maternal criticism, mother-child interaction, and bronchial asthma. *Journal of Psychosomatic Research, 33,* 469–476.

Hermanson, B., Omenn, G. S., Kronmai, R. A., & Gersh, B. J. (1988). Beneficial six-year outcome of smoking cessation in older men and women with coronary artery disease. *The New England Journal of Medicine, 319,* 1365–1369.

Hernandez, A. C. R., & Rabow, J. (1987). Passive and assertive student interventions in public and private drunken driving situations. *Journal of Studies on Alcohol, 48,* 269–271.

Herzog, A. R., Brown, M. B., Diokno, A. C., Normolle, D. P., & Brock, B. M. (1990). Two-year incidence, remission, and change patterns of urinary incontinence in noninstitutionalized older adults. *Journal of Gerontology, 45,* 67–74.

Heyden, S. (1981). *The heart book.* New York: Delair.

Hill, R. D., Storandt, M., & Malley, M. (1993). The impact of long-term exercise training on psychological function in older adults. *Journal of Gerontology: Psychological Sciences, 48,* P12–P17.

Hingson, R. W., Strunin, L., Berlin, B. M., & Heeren, T. (1990). Beliefs about AIDS, use of alcohol and drugs, and unprotected sex among Massachusetts adolescents. *The American Journal of Public Health March, 80,* 295–299.

Hinson, R. E., & Siegel, S. (1986). Pavlovian inhibitory conditioning and tolerance to pentobarbital-induced hypothermia in rats. *Journal of Experimental Psychology: Animal Behavior Processes, 12,* 363–370.

Hinson, R. E., Poulos, C. X., Thomas, W., & Cappell, H. (1986). Pavlovian conditioning and addictive behavior: Relapse to oral self-administration of morphine. *Behavioral Neuroscience, 100,* 368–375.

Hippocrates. (1923). *Hippocrates* (with Eng. trans. by W. H. S. Jones) (Vol. IV, Loeb Classical Library). New York, G. P. Putnam's Sons.

Hippocrates. (1952). On the sacred disease. In F. Adams (Trans.), *Great books of the western world* (Vol. 10, pp. 154–160). Chicago, IL: Encyclopaedia Britannica, Inc.

Holahan, C. J., & Moos, R. (1987). Personal and contextual determinants of coping strategies. *Journal of Personality and Social Psychology, 52,* 946–955.

Holleb, A. I. (Ed.). (1986). *The American Cancer Society cancer book.* Garden City, NY: Doubleday.

Hollon, S. D., & Beck, A. T. (1986). Cognitive and cognitive-behavioral therapies. In S. L. Garfield & A. E. Bergin (Eds.). *Handbook of psychotherapy and behavior change* (3rd ed., pp. 443–482). New York: Wiley.

Holmes, J. A., & Stevenson, C. A. Z. (1990). Differential effects of avoidant and attentional coping strategies on adaptation to chronic and recent-onset pain. *Health Psychology, 9,* 577–584.

Holmes, T. H., & Masuda, M. (1974). Life change and illness susceptibility. In B. S. Dohrenwend & B. P. Dohrenwend (Eds.), *Stressful life events: Their nature and effect* (pp. 45–72). New York: Wiley.

Holmes, T. H., & Rahe, R. H. (1967). The social readjustment rating scale. *Psychosomatic Medicine, 11,* 213–218.

Holroyd, K. A., & Penzien, D. B. (1990). Pharmacological versus non-pharmacological prophylaxis of recurrent migraine headache: A meta-analytic review of clinical trials. *Pain, 42,* 1–13.

Holtgrave, D. R., Doll, L. S., & Harrison, J. (1997). Influence of behavioral and social science on public health policymaking. *American Psychologist, 52,* 167–173.

Hoon, P. W., Feuerstein, M., & Papciak, A. S. (1985). Evaluation of the chronic low back pain patient: Conceptual and clinical considerations. *Clinical Psychology Review, 5,* 377–401.

Hopkins, B. L., Conard, R. J., Dangel, R. F., Fitch, H. G., Smith, M. J., & Anger, W. K. (1986). Behavioral technology for reducing occupational exposures to styrene. *Journal of Applied Behavioral Analysis, 19,* 3–11.

Hopkins, G. M. (1967). *The poems of Gerard Manley Hopkins* (4th ed.). London: Oxford University Press.

Horovitz, E. (1988). *Heart beat: A complete guide to understanding and preventing heart disease.* Encino, CA: Health Trend Publishing.

Howard, J. (1984). *Margaret Mead: A life.* New York: Simon and Schuster.

Howard, J. H., Cunningham, D. A., & Rechnitzer, P. A. (1976). Health patterns associated with Type A behavior: A managerial population. *Journal of Human Stress, 2,* 24–31.

Hudson, R. P. (1983). *Disease and its control: The*

shaping of modern thought. Westport, CN: Green-wood.

Hughes, J. R. (1992). Tobacco withdrawal in self-quitters. *Journal of Consulting and Clinical Psychology, 60,* 689–697.

Hughes, J. R. (1993). Pharmacotherapy for smoking cessation: Unvalidated assumptions, anomalies, and suggestions for future research. *Journal of Consulting and Clinical Psychology, 61,* 751–760.

Hunter, D. J., Manson, J. E., Colditz, G. A., Stampfer, M. J., Rosner, B., Hennekens, C. H., Speizer, F. E., & Willett, W. C. (1993). A prospective study of the intake of vitamins C, E, and A and the risk of breast cancer. *The New England Journal of Medicine, 329,* 234–240.

International Association for the Study of Pain Subcommittee on Taxonomy. (1986). *Classification of chronic pain: Descriptions of chronic pain syndromes and definitions of pain terms.* Amsterdam: Elsevier.

Institute of Medicine (United States). (1979). *Healthy people: The surgeon general's report on health promotion and disease prevention.* (Government Document No. HE20.2:H34/5). Rockville, MD: U.S Government Printing Office.

Institute of Medicine. (1992). Prevention and treatment of alcohol-related problems: Research opportunities. *Journal of Studies on Alcohol, 53,* 5–16.

Irvine, A. A., Cox, D., & Gonder-Frederick, L. (1992). Fear of hypoglycemia: Relationship to physical and psychological symptoms in patients with insulin-dependent diabetes mellitus. *Health Psychology, 11,* 135–138.

Irvine, J., Lyle, R. C., & Allon, R. (1982). Type A personality as psychopathology: Personality correlates and an abbreviated scoring system. *Journal of Psychosomatic Research, 26,* 183–189.

Irwin, J., & Livnat, S. (1987). Behavioral influences on the immune system: Stress and conditioning. *Progress in Neuro-Psychopharmacology & Biological Psychiatry, 11,* 137–143.

Ito, T. A., Miller, N., Pollock, V. E. (1996). Alcohol and aggression: A meta-analysis on the moderating effects of inhibitory cues, triggering events, and self-focused attention. *Psychological Bulletin, 120,* 60–82.

Jackson, S. W. (1969). Galen—on mental disorders. *Journal of History of Behavioral Science, 5,* 365–385.

Jackson, P. L. (1992). The primary care provider and children with chronic conditions. In P. L. Jackson & J. A. Vessey (Eds.), *Primary care of the child with a chronic condition* (pp. 3–11). St. Louis: C. V. Mosby.

Jacobsen, P. B., Bovbjerg, D. H., & Redd, W. H. (1993). Anticipatory anxiety in women receiving chemotherapy for breast cancer. *Health Psychology, 12,* 469–475.

Jacobson, E. (1938). *Progressive relaxation* (2nd ed.). Chicago: University of Chicago Press.

Jamieson, A. O., & Becker, P. M. (1992). Management of the 10 most common sleep disorders. *American Family Physician, 45,* 1262–1268.

Jamison, K., Ferrer-Brechner, M. T., Brechner, V. L., & McCreary, C. P. (1976). Correlation of personality profile with pain syndrome. *Advances in Pain Research and Therapy, 1,* 317–321.

Janz, N. K., & Becker, M. H. (1984). The Health Belief Model: A decade later. *Health Education Quarterly, 11,* 1–47.

Jaret, P. (1986). Our immune system: The wars within. *National Geographic, 169,* 702–735.

Jason, L. A., Ji, P. Y., Anes, M. D., & Birkhead, S. H. (1991). Active enforcement of cigarette control laws in the prevention of cigarette sales to minors. *Journal of the American Medical Association, 266,* 3159–3161.

Jay, S. M., Elliott, C. H., Woody, P. D., & Siegel, S. (1991). An investigation of cognitive-behavior therapy combined with oral Valium for children undergoing painful medical procedures. *Health Psychology, 10,* 317–322.

Jeffery, R. W., Adlis, S. A., & Forster, J. L. (1991). Prevalence of dieting among working men and women: The healthy worker project. *Health Psychology, 10,* 274–281.

Jeffrey, T. B., & Lemnitzer, N. (1981). Diet, exercise, obesity, and related health problems: A macroenvironmental analysis. In J. M. Ferguson & C. B. Taylor (Eds.), *The comprehensive handbook of behavioral medicine: Vol. 2—Syndromes and special areas* (pp. 47–66). New York: SP Medical & Scientific.

Jemmott, J. B., III. (1985). Psychoneuroimmunology: The new frontier. *American Behavioral Scientist, 28,* 497–509.

Jemmott, J. B., III, & Locke, S. E. (1984). Psychosocial factors, immunologic mediation, and human susceptibility to infectious diseases: How much do we know? *Psychological Bulletin, 95,* 78–108.

Jemmott, J. B., III, Borysenko, J. Z., Borysenko, M., McClelland, D. C., Chapman, R., Meyer, D., & Benson, H. (1983). Academic stress, power motivation, and decrease in salivary secretory immunoglobulin A secretion rate. *Lancet, 1,* 1400–1402.

Jenkins, C. D. (1988). Epidemiology of cardiovascular diseases. *Journal of Consulting and Clinical Psychology, 56,* 324–332.

Jenkins, C. D., Zyzanski, S. J., & Rosenman, R. H. (1965). *Jenkins Activity Survey.* New York: The Psychological Corporation.

Jenkins, D. J. A., Wolever, T. M. S., Vuksan, V., Brighenti, F., Cunnane, S. C., Rao, A. V., Jenkins, A. L., Buckley, G., Patten, R., Singer, W., Corey, P., & Josse, R. G. (1989). Nibbling versus gorging: Metabolic advantages of increased meal frequency. *The New England Journal of Medicine, 321,* 929–934.

Jensen, G. D., & Oakley, F. B. (1982–83). Ageism across cultures and in perspective of sociobiological and psychodynamic theories. *International Journal of Aging and Human Development, 15,* 17–26.

Jensen, M. A. (1992). School programming for the prevention of addictions. *School Counselor, 39,* 202–210.

Jensen, O. M., Wahrendorf, J., Rosenquisit, A., & Geser, A. (1984). The reliability of questionnaire-derived historic dietary information and temporal stability of food habits in individuals. *American Journal of Epidemiology, 120,* 281–290.

Jensen, T. S., & Rasmussen, P. (1989). Phantom pain and related phenomena after amputation. In P. D. Wall & R. Melzack (Eds.), *Textbook of pain* (pp. 508–521). New York: Churchill & Livingstone.

John, E. R. (1967). *Mechanisms of memory.* New York: Academic Press.

Johnson, B. T. (1989). *DSTAT: Software for the meta-analytic review of research literatures.* Lawrence Erlbaum Associates.

Johnson, C. (1987). *The etiology and treatment of bulimia nervosa.* New York: Basic Books.

Johnson, D. (1990). Animal rights and human lives. Time for scientists to right the balance. *Psychological Science, 1,* 213–214.

Johnston, R. B. (1988). Immunology: Monocytes and macrophages. *The New England Journal of Medicine, 318,* 747–752.

Johnston, V. S. (1979). Stimuli with biological significance. In H. Begleiter (Ed.), *Evoked brain potentials and behavior* (pp. 1–12). New York: Plenum.

Jonas, J. M., & Gold, M. S. (1988). The use of opiate antagonists in treating bulimia: A study of low-dose versus high-dose naltrexone. *Psychiatry Research, 24,* 194–199.

Jones, J. F., Ritenbaugh, C. K., Spence, M. A., & Hayward, A. (1991). Severe combined immunodeficiency among the Navajo. I. Characterization of phenotypes, epidemiology, and population genetics. *Human Biology, 63,* 669–682.

Jones, K. H., & Nagel, K. L. (1992, Winter). Eating disorders: A theoretical review. *Journal of Home Economics, 84,* 52–55, 64.

Jones, M. C. (1924). The elimination of children's fears. *Journal of Experimental Psychology, 7,* 382–390.

Jorgensen, R. S., & Houston, B. K. (1989). Reporting of life events, family history of hypertension, and cardiovascular activity at rest and during psychological stress. *Biological Psychology, 28,* 135–148.

Jorgensen, R. S., Johnson, B. T., Kolodziej, M. E., & Schreer, G. E. (1996). Elevated blood pressure and personality: A meta-analytic review. *Psychological Bulletin, 120,* 293–320.

Joseph, S., Yule, W., Williams, R., & Hodgkinson, P. (1993). Increased substance use in survivors of the Herald of Free Enterprise disaster. *British Journal of Medical Psychology, 66,* 185–191.

Judson, H. F. (1986, January). Annals of Science: The legend of Rosalind Franklin. *Science Digest, 94,* 56–59, 78–83.

Jung, J., & Khalsa, H. K. (1989). The relationship of daily hassles, social support, and coping to depression in black and white students. *Journal of General Psychology, 116,* 407–417.

Junqueira, L. C., Carneiro, J., & Long, J. A. (1986). *Basic histology* (5th ed.). East Norwalk, CT: Appleton & Lange.

Kabat-Zinn, J., Lipworth, L., & Burney, R. (1985). The clinical use of mindfulness meditation for the self-regulation of chronic pain. *Journal of Behavioral Medicine, 8,* 163–190.

Kail, B., & Litwak, E. (1989). Family, friends and neighbors: The role of primary groups in preventing the misuse of drugs. *The Journal of Drug Issues, 19,* 261–281.

Kalat, J. W. (1992). *Biological psychology* (4th ed.). Belmont, CA: Wadsworth.

Kalat, J. W. (1993). *Introduction to psychology* (3rd ed.). Pacific Grove, CA: Brooks/Cole.

Kalat, J. W. (1995). *Biological psychology* (5th ed.). Pacific Grove, CA: Brooks/Cole.

Kalichman, S. C., Hunter, T. L., & Kelly, J. A. (1992).

Perceptions of AIDS susceptibility among minority and nonminority women at risk for HIV infection. *Journal of Consulting and Clinical Psychology, 60,* 725–732.

Kalichman, S. C., Kelly, J. A., Hunter, T. L., Murphy, D. A., & Tyler, R. (1993). Culturally tailored HIV-AIDS risk-reduction messages targeted to African-American urban women: Impact on risk sensitization and risk reduction. *Journal of Consulting and Clinical Psychology, 61,* 291–295.

Kalichman, S. C., Rompa, D., & Coley, B. (1996). Experimental component analysis of a behavioral HIV-AIDS prevention intervention for inner-city women. *Journal of Consulting and Clinical Psychology, 64,* 687–693.

Kalichman, S. C., Russell, R. L., Hunter, T. L., & Sarwer, D. B. (1993). Earvin "Magic" Johnson's HIV serostatus disclosure: Effects on men's perceptions of AIDS. *Journal of Consulting and Clinical Psychology, 61,* 887–891.

Kalsher, M. J., Cataldo, M. F., Deal, R. M., Traughber, B., & Jankel, W. R. (1985). Behavioral covariation in the treatment of chronic pain. *Journal of Behavior Therapy and Experimental Psychiatry, 16,* 331–339.

Kamarck, T., & Jennings, J. R. (1991). Biobehavioral factors in sudden cardiac death. *Psychological Bulletin, 109,* 42–75.

Kamiya, J. (1969). Operant control of the EEG alpha rhythm and some of its reported effects on consciousness. In C. T. Tart (Ed.), *Altered states of consciousness* (pp.519–529). Garden City, NY: Anchor Books.

Kannel, W. B., & Gordon, T. (1976). Obesity and some physiological and medical concomitants: The Framingham study. In G. A. Bray (Ed.), *Obesity in America* (pp. 125–163). NIH Publication no. 79–359. Washington, DC: U.S Government Printing Office.

Kanner, A. D., Coyne, J. C., Schaefer, C., & Lazarus, R. S. (1981). Comparison of two modes of stress measurement: Daily hassles and uplifts versus major life events. *Journal of Behavioral Medicine, 4,* 1–39.

Kant, G. J., Meyerhoff, J. L., Bunnell, B. N., & Lenox, R. H. (1982). Cyclic AMP and cyclic GMP response to stress in brain and pituitary: Stress elevates pituitary cyclic AMP. *Pharmacology Biochemistry & Behavior, 17,* 1067–1072.

Kaplan, R. M. (1989). Models of health outcome for policy analysis. *Health Psychology, 8,* 723–735.

Kaplan, R. M. (1990). Behavior as the central outcome in health care. *American Psychologist, 45,* 1211–1220.

Kaplan, R. M. (1992). Health psychology during the Clinton administration. *The Health Psychologist, 14*(3), 1.

Kaplan, R. M., Anderson, J. P., & Wingard, D. L. (1991). Gender differences in health-related quality of life. *Health Psychology, 10,* 86–93.

Karoly, P. (1985). *Measurement strategies in health psychology.* New York: Wiley.

Karoly, P. (Ed.). (1988). *Handbook of child health assessment: Biopsychosocial perspectives.* New York: Wiley.

Kasl, S. V., & Cobb, S. (1966). Health behavior, illness behavior, and sick role behavior: II. Sick-role behavior. *Archives of Environmental Health, 12,* 531–541.

Kasl, S. V., & Cooper, C. L. (1987). *Stress and health: Issues in research methodology.* New York: Wiley.

Kasl, S. V., Evans, A. S., & Niederman, J. C. (1979). Psychosocial risk factors in the development of infectious mononucleosis. *Psychosomatic Medicine, 41,* 445–466.

Katz, E. R., Kellerman, J., & Siegel, S. E. (1980). Behavioral distress in children with cancer undergoing medical procedures: Developmental considerations. *Journal of Consulting and Clinical Psychology, 48,* 356–365.

Keefe, F. J., Crisson, J. E., Urban, B. J., & Williams, D. A. (1990). Analyzing chronic low back pain: The relative contribution of pain coping strategies. *Pain, 40,* 293–301.

Keefe, F., Brown, G., Wallston, K., & Caldwell, D. (1989). Coping with rheumatoid arthritis pain: Catastrophizing as a maladaptive strategy. *Pain, 37,* 51–56.

Keil, J. E., Sutherland, S. E., Knapp, R. G., Lackland, D. T., Gazes, P. C., & Tyroler, H. A. (1993). Mortality rates and risk factors for coronary disease in black as compared with white men and women. *The New England Journal of Medicine, 329,* 73–78.

Keillor, G. (1985). *Lake Wobegon days.* New York: Viking.

Keithly, L. J., Samples, S. J., & Strupp, H. H. (1980). Patient motivation as a predictor of process and outcome in psychotherapy. *Psychotherapy and Psychosomatics, 33,* 87–97.

Kelder, S. H., Perry, C. L., & Klepp, K. I. (1993). Community-wide youth exercise promotion: Long-term outcomes of the Minnesota Heart

Health Program and the Class of 1989 study. *Journal of School Health, 63,* 218–223.

Keller, S. E., Weiss, J. M., Schleifer, S. J., Miller, N. E., & Stein, M. (1981). Suppression of immunity by stress: Effect of a graded series of stressors on lymphocyte stimulation in the rat. *Science, 213,* 1397–1400.

Kelly, J. A., & Murphy, D. A. (1992). Psychological interventions with AIDS and HIV: Prevention and treatment. *Journal of Consulting and Clinical Psychology, 60,* 576–585.

Kemeny, M. E., Weiner, H., Taylor, S. E., Schneider, S., Visscher, B., & Fahey, J. L. (1994). Repeated bereavement, depressed mood, and immune parameters in HIV seropositive and seronegative gay men. *Health Psychology, 13,* 14–24.

Kenny, A. J. P. (1989). *The metaphysics of mind.* Oxford: Clarendon Press.

Kent, J. S., & Clopton, J. R. (1992). Bulimic women's perceptions of their family relationships. *Journal of Clinical Psychology, 48,* 281–292.

Kern, F. (1991). Normal plasma cholesterol in an 88-year-old man who eats 25 eggs a day. *The New England Journal of Medicine, 324,* 896–899.

Kern, P. A., Ong, J. M., Saffari, B., & Carty, J. (1990). The effects of weight loss on the activity and expression of adipose-tissue lipoprotein lipase in very obese humans. *The New England Journal of Medicine, 322,* 1053–1059.

Kettlewell, P. W., Mizes, J. S., & Wasylyshyn, N. A. (1992). A cognitive-behavioral group treatment of bulimia. *Behavior Therapy, 23,* 657–670.

Khoury, M. J., Newill, C. A., & Chase, G. A. (1985). Epidemiologic evaluation of screening for risk factors: Application to genetic screening. *American Journal of Public Health, 75,* 1204–1208.

Kiecolt-Glaser, J. K., Glaser, R., Williger, D., Stout, J., Messick, G., Sheppard, S., Ricker, D., Romisher, S. C., Briner, W., Bonnell, G., & Donnerberg, R. (1985). Psychosocial enhancement of immunocompetence in a geriatric population. *Health Psychology, 4,* 25–41.

Kiesler, C. A., & Morton, T. L. (1988). Psychology and public policy in the "health care revolution." *American Psychologist, 43,* 993–1003.

Kimball, C. P. (1986). Psychosomatic medicine and the biopsychosocial approach: The problem of synthesis and restoration. *Psychiatria Fennica, 17,* 81–101.

Kimble, D. P. (1988). *Biological psychology.* New York: Holt, Rinehart, & Winston.

Kingsbury, S. J. (1992). Some effects of prescribing privileges. *American Psychologist, 47,* 426–427.

Kirschenbaum, D. S., Fitzgibbon, M. L., Martino, S., Conviser, J. H., Rosendahl, E. H., & Laatsch, L. (1992). Stages of change in successful weight control: A clinically derived model. *Behavior Therapy, 23,* 623–635.

Kirschstein, R. (1993). Largest US clinical trial ever gets under way. *Journal of the American Medical Association, 270,* 1521.

Kirscht, J. P., Haefner, D. P., Kegeles, S. S., & Rosenstock, I. M. (1966). A national study of health beliefs. *Journal of Health and Human Behavior, 7,* 248–254.

Kivlahan, D. R., Marlatt, A., Fromme, K., Coppel, D. B., & Williams, E. (1990). Secondary prevention with college drinkers: Evaluation of an alcohol skills training program. *Journal of Consulting and Clinical Psychology, 58,* 805–811.

Klag, M. J., Ford, D. E., Mead, L. A., He, J., Whelton, P. K., Liang, K., & Levine, D. M. (1993). Serum cholesterol in young men and subsequent cardiovascular disease. *The New England Journal of Medicine, 328,* 313–318.

Kleinbaum, D. G., Kupper, L. L., & Morgenstern, H. (1982). *Epidemiologic research: Principles and quantitative methods.* New York: Van Nostrand Reinhold Company.

Klerman, G. L. (1988). Drugs and psychotherapy. In S. L. Garfield & A. E. Bergin (Eds.). *Handbook of psychotherapy and behavior change* (pp. 777–818). New York: Wiley.

Klesges, R. C., & Shumaker, S. A. (1992). Understanding the relations between smoking and body weight and their importance to smoking cessation and relapse. *Health Psychology, 11* (Suppl.), 1–3.

Klesges, R. C., Haddock, C. K., Stein, R. J., Klesges, L. M., Eck, L. H., & Hanson, C. L. (1992). Relationship between psychosocial functioning and body fat in preschool children: A longitudinal investigation. *Journal of Consulting and Clinical Psychology, 60,* 793–796.

Kline, A., & Strickler, J. (1993). Perceptions of risk for AIDS among women in drug treatment. *Health Psychology, 12,* 313–323.

Klohn, L. S., & Rogers, R. W. (1991). Dimensions of the severity of a health threat: The persuasive effects of visibility, time of onset, and rate of onset on young women's intentions to prevent osteoporosis. *Health Psychology, 10,* 323–329.

Kobasa, S. C. (1979a). Personality and resistance to

illness. *American Journal of Community Psychology, 7,* 413–423.

Kobasa, S. C. (1979b). Stressful life events, personality and health: An inquiry into hardiness. *Journal of Personality and Social Psychology, 37,* 1–11.

Kodish, E., Lantos, J., Stocking, C., Singer, P. A., Siegler, M., & Johnson, F. L. (1991). Bone marrow transplantation for sickle cell disease: A study of parents' decisions. *The New England Journal of Medicine, 325,* 1349–1353.

Kohn, P. M., Lafreniere, K., & Gurevich, M. (1991). Hassles, health, and personality. *Journal of Personality and Social Psychology, 61,* 478–482.

Kohn, R. R. (1978). *Principles of mammalian aging.* Englewood Cliffs: Prentice-Hall.

Koopman, W. J. (1991). Rheumatology. *Journal of the American Medical Association, 265,* 3169–3170.

Koralnik, I. J., Beaumanoir, A., Hausler, R., & Kohler, A. (1990). A controlled study of early neurologic abnormalities in men with asymptomatic human immunodeficiency virus infection. *The New England Journal of Medicine, 323,* 864–870.

Krantz, D. S., & Manuck, S. B. (1984). Acute psychophysiologic reactivity and risk of cardiovascular disease: A review and methodologic critique. *Psychological Bulletin, 96,* 435–464.

Kreiss, J. K., Koech, D., Plummer, F. A., Holmes, K. K., Lightfoote, M., Piot, P., Ronald, A. R., Ndinya-Achola, J. O., D'Costa, L. J., Roberts, P., Ngugi, E. N., & Quinn, T. C. (1986). AIDS virus infection in Nairobi prostitutes. *The New England Journal of Medicine, 314,* 414–418.

Krinsky, N. I. (1989). Carotenoids and cancer in animal models. *The Journal of Nutrition, 119,* 123–126.

Kris-Etherton, P. M., & Krummel, D. (1993). Role of nutrition in the prevention and treatment of coronary heart disease in women. *Journal of the American Dietetic Association, 93,* 987–993.

Kubler-Ross, E. (1969). *On death and dying.* New York: Macmillan.

Kuhn, T. S. (1972). *The structure of scientific revolutions.* Chicago: University of Chicago Press.

Kuller, L., Neaton, J., Caggiula, A., & Falvo-Gerard, L. (1980). Primary prevention of heart attacks: The Multiple Risk Factor Intervention Trial. *American Journal of Epidemiology, 112,* 185–199.

Kumpfer, K. L., & DeMarsh, J. (1985). Family environmental and genetic influences on children's future chemical dependency. *Journal of Children in Contemporary Society, 18,* 49–91.

Kupfer, D. J., & Reynolds, C. F. (1997). Management of

insomnia. *The New England Journal of Medicine, 336,* 341–346.

Labbe, E. E. (1988). Childhood muscle contraction headache: Current issues in assessment and treatment. *Headache, 28,* 430–434.

Lackner, J. M., Carosella, A. M., & Feuerstein, M. (1996). Pain expectancies, pain, and functional self-efficacy expectancies as determinants of disability in patients with chronic low back disorders. *Journal of Consulting and Clinical Psychology, 64,* 212–220.

Lackritz, E. M., Satten, G. A., Aberle-Grasse, J., Dodd, R. Y., Raimondi, V. P., Janssen, R. S., Lewis, W. F., Notari, E. P., & Petersen, L. R. (1995). Estimated risk of transmission of the human immunodeficiency virus by screened blood in the United States. *The New England Journal of Medicine, 333,* 1721–1725.

LaCroix, A. Z., Lang, J., Scherr, P., Wallace, R. B., Cornoni-Huntley, J., Berkman, L., Curb, D., Evans, D., & Hennekens, C. H. (1991). Smoking and mortality among older men and women in three communities. *The New England Journal of Medicine, 324,* 1619–1625.

Lalonde, M. (1974). *A new perspective on the health of Canadians: A working document.* Ottawa: Government of Canada.

Lambert, M. J. (1976). Spontaneous remission in adult neurotic disorders: A revision and summary. *Psychological Bulletin, 83,* 107–119.

Lambert, M. J., Shapiro, D. A., & Bergin, A. E. (1988). The effectiveness of psychotherapy. In S. L. Garfield & A. E. Bergin (Eds.). *Handbook of psychotherapy and behavior change* (3rd ed., pp. 157–211). New York: Wiley.

Lambley, P. (1993). The role of psychological processes in the aetiology and treatment of cervical cancer: A biopsychological perspective. *British Journal of Medical Psychology, 66,* 43–60.

Lamping, D. L. (1985). Assessment in health psychology. *Canadian Psychology, 26,* 121–139.

Landis, S. E., Earp, J. L., & Koch, G. G. (1992). Impact of HIV testing and counseling on subsequent sexual behavior. *AIDS Education and Prevention, 4,* 61–70.

Landis, S. E., Schoenbach, V. J., Weber, D. J., Mittal, M., Krishan, B., Lewis, K., & Koch, G. G. (1992). Results of a randomized trial of partner notification in cases of HIV infection in North Carolina. *The New England Journal of Medicine, 326,* 101–106.

Landon, C., Rosenfeld, R., Northcraft, G., & Lewiston,

N. (1980). Self-image of adolescents with cystic fibrosis. *Journal of Youth and Adolescence, 9,* 521–528.

Langer, E. J., & Rodin, J. (1976). The effects of choice and enhanced personal responsibility for the aged: A field experiment in an institutional setting. *Journal of Personality and Social Psychology, 34,* 191–198.

Langreth, R. N. (1991). Pediatric pain. *Science News, 139,* 74–75.

Larsen, G. L. (1992). Asthma in children. *The New England Journal of Medicine, 326,* 1540–1545.

Larter, N. L., & Kieckhefer, G. (1992). Asthma. In P. L. Jackson & J. A. Vessey (Eds.), *Primary care of the child with a chronic condition* (pp. 63–80). St. Louis: C. V. Mosby.

Lau, J., Antman, E. M., Jimenez-Silva, J., Kupelnick, B., Mosteller, F., & Chalmers, T. C. (1992). Cumulative meta-analysis of therapeutic trials for myocardial infarction. *The New England Journal of Medicine, 327,* 248–254.

Laws, A., Terry, R. B., & Barrett-Connor, E. (1990). Behavioral covariates of waist-to-hip ratio in Rancho Bernardo. *The American Journal of Public Health, 80,* 1358–1362.

Lazarus, R. S. (1991a). *Emotion and adaptation.* Oxford: Oxford University Press.

Lazarus, R. S. (1991b). Progress on a cognitive-motivational-relational theory of emotion. *American Psychologist, 46,* 819–834.

Lazarus, R. S. (1993). Why we should think of stress as a subset of emotion. In L. Goldberger & S. Breznitz (Eds.), *Handbook of stress: Theoretical and clinical aspects* (2nd ed., pp. 21–39). New York: Free Press.

Lazarus, R. S., & Folkman, S. (1984). *Stress, appraisal, and coping.* New York: Springer.

Lazarus, R. S., & Launier, R. (1978). Stress-related transactions between person and environment. In L. A. Pervin & M. Lewis (Eds.), *Perspectives in interactional psychology* (pp. 287–327). New York: Plenum Press.

Le, A. D. (1990). Factors regulating ethanol tolerance. *Annals of Medicine, 22,* 265–268.

Leaf, D. A. (1991). *Exercise & nutrition in preventive cardiology.* Dubuque, IA: Brown & Benchmark.

Leape, L. L., Brennan, T. A., Laird, N., Lawthers, A. G., Localio, A. R., Barnes, B. A. Hebert, L., Newhouse, J. P., Weiler, P. C., & Hiatt, H. (1991). The nature of adverse events in hospitalized patients: Results of the Harvard medical practice study II. *The New England Journal of Medicine, 324,* 377–384.

Lee, C. (1989). The clinical aspects of AIDS/HIV. In R. Miller & R. Bor, *AIDS: A guide to clinical counseling* (pp. 29–34). London: Science Press.

Lefcourt, H. M. (1976). *Locus of control: Current trends in theory and research.* Hillsdale, NJ: Lawrence Erlbaum.

Leffert, F. (1985). Asthma. In N. Hobbs & J. M. Perrin (Gen. Eds.), *Issues in the care of children with chronic illness* (pp. 366–379). San Francisco: Jossey-Bass.

Legato, M. J., & Colman, C. (1991). *The female heart.* New York: Simon & Schuster.

Leigh, H., & Reiser, M. F. (1980). *The patient: Biological, psychological, and social dimensions of medical practice.* New York: Plenum Medical.

Lejeune, J., Gautier, M., & Turpin, R. (1959). Les chromosimes humains en culture de tissus. *C. R. Academy of Science, 248,* 602–603.

Lenderking, W. R., Gelber, R. D., Cotton, D. J., Cole, B. F., Goldhirsch, A., Volberding, P. A., & Testa, M. A. (1994). Evaluation of the quality of life associated with zidovudine treatment in asymptomatic human immunodeficiency virus infection. *The New England Journal of Medicine, 330,* 738–743.

Leon, A. S., Connett, J., Jacobs, D. R., Jr., & Rauramaa, R. (1987). Leisure-time physical activity and risk of coronary heart disease and death: The MRFIT. *Journal of the American Medical Association, 258,* 2388–2395.

Lepore, S. J., Evans, G. W., & Palsane, M. N. (1991). Social hassles and psychological health in the context of chronic crowding. *Journal of Health and Social Behavior, 32,* 357–367.

Lepore, S. J., Palsane, M. N., & Evans, G. W. (1991). Daily hassles and chronic strains: A hierarchy of stressors? *Social Science & Medicine, 33,* 1029–1036.

Lerman, C. E. (1987). Rheumatoid arthritis: Psychological factors in the etiology, course, and treatment. *Clinical Psychology Review, 7,* 413–425.

Lerman, C., Trock, B., Rimer, B. K., Jepson, C., Brody, D., & Boyce, A. (1991). Psychological side effects of breast cancer screening. *Health Psychology, 10,* 259–267.

Lester, D. (1990). Galen's four temperaments and four-factor theories of personality: A comment on "Toward a four-factor theory of temperament and/or personality." *Journal of Personality Assessment, 54,* 423–426.

Levav, I., Friedlander, Y., Kark, J. D., & Peritz, E. (1988). An epidemiologic study of mortality among bereaved parents. *The New England Journal of Medicine, 319,* 457–461.

Leventhal, H., & Cleary, P. D. (1980). The smoking problem: A review of the research and theory in behavioral risk modification. *Psychological Bulletin, 88,* 370–405.

Levi, L. (1990). Occupational stress: Spice of life or kiss of death? *American Psychologist, 45,* 1142–1145.

Levin, I. P., & Chapman, D. P. (1993). Risky decision making and allocation of resources for leukemia and AIDS programs. *Health Psychology, 12,* 110–117.

Levine, C., & Bayer, R. (1989). The ethics of screening for early intervention in HIV disease. *American Journal of Public Health, 79,* 1661–1667.

Levit, K. R., Lazenby, H. C., Cowan, C. A., & Letsch, S. W. (1991). National health expenditures, 1990. *Health Care Financing Review, 13,* 29–54.

Levy, D. (1993). Genetic influence on smoking. *The New England Journal of Medicine, 328,* 353–354.

Levy, M. H. (1996). Pharmacological treatment of cancer pain. *The New England Journal of Medicine, 335,* 1124–1132.

Levy, S. M., & Wise, B. D. (1987). Psychosocial risk factors, natural immunity, and cancer progression: Implications for intervention. *Current Psychological Research & Reviews, 6,* 229–243.

Levy, S. M., Haynes, L. T., Herberman, R. B., Lee, J., McFeeley, S., & Kirkwood, J. (1992). Mastectomy versus breast conservation surgery: Mental health effects at long-term follow-up. *Health Psychology, 11,* 349–354.

Lewis, C. E., Rachelefsky, G., Lewis, M. A., de la Suta, A., & Kaplan, M. (1984). A randomized trial of A.C.T. (Asthma Care Training) for kids. *Pediatrics, 74,* 478–486.

Lewis, C. S. (1955). *Surprised by joy.* New York: Harcourt, Brace.

Lewis, F. M., Ellison, E. S., & Woods, N. F. (1985). The impact of breast cancer on the family. *Seminars in Oncology Nursing, 1,* 106–213.

Lewis, M. J. (1990). Alcohol: Mechanisms of addiction and reinforcement. *Advances in Alcohol and Substance Abuse, 9,* 47–66.

Lewiston, N. J. (1985). Cystic fibrosis. In N. Hobbs & J. M. Perrin (Gen. Eds.), *Issues in the care of children with chronic illness* (pp. 196–213). San Francisco: Jossey-Bass.

Lex, B. W. (1991). Some gender differences in alcohol and polysubstance users. *Health Psychology, 10,* 121–132.

Lichtman, R. R., Taylor, S. E., & Wood, J. V. (1988). Social support and marital adjustment after breast cancer. *Journal of Psychosocial Oncology, 5,* 47–74.

Lichtman, S. W., Pisarska, K., Berman, E. R., Pestone, M., Dowling, H., Offenbacher, E., Weisel, H., Heshka, S., Matthews, D. E., & Heymsfield, S. B. (1992). Discrepancy between self-reported and actual caloric intake and exercise in obese subjects. *The New England Journal of Medicine, 327,* 1893–1898.

Liebman, M. (1979). *Neuroanatomy made easy and understandable.* Baltimore: University Park Press.

Light, R. J., & Pillemer, D. B. (1984). *Summing up: The science of reviewing research.* Cambridge, MA: Harvard University Press.

Lilienfeld, A. M., & Lilienfeld, D. E. (1980). *Foundations of epidemiology* (2nd ed.). New York: Oxford University Press.

Lindsley, O. R. (1956). Operant conditioning methods applied to research in chronic schizophrenia. *Psychiatric Research Reports, 5,* 118–139.

Lindsley, O. R., Skinner, B. F., & Solomon, H. C. (1953). *Studies in behavior therapy. Status report I.* Waltham, MA: Metropolitan State Hospital.

Lipid Research Clinics Program. (1984). The Lipid Research Clinics Coronary Primary Prevention Trial results. II. The relationship of reduction in incidence of coronary heart disease to cholesterol lowering. *Journal of the American Medical Association, 251,* 365–374.

Lipowski, Z. J. (1977). Psychosomatic medicine in the seventies: An overview. *The American Journal of Psychiatry, 134,* 233–244.

Lissner, L., Odell, P. M., D'Agostino, R. B., Stokes, J., Kreger, B. E., Belanger, A. J., & Brownell, K. D. (1991). Variability of body weight and health outcomes in the Framingham population. *The New England Journal of Medicine, 324,* 1839–1844.

Lobato, D., Faust, D., & Spirito, A. (1988). Examining the effects of chronic disease and disability on children's sibling relationships. *Journal of Pediatric Psychology, 13,* 389–407.

Locke, S. E. (1982). Stress, adaptation, and immunity: Studies in humans. *General Hospital Psychiatry, 4,* 49–58.

Locke, S. E., Hurst, M. W., Heisel, J. S., et al. (1978, April). *The influence of stress on the immune response.* Paper presented at the annual meeting of the American Psychosomatic Society, Washington, DC.

Loeser, J. D. (1980). Perspectives on pain. In *Proceed-*

ings of the First World Conference on clinical pharmacology and therapeutics (pp. 313–316). London: Macmillan.

London, P. (1972). An end of ideology in behavior modification. *American Psychologist, 27,* 913–920.

Lopez, A. D. (1992, December). Epidemiologic surveillance of the tobacco epidemic. *Mortality and Morbidity Weekly Reports, 41* (Suppl.), 157–166.

Lorge, B. (1992, April 12). Tennis world's conspiracy of compassion for Arthur Ashe. *The New York Times, 141(Sec. 1),* N32.

Lorion, R. P. (1991). Prevention and public health: Psychology's response to the nation's health care crisis. *American Psychologist, 46,* 516–519.

Lovallo, W. R., & Pishkin, V. (1980). A psychophysiological comparison of Type A and B men exposed to failure and uncontrollable noise. *Psychophysiology, 17,* 29–36.

Love, A. W., & Peck, C. L. (1987). The MMPI and psychological factors in chronic low back pain: A review. *Pain, 28,* 1–12.

Lowe, M. R. (1993). The effects of dieting on eating behavior: A three-factor model. *Psychological Bulletin, 114,* 100–121.

Lu, L. (1991). Daily hassles and mental health: A longitudinal study. *British Journal of Psychology, 82,* 441–447.

Luborsky, L., Singer, B., & Luborsky, L. (1975). Comparative studies of psychotherapy. *Archives of General Psychiatry, 32,* 995–1008.

Ludwick-Rosenthal, R., & Neufeld, R. W. J. (1993). Preparation for undergoing an invasive medical procedure: Interacting effects of information and coping style. *Journal of Consulting and Clinical Psychology, 61,* 156–164.

Lueger, R. J., & McDonald, R. T. (1992, April). *Life change and success in a smoking cessation program.* Paper presented at the Midwestern Psychological Association Annual Conference, Chicago, IL.

Lumley, M. A., Abeles, L. A., Melamed, B. G., Pistone, L. M., & Johnson, J. H. (1990). Coping outcomes in children undergoing stressful medical procedures: The role of child-environment variables. *Behavioral Assessment, 12,* 223–238.

Lumsden, C. J., & Wilson, E. O. (1981). *Genes, mind, and culture: The coevolutionary process.* Cambridge, MA: Harvard University Press.

Lustman, P. J., & Sowa, C. J. (1983). Comparative efficacy of biofeedback and stress inoculation for stress reduction. *Journal of Clinical Psychology, 39,* 191–197.

Lynch, J. J., Paskewitz, D. A., Gimbel, K. S., & Thomas, S. A. (1977). Psychological aspects of cardiac arrhythmia. *American Heart Journal, 93,* 645–657.

Lyness, S. A. (1993). Predictors of differences between Type A and Type B individuals in heart rate and blood pressure reactivity. *Psychological Bulletin, 114,* 266–295.

Lyons, A. S., & Petrucelli, R. J. (1978). *Medicine: An illustrated history.* New York: Harry N. Abrams.

Lyter, D. W., Valdiserri, R. O., Kingsley, L. A., Amoroso, W. P., & Rinaldo, C. R. (1987). The HIV antibody test: Why gay and bisexual men want or do not want to know their results. *Public Health Reports, 102,* 468–474.

Macallan, D. C., Noble, C., Baldwin, C., Jebb, S. A., Prentice, A. M., Coward, W. A., Sawyer, M. B., McManus, T. J., & Griffin, G. E. (1995). Energy expenditure and wasting in human immunodeficiency virus infection. *The New England Journal of Medicine, 333,* 83–88.

MacConnie, S. E., Gilliam, T. B., Geenen, D. L., & Pels, A. E. (1982). Daily physical activity patterns of prepubertal children involved in a vigorous exercise program. *International Journal of Sports Medicine, 3,* 202–207.

MacCoun, R. J. (1993). Drugs and the law: A psychological analysis of drug prohibition. *Psychological Bulletin, 113,* 497–512.

MacDougall, J. M., Dembroski, T. M., Slaats, S., Herd, J. A., & Eliot, R. S. (1983). Selective cardiovascular effects of stress and cigarette smoking. *Journal of Human Stress, 9,* 13–21.

MacMurray, J. P., Nessman, D. G., Haviland, M. G., & Anderson, D. L. (1987). Depressive symptoms and persistence in treatment for alcohol dependence. *Journal of Studies on Alcohol, 48,* 277–280.

Mahoney, M. J. (1993). Introduction to special section: Theoretical developments in the cognitive psychotherapies. *Journal of Consulting and Clinical Psychology, 61,* 187–193.

Majno, G. (1975). *The healing hand: Man and wound in the ancient world.* Cambridge, MA: Harvard University Press.

Malasanos, L., Barkauskas, V., & Stoltenberg-Allen, K. (1990). *Health assessment* (4th ed.). St. Louis: Mosby.

Malonebeach, E. E., & Zarit, S. H. (1991). Current research issues in caregiving to the elderly. *International Journal of Aging & Human Development, 32,* 103–114.

Mann, J. M. (1991). Global AIDS: Critical issues for

prevention in the 1990's. *International Journal of Health Sciences, 21,* 553–559.

Manne, S. L., & Zautra, A. J. (1989). Spouse criticism and support: Their association with coping and psychological adjustment among women with rheumatoid arthritis. *Journal of Personality and Social Psychology, 56,* 608–617.

Manne, S. L., Redd, W. H., Jacobsen, P. B., Gorfinkle, K., Schorr, O., & Rapkin, B. (1990). Behavioral intervention to reduce child and parent distress during venipuncture. *Journal of Consulting and Clinical Psychology, 58,* 565–572.

Manson, J. E., Tosteson, H., Ridker, P. M., Satterfield, S., Hebert, P., O'Connor, G. T., Buring, J. E., & Hennekens, C. H. (1992). The primary prevention of myocardial infarction. *The New England Journal of Medicine, 326,* 1406–1416.

Marcus, B. H., Rakowski, W., & Rossi, J. S. (1992). Assessing motivational readiness and decision making for exercise. *Health Psychology, 11,* 257–261.

Marenberg, M. E., Risch, N., Berkman, L. F., Floderus, B., & de Faire, U. (1994). Genetic susceptibility to death from coronary heart disease in a study of twins. *The New England Journal of Medicine, 330,* 1041–1046.

Markham, B. (1983). *West with the night.* San Francisco: North Point Press.

Marks, G., Bundek, N. I., Richardson, J. L., Ruiz, M. S., Maldonado, N., & Mason, H. R. C. (1992). Self-disclosure of HIV infection: Preliminary results from a sample of Hispanic men. *Health Psychology, 11,* 300–306.

Marks, M. J., Burch, J. B., & Collins, A. C. (1983). Genetics of nicotine response in four inbred strains of mice. *Journal of Pharmacology and Experimental Therapy, 226,* 291–302.

Martin, J. L., & Dean, L. (1993). Effects of AIDS-related bereavement and HIV-related illness on psychological distress among gay men: A 7-year longitudinal study, 1985–1991. *Journal of Consulting and Clinical Psychology, 61,* 94–103.

Martin, R. A., & Lefcourt, H. M. (1983). Sense of humor as a moderator of the relation between stressors and moods. *Journal of Personality and Social Psychology, 45,* 1313–1324.

Mason, J. W. (1993). Cardiac arrhythmias and clinical electrophysiology. In R. P. Lewis (Ed.), *Adult clinical cardiology self-assessment program* (Section 5), Bethesda, MD: American College of Cardiology.

Masserman, J. H. (1943). *Behavior and neurosis.* Chicago: University of Chicago Press.

Masters, J. C., Burish, T. G., Hollon, S. D., & Rimm, D. C. (1987). *Behavior therapy: Techniques and empirical findings* (3rd ed.). New York: Harcourt, Brace, Jovanovich.

Matarazzo, J. (1982). Behavioral health's challenge to academic scientific and professional psychology. *American Psychologist, 37,* 1–14.

Matarazzo, J. D. (1986). Computerized clinical psychological test interpretations: Unvalidated plus all mean and no sigma. *American Psychologist, 41,* 14–24.

Matheny, K. B., Aycock, D. W., Pugh, J. L., Curlette, W. L., & Silva-Cannella, K. A. (1986). Stress coping: A qualitative and quantitative synthesis with implications for treatment. *Counseling Psychologist, 14,* 499–549.

Mathew, N. T. (1992). Cluster headache. *Neurology, 42*(3, Suppl. 2), 22–31.

Matthews, K. A. (1989). Interactive effects of behavior and reproductive hormones on sex differences in risk for coronary heart disease. *Health Psychology, 8,* 373–387.

Matthews, K. A., Shumaker, S. A., Bowen, D. J., Langer, R. D., Hunt, J. R., Kaplan, R. M., Klesges, R. C., & Ritenbaugh, C. (1997). Women's health initiative. *American Psychologist, 52,* 101–116.

Matthews, K. A., Woodall, K. L., Engebretson, T. O., McCann, B. S., Stoney, C. M., Manuck, S. B., & Saab, P. G. (1992). Influence of age, sex, and family on Type A and hostile attitudes and behaviors. *Health Psychology, 11,* 317–323.

Matthews, K. A., Glass, D. C., Rosenman, R. H., & Bortner, R. W. (1977). Competitive drive, Pattern A and coronary heart disease: A further analysis of some data from the Western Collaborative Group Study. *Journal of Chronic Diseases, 30,* 489–498.

May, W. T., & Belsky, J. (1992). Response to "Prescription privileges: Psychology's next frontier?" or, The siren call: Should psychologists medicate? *American Psychologist, 47,* 427.

Mayo Clinic, Committee on Dietetics (Eds.). (1981). *Mayo Clinic diet manual.* Philadelphia: Saunders.

Mazess, R., & Forman, S. (1979). Longevity and age by exaggeration in Vilcabamba, Ecuador. *Journal of Gerontology, 34,* 94–98.

McCaffrey, R. J., & Blanchard, E. B. (1985). Area review: Hypertension. *Annals of Behavioral Medicine, 7,* 5–12.

McCaul, K. D., Branstetter, A. D., Schroeder, D. M., & Glasgow, R. E. (1996). What is the relationship between breast cancer risk and mammography screening? A meta-analytic review. *Health Psychology, 15,* 423–429.

McCaul, K. D., Monson, N., & Maki, R. H. (1992). Does distraction reduce pain-produced distress among college students? *Health Psychology, 11,* 210–217.

McClusky, H. Y., Milby, J. B., Switzer, P. K., Williams, V., & Wooten, V. (1991). Efficacy of behavioral versus triazolam treatment in persistent sleep-onset insomnia. *American Journal of Psychiatry, 148,* 121–126.

McCord, C., & Freeman, H. P. (1990). Excess mortality in Harlem. *The New England Journal of Medicine, 322,* 173–177.

McCormack, M. K. (1981). Screening for genetic traits and diseases. *American Family Physician, 24,* 153–166.

McCoy, H. V., Dodds, S. E., & Nolan, C. (1990). AIDS intervention design for program evaluation: The Miami Community Outreach Project. *The Journal of Drug Issues, 20,* 223–243.

McCrea, C. W., Summerfield, A. B., & Rosen, B. (1982). Body image: A selective review of existing measurement techniques. *British Journal of Medical Psychology, 55,* 225–233.

McDaniel, S. A., & McKinnon, A. L. (1993). Gender differences in informal support and coping among elders: Findings from Canada's 1985 and 1990 general social surveys. *Journal of Women & Aging, 5,* 79–98.

McEwen, B. S., & Mendelson, S. (1993). Effects of stress on the neurochemistry and morphology of the brain: Counterregulation versus damage. In L. Goldberger & S. Breznitz (Eds.), *Handbook of stress: Theoretical and clinical aspects* (2nd ed., pp. 101–126). New York: Free Press.

McFadden, E. R., Jr., & Gilbert, I. A. (1992). Asthma. *The New England Journal of Medicine, 327,* 1928–1937.

McGinnis, J. M. (1991). Health objectives for the nation. *American Psychologist, 46,* 520–524.

McGinnis, J. M., & Nestle, M. (1989). The Surgeon General's report on nutrition and health: Policy implications and implementation strategies. *American Journal of Clinical Nutrition, 49,* 23–28.

McGrath, P. A. (1990). *Pain in children: Nature, assessment, and treatment.* New York: Guilford.

McGue, M., Pickens, R. W., & Svikis, D. S. (1992). Sex and age effects on the inheritance of alcohol problems: A twin study. *Journal of Abnormal Psychology, 101,* 3–17.

McGue, M., Vaupel, J. W., Holm, N., & Harvald, B. (1993). Longevity is moderately heritable in a sample of Danish twins born 1870–1880. *Journal of Gerontology, 1993, 48,* 237–244.

McLeod, B. (1984, October). In the wake of disaster. *Psychology Today, 18*(10), 54–57.

McMillen, D. L., Smith, S. M., & Wells-Parker, E. (1989). The effects of alcohol, expectancy, and sensation seeking on driving risk taking. *Addictive Behaviors, 14,* 477–483.

McMinn, M. R., & Katahn, M. (1986). Energy expenditure in obesity: Part I. *The Journal of Obesity and Weight Regulation, 5,* 89–113.

McMullen, A. H. (1992). Cystic fibrosis. In P. L. Jackson & J. A. Vessey (Eds.), *Primary care of the child with a chronic condition* (pp. 210–228). St. Louis: C. V. Mosby.

McMurry, M. P., Cerqueira, M. T., Connor, S. L., & Connor, W. E. (1991). Changes in lipid and lipoprotein levels and body weight in Tarahumara Indians after consumption of an affluent diet. *The New England Journal of Medicine, 325,* 1704–1708.

McNamara, J. J., Malot, M. A., Stemple, J. F., & Curring, R. T. (1971). Coronary heart disease in combat casualties in Viet Nam. *Journal of the American Medical Association, 216,* 1985–1987.

McReynolds, W. T. (1982). Toward a psychology of obesity: Review of research on the role of personality and level of adjustments. *International Journal of Eating Disorders, 2,* 37–57.

Mechanic, D. (1966). Response factors in illness: The study of illness behavior. *Social Psychiatry, 1,* 11–20.

Meehl, P. E. (1962). Schizotaxia, schizotypy, schizophrenia. *American Psychologist, 17,* 827–838.

Mehra, J. (Ed.). (1973). *The physicist's conception of nature.* Boston: Reidel.

Meichenbaum, D. (1977). *Cognitive-behavior modification: An integrative approach.* New York: Plenum.

Meichenbaum, D. (1985). *Stress inoculation training.* New York: Pergamon.

Melamed, B. G. (1978). Effects of film modeling on the reduction of anxiety-related behaviors in individuals varying in level of previous experience in the stress situation. *Journal of Consulting and Clinical Psychology, 46,* 1357–1367.

Melamed, B. G., & Siegel, L. J. (1975). Reduction of

anxiety in children facing hospitalization and surgery by use of filmed modeling. *Journal of Consulting and Clinical Psychology, 43,* 511–521.

Melzack, R. (1975). The McGill Pain Questionnaire: Major properties and scoring methods. *Pain, 1,* 277–299.

Melzack, R. (1990). Phantom limbs and the concept of a neuromatrix. *Trends in Neurosciences, 13,* 88–92.

Melzack, R. (1992, April). Phantom limbs. *Scientific American, 266,* 120–126.

Melzack, R. (1993). Pain: Past, present and future. *Canadian Journal of Experimental Psychology, 47,* 615–629.

Melzack, R., & Torgersen, W. R. (1971). The language of pain. *Anesthesiology, 34,* 50–59.

Melzack, R., & Wall, P. (1965). Pain mechanisms: A new theory. *Science, 50,* 971–979.

Memmler, R. L., & Wood, D. L. (1977). *The human body in health and disease* (4th ed.) Philadelphia: J. B. Lippincott.

Mendes-de-Leon, C. F., Powell, L. H., & Kaplan, B. H. (1991). Change in coronary-prone behaviors in the Recurrent Coronary Prevention Project. *Psychosomatic Medicine, 53,* 407–419.

Merenda, P. F. (1987). Toward a four-factor theory of temperament and/or personality. *Journal of Personality Assessment, 51,* 367–374.

Merimee, T. J. (1990). Diabetic retinopathy. *The New England Journal of Medicine, 322,* 978–983.

Mermelstein, R. J., & Riesenberg, L. A. (1992). Changing knowledge and attitudes about skin cancer risk factors in adolescents. *Health Psychology, 11,* 371–376.

Merskey, H. (1979). Pain terms. *Pain, 6,* 249–252.

Meyer, J. D., Fink, C. M., & Carey, P. F. (1988). Medical views of psychological consultation. *Professional Psychology: Research and Practice, 19,* 356–358.

Meyerowitz, B. E., Burish, T. G., & Wallston, K. A. (1986). Health psychology: A tradition of integration of clinical and social psychology. *Journal of Social and Clinical Psychology, 4,* 375–392.

Milan, A. R. (1980). *Breast self-examination.* New York: Liberty.

Miller, M. W. (1986). Effects of alcohol on the generation and migration of cerebral cortical neurons. *Science, 233,* 1308–1311.

Miller, N. E. (1985). The value of behavioral research on animals. *American Psychologist, 40,* 423–440.

Miller, N. S., & Giannini, A. J. (1990). The disease model of addiction: A biopsychiatrist's view. *Journal of Psychoactive Drugs, 22,* 83–85.

Miller, N. S., Dackis, C. A., & Gold, M. S. (1987). The relationship of addiction, tolerance, and dependence to alcohol and drugs: A neurochemical approach. *Journal of Substance Abuse Treatment, 4,* 197–207.

Miller, R., & Bor, R. (1989). *AIDS: A guide to clinical counseling.* London: Science Press.

Miller, T. Q., Smith, T. W., Turner, C. W., Guijarro, M. L., & Hallet, A. J. (1996). A meta-analytic review of research on hostility and physical health. *Psychological Bulletin, 119,* 322–348.

Miller, T. Q., Turner, C. W., Tindale, R. S., Posavac, E. J., & Dugoni, B. L. (1991). Reasons for the trend toward null findings in research on Type A behavior. *Psychological Bulletin, 110,* 469–485.

Miller, T. W. (1981). Professional services evaluation in a medical setting. In C. K. Prokop & L. A. Bradley (Eds.), *Medical psychology: Contributions to behavioral medicine* (pp. 471–483). New York: Academic Press.

Miller-Johnson, S., Emery, R. F., Marvin, R. S., Clarke, W., Lovinger, R., & Martin, M. (1994). Parent-child relationships and the management of insulin-dependent diabetes mellitus. *Journal of Consulting and Clinical Psychology, 62,* 603–610.

Millon, T., Green, C. J., & Meagher, R. (1982). *Handbook of clinical health psychology.* New York: Plenum.

Mills, J. K. (1992). Control orientation as a personality dimension among alcoholic and obese adult men undergoing addictions treatment. *Journal of Psychology, 125,* 537–542.

Millstein, S. G. (1989). Adolescent health: Challenges for behavioral scientists. *American Psychologist, 44,* 837–842.

Millstein, S. G., & Irwin, C. E. (1987). Concepts of health and illness: Different constructs or variations on a theme? *Health Psychology, 6,* 515–524.

Milner, B. (1966). Amnesia following operation on the temporal lobes. In C. W. M. Whitty & O. Zangwill (Eds.), *Amnesia* (pp. 109–133). London: Butterworth.

Milner, B., Corkin, S., & Teuber, H. L. (1968). Further analysis of the hippocampal amnesic syndrome: 14-year follow-up study of H. M. *Neuropsychologia, 6,* 215–234.

Mintz, L. B., O'Halloran, M. S., Mulholland, A. M., & Schneider, P. A. (1997). Questionnaire for eating disorder diagnoses: Reliability and validity of operationalizing DSM-IV criteria into a self-report format. *Journal of Counseling Psychology, 44,* 63–79.

Minuchin, S., Rosman, B. L., & Baker, L. (1978). *Psychosomatic families: Anorexia nervosa in context*. Cambridge, MA: Harvard University Press.

Mitchell, J. M., & Sunshine, J. H. (1992). Consequences of physicians' ownership of healthcare facilities—Joint ventures in radiation therapy. *The New England Journal of Medicine, 327*, 1497–1501.

Mohs, R. C., Breitner, J. C. S., Silverman, J. M., & Davis, K. L. (1987). Alzheimer's Disease: Morbid risk among first-degree relatives approximates 50% by 90 years of age. *Archives of General Psychiatry, 44*, 405–408.

Monroe, S. M., & Simons, A. D. (1991). Diathesis-stress theories in the context of life stress research: Implications for the depressive disorders. *Psychological Bulletin, 110*, 406–425.

Montano, D. E., & Taplin, S. H. (1991). A test of an expanded theory of reasoned action to predict mammography participation. *Social Science & Medicine, 32*, 733–741.

Monti, P. M., Rohsenow, D. J., Rubonis, A. V., Niaura, R. S., Sirota, A. D., Colby, S. M., Goddard, P., & Abrams, D. B. (1993). Cue exposure with coping skills treatment for male alcoholics: A preliminary investigation. *Journal of Consulting and Clinical Psychology, 61*, 1011–1019.

Moore, R. D., Stanton, D., Gopalan, R., & Chaisson, R. E. (1994). Racial differences in the use of drug therapy for HIV disease in an urban community. *The New England Journal of Medicine, 330*, 763–768.

Morgan, W. P., & Goldston, S. E. (Eds.). (1987). *Exercise and Mental Health*. Washington, DC: Hemisphere.

Morin, C. M., & Azrin, N. H. (1988). Behavioral and cognitive treatments of geriatric insomnia. *Journal of Consulting and Clinical Psychology, 56*, 748–753.

Morin, C. M., Kowatch, R. A., Barry, T., & Walton, E. (1993). Cognitive-behavior therapy for late-life insomnia. *Journal of Consulting and Clinical Psychology, 61*, 137–146.

Morin, S. F. (1988). AIDS: The challenge to psychology. *American Psychologist, 43*, 838–842.

Morin, S. F., Charles, K. A., & Malyon, A. K. (1984). The psychological impact of AIDS on gay men. *American Psychologist, 39*, 1288.

Moritz, D. J., & Ostfeld, A. M. (1990). The epidemiology and demography of aging. In W. R. Hazzard, R. Andres, E. L. Bierman, & J. P. Blass (Eds.), *Principles of geriatric medicine and gerontology* (2nd ed., pp. 146–156). New York: McGraw-Hill.

Morris, R. D., & Rimm, A. A. (1991). Association of waist to hip ratio and family history with the prevalence of NIDDM among 25,272 adult, white females. *The American Journal of Public Health, 81*, 507–509.

Morrison, F. R., & Paffenbarger, R. A. (1981). Epidemiological aspects of biobehavior in the etiology of cancer: A critical review. In S. M. Weiss, J. A. Herd, & B. H. Fox (Eds.), *Perspectives on behavioral medicine* (pp. 135–161). New York: Academic Press.

Morrow, G. R., & Morrell, C. (1982). Behavioral treatment for the anticipatory nausea and vomiting induced by cancer chemotherapy. *The New England Journal of Medicine, 307*, 1476–1480.

Morrow, G. R., Asbury, R., Hammon, S., Dobkin, P., Caruso, L., Pandya, K., & Rosenthal, S. (1992). Comparing the effectiveness of behavioral treatment for chemotherapy-induced nausea and vomiting when administered by oncologists, oncology nurses, and clinical psychologists. *Health Psychology, 11*, 250–256.

Morse, R. M., & Flavin, D. K. (1992). The definition of alcoholism. *Journal of the American Medical Association, 268*, 1012–1014.

Mossberg, H. (1989). 40-year follow-up of overweight children. *The Lancet, 1989, 2*, 491–493.

Mount, R., Neziroglu, F., & Taylor, C. J. (1990). An obsessive-compulsive view of obesity and its treatment. *Journal of Clinical Psychology, 46*, 68–78.

Mumford, E. (1983). *Medical sociology: Patients, providers, and policies*. New York: Random House.

Murphy, S. A. (1984). Stress levels and health status of victims of a natural disaster. *Research in Nursing and Health, 7*, 205–215.

Murray, D. M., Davis-Hearn, M., Goldman, A. I., Pirie, P., & Luepker, R. V. (1988). Four- and five-year follow-up results from four seventh-grade smoking prevention strategies. *Journal of Behavioral Medicine, 11*, 395–405.

Murray, D. M., Luepker, R. V., Johnson, C. A., & Mittelmark, M. B. (1984). The prevention of cigarette smoking in children: A comparison of four strategies. *Journal of Applied Social Psychology, 14*, 274–288.

Must, A., Jacques, P. F., Dallal, G. E., Bajema, C. J., & Dietz, W. H. (1992). Long-term morbidity and mortality of overweight adolescents. *The New England Journal of Medicine, 327*, 1350–1355.

Myers, J. K., Weissman, M. M., Tischler, G. L., Holzer, C. E., Leaf, P. J., Orvaschel, H., Anthony, J. C., Boyd, J. H., Burke, J. D., Kramer, M., & Stoltzman, R. (1984). Six-month prevalence of psychiatric disorders in three communities: 1980 to 1982. *Archives of General Psychiatry, 41,* 959–967.

Nagy, M. H. (1948). The child's theories concerning death. *Journal of Genetic Psychology, 73,* 3–27.

Nakano, K. (1989). Intervening variables of stress, hassles, and health. *Japanese Psychological Research, 31,* 143–148.

Natelson, B. H. (1983). Stress, predisposition and the onset of serious disease: Implications about psychosomatic etiology. *Neuroscience & Biobehavioral Reviews, 7,* 511–527.

Nathan, D. M. (1993). Long-term complications of diabetes mellitus. *The New England Journal of Medicine, 328,* 1676–1685.

National Center for Health Statistics. (1988). *Monthly vital statistics report, 37,* 1–10.

National Center for Health Statistics. (1992). Prevention profile. *Health, United States, 1991.* Hyattsville, MD: Public Health Service.

National Center for Health Statistics. (1996). *Health, United States, 1995.* Hyattsville, MD: Public Health Services.

National Cholesterol Education Program. (1992). Highlights of the report of the expert panel on blood cholesterol levels in children and adolescents. *American Family Physician, 45,* 2127–2136.

NCEP: National Cholesterol Education Program. (1993). Summary of the second report of the National Cholesterol Education Program (NCEP) expert panel on detection, evaluation, and treatment of high blood cholesterol in adults (adult treatment panel II). *Journal of the American Medical Association, 269,* 3015–3023.

National Commission on Aids. (1993). *Behavioral and Social Sciences and the HIV/AIDS Epidemic.* Rockville, MD: CDC National AIDS Clearinghouse.

National Research Council, National Academy of Sciences. (1989). *Diet and Health: Implications for Reducing Chronic Disease Risk.*

National Safety Council. (1986). *Accident facts— 1986.* Chicago: National Safety Council.

Nebes, R. D. (1989). Semantic memory in Alzheimer's Disease. *Psychological Bulletin, 106,* 377–394.

Nelson, K. E., Celentano, D. D., Eiumtrakol, S., Hoover, D. R., Beyrer, C., Supraset, S., Kuntolbutra, S., & Khamboonruang, C. (1996). Changes in sexual behavior and a decline in HIV infection among young men in Thailand. *The New England Journal of Medicine, 335,* 297–303.

Nelson, P. D. (1974). Comment. In E. K. E. Gunderson & R. H. Rahe (Eds.), *Life stress and illness* (pp. 79–89). Springfield, IL: Charles C Thomas.

Nerviano, V. J., & Gross, H. W. (1983). Personality types of alcoholics on objective inventories: A review. *Journal of Studies on Alcohol, 44,* 837–851.

Newall, D. J., Gadd, E. M., & Priestman, T. J. (1987). Presentation of information to cancer patients: A comparison of two centres in the UK and USA. *British Journal of Medical Psychology, 60,* 127–131.

Newlin, D. B. (1989). The skin flushing response: Autonomic, self-report, and conditioned responses to repeated administrations of alcohol in Asian men. *Journal of Abnormal Psychology, 98,* 421–425.

Nicholas, P., & Dwyer, J. (1986). Diets for weight reduction: Nutritional considerations. In K. D. Brownell & J. P. Foreyt (Eds.), *Handbook of eating disorders: Physiology, psychology, and treatment of obesity, anorexia, and bulimia* (pp. 122–144). New York: Basic Books.

Nilsson, B. E., Anderson, S. M., Havdrup, R., & Westlin, N. E. (1978). Ballet-dancing and weight-lifting: Effects on BMC. *American Journal of Roetengraphy, 131,* 541–542.

Noel, N. E., McCrady, B. S., Stout, R. L., & Fisher-Nelson, H. (1987). Predictors of attrition from an outpatient alcoholism treatment program for couples. *Journal of Studies on Alcohol, 48,* 229–237.

Norman, N. M., & Tedeschi, J. T. (1989). Self-presentation, reasoned action, and adolescents' decisions to smoke cigarettes. *Journal of Applied Social Psychology, 19,* 543–558.

Nossal, G. J. V. (1987). The basic components of the immune system. *The New England Journal of Medicine, 316,* 1320–1325.

Novello, A. (1991, Feb). Quoted in *The APA Monitor, 22(2),* 30.

O'Brien, C. P. (1996). Recent developments in the pharmacotherapy of substance abuse. *Journal of Consulting and Clinical Psychology, 64,* 677–686.

O'Brien, C. P., Childress, A. R., McLellan, A. T., Ehrman, R., & Ternes, J. W. (1988). Types of Conditioning Found in Drug-Dependent Humans. In *Learning factors in substance abuse* (pp.

44–61), NIDA Research Monograph 84, U.S Department of Health and Human Services.

O'Keeffe, M. K., Nesselhof-Kendall, S., & Baum, A. (1990). Behavior and prevention of AIDS: Bases of research and intervention. *Personality and Social Psychology Bulletin, 16,* 166–180.

O'Leary, A. (1990). Stress, emotion, and human immune function. *Psychological Bulletin, 108,* 363–382.

O'Leary, A., Shoor, S., Lorig, K., & Holman, H. R. (1988). A cognitive-behavioral treatment for rheumatoid arthritis [Special issue: Clinical health psychology]. *Health Psychology, 7,* 527–544.

O'Leary, K. D., & Borkovec, T. D. (1978). Conceptual, methodological, and ethical problems of placebo groups in psychotherapy research. *American Psychologist, 33,* 821–830.

Oetting, E., & Beauvais, F. (1987). Common elements in youth drug abuse: Peer clusters and other psychosocial factors. *Journal of Drug Issues, 17,* 133–151.

Office of Technology Assessment, U.S. Congress. (1990). *Genetic monitoring and screening in the workplace* (OTA-BA-455). Washington, DC: U.S. Government Printing Office.

Office of Technology Assessment, U.S. Congress. (1992). *Cystic Fibrosis and DNA tests: Implications of carrier screening* (OTA-BA-532). Washington, DC: U.S. Government Printing Office.

Olds, J., & Milner, P. (1954). Positive reinforcement produced by electrical stimulation of the septal area and other regions of the rat brain. *Journal of Comparative and Physiological Psychology, 47,* 419–427.

Orford, J., & Velleman, R. (1991). The environmental intergenerational transmission of alcohol problems: A comparison of two hypotheses. *British Journal of Medical Psychology, 64,* 189–200.

Orleans, C. T., Rimer, B. K., Cristinzio, S., Keintz, M. K., & Fleisher, L. (1991). A national survey of older smokers: Treatment needs of a growing population. *Health Psychology, 10,* 343–351.

Ornish, D., Brown, S. E., Scherwitz, L. W., Billings, J. H., Armstrong, W. T., Ports, T. A., McLanahan, S. M., Kirkeeide, R. L., Brand, R. J., & Gould, K. L. (1990). Can lifestyle changes reverse coronary heart disease? *Lancet, 336,* 129–133.

Osler, W. (1901/1984). *The principles and practice of medicine.* Norwalk, CT: Appleton-Century-Crofts.

Osterweis, M., Solomon, F., & Green, M. (Eds.). (1984). *Bereavement: Reactions, consequences, and care.* Washington, DC: National Academy Press.

Ostlund, R. E. Jr., Staten, M., Kohrt, W. M., Schultz, J., & Malley, M. (1990). The ratio of waist-to-hip circumference, plasma insulin level, and glucose intolerance as independent predictors of the HDL2 cholesterol level in older adults. *The New England Journal of Medicine, 322,* 229–234.

Ots, T. (1990). The angry liver, the anxious heart and the melancholy spleen. *Culture, Medicine and Psychiatry, 14,* 21–58.

Owen, N., Wakefield, M., Roberts, L., & Esterman, A. (1992). Stages of readiness to quit smoking: Population prevalence and correlates. *Health Psychology, 11,* 413–417.

Pace, P. W., Bolton, M. P., & Reeves, R. S. (1991). Ethics of obesity treatment: Implications for dietitians. *Journal of the American Dietetic Association, 91,* 1258–1260.

Pandina, R. J., & Johnson, V. (1989). Familial drinking history as a predictor of alcohol and drug consumption among adolescent children. *Journal of Studies on Alcohol, 50,* 245–253.

Pang, M. G., Wells-Parker, E., & McMillen, D. L. (1989). Drinking reasons, drinking locations, and automobile accident involvement among collegians. *The International Journal of the Addictions, 24,* 215–227.

Pantaleo, G., Graziosi, C., & Fauci, A. S. (1993). The immunopathogenesis of human immunodeficiency virus infection. *The New England Journal of Medicine, 328,* 327–335.

Pappas, G., Gergen, P. J., & Carroll, M. (1990). Hypertension prevalence and the status of awareness, treatment, and control in the Hispanic Health and Nutrition Examination Survey (HHANES), 1982–1984. *American Journal of Public Health, 80,* 1431–1436.

Parker, D. A., & Harford, T. C. (1987). Alcohol-related problems of children of heavy-drinking parents. *Journal of Studies on Alcohol, 48,* 265–268.

Parsons, T. (1951). *The social system.* New York: Free Press.

Patterson, D. R., Everett, J. J., Burns, G. L., & Marvin, J. A. (1992). Hypnosis for the treatment of burn pain. *Journal of Consulting and Clinical Psychology, 60,* 713–717.

Patterson, D. R., Everett, J. J., Bombardier, C. H., Questad, K. A., Lee, V. K., & Marvin, J. A. (1993).

Psychological effects of severe burn injuries. *Psychological Bulletin, 113,* 362–378.

Patterson, J. M. (1985). Critical factors affecting family compliance with home treatment for children with cystic fibrosis. *Family Relations, 34,* 79–89.

Pavlov, I. P. (1927). *Conditioned reflexes: An investigation of the physiological activity of the cerebral cortex* (G. V. Anrep, Trans.). London: Oxford University Press.

Pekkanen, J., Linn, S., Heiss, G., Suchindran, C. M., Leon, A., Rifkind, B. M., & Tyroler, H. A. (1990). Ten-year mortality from cardiovascular disease in relation to cholesterol level among men with and without preexisting cardiovascular disease. *The New England Journal of Medicine, 322,* 1700–1707.

Pelleymounter, M. A., Cullen, M. J., Baker, M. B., Hecht, R., Winters, D., Boone, T., & Collins, F. (1995). Effects of the obese gene product on body weight regulation in ob/ob mice. *Science, 269,* 540–543.

Pelligrino, E. D. (1963). Medicine, history, and the idea of man. In J. A. Clausen & R. Straus (Eds.), *Medicine and Society* (pp. 9–20). The Annals of the American Academy of Political and Social Science.

Pepper, S. C. (1942). *World hypothesis.* Berkeley: University of California Press.

Perkins, K. A. (1989). Interactions among coronary heart disease risk factors. *Annals of Behavioral Medicine, 11,* 3–11.

Perls, F., Hefferline, R., & Goodman, P. (1951). *Gestalt therapy.* New York: Dell.

Perrone, B., Stockel, H. H., Krueger, V. (1989). *Medicine women,* curanderos, *and women doctors.* Norman, OK: University of Oklahoma Press.

Perry, C. L., Kelder, S. H., Murray, D. M., & Klepp, K. I. (1992). Communitywide smoking prevention: Long-term outcomes of the Minnesota Heart Health Program and the Class of 1989 Study. *The American Journal of Public Health, 82,* 1210–1216.

Perry, C. L., Klepp, K. I., & Shultz, J. M. (1988). Primary prevention of cardiovascular disease: Community-wide strategies for youth. *Journal of Consulting and Clinical Psychology, 56,* 358–364.

Perry, C., Klepp, K., & Sillers, C. (1989). Communitywide strategies for cardiovascular health: The Minnesota heart health program youth program. *Health Education Research, 4,* 87–101.

Peters, R. K., Benson, H., & Peters, J. M. (1977). Daily relaxation response breaks in a working population: II. Effects on blood pressure. *The American Journal of Public Health, 67,* 954–959.

Peterson, C., & Seligman, M. E. P. (1987). Explanatory style and illness. Special issue: Personality and physical health. *Journal of Personality, 55,* 237–265.

Peterson, J. L., & Marín, G. (1988). Issues in the prevention of AIDS among Black and Hispanic men. *American Psychologist, 43,* 871–877.

Peterson, L., & Harbeck, C. (1988). *The pediatric psychologist.* Champaigne, IL: Research Press.

Pichot, P. (1989). The historical roots of behavior therapy. *Journal of Behavioral & Experimental Psychiatry, 20,* 107–114.

Pickens, R. W., Svikis, D. S., McGue, M., Lykken, D. T., Heston, L. L., & Clayton, P. J. (1991). Heterogeneity in the inheritance of alcoholism. *Archives of General Psychiatry, 48,* 19–28.

Pihl, R. O., Young, S. N., Ervin, F. R., & Plotnick, S. (1987). Influence of tryptophan availability on selection of alcohol and water by men. *Journal of Studies on Alcohol, 48,* 260–264.

Pinel, J. P. J. (1993). *Biopsychology* (2nd ed.). Boston: Allyn & Bacon.

Pinkerton, S. S., Hughes, H., & Wenrich, W. W. (1982). *Behavioral medicine: Clinical applications.* New York: Wiley.

Piper, W. E., Joyce, A. S., McCallum, M., & Azim, H. F. A. (1993). Concentration and correspondence of transference interpretations in short-term psychotherapy. *Journal of Consulting and Clinical Psychology, 61,* 586–595.

Platt, O. S., Thorington, B. D., Brambilla, D. J., Milner, P. F., Rosse, W. F., Vichinsky, E., & Kinney, T. R. (1991). Pain in sickle cell disease: Rates and risk factors. *The New England Journal of Medicine, 325,* 11–16.

Plaut, S. M., & Friedman, S. B. (1981). Psychosocial factors, stress, and disease processes. In R. Ader (Ed.), *Psychoneuroimmunology* (pp. 3–29). New York: Academic Press.

Plomin, R. (1990). The role of inheritance in behavior. *Science, 248,* 183–188.

Plomin, R., DeFries, J. C., & McClearn, G. E. (1980). *Behavioral genetics: A primer.* San Francisco: Freeman.

Pohorecky, L. A. (1990). Interaction of ethanol and stress: Research with experimental animals—an update. *Alcohol & Alcoholism, 25,* 263–276.

Polich, J., Pollock, V. E., & Bloom, F. E. (1994). Meta-analysis of P300 amplitude from males at risk for alcoholism. *Psychological Bulletin, 115,* 55–73.

Polivy, J., Garner, D. M., & Garfinkel, P. E. (1986). Causes and consequences of the current preference for thin female physiques. In C. P. Herman, M. P. Zanna, & E. T. Higgins (Eds.), *Physical appearance, stigma, and social behavior: The Ontario Symposium, Volume 3* (pp. 89–112). Hillsdale, NJ: Erlbaum.

Pollack, A. (1991, April 29). Medical technology "arms race." *The New York Times, 140,* A1.

Pons, T. P., Garraghty, P. E., Ommaya, A. K., Kaas, J. H., Taub, E., & Mishkin, M. (1991). Massive cortical reorganization after sensory deafferentation in adult macaques. *Science, 252,* 1857–1861.

Popkin, B. M., Siega-Riz, A. M., & Haines, P. S. (1996). A comparison of dietary trends among racial and socioeconomic groups in the United States. *The New England Journal of Medicine, 335,* 716–720.

Potter, W. Z., Rudorfer, M. V., & Manji, H. (1991). The pharmacologic treatment of depression. *The New England Journal of Medicine, 325,* 633–642.

Poulos, C. X., & Cappell, H. (1991). Homeostatic theory of drug tolerance: A general model of physiological adaptation. *Psychological Review, 98,* 390–408.

Preston, D. S., & Stern, R. S. (1992). Nonmelanoma cancers of the skin. *The New England Journal of Medicine, 327,* 1649–1662.

Price, V. A. (1988). Research and clinical issues in treating Type A behavior. In B. K. Houston & C. R. Snyder (Eds.), *Type A behavior pattern: Research, theory and intervention* (pp. 275–311). New York: Wiley.

Prinz, P. N., Vitiello, M. V., Raskind, M. A., & Thorpy, M. J. (1990). Geriatrics: Sleep disorders and aging. *The New England Journal of Medicine, 323,* 520–526.

Prochaska, J. O., & DiClemente, C. C. (1983). Stages and processes of self-change of smoking: Toward an integrative model of change. *Journal of Consulting and Clinical Psychology, 51,* 390–395.

Prochaska, J. O., DiClemente, C. C., & Norcross, J. C. (1992). In search of how people change: Applications to addictive behaviors. *American Psychologist, 47,* 1102–1114.

Prokop, C. K., & Bradley, L. A. (Eds.). (1981). *Medical psychology: Contributions to behavioral medicine.* New York: Academic Press.

Puglisi-Allegra, S., Kempf, E., & Cabib, S. (1990). Role of genotype in the adaptation of the brain dopamine system to stress. *Neurosciences & Biobehavioral Review, 14,* 523–528.

Quinton, P. M. (1989). Defective epithelial ion transport in cystic fibrosis. *Clinical Chemistry, 35,* 726–730.

Rabin, B. S., Cohen, S., Ganguli, R., Lysle, D. T., & Cunnick, J. E. (1989). Bidirectional interaction between the central nervous system and the immune system. *Critical Reviews in Immunology, 9,* 279–312.

Rabkin, J. G., & Struening, E. L. (1976). Life events, stress, and illness. *Science, 194,* 1013–1020.

Rabkin, J. G., Williams, J. B. W., Remien, R. H., Goetz, R., Kertzner, R., & Gorman, G. M. (1991). Depression, distress, lymphocyte subsets, and human immunodeficiency virus symptoms on two occasions in HIV-positive homosexual men. *Archives of General Psychiatry, 48,* 111–119.

Rachman, S. J., & Wilson, G. T. (1980). *The effects of psychological therapy* (2nd ed.). New York: Pergamon.

Ragland, D. R., & Brand, R. J. (1988). Type A behavior and mortality from coronary heart disease. *The New England Journal of Medicine, 318,* 65–69.

Rahe, R. H., & Arthur, R. J. (1978). Life change and illness studies: Past history and future directions. *Journal of Human Stress, 4,* 3–15.

Rainwater, N., & Alexander, A. B. (1982). Respiratory disorders: Asthma. In D. M. Doleys, R. L. Meredith, & A. R. Ciminero (Eds.), *Behavioral medicine: Assessment and treatment strategies* (pp. 435–446). New York: Plenum.

Raithel, K. S. (1987). 20 years after first human heart transplant, 1987 may see 4000 procedures performed worldwide. *Journal of the American Medical Association, 258,* 3084–3085.

Rakover, S. (1989). Incommensurability: The scaling of mind-body theories as a counter example. *Behaviorism, 17,* 103–118.

Rakowski, W., Fulton, J. P., & Feldman, J. P. (1993). Women's decision making about mammography: A replication of the relationship between stages of adoption and decisional balance. *Health Psychology, 12,* 209–214.

Ramsay, D. S., & Woods, S. C. (1997). Biological consequences of drug administration: Implications for acute and chronic tolerance. *Psychological Review, 104,* 170–193.

Raskin, P., & Rosenstock, J. (1987). Hyperglycemia, genetic susceptibility, and diabetic complications. *Clinical Diabetes, 5,* 135–141.

Ravussin, E., & Swinburn, B. A. (1992). Pathophysiology of obesity. *Lancet, 340,* 404–408.

Ravussin, E., Lillioja, S., Knowler, W. C., Christin, L., Freymond, D., Abbott, W. G. H., Boyce, V., Howard, B. V., & Bogardus, C. (1988). Reduced rate of energy expenditure as a risk factor for body-weight gain. *The New England Journal of Medicine, 318,* 467–472.

Redline, S. (1991). The epidemiology of COPD. In N. S. Cherniack (Ed.), *Chronic obstructive pulmonary disease* (pp. 225–234). Philadelphia: Saunders.

Reich, T. (1988). Biological-marker studies in alcoholism. *The New England Journal of Medicine, 318,* 180–182.

Reid, J. D., & Willis, S. L. (1991). Doctoral training in the psychology of adult development and aging: 1989–1990 survey results. *Educational Gerontology, 17,* 247–256.

Reif, A. E. (1981). The causes of cancer. *American Scientist, 69,* 437–446.

Reisman, L. E., & Matheny, A. P. (1969). *Genetics and counseling in medical practice.* St. Louis: Mosby.

Relman, A. S. (1991). Shattuck lecture—The health care industry: Where is it taking us? *The New England Journal of Medicine, 325,* 854–859.

Rescorla, R. A., & Wagner, A. R. (1972). A theory of Pavlovian conditioning: Variation in the effectiveness of reinforcement and nonreinforcement. In A. H. Black & W. F. Prokasy (Eds.), *Classical conditioning II: Current research and theory* (pp. 64–99). New York: Appleton-Century-Crofts.

Rest, J., Power, C., & Brabeck, M. (1988). Lawrence Kohlberg (1927–1987). *American Psychologist, 43,* 399–400.

Retchin, S. M., Wells, J. A., Valleron, A. J., & Albrecht, G. L. (1992). Health behavior changes in the United States, the United Kingdom, and France. *Journal of General Internal Medicine, 7,* 615–622.

Revenson, T. A., Schiaffino, K. M., Mjerovitz, D., & Gibofsky, A. (1991). Social support as a double-edged sword: The relation of positive and problematic support to depression among rheumatoid arthritis patients. *Social Science & Medicine, 33,* 807–813.

Revenson, T. A., Wollman, C. A., & Felton, B. J. (1983). Social supports as stress buffers for adult cancer patients. *Psychosomatic Medicine, 45,* 321–331.

Reynolds, D. V. (1969). Surgery in the rat during electrical analgesia induced by focal brain stimulation. *Science, 164,* 444–445.

Riad, J. K., & Norris, F. H. (1996). The influence of relocation on the environmental, social, and psychological stress experienced by disaster victims. *Environment and Behavior, 28,* 163–183.

Rice, D. P., Kelman, S., & Miller, L. S. (1991). Estimates of economic costs of alcohol and drug abuse and mental illness, 1985 and 1988. *Public Health Reports, 106,* 280–292.

Rice, P. L. (1992). *Stress and health* (2nd ed.). Pacific Grove, CA: Brooks/Cole.

Riche, J. M., & Thelen, M. H. (1989, May). *Individuals' health comparisons with specific others.* Paper presented at the Annual Midwestern Psychological Association Conference, Chicago, IL.

Rich-Edwards, J. W., Hennekens, C. H., & Buring, J. E. (1995). The primary prevention of coronary heart disease in women. *The New England Journal of Medicine, 332,* 1758–1766.

Rickels, K., Schweizer, E., Csanalosi, I., Case, G., & Chung, H. (1988). Long-term treatment of anxiety and risk of withdrawal: Prospective comparison of clorazepate and buspirone. *Archives of General Psychiatry, 45,* 444–450.

Ried, L. D., Christensen, D. B., & Stergachis, A. (1990). Medical and psychosocial factors predictive of psychotropic drug use in elderly patients. *The American Journal of Public Health, 80,* 1349.

Rigby, K., Brown, M., Anagnostou, P., Ross, M. W., & Rosser, B. R. S. (1989). Shock tactics to counter AIDS: The Australian experience. *Psychology and Health, 3,* 145–159.

Riley, V. (1981). Psychoneuroendocrine influences on immunocompetence and neoplasia. *Science, 212,* 1100–1109.

Rimm, E. B., Stampfer, M. J., Ascherio, A., Giovannucci, E., Colditz, G. A., & Willett, W. C. (1993). Vitamin E consumption and the risk of coronary disease in men. *The New England Journal of Medicine, 328,* 1450–1456.

Riscalla, L. M. (1983). A holistic concept of the immune system. *Journal of the American Society of Psychosomatic Dentistry and Medicine, 30,* 97–101.

Ritz, M. C., George, F. R., de Fiebre, C. M., & Meisch, R. A. (1986). Genetic differences in the establishment of ethanol as a reinforcer. *Pharmacology, Biochemistry and Behavior, 24,* 1089–1094.

Roberts, J. A., Roberts, J. A. F., & Pembrey, M. E. (1985). *An introduction to medical genetics* (8th ed.). Oxford: Oxford University Press.

Roberts, S. B., Savage, J., Coward, W. A., Chew, B., & Lucas, A. (1988). Energy expenditure and intake in infants born to lean and overweight mothers.

The New England Journal of Medicine, 318, 461–466.

Robins, L. N., Helzer, J. E., & Davis, D. H. (1975). Narcotic use in Southeast Asia and afterward: An interview study of 898 Vietnam returnees. *Archives of General Psychiatry, 32,* 955–961.

Rodin, J. (1981). Current status of the internal-external hypothesis for obesity: What went wrong? *American Psychologist, 36,* 361–372.

Rodin, J. (1987). Weight change following smoking cessation: The role of food intake and exercise. *Addictive Behaviors, 12,* 303–317.

Rodin, J., & Ickovics, J. R. (1990). Women's health: Review and research agenda as we approach the 21st century. *American Psychologist, 45,* 1018–1034.

Rodin, J., & Salovey, P. (1989). Health psychology. *Annual Review of Psychology, 40,* 533–579.

Rodin, J., Elias, M., Silberstein, L. R., & Wagner, A. (1988). Combined behavioral and pharmacologic treatment for obesity: Predictors of successful weight maintenance. *Journal of Consulting and Clinical Psychology, 56,* 399–404.

Rogers, C. R. (1951). *Client-centered therapy.* Boston: Houghton Mifflin.

Rogers, R. W., Rogers, J. S., Bailey, J. S., Runkle, W., & Moore, B. (1988). Promoting safety belt use among state employees: The effects of prompting and a stimulus-control intervention. *Journal of Applied Behavior Analysis, 21,* 263–269.

Rohsenow, D. J., Monti, P. M., Rubonis, A. V., Sirota, A. D., Niaura, R. S., Colby, S. M., Wunschel, S. M., & Abrams, D. B. (1994). Cue reactivity as a predictor of drinking among male alcoholics. *Journal of Consulting and Clinical Psychology, 62,* 620–626.

Rohsenow, D. J., Monti, P. M., Zwick, W. R., Nirenberg, T. D., Liepman, M. R., Binkoff, J. A., & Abrams, D. B. (1989). Irrational beliefs, urges to drink and drinking among alcoholics. *Journal of Studies on Alcohol, 50,* 461–464.

Rolls, B. J., Fedoroff, I. C., & Guthrie, J. F. (1991). Gender differences in eating behavior and body weight regulation. *Health Psychology, 10,* 133–142.

Romano, J. M., Turner, J. A., Friedman, L. S., Bulcroft, R. A., Jensen, M. P., Hops, H., & Wright, S. F. (1992). Sequential analysis of chronic pain behaviors and spouse responses. *Journal of Consulting and Clinical Psychology, 60,* 777–782.

Rommens, J. M., Iannuzzi, M. C., Kerem, B., Drumm, M. L., Melmer, G., Dean, M., Rozmahel, R., Cole, J.

L., Kennedy, D., Hidaka, N., Zsiga, M., Buchwald, M., Riordan, J. R., Tsui, L., & Collins, F. S. (1989). Identification of the cystic fibrosis gene: Chromosome walking and jumping. *Science, 245,* 1059–1065.

Roper, W. L. (1991). Current approaches to prevention of HIV infections. *Public Health Reports, 106,* 111–115.

Roque, G. M., & Roberts, M. C. (1989). A replication of the use of public posting in traffic speed control. *Journal of Applied Behavior Analysis, 22,* 325–330.

Rose, R. J. (1988). Genes, stress and the heart. *Stress Medicine, 4,* 265–271.

Rose, R. J., & Chesney, M. A. (1986). Cardiovascular stress reactivity: A behavior-genetic perspective. *Behavior Therapy, 17,* 314–323.

Rosen, B. (1979). A method of structured brief psychotherapy. *British Journal of Medical Psychology, 52,* 157–162.

Rosen, J. C., & Leitenberg, H. (1982). Bulimia nervosa: Treatment with exposure and response prevention. *Behavior Therapy, 13,* 117–124.

Rosenberg, H. (1993). Prediction of controlled drinking by alcoholics and problem drinkers. *Psychological Bulletin, 113,* 129–139.

Rosenberg, L., Palmer, J. R., & Shapiro, S. (1990). Decline in the risk of myocardial infarction among women who stop smoking. *The New England Journal of Medicine, 322,* 213–217.

Rosenhan, D. L., & Seligman, M. E. P. (1989). *Abnormal psychology* (2nd ed.). New York: Norton.

Rosenman, R. H., & Friedman, M. (1961). Association of specific behavior pattern in women with blood and cardiovascular findings. *Circulation, 24,* 1173–1184.

Rosenman, R. H., Friedman, M., Straus, R., Jenkins, C. D., Zyzanski, S. J., & Wurm, M. (1970). Coronary heart disease in the Western Collaborative Group Study: A follow-up experience of 4½ years. *Journal of Chronic Disease, 23,* 173–190.

Rosenman, R. H., Friedman, M., Straus, R., Wurm, M., Kositcheck, R., Hahn, W., & Werthessen, N. T. (1964). A predictive study of coronary heart disease: the Western Collaborative Group Study. *Journal of the American Medical Association, 189,* 15–22.

Rosenstock, I. M. (1966). Why people use health services. *Milbank Memorial Fund Quarterly, 44,* 94–124.

Rosenthal, R. (1966). *Experimenter effects in behavioral research.* New York: Appleton-Century-Crofts.

Rosenthal, R., & Rosnow, R. L. (1991). *Essentials of behavioral research: Methods and data analysis* (2nd ed.). New York: McGraw-Hill.

Roskies, E., Seraganian, P., Oseasohn, R., Hanley, J. A., Collu, R., Martin, N., & Smilga, C. (1986). The Montreal Type A Intervention Project: Major findings. *Health Psychology, 5,* 45–70.

Rosner, F. (1977). *Medicine in the Bible and the Talmud.* New York, NY: Ktav Publishing.

Ross, R. (1986). The pathogenesis of atherosclerosis—an update. *The New England Journal of Medicine, 314,* 488–500.

Rostand, S. G. (1989). Diabetic renal disease in blacks—inevitable or preventable? *The New England Journal of Medicine, 321,* 1121–1122.

Rothman, A. J., & Salovey, P. (1997). Shaping perceptions to motivate healthy behavior: The role of message framing. *Psychological Bulletin, 121,* 3–19.

Rotter, J. B. (1966). Generalized expectancies for internal versus external control of reinforcement. *Psychological Monographs, 80.*

Rotter, J. B. (1990). Internal versus external control of reinforcement: A case history of a variable. *American Psychologist, 45,* 489–493.

Rounsaville, B. J., Weissman, M. M., Crits-Christoph, K., Wilber, C., & Kleber, H. (1982). Diagnosis and symptoms of depression in opiate addicts. *Archives of General Psychiatry, 39,* 151–156.

Rowe, J. W., & Kahn, R. L. (1987). Human aging: Usual and successful. *Science, 237,* 143–149.

Royce, J. E. (1989). *Alcohol problems and alcohol* (rev. ed.). New York: Free Press.

Royer, H. D., & Reinherz, E. L. (1987). T lymphocytes: Ontogeny, function, and relevance to clinical disorders. *The New England Journal of Medicine, 317,* 1136–1142.

Rubin, B. K. (1990). Exposure of children with cystic fibrosis to environmental tobacco smoke. *The New England Journal of Medicine, 323,* 782–788.

Rubin, R. T. (1974). Biochemical and neuroendocrine responses to severe psychological stress. In E. K. E. Gunderson & R. H. Rahe (Eds.), *Life stress and illness* (pp. 227–241). Springfield, IL: Charles C. Thomas.

Rudolph, K. D., Dennig, M. D., & Weisz, J. R. (1995). Determinants and consequences of children's coping in the medical setting: Conceptualization, review, and critique. *Psychological Bulletin, 118,* 328–357.

Rushton, J. P. (1987). An evolutionary theory of health, longevity, and personality: Sociobiology and r/K reproductive strategies. *Psychological Reports, 60,* 539–549.

Russell, G. F. M. (1979). Bulimia nervosa: An ominous variant of anorexia nervosa. *Psychological Medicine, 9,* 429–448.

Rychtarik, R. G., Prue, D. M., Rapp, S. R., & King, A. C. (1992). Self-efficacy, aftercare and relapse in a treatment program for alcoholics. *Journal of Studies on Alcohol, 53,* 435–440.

Ryle, G. (1949). *The concept of mind.* New York: Barnes & Noble.

Saad, M. F., Lillioja, S., Nyomba, B. L., Castillo, C., Ferraro, R., De Gregorio, M., Ravussin, E., Knowler, W. C., Bennett, P. H., Howard, B. V., & Bogardus, C. (1991). Racial differences in the relation between blood pressure and insulin resistance. *The New England Journal of Medicine, 324,* 733–739.

Saile, H., Burgmeier, R., & Schmidt, L. R. (1988). A meta-analysis of studies on psychological preparation of children facing medical procedures. *Psychology and Health, 2,* 107–132.

Salovey, P., Sieber, W. J., Smith, A. F., Turk, D. C., Jobe, J. B., & Willis, G. B. (1992). Reporting chronic pain episodes on health surveys (PHS 92-1081). Hyattsville, MD: U.S. Department of Health and Human Services.

Salzman, C. (1991). The APA task force report on benzodiazepine dependence, toxicity, and abuse. *American Journal of Psychiatry, 148,* 151–152.

Sanders, M. R., Patel, R. K., Le Grice, B., & Shepherd, R. W. (1993). Children with persistent feeding difficulties: An observational analysis of the feeding interactions of problem and non-problem eaters. *Health Psychology, 12,* 64–73.

Sanders, M. R., Rebgetz, M., Morrison, M., Bor, W., Gordon, A., Dadds, M., & Shepherd, R. (1989). Cognitive-behavioral treatment of recurrent nonspecific abdominal pain in children: An analysis of generalization, maintenance, and side effects. *Journal of Consulting and Clinical Psychology, 57,* 294–300.

San Francisco notes 10,000th AIDS death. (1993, Jan. 11). *The New York Times, 142,* p. B7(L), col. 5.

Saunders, C. (1976). St. Christopher's Hospice. In E. Shneidman (Ed.), *Death: Current perspectives* (pp. 356–361). Palo Alto: Mayfield.

Sauter, S. L., Murphy, L. R., & Hurrell, J. J. (1990). Prevention of work-related psychological disorders. *American Psychologist, 45,* 1146–1158.

Sawada, Y., & Steptoe, A. (1988). The effects of brief meditation on cardiovascular stress response. *Journal of Psychophysiology, 2,* 249–257.

Saxon, A. J., & Calsyn, D. A. (1992). Alcohol use and high-risk behavior by intravenous drug users in an AIDS education paradigm. *Journal of Studies on Alcohol, 53,* 611–618.

Sayre, A. (1975). *Rosalind Franklin and DNA.* New York: Norton.

Scanlon, E. F., & Strax, P. (1986). Breast cancer. In *The American Cancer Society Book* (pp. 297–340). Garden City, NJ: Doubleday.

Schacter, S., & Rodin, J. (1974). *Obese humans and rats.* Washington, DC: Erlbaum/Wiley.

Schapira, D. V. (1992). Nutrition and cancer prevention. *Cancer Epidemiology, Prevention, and Screening, 19,* 481–491.

Schatzberg, A. F., & Cole, J. O. (1991). *Manual of clinical psychopharmacology* (2nd ed.). Washington, DC: American Psychiatric Press.

Schatzkin, A., Jones, Y., Hoover, R. N., Taylor, P. R., Brinton, L. A., Ziegler, R. G., Harvey, E. B., Carter, C., Licitra, L. M., Dufour, M. C., & Larson, D. B. (1987). Alcohol consumption and breast cancer in the epidemiologic follow-up study of the first national health and nutrition examination survey. *The New England Journal of Medicine, 316,* 1169–1173.

Scheier, M., & Carver, C. S. (1987). Dispositional optimism and physical well-being: The influence of generalized outcome expectancies on health. *Journal of Personality, 55,* 169–210.

Scheper-Hughes, N. (1990). Three propositions for a critically applied medical anthropology. *Social Science & Medicine, 30,* 189–197.

Scherwitz, L., Graham, L. E., Grandits, G., & Billings, J. (1987). Speech characteristics and behavior-type assessment in the Multiple Risk Factor Intervention Trial (MRFIT) structured interviews. *Journal of Behavioral Medicine, 10,* 173–195.

Schobinger, R., Florin, I., Zimmer, C., Lindemann, H., & Winter, H. (1992). Childhood asthma: Paternal critical attitude and father-child interaction. *Journal of Psychosomatic Research, 36,* 743–750.

Schroeder, D. H., & Costa, P. T. (1984, May). *Do stressful life events influence objectively-measured health? A prospective evaluation.* Paper presented at the Midwestern Psychological Association Annual Conference, Chicago, IL.

Schuckit, M. A. (1985). Genetics and the risk for alcoholism. *Journal of the American Medical Association, 254,* 2614–2617.

Schuckit, M. A. (1996). Recent developments in the pharmacotherapy of alcohol dependence. *Journal of Consulting and Clinical Psychology, 64,* 669–676.

Schultz, J., & Luthe, W. (1959). *Autogenic training: A psychophysiological approach to psychotherapy.* New York: Grune & Stratton.

Schwab, J. J. (1985). Psychosomatic medicine: Its past and present. *Psychosomatics, 26,* 583–593.

Schwartz, G. E. (1982). Testing the biopsychosocial model: The ultimate challenge facing behavioral medicine? *Journal of Consulting and Clinical Psychology, 50,* 1040–1053.

Schwartz, G. E., & Weiss, S. M. (1978a). *Proceedings of the Yale Conference on Behavioral Medicine.* DHEW Publication No. (NIH) 78-1424. Washington, DC: U.S Government Printing Office.

Schwartz, G. E., & Weiss, S. M. (1978b). Behavioral Medicine revisited: An amended definition. *Journal of Behavioral Medicine, 1,* 249–251.

Searle, J. R. (1984). *Minds, brains and science.* Cambridge, MA: Harvard University Press.

Searles, J. S. (1988). The role of genetics in the pathogenesis of alcoholism. Special Issue: Models of addiction. *Journal of Abnormal Psychology, 97,* 153–167.

Searles, J. S. (1991). The genetics of alcoholism: Impact on family and sociological models of addiction. *Family Dynamics of Addiction Quarterly, 1,* 8–21.

Sears, M. R., Burrows, B., Flannery, E. M., Herbison, G. P., Hewitt, C. J., & Holdaway, M. D. (1991). Relation between airway responsiveness and serum IgE in children with asthma and in apparently normal children. *The New England Journal of Medicine, 325,* 1067–1071.

Sechrest, L., & Figueredo, A. J. (1993). Program evaluation. *Annual Review of Psychology, 44,* 645–674.

Seeman, J. (1989). Toward a model of positive health. *American Psychologist, 44,* 1099–1109.

Selby, J. V., Friedman, G. D., Quesenberry, C. P., & Weiss, N. S. (1992). A case-control study of screening sigmoidoscopy and mortality from colorectal cancer. *The New England Journal of Medicine, 326,* 653–657.

Seligman, J. (1992, February 3). The new age of aquarius. *Newsweek, 119*(5), 65–67.

Seligmann, M., Chess, L., Fahey, J. L., Fauci, A. S.,

Lachmann, P. J., L'Age-Stehr, J., Ngu, J., Pinching, A. J., Rosen, F. S., Spira, T. J., & Wybran, J. (1984). AIDS—an immunologic reevaluation. *The New England Journal of Medicine, 311,* 1286–1292.

Selwyn, P. A., Alcabes, P., Hartel, D., Buono, D., Schoenbaum, E. E., Klein, R. S., Davenny, K., & Friedland, G. H. (1992). Clinical manifestations and predictors of disease progression in drug users with human immunodeficiency virus infection. *The New England Journal of Medicine, 327,* 1697–1703.

Selye, H. (1974). *The stress of life.* New York: McGraw-Hill.

Selye, H. (1976). *Stress in health and disease.* Reading, MA: Butterworth.

Selye, H. (1980). The stress concept today. In I. L. Kutash, L. B. Schlesinger, & Associates (Eds.), *Handbook on stress and anxiety* (pp. 127–143). San Francisco: Jossey-Bass.

Shadish, W. R., Cook, T. D., & Leviton, L. C.. (1991). *Foundations of program evaluation: Theories of practice.* Newbury Park, CA: Sage.

Shaffer, M. (1993). Women's health study under gun: Critics say dietary arm should focus on heart disease. *Medical World News, 34,* 19.

Shah, I. (1970). *The way of the Sufi.* New York: Dutton.

Shapiro, D., & Goldstein, I. B. (1982). Biobehavioral perspectives on hypertension. *Journal of Consulting and Clinical Psychology, 50,* 841–858.

Shapiro, D., Tursky, B., Schwartz, G. E., & Shnidman, S. R. (1971). Smoking on cue: A behavioral approach to smoking reduction. *Journal of Health and Social Behavior, 12,* 108–113.

Shapiro, J. (1983). Family reactions and coping strategies in response to the physically ill or handicapped child: A review. *Social Science & Medicine, 17,* 913–931.

Shavit, Y., Lewis, J. W., Terman, G. W., Gale, R. P., & Liebeskind, J. C. (1984). Opiod peptides mediate the suppressive effect of stress on natural killer cell cytotoxicity. *Science, 223,* pp. 188–190.

Shedler, J., & Block, J. (1990). Adolescent drug use and psychological health. *American Psychologist, 45,* 612–630.

Shekelle, R. B., Gale, M., Ostfeld, A. M., & Paul, O. (1983). Hostility, risk of coronary heart disease, and mortality. *Psychosomatic Medicine, 45,* 109–114.

Sheley, J. F., Kinchen, E. W., Morgan, D. H., & Gordon, D. F. (1991). Limited impact of testicular self-examination promotion. *Journal of Community Health, 16,* 117–124.

Shepherd, M. (1978). Epidemiological perspective of psychosomatic medicine. *International Journal of Epidemiology, 7,* 201–204.

Sher, K. J., Walitzer, K. S., Wood, P. K., & Brent, E. E. (1991). Characteristics of children of alcoholics: Putative risk factors, substance use and abuse, and psychopathology. *Journal of Abnormal Psychology, 100,* 427–448.

Sheridan, C. L., & Radmacher, S. A. (1992). *Health psychology: Challenging the biomedical model.* New York: Wiley.

Sheridan, E. P., Matarazzo, J. D., Boll, T. J., Perry, N. W. Jr., Weiss, S. M., & Belar, C. D. (1988). Postdoctoral education and training for clinical service providers in health psychology. *Health Psychology, 7,* 1–17.

Sherman, S. (1975). Mutual assistance and support in retirement housing. *British Journal of Gerontology, 30,* 479–483.

Shiffman, S. (1989). Tobacco "chippers"—individual differences in tobacco dependence. *Psychopharmacology, 97,* 539–547.

Shiffman, S. (1993). Smoking cessation treatment: Any progress? *Journal of Consulting and Clinical Psychology, 61,* 718–722.

Shneidman, E. (1989). The Indian Summer of life: A preliminary study of septuagenarians. *American Psychologist, 44,* 684–694.

Shumaker, S. A., & Hill, D. R. (1991). Gender differences in social support and physical health. *Health Psychology, 10,* 102–111.

Shuval, J. T. (1990). Health in Israel: Patterns of equality and inequality. *Social Science & Medicine, 31,* 291–303.

Sicuteri, F. (1986). Changing trends in migraine and cluster headache: The concept of functional deafferentation. *IRCS Medical Science Psychology and Psychiatry, 14,* 1062–1065.

Sicuteri, F., Fanciullacci, M., Nicolodi, M., Geppetti, P., Fusco, B. M., Marabini, S., Alessandri, M., & Campagnolo, V. (1990). Substance P theory: A unique focus on the painful and painless phenomena of cluster headaches. *Headache, 30,* 69–79.

Siegal, M. (1988). Children's knowledge of contagion and contamination as causes of illness. *Child Development, 59,* 1353–1359.

Siegel, K., Mesagno, F. P., & Christ, G. (1990). A prevention program for bereaved children. *American Journal of Orthopsychiatry, 60,* 168–175.

Siegel, K., Mesagno, F. P., Karus, D., Christ, G., Banks, K., & Moynihan, R. (1992). Psychosocial adjustment of children with a terminally ill parent. *Journal of the American Academy of Child and Adolescent Psychiatry, 31,* 327–333.

Siegel, S. (1988). Drug anticipation and the treatment of dependence. In *Learning factors in substance abuse* (pp 1–24), NIDA Research Monograph 84. Washington, DC: U. S. Department of Health and Human Services.

Siegel, S., & Sdao-Jarvie, K. (1986). Attenuation of ethanol tolerance by a novel stimulus. *Psychopharmacology, 88,* 258–261.

Siegel, S., Hinson, R. E., Krank, M. D., & McCully, J. (1982). Heroin "overdose" death: Contribution of drug-associated environmental cues. *Science, 216,* 436–437.

Sigerist, H. E. (1971). *The great doctors: A biographical history of medicine.* Freeport, NY: Books for Libraries Press.

Silverman, M. M., Eichler, A., & Williams, G. D. (1987). Self-reported stress: Findings from the 1985 National Health Interview Survey. *Public Health Reports, 102,* 47–53.

Silverman, P. (1978). *Animal behaviour in the laboratory.* New York: Pica.

Singer, C. (1959). *A history of biology* (3rd ed.). New York: Abelard-Schuman.

Singh, D. (1993). Adaptive significance of female physical attractiveness: Role of waist-to-hip ratio. *Journal of Personality and Social Psychology, 65,* 293–307.

Sjaastad, O., Salvesen, R., Fredriksen, T. A., & Antonaci, F. (1989). Cluster headache: Do the autonomic signs have an organic or a mental basis? *Giornale di Neuropsicofarmacologia, 11,* 87–88.

Sklar, L. S., & Anisman, H. (1980). Social stress influences tumor growth. *Psychosomatic Medicine, 42,* 347–365.

Skrabanek, P. (1988). Cervical cancer in nuns and prostitutes: A plea for scientific continence. *Journal of Clinical Epidemiology, 6,* 577–582.

Smith, C. A., & Wallston, K. A. (1992). Adaptation in patients with Chronic Rheumatoid Arthritis: Application of a general model. *Health Psychology, 11,* 151–162.

Smith, G. (1993, October 4). We're going to beat this thing. *Sports Illustrated, 79(14),* 16–29.

Smith, J. C. (1988). Steps toward a cognitive-behavioral model of relaxation. *Biofeedback and Self-Regulation, 13,* 307–329.

Smith, M. S., & Womack, W. M. (1987). Stress management techniques in childhood and adolescence: Relaxation training, meditation, hypnosis, and biofeedback: Appropriate clinical applications. *Clinical Pediatrics, 26,* 581–585.

Smith, S. L. (1984). Significant research findings in the etiology of child abuse. *Social Casework, 65,* 665–683.

Smith, T. W., & Leon, A. S. (1992). *Coronary heart disease: A behavioral perspective.* Champaign, IL: Research Press.

Smith, T. W., Peck, J. R., & Ward, J. R. (1990). Helplessness and depression in Rheumatoid Arthritis. *Health Psychology, 9,* 377–389.

Smyer, M. A. (1989, August). *Drugs and the elderly: Risks, benefits, and alternatives.* Paper presented at the 97th Annual Meeting of the American Psychological Association.

Sobal, J. (1990, Spring). The social epidemiology of obesity. *Human Ecology,* 17–18.

Sobell, M. B., & Sobell, L. C. (1978). *Behavioral treatment of alcohol problems: Individualized therapy and controlled drinking.* New York: Plenum.

Sobell, M. B., & Sobell, L. C. (1987). *Moderation as a goal or outcome of treatment for alcohol problems.* New York: Haworth.

Solarz, A. L. (1990). Rehabilitation psychologists: A place in the policy process? *American Psychologist, 45,* 766–770.

Solomon, R. L. (1977). An opponent process theory of acquired motivation: The affective dynamics of addiction. In J. Maser & M. Seligman (Eds.), *Psychopathology: Experimental models* (pp. 66–103). San Francisco: Freeman.

Solomon, R. L. (1980). The opponent process theory of acquired motivation: The costs of pleasure and the benefits of pain. *American Psychologist, 35,* 691–712.

Solomon, R. L., & Corbit, J. D. (1974). An opponent-process theory of motivation: I. The temporal dynamics of affect. *Psychological Review, 81,* 119–145.

Solomon, S. (1993). Migraine diagnosis and clinical symptomatology. *Headache, 34,* S8–S12.

Sommer, A., Tielsch, J. M., Katz, J., Quigley, H. A., Gottsch, J. D., Javitt, J. C., Martone, J. F., Royall, R. M., Witt, K. A., & Ezrine, S. (1991). Racial differences in the cause-specific prevalence of blindness in East Baltimore. *The New England Journal of Medicine, 325,* 1412–1417.

Sorbi, M., & Tellegen, B. (1988). Stress-coping in

migraine. Special Issue: Stress and coping in relation to health and disease. *Social Science and Medicine, 26,* 351–358.

Sorbi, M., Tellegen, B., & du Long, A. (1989). Long-term effects of training in relaxation and stress-coping in patients with migraine: A 3-year follow-up. *Headache, 29,* 111–121.

Sowers-Hoag, K. M., Thyer, B. A., & Bailey, J. S. (1987). Promoting automobile safety belt use by young children. *Journal of Applied Behavior Analysis, 20,* 133–138.

Special Committee on Aging. (1993). *Cataract surgery: Guidelines and outcomes.* Washington, DC: U.S. Government Printing Office.

Spence, A. P. (1989). *Biology of human aging.* Englewood Cliffs, NJ: Prentice-Hall.

Spiegel, D. (1986). Psychosocial interventions with cancer patients. *Journal of Psychosocial Oncology, 3,* 83–95.

Spiegel, D., Kraemer, H. C., Bloom, J. R., & Gottheil, E. (1989). Effect of psychosocial treatment on survival of patients with metastatic breast cancer. *The Lancet, 2,* 888–891.

Spielberger, C. D., & Jacobs, G. A. (1982). Personality and smoking behavior. *Journal of Personality Assessment, 46,* 396–403.

Spielman, A. J., Saskin, P., & Thorpy, M. J. (1987). Treatment of chronic insomnia by restriction of time in bed. *Sleep, 10,* 45–56.

Spitzer, L., & Rodin, J. (1981). Human eating behavior: A critical review of studies in normal weight and overweight individuals. *Appetite: Journal for Intake Research, 2,* 293–329.

St. Lawrence, J. S. (1993). African-American adolescents' knowledge, health-related attitudes, sexual behavior, and contraceptive decisions: Implications for the prevention of adolescent HIV infection. *Journal of Consulting and Clinical Psychology, 61,* 104–112.

Stacy, A. W., Sussman, S., Dent, C. W., Burton, D., & Flay, B. R. (1992). Moderators of peer social influence in adolescent smoking. *Personality and Social Psychology Bulletin, 18,* 163–172.

Stall, R. D., Coates, T. J., & Hoff, C. (1988). Behavioral risk reduction for HIV infection among gay and bisexual men: A review of results from the United States. *American Psychologist, 43,* 878–885.

Stampfer, M. J., Colditz, G. A., Willett, W. C., Speizer, F. E., & Hennekens, C. H. (1988). A prospective study of moderate alcohol consumption and the risk of coronary disease and stroke in women. *The New England Journal of Medicine, 319,* 267–273.

Stampfer, M. J., Hennekens, C. H., Manson, J. E., Colditz, G. A., Rosner, B., & Willett, W. C. (1993). Vitamin E consumption and the risk of coronary disease in women. *The New England Journal of Medicine, 328,* 1444–1449.

Stark, L. J., Powers, S. W., Jelalian, E., Rape, R. N., et al. (1994). Modifying problematic mealtime interactions of children with cystic fibrosis and their parents via behavioral parent training. *Journal of Pediatric Psychology, 19,* 751–768.

Starr, C., & Taggart, R. (1984). *Biology: The unity and diversity of life* (3rd ed.). Belmont, CA: Wadsworth.

Steele, C. M., & Josephs, R. A. (1990). Alcohol myopia: Its prized and dangerous effects. *American Psychologist, 45,* 921–933.

Steenland, K., Stayner, L., Greife, A., Halperin, W., Hayes, R., Hornung, R., & Nowlin, S. (1991). Mortality among workers exposed to ethylene oxide. *The New England Journal of Medicine, 324,* 1402–1407.

Steering Committee of the Physicians' Health Study Research Group. (1988). Preliminary report: Findings from the aspirin component of the ongoing Physicians' Health Study. *The New England Journal of Medicine, 318,* 262–264.

Stein, M. (1982). Biopsychosocial factors in asthma. In L. J. West & M. Stein (Eds.), *Critical issues in behavioral medicine* (pp. 159–182). Philadelphia: Lippincott.

Stein, M., & Miller, A. H. (1993). Stress, the immune system, and health and illness. In L. Goldberger & S. Breznitz (Eds.), *Handbook of stress: Theoretical and clinical aspects* (2nd ed., pp. 127–141). New York: Free Press.

Steingart, R. M., Packer, M., Hamm, P., Coglianese, M. E., Gersh, B., Geltman, E. M., Solano, J., Katz, S., Moyé, L., Basta, L. L., Lewis, S. J., Gottlieb, S. S., Bernstein, V., McEwan, P., Jacobson, K., Brown, E. J., Kukin, M. L., Kantrowitz, N. E., & Pfeffer, M. A. (1991). Sex differences in the management of coronary artery disease. *The New England Journal of Medicine, 325,* 226–230.

Stephens, G. J. (1980). *Pathophysiology for health practitioners.* New York: Macmillan.

Stephens, R. C., Feucht, T. E., & Roman, S. W. (1991). Effects of an intervention program on AIDS-related drug and needle behavior among intravenous drug users. *American Journal of Public Health, 81,* 568–571.

Stern, R. C. (1997). The diagnosis of cystic fibrosis. *The New England Journal of Medicine, 336,* 487–491.

Sternbach, R. A. (1986). Pain and "hassles" in the United States: Findings of the Nuprin pain report. *Pain, 27,* 69–80.

Stitzer, M. L., Rand, C. S., Bigelow, G. E., & Mead, A. M. (1986). Contingent payment procedures for smoking reduction and cessation. *Journal of Applied Behavior Analysis, 19,* 197–202.

Stone, A. A., Cox, D. S., Valdimarsdottir, H., Jandorf, L., & Neale, J. M. (1987). Evidence that secretory IgA antibody is associated with daily mood. *Journal of Personality and Social Psychology, 52,* 988–993.

Stone, G. C. (1991). Foreword. In J. J. Sweet, R. H. Rozensky, & S. M. Tovian (Eds.), *Handbook of clinical psychology in medical settings* (pp. xi–xii). New York: Plenum.

Stone, G. C., Cohen, F., & Adler, N. (1979). *Health psychology—A handbook.* San Francisco: Jossey-Bass.

Stoney, C. M., Davis, M. C., & Matthews, K. A. (1987). Sex differences in physiological responses to stress and in coronary heart disease: A causal link? *Psychophysiology, 24,* 127–131.

Story, M., & Faulkner, P. (1990). The prime time diet: A content analysis of eating behavior and food messages in television program content and commercials. *The American Journal of Public Health, 80,* 738–740.

Strauss, R. P., Corless, I. B., Luckey, J. W., van der Horst, C. M., & Dennis, B. H. (1992). Cognitive and attitudinal impacts of a university AIDS course: Interdisciplinary education as a public health intervention. *American Journal of Public Health, 82,* 569–572.

Streilein, J. W. (1991). Immunogenetic factors in skin cancer. *The New England Journal of Medicine, 325,* 884–887.

Streissguth, A. P., Aase, J. M., Clarren, S. K., Randels, S. P., LaDue, R. A., & Smith, D. F. (1991). Fetal alcohol syndrome in adolescents and adults. *Journal of the American Medical Association, 265,* 1961–1967.

Streissguth, A. P., Barr, H. M., & Martin, D. C. (1983). Maternal alcohol use and neonatal habituation assessed with the Brazelton Scale. *Child Development, 54,* 1109–1118.

Strickland, B. (1988). Sex-related differences in health and illness. *Psychology of Women Quarterly, 12,* 381–399.

Strickland, B. (1989). Internal-external control expectancies: From contingency to creativity. *American Psychologist, 44,* 1–12.

Striegel-Moore, R., & Rodin, J. (1985). Prevention of obesity. In J. C. Rosen & L. J. Solomon (Eds.), *Prevention in health psychology* (pp. 72–110). Hanover, NH: University Press of New England.

Striegel-Moore, R., & Rodin, J. (1986). The influence of psychological variables in obesity. In K. D. Brownell & J. P. Foreyt (Eds.), *Handbook of eating disorders: Physiology, psychology, and treatment of obesity, anorexia, and bulimia* (pp. 99–121). New York: Basic Books.

Striegel-Moore, R. H., Silberstein, L. R., and Rodin, J. (1986). Toward an understanding of risk factors for bulimia. *American Psychologist, 41,* 246–263.

Strober, M., Morrell, W., Burroughs, J., Salkin, B., & Jacobs, C. (1985). A controlled family study of anorexia nervosa. *Journal of Psychiatric Research, 19,* 239–246.

Strube, M. J., Smith, J. A., Rothbaum, R., & Sotelo, A. (1991). Measurement of health care attitudes in cystic fibrosis patients and their parents. *Journal of Applied Social Psychology, 21,* 397–408.

Strunin, L., & Hingson, R. (1993, Winter). Alcohol use and risk for HIV infection. *Alcohol Health & Research World, 17,* 35–38.

Strupp, H. H., Butler, S. F., & Rosser, C. L. (1988). Training in psychodynamic therapy. *Journal of Consulting and Clinical Psychology, 56,* 689–695.

Stunkard, A. J. (1976). *The pain of obesity.* Palo Alto, CA: Bull.

Stunkard, A. J., Foch, T. T., & Hrubec, Z. (1986). A twin study of human obesity. *Journal of the American Medical Association, 256,* 51–54.

Stunkard, A. J., Harris, J. R., Pederson, N. L., & McClearn, G. E. (1990). The body-mass index of twins who have been reared apart. *The New England Journal of Medicine, 322,* 1483–1487.

Stunkard, A. J., Sorensen, T. I. A., Hanis, C., Teasdale, T. W., Chakraborty, R., Schull, W. J., Schulsinger, F. (1986). An adoption study of human obesity. *The New England Journal of Medicine, 314,* 193–198.

Sturgis, E. T., & Gramling, S. (1988). Psychophysiological assessment. In A. S. Bellack & M. Hersen (Eds.), *Behavioral assessment: A practical handbook* (3rd ed., pp. 213–251). New York: Pergamon.

Suinn, R. M. (1975). The cardiac stress management program for Type A patients. *Cardiac Rehabilitation, 5,* 13–15.

Sulik, K. K., Johnston, M. C., & Webb, M. A. (1981). Fetal alcohol syndrome: Embryogenesis in a mouse model. *Science, 214,* 936–938.

Sullivan, L. (1990). Sounding board: Healthy people

2000. *The New England Journal of Medicine, 323,* 1065–1067.

Sullivan, M. J. L., Reesor, K., Mikail, S., & Fisher, R. (1992). The treatment of depression in chronic low back pain: Review and recommendations. *Pain, 50,* 5–13.

Sullivan, M. K. (1990). Organic or functional? Why psychiatry needs a philosophy of mind. *Psychiatric Annals, 20,* 271–277.

Sunderwirth, S. G., & Milkman, H. (1991). Behavioral and neurochemical commonalities in addiction [Special issue: Addictions and the family]. *Contemporary Family Therapy: An International Journal, 13,* 421–433.

Surwit, R. S., & Feinglos, M. N. (1988). Stress and autonomic nervous system in Type II diabetes: A hypothesis. *Diabetes Care, 11,* 83–85.

Suter, P. M., Schutz, Y., & Jequier, E. (1992). The effect of ethanol on fat storage in healthy subjects. *The New England Journal of Medicine, 326,* 983–987.

Svartberg, M., & Stiles, T. C. (1991). Comparative effects of short-term psychodynamic psychotherapy: A meta-analysis. *Journal of Consulting and Clinical Psychology, 59,* 704–714.

Swedish Aspirin Low-Dose Trial (SALT). (1991). Swedish Aspirin Low-Dose Trial (SALT) of 75 mg aspirin as secondary prophylaxis after cerebrovascular ischemic events. *The Lancet, 338,* 1345–1349.

Sytkowski, P. A., Kannel, W. B., & D'Agostino, R. B. (1990). Changes in risk factors and the decline in mortality from cardiovascular disease. *The New England Journal of Medicine, 322,* 1635–1641.

Tanaka, M., Kohno, Y., Nakagawa, R., Ida, Y., Takeda, S., Nagasaki, N., & Noda, Y. (1983). Regional characteristics of stress-induced increases in brain noradrenaline release in rats. *Pharmacology, Biochemistry & Behavior, 19,* 543–547.

Tarter, R. E., Arria, A. M., Moss, H., Edwards, N. J., & van Thiel, D. H. (1987). DSM-III criteria for alcohol abuse: Associations with alcohol consumption behavior. *Alcoholism Clinical and Experimental Research, 11,* 541–543.

Taylor, A. L., & Fishman, L. M. (1988). Corticotropin-releasing hormone. *The New England Journal of Medicine, 319,* 213–222.

Taylor, C. B., & Fortmann, S. P. (1983). Essential hypertension. *Psychosomatics, 24,* 433–448.

Taylor, C. B., Houston-Miller, N., Haskell, W. L., & Debusk, R. F. (1988). Smoking cessation after acute myocardial infarction: The effects of exercise training. *Addictive Behaviors, 13,* 331–335.

Taylor, G. K. (1981). Disease concepts and the logic of classes. *British Journal of Medical Psychology, 54,* 277–286.

Taylor, M. R. H., & O'Connor, P. (1989). Resident parents and shorter hospital stay. *Archives of Disease in Psychology, 64,* 274–276.

Taylor, P., Abrams, D., & Hewstone, M. (1988). Cancer, stress and personality: A correlational investigation of life-events, repression-sensitization and locus of control. *British Journal of Medical Psychology, 61,* 179–183.

Taylor, S. E. (1986). Implications of health psychology for mental health services. *Administration in mental health, 14,* 44–59.

Taylor, S. E. (1990). Health psychology: The science and the field. *American Psychologist, 45,* 40–50.

Taylor, S. E., & Aspinwall, L. G. (1993). Coping with chronic illness. In L. Goldberger & S. Breznitz (Eds.), *Handbook of stress: Theoretical and clinical aspects* (2nd ed., pp. 511–531). New York: Free Press.

Taylor, W. J. (1986). Radiation therapy. In A. I. Holleb (Ed.), *The American Cancer Society Cancer Book* (pp. 140–150). Garden City, NJ: Doubleday.

Tayman, J., & Pennell, S. (1992). Toward a causal model of drug use. *Crime & Delinquency, 38,* 583–601.

Teichman, Y., Rafael, M. B., & Lerman, M. (1986). Anxiety reaction of hospitalized children. *British Journal of Medical Psychology, 59,* 375–382.

Temple, M. T., & Leigh, B. C. (1992). Alcohol consumption and unsafe sexual behavior in discrete events. *The Journal of Sex Research, 29,* 207–219.

Teri, L., & Wagner, A. (1992). Alzheimer's disease and depression. *Journal of Consulting and Clinical Psychology, 60,* 379–391.

Thackwray, D. E., Smith, M. C., Bodfish, J. W., & Meyers, A. W. (1993). A comparison of behavioral and cognitive-behavioral interventions for bulimia nervosa. *Journal of Consulting and Clinical Psychology, 61,* 639–645.

Thomas, L. (1980). Future prospects for basic science in medicine. *Bulletin of the American Academy of Arts and Science, 34,* 20–41.

Thompson, R. J. Jr. (1987). Psychologists in medical schools. *American Psychologist, 42,* 866–868.

Thurman, J. (1982). *Isak Dinesen: The life of a storyteller.* New York: St. Martin's Press.

Tiffany, S. T. (1990). A cognitive model of drug urges and drug-use behavior: Role of automatic and nonautomatic processes. *Psychological Review, 97,* 147–168.

Tjio, J. H., & Levan, A. (1956). The chromosome number of man. *Hereditas, 42,* 1–6.

Tønnesen, P., Nørregaard, J., Simonsen, K., & Säwe, U. (1991). A double-blind trial of a 16-hour transdermal nicotine patch in smoking cessation. *The New England Journal of Medicine, 325,* 311–315.

Tønnesen, P., Fryd, V., Hansen, M., Helsted, J., Gunnersen, A. B., Forchammer, H., & Stockner, M. (1988). Effect of nicotine chewing gum in combination with group counseling on the cessation of smoking. *The New England Journal of Medicine, 318,* 15–18.

Tobacco: Clinton proposes youth antismoking plan. (1995, August 17). *Facts on File, 55,* 594–596.

Topel, H. (1985). Biochemical basis of alcoholism: Statements and hypotheses of present research. *Alcohol, 2,* 711–788.

Torosian, T., Lumley, M. A., Pickard, S. D., & Ketterer, M. W. (1997). Silent versus symptomatic myocardial ischemia: The role of psychological and medical factors. *Health Psychology, 16,* 123–130.

Totman, R. G., & Kiff, J. (1979). Life stress and susceptibility to colds. In D. J. Oborne, M. M. Gruneberg, & J. R. Eiser (Eds.), *Research in psychology and medicine* (Vol. 1, pp. 141–148). New York: Academic Press.

Træeen, B., Lewin, B., & Sundet, J. M. (1992). Use of birth control pills and condoms among 17–19-year-old adolescents in Norway: Contraceptive versus protective behaviour? *AIDS Care, 4,* 371–380.

Travis, C. B. (1988). *Women and health psychology: Biomedical issues.* Hillsdale, NJ: Erlbaum.

Tryon, R. C. (1940). Genetic differences in maze-learning in rats. *39th Yearbook of the National Society for the Study of Education* (pp. 111–119). Bloomington, Il: Public School.

Tucker, L. A. (1985). Physical, psychological, social, and lifestyle differences among adolescents classified according to cigarette smoking intention status. *Journal of School Health, 55,* 127–131.

Tucker, L. A. (1986). The relationship of television viewing to physical fitness and obesity. *Adolescence, 21,* 797–806.

Tucker, L. A., & Friedman, G. M. (1989). Television viewing and obesity in adult males. *The American Journal of Public Health, 79,* 516–518.

Tufts University. (1993, December). A well-kept secret among the elderly: Alcoholism. *Tufts University Diet & Nutrition Letter, 11(10),* 1–2.

Turing, A. M. (1950). Computing machinery and intelligence. *Mind, 59,* 433–460.

Turk, D. C., & Rudy, T. E. (1988). Toward an empirically derived taxonomy of chronic pain patients: Integration of psychological assessment data. *Journal of Consulting and Clinical Psychology, 56,* 233–238.

Turk, D. C., Meichenbaum, D., & Genest, M. (1983). *Pain and behavioral medicine: A cognitive-behavioral perspective.* New York: Plenum.

Turk, D. C., Wack, J. T., & Kerns, R. D. (1985). An empirical examination of the "pain behavior" construct. *Journal of Behavioral Medicine, 9,* 119–130.

Turner, J. A., & Clancy, S. (1988). Comparison of operant behavioral and cognitive-behavioral group treatment for chronic low back pain. *Journal of Consulting and Clinical Psychology, 56,* 261–266.

U.S. Bureau of the Census. (1990). *Statistical Abstract of the United States: 1991.* Washington, DC: U.S. Government Printing Office.

U.S. Bureau of the Census. (1991). *Statistical Abstract of the United States: 1991.* Washington, DC: U.S. Government Printing Office.

U.S. Bureau of the Census. (1993). *Statistical Abstract of the United States: 1991.* Washington, DC: U.S. Government Printing Office.

Ullmann, L. P., & Krasner, L. (Eds.). (1965). *Case studies in behavior modification.* New York: Holt, Rinehart & Winston.

Umberson, D. (1987). Family status and health behaviors: Social control as a dimension of social integration. *Journal of Health and Social Behavior, 28,* 306–319.

Urba, W. J., & Longo, D. L. (1992). Hodgkin's disease. *The New England Journal of Medicine, 326,* 678–687.

Uttal, W. R. (1978). *The psychobiology of mind.* Hillsdale, NJ: Lawrence Erlbaum.

Vaernes, R., Ursin, H., Darragh, A., & Lambe, R. (1982). Endocrine response patterns and psychological correlates. *Journal of Psychosomatic Research, 26,* 123–131.

VandenBos, G. R., & Costa, P. T. Jr. (Eds.). (1990). *Psychological aspects of serious illness.* Washington, DC: American Psychological Association.

van Doornen, L. J. P. (1980). The coronary risk personality: Psychological and psychophysiological aspects. *Psychotherapy & Psychosomatics, 34,* 204–215.

van Hooft, I. M. S., Grobbee, D. E., Derkx, F. H. M., de Leeuw, P. W., Schalekamp, M. A. D. H., Hofman, A. (1991). Renal hemodynamics and the renin-angiotensin-aldosterone system in normotensive subjects with hypertensive and normotensive parents. *The New England Journal of Medicine, 324,* 1305–1311.

Van Houten, R., Nau, P., & Marini, Z. (1980). An analysis of public posting in reducing speeding behavior on an urban highway. *Journal of Applied Behavior Analysis, 13,* 383-395.

van Roosmalen, E. H., & McDaniel, S. A. (1989). Peer group influence as a factor in smoking behavior of adolescents. *Adolescence, 24,* 801–816.

Velicer, W. F., DiClemente, C. C., Prochaska, J., & Brandenburg, N. (1985). A decisional balance measure for assessing and predicting smoking status. *Journal of Personality and Social Psychology, 48,* 1279–1289.

Velicer, W. F., Prochaska, J. O., Rossi, J. S., & Snow, M. G. (1992). Assessing outcome in smoking cessation studies. *Psychological Bulletin, 111,* 23–41.

Veniga, R. L., & Spradley, J. P. (1981). *The work/STRESS connection.* Boston: Little, Brown.

Verbrugge, L. M. (1985). Gender and health: An update on hypotheses and evidence. *Journal of Health and Social Behavior, 26,* 156–182.

Verbrugge, L. M. (1986). Role burdens and physical health of women and men. *Women & Health, 11,* 47–77.

Vichinsky, E. P., Johnson, R., & Lubin, B. H. (1982). Multidisciplinary approach to pain management in sickle cell disease. *The American Journal of Pediatric Hematology/Oncology, 4,* 328–333.

Viney, L. L., & Westbrook, M. T. (1982). Patients' psychological reactions to chronic illness: Are they associated with rehabilitation. *Journal of Applied Rehabilitation Counseling, 13,* 38–44.

Vitaliano, P. P., Maiuro, R. D., Russo, J., Katon, W., DeWolfe, D., & Hall, G. (1990). Coping profiles associated with psychiatric, physical health, work, and family problems. *Health Psychology, 9,* 348–376.

Volberding, P. A., Lagakos, S. W., Koch, M. A., Peltinelli, C., Meyers, M. W., Booth, D. K., Balfour, H. H., Reichman, R. C., Bartlett, J. A., Hirsch, M. S., Murphy, R. L., Hardy, W. D., Soeiro, R., Fischl, M. A., Bartlett, J. G., Merigan, T. C., Hyslop, N. E., Richman, D. D., Valentine, F. T., Corey, L., & the

AIDS Clinical Trials Group. (1990). Zidovudine in asymptomatic human immunodeficiency virus infection: A controlled trial in persons with fewer than 500 CD4-positive cells per cubic millimeter. *The New England Journal of Medicine, 322,* 941–949.

Wadden, T. A., & Brownell, K. D. (1984). The development and modification of dietary practices in individuals, groups, and large populations. In J. D. Matarazzo, S. M. Weiss, J. A. Herd, N. E. Miller, & S. M. Weiss (Eds.). *Behavioral health: A handbook of health enhancement and disease prevention* (pp. 608–631). New York: Wiley.

Wadden, T. A., Foster, G. D., Letizia, K. A., & Stunkard, A. J. (1992). A multicenter evaluation of a proprietary weight reduction program for the treatment of marked obesity. *Archives of Internal Medicine, 152,* 961–966.

Wahlqvist, M. L., & Kouris, A. (1990). Trans-cultural aspects of nutrition in old age. *Age and Aging, 19,* S43–S52.

Wahrendorf, J. (1986). The changing face of cancer epidemiology. *Statistics in Medicine, 5,* 547–553.

Waldstein, S. R., Manuck, S. B., Ryan, C. M., & Muldoon, M. F. (1991). Neuropsychological correlates of hypertension: Review and methodologic considerations. *Psychological Bulletin, 110,* 451–468.

Walker, D. K., Stein, R. E., Perrin, E. C., & Jessop, D. J. (1990). Assessing psychosocial adjustment of children with chronic illnesses: A review of the technical properties of PARS III. *Journal of Developmental and Behavioral Pediatrics, 11,* 116–121.

Wall, P. D., & Jones, M. (1991). *Defeating pain.* New York: Plenum Press.

Wall, P. D., & Melzack, R. (Eds.). (1989). *Textbook of pain* (2nd ed.). New York: Churchill & Livingstone.

Wallhagen, M. I. (1993). Perceived control and adaptation in elder caregivers: Development of an explanatory model. *International Journal of Aging & Human Development, 36,* 219–237.

Walsh, D. C., Hingson, R. W., Merrigan, D. M., Levenson, S. M., Cupples, A., Heeren, T., Coffman, G. A., Becker, C. A., Barker, T. A., Hamilton, S. K., McGuire, T. G., & Kelly, C. A. (1991). A randomized trial of treatment options for alcohol-abusing workers. *The New England Journal of Medicine, 325,* 775–782.

Walsh, P., Dale, A., & Anderson, D. E. (1977). Comparison of biofeedback, pulse wave velocity and progressive relaxation in essential hypertensives. *Perceptual and Motor Skills, 44,* 839–843.

Walter, H., Hofman, A., Vaughan, R. D., & Wynder, E. L. (1988). Modification of risk factors for coronary disease: Five-year results of a school-based intervention trial. *The New England Journal of Medicine, 318,* 1093–1100.

Wambach, K. G., Byers, J. B., Harrison, D. F., Levine, P., Imershein, A. W., Quadagno, D. M., & Maddox, K. (1992). Substance use among women at risk for HIV infection. *Journal of Drug Education, 22,* 131–146.

Ward, M. M., Mefford, I. N., Parker, S. D., Chesney, M. A., Taylor, C. B., Keegan, D. L., & Barchas, J. D. (1983). Epinephrine and norepinephrine responses in continuously collected human plasma to a series of stressors. *Psychosomatic Medicine, 45,* 471–486.

Warram, J. H., Rich, S. S., & Krolewski, A. S. (1994). Epidemiology and genetics of diabetes mellitus. In C. R. Kahn & G. C. Weir (Eds.), *Joslin's diabetes mellitus—13th.* (pp. 193–200). Malvern, PA: Lea & Febiger.

Watson, J. B., & Rayner, R. (1920). Conditioned emotional reactions. *Journal of Experimental Psychology, 3,* 1–14.

Watson, J. D., & Crick, F. H. C. (1953). A structure for deoxyribose nucleic acid. *Nature, 171,* 737–738.

Watzl, B., & Watson, R. R. (1992). Role of alcohol abuse in nutritional immunosuppression. *The Journal of Nutrition, 122,* 733–737.

Weinstein, A. G., Faust, D. S., McKee, L., & Padman, R. (1992). Outcome of short-term hospitalization for children with severe asthma. *Journal of Allergy and Clinical Immunology, 90,* 66–75.

Weinstein, N. D. (1993). Testing four competing theories of health-protective behavior. *Health Psychology, 12,* 324–333.

Weir, G. C., & Leahy, J. L. (1994). Pathogenesis of non-insulin-dependent (Type II) diabetes mellitus. In C. R. Kahn & G. C. Weir (Eds.), *Joslin's diabetes mellitus—13th.* (pp. 240–264). Malvern, PA: Lea & Febiger.

Weiss, J. M. (1968). Effects of coping responses on stress. *Journal of Comparative Physiological Psychology, 65,* 251–260.

Weiss, J. M. (1971a). Effects of coping behavior in different warning signal conditions on stress pathology in rats. *Journal of Comparative Physiological Psychology, 77,* 1–13.

Weiss, J. M. (1971b). Effects of coping behavior with

and without feedback signal on stress pathology in rats. *Journal of Comparative Physiological Psychology, 77,* 22–30.

Weiss, K. B., Gergen, P. J., & Hodgson, T. A. (1992). An economic evaluation of asthma in the United States. *The New England Journal of Medicine, 326,* 862–866.

Weisz, J. R., Weiss, B., & Donenberg, G. R. (1992). The lab versus the clinic: Effects of child and adolescent psychotherapy. *American Psychologist, 47,* 1578–1585.

Welch, K. M. A. (1993). Drug therapy of migraine. *The New England Journal of Medicine, 329,* 1476–1483.

Wells, R. A., & Ginnetti, V. J. (Eds.). (1990). *Handbook of the brief psychotherapies.* New York: Plenum.

Wells, R. A., & Phelps, P. A. (1990). The brief psychotherapies: A selective overview. In R. A. Wells & V. J. Giannetti (Eds.), *Handbook of the brief psychotherapies* (pp. 3–26). New York: Plenum.

Wenger, N. K., Speroff, L., & Packard, B. (1993). Cardiovascular health and disease in women. *The New England Journal of Medicine, 329,* 247–256.

West, J. R. (1993). Use of pup in a cup model to study brain development. *The Journal of Nutrition, 123,* 382–385.

Whipple, B. (1987, Fall). Methods of pain control: Review of research and literature. *IMAGE: Journal of Nursing Scholarship, 19*(3), 142–146.

White, L., Tursky, B., & Schwartz, G. E. (Eds.). (1985). *Placebo: Theory, research, and mechanisms.* New York: Guilford Press.

Whittle, J., Conigliaro, J., Good, C. B., & Lofgren, R. P. (1993). Racial differences in the use of invasive cardiovascular procedures in the department of veterans affairs medical system. *The New England Journal of Medicine, 329,* 621–627.

Wicherski, M., & Kohout, J. (1995). *1993 doctorate employment survey.* Washington, DC: American Psychological Association.

Wieczorek, W. F., & Miller, B. A. (1992). Preliminary typology designed for treatment matching of driving-while-intoxicated offenders. *Journal of Consulting and Clinical Psychology, 60,* 757–765.

Willard, M. D. (1991). Obesity: Types and treatments. *American Family Physician, 43,* 2099–2108.

Willett, W. C., Green, A., Stampfer, M. J., Speizer, F. E., Colditz, G. A., Rosner, B., Monson, R. R., Stason, W., & Hennekens, C. H. (1987). Relative and absolute excess risks of coronary heart disease among women who smoke cigarettes. *The New England Journal of Medicine, 317,* 1303–1309.

Williams, A. F., & Lund, A. K. (1992). Injury control: What psychologists can contribute. *American Psychologist, 47,* 1036–1039.

Williams, D. A., & Keefe, F. J. (1991). Pain beliefs and the use of cognitive-behavioral coping strategies. *Pain, 46,* 185–190.

Williams, M., Thyer, B. A., Bailey, J. S., & Harrison, D. F. (1989). *Journal of Applied Behavior Analysis, 22,* 71–76.

Williams, R., Zyzanski, S. J., & Wright, A. L. (1992). Life events and daily hassles and uplifts as predictors of hospitalization and outpatient visitation. *Social Science and Medicine, 34,* 763–768.

Williamson, D. A., Davis, C. J., & Prather, R. C. (1988). Assessment of health-related disorders. In A. S. Bellack, & M. Hersen (Eds.), *Behavioral assessment: A practical handbook* (3rd. ed., pp. 396–440). New York: Pergamon.

Wilson, B. R. A. (1989). Cardiovascular risk reduction. *International Psychologist, 29,* 49–54.

Wilson, E. O. (1975). *Sociobiology: The new synthesis.* Cambridge: Harvard University Press.

Wing, R. R., Lamparski, D. M., Zaslow, S., Betschart, J., Siminerio, L., & Becker, D. (1985). Frequency and accuracy of self-monitoring of blood glucose in children: Relationship to glycemic control. *Diabetes Care, 8,* 214–218.

Wingard, D. L., & Cohn, B. A. (1990). Variations in disease-specific sex morbidity and mortality ratios in the United States. In M. G. Ory, & H. R. Warner (Eds.). *Gender health and longevity: Multidisciplinary perspectives* (pp. 25–27). New York: Springer.

Winter, L., & Goldy, A. S. (1993). Effects of prebehavioral cognitive work on adolescents' acceptance of condoms. *Health Psychology, 12,* 308–312.

Winters, R. (1985). Behavioral approaches to pain. In N. Schneiderman & J. T. Tapp (Eds.), *Behavioral medicine: The biopsychosocial approach* (pp. 565–587). Hillsdale, NJ: Erlbaum.

Wise, R. A. (1988). The neurobiology of craving: Implications for the understanding and treatment of addiction. *Journal of Abnormal Psychology, 97,* 118–132.

Wise, R. A., & Bozarth, M. A. (1987). A psychomotor stimulant theory of addiction. *Psychological Review, 94,* 469–492.

Witkin, H. A., Mednick, S. A., Schulsinger, F., Bakkestrom, E., Christiansen, K. O., Goodenough, D. R., Hirschhorn, K., Lundsteen, C., Owen, D. R., Philip, J., Rubin, D. B., & Stocking, M. (1976). Criminality in XYY and XXY men: The elevated crime rate of XYY males is not related to aggression. *Science, 193,* 547–555.

Witkowska, H. E., Lubin, B. H., Beuzard, Y., Baruchel, S., Esseltine, D., Vichinsky, E. P., et al. (1991). Sickle cell disease in a patient with sickle cell trait and compound heterozygosity for hemoglobin S and hemoglobin Quebec-Chori. *The New England Journal of Medicine, 325,* 1150–1154.

Wolpe, J. (1958). *Psychotherapy by reciprocal inhibition.* Stanford, CA: Stanford University Press.

Wonderlich, S., Klein, M. H., & Council, J. R. (1996). Relationship of social perceptions and self-concept in bulimia nervosa. *Journal of Consulting and Clinical Psychology, 64,* 1231–1237.

Woodruff-Pak, D. S. (1988). *Psychology and aging.* Englewood Cliffs, NJ: Prentice-Hall.

Woods, S. C. (1991). The eating paradox: How we tolerate food. *Psychological Review, 98,* 488–505.

Woodward, R., & Jones, R. B. (1980). Cognitive restructuring treatment: A controlled trial with anxious patients. *Behavioral Research and Therapy, 18,* 401–407.

Worth, D. (1990). Sexual decision-making and AIDS: Why condom promotion among vulnerable women is likely to fail. *Studies in Family Planning, 20,* 297–307.

Wray, L. A. (1992). Cross-cultural medicine: A decade later. *Western Journal of Medicine, 157,* 357–361.

Wright, L. (1988). The Type A Behavior Pattern and coronary artery disease. *American Psychologist, 43,* 2–14.

Wright, L., Carbonari, J., & Voyles, W. (1992). A factor analytic study of physical risk variables for CHD. *Journal of Clinical Psychology, 48,* 165–170.

Wu, T., Tashkin, D. P., Djahed, B., & Rose, J. E. (1988). Pulmonary hazards of smoking marijuana as compared with tobacco. *The New England Journal of Medicine, 318,* 347–351.

Wynder, E. L., Kajitani, T., Kuno, J., Lucas, J. C., Depalo, A., & Farrow, J. A. (1963). A comparison of survival rates between American and Japanese patients with breast cancer. *Surgery, Gynecology and Obstetrics, 117,* 196.

Wynder, E. L., Weisburger, J. H., & Ng, S. K. (1992). Nutrition: The need to define "optimal" intake as a basis for public policy decisions. *The American Journal of Public Health, 82,* 346–350.

Wysocki, T., Green, L., & Huxtable, K. (1989). Blood glucose monitoring by diabetic adolescents: Compliance and metabolic control. *Health Psychology, 8,* 267–284.

Yan, S. D., Chen, X., Fu, J., Chen, M., Zhu, H., Roher, A., Slattery, T., Zhao, L., Nagashima, M., Morser, J., Migheli, A., Nawroth, P., Stern, D., & Schmidt, A. M. (1996). RAGE and amyloid-B peptide neurotoxicity in Alzheimer's disease. *Nature, 382,* 685–691.

Yates, A. (1989). Current perspectives on the eating disorders: II. Treatment, outcome, and research direction. *Journal of the American Academy of Child and Adolescent Psychiatry, 29,* 1–9.

Yeung, A. C., Vekshtein, V. I., Krantz, D. S., Vita, J. A., Ryan, T. J., Ganz, P., & Selwyn, A. P. (1991). The effect of atherosclerosis on the vasomotor response of coronary arteries to mental stress. *The New England Journal of Medicine, 325,* 1551–1556.

Zarit, S. H., Zarit, J. M., & Reever, K. E. (1982). Memory training for severe memory loss: Effects on senile dementia patients and their families. *The Gerontologist, 22,* 373–377.

Zedeck, S., & Mosier, K. L. (1990). Work in the family and employing organizations. *American Psychologist, 45,* 240–251.

Zelman, D. C., Brandon, T. H., Jorenby, D. E., & Baker, T. B. (1992). Measures of affect and nicotine dependence predict differential response to smoking cessation treatments. *Journal of Consulting and Clinical Psychology, 60,* 943–952.

Zhang, Y., Proenca, R., Maffel, M., Barone, M., Leopold, L., & Friedman, J. M. (1994). Positional cloning of the mouse *obese gene* and its human homologue. *Nature, 372,* 425–432.

Zheng, Z., Wang, Z., Zhu, H., Yang, J., Peng, H., Wang, L., Li, J., Jiang, X., & Yu, Y. (1993). Survey of 160 centenarians in Shanghai. *Age and Ageing, 22,* 16–19.

Ziegler, P. (1969). *The black death*. New York: John Day.

Ziegler, R. G. (1988). A review of epidemiologic evidence that carotenoids reduce the risk of cancer. *Journal of Nutrition, 119,* 116–122.

Zilboorg, G. (1941). *A history of medical psychology*. New York: Norton.

Zuckerman, M. (1971). Dimensions of sensation seeking. *Journal of Consulting and Clinical Psychology, 36,* 35–52.

Name Index

Subject Index

Credits

This page constitutes an extension of the copyright page. We have made every effort to trace the ownership of all copyrighted material and to secure permission from copyright holders. In the event of any question arising as to the use of any material, we will be pleased to make the necessary corrections in future printings. Thanks are due to the following authors, publishers, and agents for permission to use the material indicated.

Chapter 2: 48: Table 2.3 adapted from *Basic Pathophysiology: A Conceptual Approach,* Third Edition, by M. W. Groër and M. E. Shekleton. Copyright © 1989 The C. V. Mosby Company. Reprinted by permission. **49:** Figure 2.10 from *Basic Pathophysiology: A Conceptual Approach,* by M. W. Groër and M. E. Shekleton, p. 30. Copyright © 1983 Mosby-Year Book. Reprinted by permission. **50:** Figure 2.11 from *Understanding Physical, Sensory, & Health Impairments,* by K. W. Heller, P. A. Alberto, P. E. Forney, and M. N. Schwartzman. Copyright © 1996 Brooks/Cole Publishing Co. Reprinted by permission of Wadsworth Publishing Co.

Chapter 3: 61: Figure 3.2 adapted from *The Mind-Body Problem: A Psychobiological Approach,* by M. Bunge, p. 9. Copyright © 1980 Pergamon Press. Adapted by permission. **70:** Table 3.1 from "The Patient: Biological, Psychological, and Social Dimensions of Medical Practice," by H. Leigh and M. Reiser, Figure 1-5. Copyright © 1980 Plenum Medical. Reprinted by permission. **73:** Figure 3.5 from *Biology: The Unity and Diversity of Life,* 4th Edition, by C. Starr and R. Taggart. Copyright © 1987 Wadsworth Publishing Company. Reprinted by permission.

Chapter 4: 83: Table 4.1 adapted from "Unconventional Medicine in the United States," by D. M. Eisenberg, R. C. Kessler, et al., *New England Journal of Medicine,* 1993, *328,* pp. 246–252. Copyright © 1993. Massachusetts Medical Society. All rights reserved. **87:** Table 4.3 from *Women's Health: Review and Research Agenda As We Approach the 21st Century,* by J. Rodin and J. Ickovics, pp. 1021. Copyright © 1990 American Psychological Association. Reprinted by permission. **91:** Table 4.4 reprinted by permission of *The New England Journal of Medicine,* from "Changes in Lipid and Lipoprotein Levels and Body Weight in Tarahumara Indians After Consumption of an Affluent Diet," by M. P. McMurry, M. T. Cerqueira, S. L. Connor, and W. E. Connor, 1991, *The New England Journal of Medicine, 325,* pp. 1704–1708. Copyright © 1991 Massachusetts Medical Society. **95:** Figure 4.5 from "Sociobehavioral Determinants of Compliance with Health and Medical Care Recommendations," by M. H. Becker and L. A. Maiman, 1975, *Medical Care, 13,* p. 12. Copyright © 1975 Lippincott-Raven Publishers. Reprinted by permission. **101:** Figure 4.10 from "Excess Mortality in Harlem," by C. McCord & H. Freeman, 1990, *New England Journal of Medicine, 322,* pp. 173–177. Copyright © 1990 Massachusetts Medical Society. All rights reserved. Adapted with permission.

Chapter 5: 113: Figure 5.2 from *National Health Expenditures, 1990,* by K. Levit, H. Lazenby, C. Cowan and S. Letsch, pp. 29–54. Copyright © 1991 Office of National Health Statistics. Reprinted by permission. **117:** Figure 5-3 from "The Lab Versus the Clinic: Effects of Child and Adolescent Psychotherapy," by J. R. Weisz, B. Weiss, and G. R. Donenberg, 1992,

1992, pp. 435–440, 1992. Copyright by Alcohol Research Documentation, Inc., Rutgers Center of Alcohol Studies, Piscataway, NJ 08855. **260:** Figure 9.8 reprinted by permission of *The New England Journal of Medicine* from "A Randomized Trial of Treatment Options for Alcohol-Abusing Workers," by D. C. Walsh, R. W. Hingson, D. M. Merrigan, S. M. Levenson, A. Cupples, T. Heeren, G. A. Coffman, C. A. Becker, T. A. Barker, S. K. Hamilton, T. G. McGuire, and C. A. Kelly, 1991, *The New England Journal of Medicine, 325,* pp. 775–782. Copyright © 1991, Massachusetts Medical Society.

Chapter 10: 268: Figure 10.2 from "Do We Fatten Our Children at the Television Set?" by W. Dietz Jr., and S. Gortmaker. Reproduced by permission of *Pediatrics, 75,* pp. 807–812. Copyright © 1985. **272:** Figure 10.5 reprinted by permission of Dr. George Bray, Pennington Biomedical Research Center, 6400 Perkins Road, Baton Rouge, LA 90808-4124. **272:** Figure 10.6 from "Treatment of Obesity," by J. S. Garrow, 1992, *The Lancet, 340,* p. 409. Copyright © 1992 by The Lancet Ltd. Reprinted by permission. **274:** Figure 10.8 from "Effects of Obesity on Health & Happiness," from *Handbook of Eating Disorders* by Kelly D. Brownell and John P. Foreyt et al. Copyright © 1986 by Basic Books, Inc. Reprinted by permission of BasicBooks, a division of HarperCollins Publishers, Inc. **276:** Figure 10.9 adpated from "Obesity, Types and Treatments," by M. D. Willard, drawing by Rebekah Dodson, 1991, *American Family Physician, 43,* pp. 2099–2108. Copyright © 1991 American Academy of Family Physicians. Reprinted by permission of the artist.

Chapter 11: 297: Figure 11.2 from "Immuno-pathogenic Mechanisms of HIV Infection," by A. S. Fauci, G. Pantaleo, S. Stanley, and D. Weissman, April 1996, *Annals of Internal Medicine, 127*(7), p. 655. Copyright © 1996 American College of Physicians. Reprinted by permission. **302:** Table 11.2 from "Behavioral Factors in HIV Infection," by T. J. Coates, R. D. Stall, J. A. Catania, and S. Kegeles, *AIDS 1988, 2*(Suppl.1), S239–S246. Reprinted by permission of the author. **309:** Figure 11.5 from "Use of Birth Control Pills and Condoms Among 17-19 Year Old Adolescents in Norway: Contraceptive Versus Protective Behaviour?" by B. Træeen, B. Lewin, and J. Sundet, 1992, *AIDS Care, 4,* pp. 371–380. Copyright © 1992 Carfax Publishing Company, 875-81 Massachusetts Avenue, Cambridge, MA 02139. Reprinted by permission. **311:** Figure 11.6 from "Effects of AIDS-Related Bereavement and HIV-Related Illness on Psychological Distress Among Gay Men: A 7-Year Longitudinal Study," by J. L. Martin and L. Dean, 1993, *Journal of Consulting and Clinical Psychology, 61,* pp. 94–103. Copyright © 1993 by the American Psychological Association. Reprinted by permission. **317:** Figure 11.8 from "Changing AIDS-Risk Behavior," by J. D. Fisher and W. A. Fisher, *Psychological Bulletin, 111,* pp. 455–474. Copyright © 1992 by the American Psychological Association. Reprinted by permission.

Chapter 12: 331: Figure 12.3 from *Understanding Physical, Sensory, & Health Impairments,* by K. W. Heller, P. A. Alberto, P. E. Forney, and M. N. Schwartzman. Copyright © 1996 Brooks/Cole Publishing Co. Reprinted by permission of Wadsworth Publishing Co. **337:** Figure 12.6 reprinted by permission of *The New England Journal of Medicine* from "Racial Differences in the Incidence of Cardiac Arrest and Subsequent Survival," by L. B. Becker, B. H. Han, P. M. Meyer, F. A. Wright, K. V. Rhodes, D. W. Smith, J. Barrett, and the Chicago CPR Project, 1993, *The New England Journal of Medicine, 329,* pp. 600–606. Copyright © 1993, Massachusetts Medical Society. Reprinted by permission of The New England Journal of Medicine.

Chapter 13: 361: Figure 13.3 from "Toward An Empirically Derived Taxonomy of Chronic Pain Patients: Integration of Psychological Assessment Data," by D. C. Turk and T. E. Rudy, 1988, *Journal of Consulting and Clinical Psychology,*

Photo Credits

Chapter 1: 4, AP / Wide World Photos; **7**, © A. Ramey / PhotoEdit; **8**, photo used with permission of Joe Matarazzo; **18**, photo used with permission of Cynthia Belar. **Chapter 2: 30**, The National Library of Medicine; **32**, bottom, courtesy of Nationalmuseet, Copenhagen, Denmark; **36**, World Publishing Co.; **38**, courtesy of Bibliotheque Nationale, Paris, France; **39**, Ayer Company Publishers, Inc.; **41**, courtesy of the Pasteur Institute; **43**, Corbis-Bettmann; **47**, reprinted by permission of CV Mosby Co. **Chapter 3: 57**, National Library of Medicine; **61**, National Library of Medicine; **76**, courtesy of Janice Kiecolt-Glaser. **Chapter 4: 84**, © Diane Alexander White / The Field Museum of Natural History Chicago, IL; **90**, Corbis-Bettmann; **94**, AP / Wide World Photos; **96**, Reuters / Corbis-Bettmann; **99**, © Mark Richards / PhotoEdit; **102**, AP / Wide World Photos. **Chapter 5: 112**, courtesy of Newsweek; **121**, Courtesy of Aaron Beck / Aaron Beck Institute; **124**, Archives of the History of American Psychology, University of Akron; **125**, courtesy of Joseph Wolpe / Pepperdine University; **127**, © Mark Richards / PhotoEdit. **Chapter 6: 154**, reprinted by permission of the Society for Experimental Analysis for Behavior, Department of Human Development, University of Kansas. **Chapter 7: 172**, © John Lopinot / The Palm Beach Post; **175**, AP / Wide World Photos; **178**, © Jonathan Nourok / PhotoEdit; **193**, reprinted by permission of McGraw-Hill, Inc.; **194**, Courtesy of Andrew Baum, Division of Behavioral Medicine and Oncology, University of Pittsburgh Cancer Institute; **198**, courtesy of Susan Folkman, Center for AIDS Prevention Studies, University of California San Francisco. **Chapter 8: 206**, © ARCHIV/Photo Researchers, Inc.; **225**, © Robert Brenner / PhotoEdit; **228**, © Tony Freeman / PhotoEdit. **Chapter 9: 238**, Corbis-Bettmann; **241**, © James Schaffer / PhotoEdit. **Chapter 10: 269**, Reuters / Corbis-Bettmann; **270**, UPI / Corbis-Bettmann; **278**, courtesy of Judith Rodin, University of Pennsylvania; **283**, left, UPI / Corbis-Bettmann, right, Glenn Waggner / UPI / Corbis-Bettmann. **Chapter 11: 294**, © Peter Southwick / Stock Boston; **316**, courtesy of Margaret Chesney, Clinical Epidemiology Program School of Medicine, University of California, San Francisco. **Chapter 12: 328**, UPI / Corbis-Bettmann; **329**, © Mark Richards / PhotoEdit; **333**, © Tom McCarthy / PhotoEdit; **345**, courtesy of Karen Matthews, Psychiatry Dept., University of Pittsburgh. **Chapter 13: 356**, Bettmann Archive; **375**, © West Rim Enterprises. **Chapter 14: 388**, courtesy of Shelly Taylor, Department of Psychology, University of California, Los Angeles. **Chapter 15: 414**, © Michael O'Neill / S.I. Picture Collection; **417**, © David Young-Wolf / PhotoEdit; **419**, © Tom McCarthy / PhotoEdit; **427**, courtesy of Barbara Melamed, Dept. of Clinical Psychology, University of Florida; **431**, Reuters / Corbis-Bettmann. **Chapter 16: 446**, courtesy of Phillip Rice; **447**, courtesy of Phillip Rice; **452**, photos courtesy of Dr. Robert D. Terry; **455**, from DeBusk, 1972; **458**, White House Photo; **459**, after Scheibel, 1983; **461**, Union-Tribune Publishing Co.; **469**, AP / Wide World Photos; **470**, © A. Ramey / PhotoEdit.

TO THE OWNER OF THIS BOOK:

I hope that you have found *Health Psychology* useful. So that this book can be improved in a future edition, would you take the time to complete this sheet and return it? Thank you.

School and address: _____

Department: _____

Instructor's name: _____

1. What I like most about this book is: _____

_____

_____

2. What I like least about this book is: _____

_____

_____

3. My general reaction to this book is: _____

_____

4. The name of the course in which I used this book is: _____

_____

5. Were all of the chapters of the book assigned for you to read? _____

 If not, which ones weren't? _____

6. In the space below, or on a separate sheet of paper, please write specific suggestions for improving this book and anything else you'd care to share about your experience in using the book.

_____

_____

_____

_____

_____

Optional:

Your name: _____ Date: _____

May Brooks/Cole quote you, either in promotion for *Health Psychology* or in future
 publishing ventures?

   Yes: _____ No: _____

   Sincerely,

   Phillip L. Rice